Fourth Edition

Nursing Outcomes Classification (NOC)

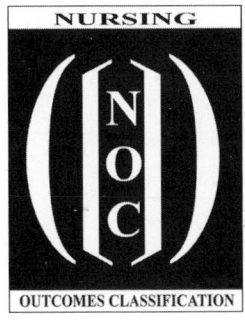

Editors

Sue Moorhead, PhD, RN
Marion Johnson, PhD, RN
Meridean L. Maas, PhD, RN, FAAN
Elizabeth Swanson, PhD, RN

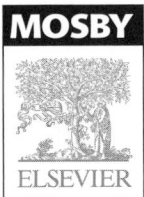

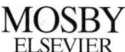

MOSBY
ELSEVIER

11830 Westline Industrial Drive
St. Louis, Missouri 63146

Notice

Neither the Publisher nor the Editors assume any responsibility for any loss or injury and/or damage to persons or property arising out of or related to any use of the material contained in this book. It is the responsibility of the treating practitioner, relying on independent expertise and knowledge of the patient, to determine the best treatment and method of application for the patient.

The Publisher

Previous editions copyrighted 1997, 2000, 2004

ISBN: 978-0-323-05408-9

Senior Acquisitions Editor: Sandra Clark Brown
Senior Developmental Editor: Cindi Anderson
Publishing Services Manager: John Rogers
Senior Project Manager: Beth Hayes
Designer: Maggie Reid

Working together to grow
libraries in developing countries

www.elsevier.com | www.bookaid.org | www.sabre.org

ELSEVIER   BOOK AID International   Sabre Foundation

Printed in the United States of America

Last digit is the print number: 9   8   7   6   5   4   3   2   1

Members of the NOC Research Team

Original Authors of the Nursing Outcomes Classification

Mary Lober Aquilino
Sandra Bellinger
Veronica Brighton
Ginette Budreau
Jeannette Daly
M. Patricia Donahue
Joyce Eland

Marion Johnson
Kathleen Kelly
Tom Kruckeberg
Anne Lewis
Meridean Maas
Leslie Marshall
Sue Moorhead

Colleen Prophet
Margaret Rankin
Deborah Perry Schoenfelder
Elizabeth A. Swanson
Bonnie L. Westra
Marilyn Willits
George Woodworth

Editors

First Edition, 1997
Marion Johnson
Meridean Maas

Second Edition, 2000
Marion Johnson
Meridean Maas
Sue Moorhead

Third Edition, 2004
Sue Moorhead
Marion Johnson
Meridean Maas

We wish to thank the following individuals who have shared their expertise by reviewing or developing specific outcomes, or contributing in other ways to this edition.

Craig Albers, MSN, RN
Clinical Manager
St. Rita's Medical Center
Lima, OH

Mary Ann Anderson, PhD, RN
Associate Professor
University of Illinois, Quad Cities Regional
  Program
College of Nursing
Moline, IL

Melchora Bartley, RN, BSN
Education Coordinator/Medical Intensive
  Care and Medicine Progressive Care Units
St. Joseph Mercy Hospital
Ann Arbor, MI

Sandra L. Bellinger, EdD, RN
Adjunct Faculty
Trinity College of Nursing & Health Sciences
Department of Nursing
Moline, IL

Veronica Brighton, MA, ARNP, CS
Assistant Professor (Clinical)
The University of Iowa
College of Nursing
Iowa City, IA

Jane Brokel, PhD, RN
Assistant Professor
The University of Iowa
College of Nursing
Iowa City, IA

Lisa Burkhart PhD, RN
Assistant Professor
Loyola University
Marcella Niehoff School of Nursing
Chicago, IL

Judy Carlson, EdD, APRN, FNP, BCIA-EEG
Nurse Researcher
Tripler Army Medical Center
Honolulu, HI

Mary Clarke, PhD, RN, BC
Director of Nursing Practice, Research
and Innovation
Genesis Medical Center
Davenport, IA

Teresa Cochran, MSN, RN
Faculty
Trinity College of Nursing & Health Sciences
Rock Island, IL

Tawna Cooksey-James, PhD, RN
Post Doctoral Fellow
The University of Iowa
College of Nursing
Iowa City, IA

Perle Slavik Cowen, PhD, RN
Associate Professor
The University of Iowa
College of Nursing
Iowa City, IA

Sister Ruth Cox, OSF, PhD, RN
Faculty
Kirkwood Community College
Cedar Rapids, IA

Martha Craft-Rosenberg, PhD, RN, FAAN
Professor Emerita
The University of Iowa
College of Nursing
Iowa City, IA

Judith Daugherty, PhD, RN
Clinical Director
EXCELCARE, Inc.
Ligonier, PA

Janice Denehy, PhD, RN
Associate Professor Emerita
The University of Iowa
College of Nursing
Iowa City, IA

Mary Ann Fahrenkrug, RN, MS
Faculty
St. Ambrose University
Davenport, IA

Carme Espinosa i Fresnedo
Professor
University of Andorra
College of Nursing

Kimberly Gray, RN, MSN, CNRN
Stroke Program Coordinator
St. Joseph Mercy Hospital
Ann Arbor, MI

Jennifer Hafner RN, BSN, PCCN, TNCC
Medical Surgical Intensive Care
Aspirus Wausau Hospital
Wausau, WI

Renae Harroun, MSN, RN
Faculty
Trinity College of Nursing & Health Sciences
Rock Island, IL

Crystal Heath, MS, RN
Doctoral Student
University of Michigan
Ann Arbor, MI

Barbara Head, PhD, RN
Assistant Professor
University of Nebraska Medical Center
College of Nursing
Omaha, NE

Marcia Hegstad, RN, MN, CS, CDE, BC-ADM
Clinical Nurse Specialist for Diabetes/CNS
  Link to Medical Intensive Care and Medicine
Progressive Care Units
St. Joseph Mercy Hospital
Ann Arbor, MI

Barbara Heilmann, RN, BSN, TNCC
Medical Surgical Intensive Care
Aspirus Wausau Hospital
Wausau, WI

Jean Hirt, RN, BSN
Education Coordinator/General Medicine,
  Older Adult, and Stroke Unit
St. Joseph Mercy Hospital
Ann Arbor, MI

Penny Hunt, MHSA, RN
Nursing Information Systems Coordinator
St. Rita's Medical Center
Lima, OH

Gail Keenan, PhD, RN
Associate Professor
Director, Nursing Informatics Initiative
University of Illinois
College of Nursing
Chicago, IL

Peg Kerr, MS, PhD, RN
Post Doctoral Fellow
The University of Iowa
College of Nursing
Iowa City, IA

Mary B. Killeen, PhD, RN, CNAA, BC
Assistant Professor
Michigan State University
College of Nursing
East Lansing, MI

Katharine Kolcaba, PhD, RN, C
Associate Professor
The University of Akron
Akron, OH

Cathy Konrad, PhD, RNC
Faculty
Trinity College of Nursing & Health Sciences
Rock Island, IL

Mary E. Kravutske, PhD, RN
Nurse Scholar
Henry Ford Hospital
Detroit, MI

Regina Holly Lange, MS, RN
Faculty
Trinity College of Nursing & Health Sciences
Rock Island, IL

Kathryn McKnight, MSN, PNP, MPH
Faculty
St. Ambrose University
Davenport, IA

Jodi Pahl, MSN, RN-C
Clinical Manager
St. Rita's Medical Center
Lima, OH

Lisa Payden, MS, TNS, RN
Manager
Trauma Center, Trinity West
Rock Island, IL

Shelley-Rae Pehler, PhD, RN
Faculty
St. Ambrose University
Davenport, IA

LesLea Pitcher, MS, RN
Nurse Educator
United Health Services
Binghamton, NY

Cindy Scherb, PhD, RN
Associate Professor
Winona State University
Rochester, MN

Corinne Snell, RN, BSN, CCRN, TNCC
Medical Surgical Intensive Care
Aspirus Wausau Hospital
Wausau, WI

Janet Specht, PhD, RN, FAAN
Associate Professor
University of Iowa
College of Nursing
Iowa City, IA

Patricia Strasser-Thomas, RN
Care Plan Coordinator
United Health Services
Binghamton, NY

Shirley Wiesman, RN, MSN, CCRN
Medical Surgical Intensive Care
Aspirus Wausau Hospital
Wausau, WI

Marilyn Willits, MS, RN, CPHQ
Standards Nurse Specialist
Genesis Medical Center East
Davenport, IA

Karen Wilson, MSN, RN
Program Coordinator, Emergency Medical
  Services
Trinity College of Nursing & Health Sciences
Rock Island, IL

Mary Zugcic, MS, RN-BC
Instructor—Clinical
Wayne State University
College of Nursing
Detroit, MI

Students

Noriko Abe
Doctoral student

Rebecca Porter
Doctoral student

Mikyoung Lee
Doctoral student, Research assistant

Molly Sandholm
Baccalaureate student, Young scientist

Melissa Lehan-Makin
Doctoral student

Maneewan Sanubol Seay
Doctoral student

Angela Oldenberg
Doctoral student

Leah Shever
Doctoral student

Eun-Jun Park
Doctoral student, Research assistant

Visiting Professor

Renate Stemmer
Catholic University of Applied Sciences
Mainz Germany
Jong Kyung Kim
South Korea

Staff

Sharon Sweeney
Coordinator, Center for Nursing Classification
  & Clinical Effectiveness
University of Iowa
College of Nursing
Iowa City, IA

Linda Curran
Secretary
University of Iowa
College of Nursing
Iowa City, IA

David Reed, PhD
Statistician
University of Iowa
College of Nursing
Iowa City, IA

Fellows—Center for Nursing Classification and Clinical Effectiveness

The Center for Nursing Classification and Clinical Effectiveness at the College of Nursing. The University of Iowa has established a fellows program. An appointment of *Fellow, Center for Nursing Classification & Clinical Effectiveness* is designated for individuals who contribute significantly to the ongoing upkeep and implementation of NIC and NOC. Fellows may be research team members, staff at cooperating agencies, retired professors, and visiting scholars. Graduate students who are within a year of finishing their doctoral dissertation and who have made substantial contributions to the work of the CNC are eligible.

Fellows donate a portion of their time to some work activity of the Center. They are available as resource persons for such activities as: ad hoc reviews of proposed new interventions and outcomes, participating in team or other meetings, serving on a planning committee for a conference, reviewing drafts of monographs, participating in grant writing activities, and advising the board of current developments related to classification work. An appointment of a fellow is for a 3-year period or shorter time depending on need (e.g., Visiting Scholar).

The following individuals are serving as Fellows as of January 1, 2007:
- Mary Ann Anderson, Associate Professor, College of Nursing, University of Illinois, Quad Cities Regional Program
- Ida Androwich, Professor, Loyola University, Chicago
- Sandra Bellinger, Adjunct Faculty, Trinity College of Nursing & Health Sciences
- Teresa Boese, Associate Professor (Clinical), College of Nursing, University of Iowa
- Veronica Brighton, Assistant Professor (Clinical), College of Nursing, University of Iowa
- Jane Brokel, Assistant Professor, College of Nursing, University of Iowa
- Kathleen Buckwalter, Professor & Director John A. Hartford Center for Geriatric Nursing Excellence, College of Nursing, University of Iowa
- Lisa Burkhart, Assistant Professor, Loyola University, Chicago
- Gloria Bulechek, Professor, College of Nursing, University of Iowa
- Howard Butcher, Associate Professor, College of Nursing, University of Iowa
- Teresa Clark, Advance Practice Nurse, Informatics, University of Iowa Hospitals and Clinics
- Mary Clarke, Director of Nursing Practice, Research, and Innovation, Genesis Medical Center, Davenport, Iowa
- Perle Slavik Cowen, Associate Professor, College of Nursing, University of Iowa
- Sister Ruth Cox, Faculty, Kirkwood Community College, Cedar Rapids
- Martha Craft-Rosenberg, Professor Emerita, College of Nursing, University of Iowa
- Jeanette Daly, Research Assistant, Family Medicine, University of Iowa
- Connie Delaney, Dean and Professor, College of Nursing, University of Minnesota
- Janice Denehy, Associate Professor Emerita, College of Nursing, University of Iowa
- Joanne Dochterman, Professor Emerita, College of Nursing, University of Iowa
- Gloria Dorr, Advance Practice Nurse, Informatics, University of Iowa Hospitals and Clinics
- Barbara Head, Assistant Professor, College of Nursing, University of Nebraska Medical Center
- Keela Herr, Professor, College of Nursing, University of Iowa
- Larry Hertel, President and Founder, Professional Home Health Services, Cedar Rapids
- Todd Ingram, Assistant Professor (Clinical), College of Nursing, University of Iowa

- Marion Johnson, Professor Emerita, College of Nursing, University of Iowa
- Gail Keenan, Associate Professor, Director Nursing Informatics Initiative, University of Illinois Chicago, College of Nursing
- Peg Kerr, Post Doctoral Fellow, College of Nursing, University of Iowa
- Cathy Konrad, Faculty, Trinity College of Nursing & Health Sciences
- Vicki Kraus, Advanced Nurse Practitioner, University of Iowa Hospital & Clinics
- Meridean Maas, Professor Emerita, College of Nursing, University of Iowa
- Paula Mobily, Associate Professor, College of Nursing, University of Iowa
- Sue Moorhead, Associate Professor, & Director, Center for Nursing Classification & Clinical Effectiveness, College of Nursing, University of Iowa
- Aleta Porcella, Clinical Nurse Specialist–Informatics, University of Iowa Hospitals and Clinics
- Barb Rakel, Assistant Professor, College of Nursing, University of Iowa
- David Reed, Director, Center for Computational Nursing, College of Nursing, University of Iowa
- Cindy Scherb, Associate Professor, Winona State University
- Debra Schutte, Assistant Professor, College of Nursing, University of Iowa
- Margaret Simons, Diabetes Nurse Specialist, Iowa City VA Medical Center
- Janet Specht, Associate Professor, College of Nursing, University of Iowa
- Elizabeth Swanson, Associate Professor, College of Nursing, University of Iowa
- Mary Tarbox, Professor and Chair, Department of Nursing, Mt. Mercy College
- Marita Titler, Senior Associate Director of Nursing & Director, Nursing Research, Quality & Outcomes Management, University of Iowa Hospital & Clinics
- Toni Tripp-Reimer, Professor, College of Nursing, University of Iowa
- Cheryl Wagner, Doctoral Student, College of Nursing, University of Iowa and Associate Professor, Kaplan University, Chicago
- Bonnie Wakefield, Research Associate Professor, Sinclair School of Nursing, University of Missouri
- Janet Williams, Professor, College of Nursing, University of Iowa
- Marilyn Willits, Standards Nurse Specialist, Genesis Health Care, Davenport, Iowa

Preface

The fourth edition of the *Nursing Outcomes Classification (NOC)* contains 385 outcomes and represents more than 16 years of work by the Iowa Outcomes team. The classification standardizes the outcome name and definitions for use in practice, education, and research. Each outcome includes a label name, a definition, a set of indicators that describe specific states, perceptions, or behaviors related to the outcome, a 5-point Likert measurement scale(s) and selected references used in the development of the outcome. The outcomes assist nurses and other health care providers to evaluate and quantify the status of the patient, caregiver, family, or community. A strength of this classification is its focus on the measurement of outcomes across a variety of specialties and settings. In addition, nurses are able to quantify the change in patient status after interventions and monitor progress. Feedback from clinicians using the outcome measures in clinical settings has been positive, and their suggestions have helped improve the classification. We have also been consulting with nursing in the area of informatics to better position this work for inclusion in an electronic health record.

Fifty-eight new outcomes have been added to the classification in this edition and are listed in Appendix A along with a list of changes in the outcomes. In the last edition comments from nurses in practice helped us improve the format of the outcomes, as well as refine definitions, measurement scales, and indicators. Changes in this edition reflect our current focus on standardizing the indicators used with each scale. There has been a conscious effort to refine the indicators based on the measurement scale they are associated within the classification. This has been a lengthy project and resulted in many indicators having minor changes so they were worded the same in outcomes using a specific scale. We have also developed a preferred verb list for scales that focus on behavior. We anticipate that the next edition will continue this work and will result in a new coding system to provide the same code for indictors that are used in more than one outcome.

This edition provides practical guidance on how to use NOC in clinical practice. Chapter 1 provides an overview of outcome research in health care and nursing and early research to develop and refine this classification. This chapter is helpful for nurses who are beginning to consider the use of outcome measures in their practice and want an overview of outcome use in nursing. Chapter 2 describes the current classification presented in this edition. Definition of terms, frequently asked questions, and new features are highlighted. Chapter 3 discusses how to use NOC in clinical practice and has useful suggestions and updated examples of how NOC has been used in a variety of settings. Chapter 4 discusses the use of NOC in education and research and highlights current work and future directions.

Linkages between the NANDA diagnoses and the NOC outcomes are included in Part IV of the book. The reader will note that the NANDA diagnoses are listed by key concept and are consistent with the terminology used in the 2007-2008 edition of the NANDA International Classification. Also included in this section are linkages with Gordon's Functional Patterns. A brief summary of a project linking NOC and the International Classification of Functioning is also included in Part IV. It is important to note that these linkages are not prescriptive and have not been validated with clinical data. They are suggested to assist nurses with identifying possible outcomes when a diagnosis is made or to develop a framework for clinical information systems. *The nurse's clinical judgment remains the most important factor in selecting outcomes.*

The need for nursing to define the patient outcomes that are responsive to nursing care has continued to increase since the first edition of this book was published. The growth of managed care, the emphasis on cost containment, and the need for evidence-based practice continue to bring concerns about effectiveness of nursing interventions and health care quality to the attention of nurses, consumers, health care organizations, payers, and policy makers. Nursing plays a key role in the delivery of cost-effective care in every health care setting; therefore it is imperative that nursing data be included in the evaluation of health care effectiveness. The NOC completes the nursing process elements of the Nursing Minimum Data Set (NMDS). NOC is a companion language to the NIC interventions and the NANDA diagnoses. Standardized nursing languages are required to ensure that the nursing elements identified in the NMDS are included in electronic patient databases. They also facilitate the study and teaching of diagnostic reasoning and the development of mid-range theory as linkages between patient characteristics, nursing diagnoses, nursing interventions, and nursing-sensitive outcomes are tested.

The editors of this book thank the many nurses who have contributed to the development of NOC. The team has worked diligently to continue to expand and evaluate the NOC outcomes. Many individuals have shared their knowledge and work with us or have agreed to review an outcome related to their specialty. Without them, this edition would not be possible.

Sue Moorhead, PhD, RN
Marion Johnson, PhD, RN
Meridean L. Maas, PhD, RN, FAAN
Elizabeth Swanson, PhD, RN

Strengths of the Nursing Outcomes Classification

Comprehensive. The NOC contains outcomes for individuals, caregivers, families, and communities that can be used with all clinical specialties in numerous settings. Although there are still outcomes to develop, the outcomes in this fourth edition are useful for the entire scope of nursing practice.

Research-based. The research, conducted by a large team of University of Iowa College of Nursing faculty and students in conjunction with clinicians from a variety of settings began in 1991. Both qualitative and quantitative strategies were used to develop the classification. Methods included content analysis, concept analysis, survey of experts, similarity analysis, hierarchical clustering analysis, multidimensional scaling, and clinical field site testing. The outcomes were evaluated for interrater reliability, validity, and usefulness in 10 clinical sites representing the care continuum.

Developed inductively and deductively. Sources of data for the initial development of outcomes and indicators were nursing textbooks, care plan guides, nursing clinical information systems, standards of practice, and research instruments. Research team focus groups reviewed outcomes in eight broad categories that were drawn from the Medical Outcomes Study and nursing literature. Based on a review of literature, outcomes were grouped in broad categories and refined through concept analysis.

Grounded in clinical practice and research. Developed initially from nursing texts, care plan guides, and clinical information systems, the outcomes were reviewed by clinical experts and many were tested in clinical field sites. Feedback from clinicians and educators is solicited through a defined feedback process. Beginning work on core NOC outcomes for specialty practice was first included in the third edition. This grounding in clinical practice continues with this edition as numerous outcomes were developed by clinical experts and forwarded to the authors.

Uses clear, clinically useful language. Throughout the development of the NOC, clarity and usefulness of the language have been emphasized. Care has been taken to ensure that the language distinguishes NOC outcomes from nursing interventions and diagnoses. The outcomes are developed for patients, caregivers, families, and communities.

Has easy to use organizing structure. The taxonomy has 5 levels: domains, classes, outcomes, indicators, and measurement scales. All 5 levels have been coded for use in practice. New outcomes are added to the taxonomy as the classification is further developed. This structure aids nurses in identifying outcomes to use in their clinical practice and provides a framework for teaching NOC to students in educational settings.

Outcomes can be shared by all disciplines. Although the NOC emphasizes outcomes that are most responsive to nursing interventions, the outcomes describe patient, family, or community states at a conceptual level. Thus the NOC provides a classification of patient outcomes that are potentially influenced by all health care disciplines. Use of the outcomes by all members of the interdisciplinary team provides standardization, yet allows the selection of indicators that are most responsive to each discipline. Field testing demonstrated that the outcomes were useful to interdisciplinary teams in practice.

Optimizes information used for the evaluation of effectiveness. The outcomes and indicators are variable concepts. They allow for measurement of the patient, family, or community outcome at any point on a continuum from most negative to most positive and at different points in time. Rather than the limited information of whether a goal is met or unmet, NOC outcomes can be used to monitor the extent of progress, or lack of progress, throughout an episode of care and across different care settings. Change in outcome ratings can be reported and recorded as a result of nursing interventions instituted across time and care setting.

Funded by extramural grants. To date, the NOC research has received 9 years of peer-reviewed grant funding: 1 year from Sigma Theta Tau International and 8 years from the National Institute of Nursing Research (NINR).

Tested in clinical field sites. Testing of the NOC has been conducted in a variety of clinical field sites, including tertiary care hospitals, intermediate care hospitals, a nursing home, home health care settings, nurse managed clinics, and a parish nursing organization. The field tests have provided important information about the clinical usefulness of the outcomes and indicators; linkages between nursing diagnoses, interventions, and outcomes; and the process of implementing the outcomes in clinical nursing information systems.

Dissemination emphasized. Information about the classification, its development, and use is available in this book published by Elsevier every 4 years and in numerous journal articles and book chapters. The NOC research is described on a University of Iowa College of Nursing World Wide Web home page (http://www.nursing.uiowa.edu/cnc), and a listserv is maintained to share information about the NOC and for dialogue with interested users. The NOC work has been disseminated in numerous national and international presentations. Although developed in the United States, nurses in other countries are finding the classification useful. Translations are complete or in process for the following languages: Chinese, Dutch, French, German, Japanese, Korean, Spanish, and Portuguese.

Linked to other nursing languages. Linkages have been developed by the NIC and NOC research teams to assist nurses with the use of the classifications and to facilitate use in clinical information systems. Linkages with NANDA-International diagnoses and Gordon's Functional Health Care Patterns are included in the book. Linkages among NANDA diagnoses, NOC outcomes, and NIC interventions are available in the book *NANDA, NIC, and NOC linkage: Nursing diagnoses, interventions and outcomes*, published by Elsevier in 2006. In addition, linkages have been developed with the International Classification of Functioning, Disability and Health (ICF) and NOC in an attempt to explore the components of ICF and identify the relevant concepts to promote language development in nursing. In addition, ICF was chosen for its international and interdisciplinary use. Work is also being done to link ICF to NNN.

Included in initiatives for electronic clinical record. Concepts for NOC will be included in SNOMED Clinical Terms, a reference terminology for use in clinical information systems. NOC has been registered with Health Level 7, a U.S. standards organization dedicated to simplifying the exchange, management, and integration of clinical and administrative data in health records. A growing number of vendors have licensed NOC for inclusion in their software development initiatives for a nursing component of an electronic clinical record.

Developed as companion to the NIC. Experience with the NIC at Iowa has aided the NOC research. Both classifications are comprehensive and research-based and reflect current clinical nursing practice. They are both housed in the Center for Nursing Classification and Clinical Effectiveness.

Recipient of national recognition. NOC is recognized by the American Nurses Association (ANA), is included in the Metathesaurus for a Unified Medical Language at the National Library of Medicine and the CINAHL index, and is listed as one of the languages that meets the standards set by ANA's Nursing Information and Data Set Evaluation Center (NIDSEC).

Structure for continued development and refinement. The classification continues to be evaluated, developed, and refined by the NOC research team. Continued refinement will be facilitated through the Center for Nursing Classification and Clinical Effectiveness, the College of Nursing, and the University of Iowa. In addition to seeking continued grant support, a $1 million endowment is being raised to ensure a solid financial foundation for supporting further development of both NIC and NOC. Revenue from the sales of the book and licensing are used to support the staff and work of the Center for Nursing Classification and Clinical Effectiveness.

Acknowledgments

Continual development of the Nursing Outcomes Classification (NOC) and this publication would not have been possible without the work and support of numerous individuals and organizations. We are indebted to the many individuals who have supported out work and encouraged us along the way. We would like to acknowledge and thank the following individuals and organizations for their efforts:

- *Sigma Theta Tau International* for a 1 year grant (1992-1993) and the Office of Nursing Research, University of Iowa, for seed grants (1992-1993). These grants partially funded the pilot work and beginning development of the NOC.
- *The National Institute of Nursing Research, National Institutes of Health*, for a 4-year grant (1993-1997) to continue the development of the classification, construct the taxonomy, and field test the outcomes and for a 4-year continuation grant (1998-2001) entitled "Evaluation of Nursing-Sensitive Patient Outcome Measures" to pilot the outcomes and evaluate the measurement scales in clinical sites.
- The *College of Nursing at the University of Iowa* for support of this work by *past Deans Geraldene Felton and Melanie Dreher and Interim Dean Martha Craft-Rosenberg*. This support for the Center for Nursing Classification and Effectiveness since it was founded in 1995 has been instrumental in the continuing development and refinement of both NIC and NOC and our work on Linkages among diagnoses, interventions, and outcomes.
- The *team members, clinicians, educators, fellows, and students* who have devoted hours of work to develop, review, and refine the outcomes, associated indicators, and measurement scales that appear in the NOC.
- The *American Nurses Association* for supporting the validation survey and the *ANA's Congress of Nursing Practice Steering Committee on Databases to Support Clinical Nursing Practice* for recognizing NOC as a classification system useful for clinical nursing practice.
- The *NANDA International* organization for its partnership through the Alliance that links NANDA, NIC, and NOC in efforts such as the NNN taxonomy structure development and NANDA, NIC, and NOC national conferences.
- The *clinical sites and their staff* who worked diligently to include the NOC outcomes and measurement scales in their clinical sites as part of our research: Alverno Health Care Facility–Clinton, IA; Mayo Clinic–Rochester, MN; Genesis Medical Center–Davenport, IA; University of Michigan Community Family Health Center–Ann Arbor, MI; North Campus Nursing Center–Ann Arbor, MI; Huron Valley Visiting Nurse Association–Ann Arbor, MI; Pontiac-Oakland Visiting Nurse Association–Waterford, MI; University of Iowa Hospitals and Clinics–Iowa City, IA; Mayo Health System–Mankato and Austin, MN
- EXCELCARE, Inc. and the clinical sites Henry Ford Hospital, Detroit, MI; St. Rita's Medical Center, Lima, OH; and United Health Services, Binghamton, NY
- *Nurses from a variety of nursing specialty organizations* who shared their expertise by completing validation surveys and core surveys to further this effort.
- The many *patients and their families* who were willing to participate in our research and complete both outcome ratings and criterion tool measures as we tested our outcomes in clinical settings.
- *Contributors to our endowment fund* to support the efforts of the Center for Nursing Classification and Clinical Effectiveness.

- Our very competent staff, *Sharon Sweeney* and *David Reed,* who believed in this work, shared in our vision, and managed the data and details of this classification to make this edition possible. A special thank you to *Linda Curran,* who helped with the manuscript submission for this edition.
- Barbara Cullen, who has facilitated the development and publication of this classification focused on outcomes. We also thank Michael Wisniewski, Director of Licensing Sales; Karen Delaney, Licensing Specialist; Sandra Clark Brown, Senior Acquistions Editor; and Cindi Anderson, Senior Development Editor for this edition.

Detailed Contents

PART THREE Outcomes, 145

PART FOUR NOC Linkages: Health Patterns: NANDA—International International Classification Functioning, 735

NOC Linkages—Health Patterns, 737

PART FIVE Core Outcomes for Nursing Specialty Areas, 841

Identifying Core Outcomes, 843

Nursing Outcomes Classification: Development, Refinement, and Use in Practice, Research, and Education

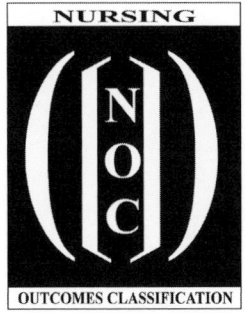

CHAPTER ONE

Outcome Development
and Significance

Despite several decades of concern about the costs and quality of health care in the United States, costs continue to increase and quality remains a prominent issue. A variety of evaluation tools that are designed to measure the outcomes of health care delivery have resulted. Although these measures have the potential to improve care delivery and to provide information about physician practice and organizational outcomes, the interventions and outcomes of nursing care are not readily apparent in most evaluation systems. More recently, patient safety emerged as a prominent and critical imperative with the publication of *To Err Is Human: Building a Safer Health System* by the Institute of Medicine (IOM).[87] Although more than 5 years have passed, to date, few health care organizations have reached the goals for patient safety and quality set forth by the IOM. Evidence indicates that patient safety and quality of care deficits persist as a result of poor communication and collaboration among interdisciplinary providers and the differing priorities of patient care among members of the health care team.[47]

Nurses have primary accountability for the monitoring and management of health care delivered to patients each day in a variety of settings.[18] Nurses are responsible for early detection of patient complications and problems and are best positioned to initiate actions that minimize negative patient outcomes.[30,31] In addition, nurses are accountable for diagnosing patient problems that are amenable to nursing interventions, such as pain, impaired skin integrity, knowledge deficit, and self-care deficits. The clinical reasoning and decision making of nurses are integral to quality health care and account for much of the health care system "safety net." Despite the critical role of nurses in maintaining quality and safety of patients; outcomes of nursing interventions have been largely neglected. As efforts to improve the quality of health care and patient safety continue, it is imperative that nursing define its interventions and outcomes and that these standardized nomenclatures be included in clinical nursing information systems and in large data sets used for systematic analysis.

OUTCOME DEVELOPMENT IN HEALTH CARE

The systematic use of patient outcomes to evaluate health care began when Florence Nightingale recorded and analyzed health care conditions and patient outcomes during the Crimean War.[95,158] Since that time, attempts to identify, measure, and use patient outcomes in the evaluation of health care delivery have been sporadic, often discipline-specific, and commonly focused on physician practice.[75,104] Efforts to evaluate physician practice began in the early 1900s when Codman, a Boston surgeon, proposed the use of outcome-based measures as indicators of medical care quality.[153] His work is considered the precursor of modern outcomes research. It wasn't until the mid-1960s, however, that a model for assessing the quality of physician practice was proposed by Donabedian.[43] The model, which emphasized structure, process, and outcome, was adopted by other health care disciplines and gained wide use as the preferred method of evaluating the quality of health care services. Still, the complexity of problems inherent in identifying and measuring patient outcomes resulted in measures of structure and process developing more rapidly than measures of patient outcomes. Until the 1980s, mortality, morbidity, and clinical signs served as traditional outcome measures. With the emphasis on effectiveness in the mid-1980s fueled by political pressure and the availability of large data sets because of advances in information technology, attention again turned to measures of patient outcomes to evaluate physician practice.

An important study of physician practice, the Medical Outcomes Study (MOS), used structure, process, and outcome elements to evaluate medical care effectiveness.[167] Outcome measures in the MOS were defined in broad categories of clinical end points, including signs and symptoms, laboratory values, and death; functional status, including physical, mental, social, and role; general well-being, which included health perceptions, energy/fatigue, pain, and life satisfaction; and satisfaction with care, including access, convenience, financial coverage, quality, and general satisfaction. Shortened versions of outcome measures,[177] such as the Medical Outcomes Study Short Form-36 (MOS-SF-36)[178] and MOS-SF-12 have gained wide acceptance as general measures of health care delivery effectiveness and quality.

As the costs of health care have continued to increase, so have concerns about the quality of care. As previously noted, patient safety became a major national concern with the publication of *To Err Is Human: Building a Safer Health System* by the Institute of Medicine (IOM).[87] A consequence has been the development of a variety of quality and performance measures by federal agencies, regulatory bodies, and public organizations. A number of standardized performance measures, referred to as *report cards,* have been developed in an attempt to quantify the quality and effectiveness of health care delivery systems and organizations. Examples are the Outcome Concept System and the Health Plan Employer Data and Information Set (HEDIS) developed for evaluating the quality of managed care plan performance (National Committee for Quality Assurance [NCQA]).[132,134] An analysis of report cards, however, noted that while some contain outcomes that are sensitive to nursing interventions, many have no nursing content.[14] Quality Compass is a report of HEDIS measures, focusing on medical care and prepared for consumers.[134] HEDIS 3.0 includes measures of effective care processes, access and availability of care, patient satisfaction, cost of care, and the health care plan.[118]

Accrediting agencies foster the use of outcomes to evaluate the effectiveness and quality of health care delivered by organizations. The Joint Commission (TJC), formerly known as The Joint Commission on Accreditation of Healthcare Organizations (JCAHO), initiated a requirement that all hospitals and long-term care organizations seeking TJC accreditation use a performance measurement system to provide data about patient outcomes and other indicators of care effective January 1, 1998.[179] Organizations can select TJC's Indicator Measurement System (IMSystem), one of the commercial systems approved by the commission, or they can develop their own system for approval.[130,179] IMSystem contains 31 measures for perioperative, obstetric, trauma, oncology, and cardiovascular patients, as well as 11 measures of medication use and infection control.[130] Currently, TJC requires home care agencies certified by CMS for Medicare and Medicaid reimbursement to submit performance indicators based on aggregated data from the federally mandated Outcome and Assessment Information Set (OASIS).[10]

The federal government has assumed an active role in outcomes research and management, primarily through the Agency for Healthcare Research and Quality (AHRQ) (formerly the Agency for Health Care Policy and Research) and the Center for Medicare and Medicaid Services (CMS), formerly the Health Care Financing Administration (HCFA). Between 1992 and 1996, AHRQ sponsored the development and dissemination of 20 clinical practice guidelines. The agency has initiated a new program called the Clinical Improvement Program with three new initiatives: the creation of evidence-based practice centers, a national guideline clearinghouse, and product research and evaluation.[118] CMS has used the work of the AHRQ to develop and test national quality indicator modules[118] and to set requirements for standardized data collection for nursing homes, home care agencies, and hospitals.

AHRQ issues an annual report, the National Healthcare Quality Report (NHQR), built each year on core measures selected from 179 measures assembled across four dimensions of quality-effectiveness, patient safety, timeliness, and patient centeredness.[174] The 179 measures are developed for specific diseases, such as breast cancer and heart failure, and focus on medical care processes. Healthcare Cost and Utilization Project Quality Indicators (HCUP QIs) were developed by AHRQ in the early 1990s in response to states' requests for a quality assessment tool that could be used with hospital administrative data. The HCUP QIs comprised a set of 33 clinical performance measures that could be used to inform hospitals' self-assessments of inpatient quality of care, as well as state and community assessments of access to primary care. Because of recognized limitations of the HCUP QIs, AHRQ contracted with Stanford University's Evidence-Based Practice Center to evaluate Healthcare Cost and Utilization Project (HCUP) QIs and develop new indicators, which became the AHRQ Quality Indicators. The AHRQ QIs now replace the original HCUP indicators. The AHRQ QIs provide a standardized measure to highlight potential quality concerns, to identify areas that need further study, and to enable tracking of changes over time. The intent is to facilitate transparency by making comparative quality information accessible, to enhance the decision making of all stakeholders, including federal, state, and local policymakers, clinicians, and purchasers.

In July 1999, CMS initiated a nursing home quality indicator (QI) system of reporting to states. The QI reporting system was developed under contract with researchers at the Center for Health Services and Research Assessment (CHSRA), the University of Wisconsin–Madison, using data from the Long Term Care Minimum Data Set (LTC-MDS). Accessed through Internet web browsers, the state reporting system provides nursing home facility-level and resident-level summary reports that can be accessed by surveyors, facilities, and consumers. The Quality Initiative was launched nationally by CMS in 2002 with the Nursing Home Quality Initiative (NHQI) and expanded in 2003 with the Home Health Quality Initiative (HHQI) and the Hospital Quality Initiative (HQI). In 2004, the Physician Focused Quality Initiative was developed and was expanded to officially include kidney dialysis facilities. The End Stage Renal Disease (ESRD) Quality Initiative promotes ongoing CMS strategies to improve the quality of care provided to ESRD patients. In 2005, CMS announced the Physician Voluntary Reporting Program to begin in 2006.[27]

Clearly, there are many federal and public efforts to develop valid and useful measures of quality for policy makers, providers, and consumers to ensure the effectiveness of health care. To enable all federal agencies with health care responsibilities to coordinate their activities to measure and improve the quality of care, to provide beneficiaries with information to assist them in making choices about their care, and to develop the infrastructure needed to improve the health care system, including knowledgeable and empowered workers, well-designed systems of care, and useful information systems, the federal government established the Quality Interagency Coordination Task Force (QuIC). In addition, AHRQ maintains the National Quality Measures Clearinghouse (www.qualitymeasures.ahrq.gov), a public repository for evidence-based quality measures and measure sets. In an attempt to develop and implement a national strategy for health care quality measurement and reporting, the National Quality Forum (NQF), a private, not-for-profit membership organization, was formed. In addition to developing performance standards and measures for medical care, the NQF reviews performance measures and QIs developed by others, such as AHRQ and CMS, and promotes national standardization of these measures of quality.

OUTCOME DEVELOPMENT IN NURSING

The use of patient outcomes to evaluate nursing care quality began in the mid-1960s, when Aydelotte[13] used changes in behavioral and physical characteristics of patients to evaluate the effectiveness of nursing care delivery systems. Since that time, additional outcome measures have been developed and tested for nursing[60] and a variety of patient outcomes have been used to evaluate the quality of nursing care and the effects of nursing interventions.[94,133,136,166]

In addition to the development and testing of outcome measures, nurses have expended considerable effort to categorize outcomes and more recently to identify "core" outcome measures.

Early work to classify nursing-sensitive patient outcomes took place in the late 1970s. Hover and Zimmer[65] identified the following five general outcome measures focused on the patient's knowledge: knowledge of illness and its treatments; knowledge of medications; self-care skills; adaptive behaviors; and health status. These broad outcome categories were based on a review of patient outcomes used by nurses at that time.

Horn and Swain[64] conducted a major research effort to identify outcome measures useful for nursing research and categorized more than 300 indicators in the broad categories of universal demands and health deviation. Daubert[34] proposed the following five categories to measure rehabilitation potential in home care: (1) recovery, (2) self-care, (3) rehabilitation, (4) maintenance, and (5) terminal care. Lalonde[93] developed and tested the following measures for home health evaluation: taking prescribed medications as instructed, general symptom distress, discharge status, caregiver status, functional status, knowledge of major health problems and diagnosis, and physiological indicators.

In the 1980s two outcome categorizations based on extensive reviews of outcomes used in nursing research were formulated. Lang and Clinton[94] identified the following six outcome categories: (1) physical health status; (2) mental health status; (3) social and physical functioning; (4) health attitudes, knowledge, and behavior; (5) use of professional health resources; and (6) patient perceptions of the quality of nursing care. Marek[110] identified 15 outcome categories describing patient status and resource use based on a review of outcomes used to evaluate nursing care. Table 1-1 lists these categories. This work by Marek[110] was the foundation on which outcomes research was based.

The increased importance placed on health care effectiveness in the 1990s resulted in a renewed emphasis on outcome development in nursing, including efforts to identify "core" patient outcomes for evaluation of nursing care effectiveness. McCormick[117] proposed a list of measurable outcomes that included process and patient outcomes as a means of evaluating nursing effectiveness, primarily in acute care settings. Patient outcomes identified as salient for nursing were normal fluid hydration, continence, mobility, and the absence of decubitus and mucous membrane ulcers. The American Nurses Association (ANA) developed a Nursing Care Report Card for hospitals. This report card identifies a core set of nursing quality indicators, which includes structure, process, and outcome indicators. Outcome indicators include mortality rate, length of stay, adverse incidents, complications such as nosocomial infections and decubitus ulcers, and patient satisfaction with nursing care. The ANA outcome indicators are aggregated measures that characterize the hospital or patient care unit rather than individual patients.

In addition to the identification of core outcome measures sensitive to nursing interventions, there has been increased emphasis on the development of conceptual models or frameworks to

---

Table 1-1   OUTCOME CATEGORIES DEVELOPED BY MAREK[110]

Physiological measures	Goal attainment
Psychosocial measures	Patient satisfaction
Functional measures	Safety
Client behaviors	Frequency of service
Client knowledge	Cost
Symptom control	Rehospitalization
Home maintenance	Resolution of nursing diagnoses
Well-being	

describe the patient outcomes relevant for nursing, and the relationships among patient outcomes, structure and process elements, and patient characteristics. An example presented by Gillette and Jenko proposes a framework generated for use in hospital settings suggested the measurement of outcomes that evaluate patient/family education, facilitation of self-care, symptom distress management, provisions for patient safety, and enhancement of patient satisfaction.[50] Brown[23] proposed a conceptual framework for quality evaluation that included physiological condition, psychological status, health knowledge, and satisfaction. Naylor and associates[136] have suggested functional status, mental status, stress level, satisfaction with care, burden of care, and cost of care as appropriate outcomes for the evaluation of nursing care effectiveness. The Quality Health Outcomes Model has been developed by an American Academy of Nursing expert panel.[123] The model incorporates structure and process elements as system characteristics and proposes a reciprocal relationship among system characteristics, interventions, outcomes, and patient characteristics.

Efforts have also focused on the development of nursing vocabularies and taxonomies. In addition to the classification described in this book, there are other classifications that contain patient outcome systems recognized by the ANA. Two of these were developed for use in home care. The Omaha System[112,113] includes a problem classification scheme, an intervention scheme, and the Problem Rating Scale for Outcomes (PRSO). The rating scale is a five-point ordinal scale measuring patient progress in relation to knowledge, behavior, and status. The scale can be applied to any of the problems identified in the classification. An initial assessment of the content validity and inter-rater reliability of the scale has been published.[114] The Home Health Care Classification, now called Clinical Care Classification, uses three discharge status measures— improved, stabilized, and deteriorated.[156,157] The measures can be assigned to any problem identified in the classification. The Patient Care Data Set[141] was developed for use in hospital settings. It provided a range of possible outcomes for specific patient problems common in acute care settings. This system was recently retired from the ANA recognition list.

Two other outcome systems important for nursing are in use or being tested. The Outcome Assessment Information Set (OASIS) was developed at the Center for Health Policy Research at the University of Colorado.[159] The system contains core measures that apply to all client groups and specific measures for client groups with a particular diagnosis or problem. Each outcome is measured on a scale specific for the outcome to determine whether the patient has improved, stabilized or deteriorated. This is the only system that has reported testing of risk adjustment factors. Beginning in 1998 the HCFA's Conditions of Participation required all Medicare-accredited home health organizations to incorporate the OASIS data set into their processes of care.[29] The OASIS data set includes information about the sensory, integumentary, respiratory, elimination, neurologic, emotional, behavioral, and functional status of the patient in addition to demographic and other information. The other classification of importance to nursing is the International Classification for Nursing Practice (ICNP). The ICNP is a multi-axial classification of nursing phenomena in which an outcome classification is replaced by nursing diagnostic judgments of patient status made at differing points in time.[15,137] The diagnostic judgments include terms such as *altered, disturbed, enhanced,* and *dysfunctional* applied to a focus of nursing practice, for example, body nutrition or sleep. A range of five measures—*extremely, substantially, moderately, mildly,* or *not*—is applied to the diagnostic judgment, for example, "mildly altered" or "extremely disturbed."

The National Quality Forum (NQF) has embarked on an ambitious initiative, the Nursing Care Quality project, to identify a framework for how to measure nursing care performance, with particular attention to the performance of nurses as teams and their contributions to the overall health care team; "endorse a set of voluntary consensus standards for evaluating the quality of nursing care (including designating consensus standards that are appropriate for public reporting); and identify and prioritize unresolved issues regarding nursing care performance measurement and research needs."[135] Fifteen national voluntary consensus standards for nursing care have been developed: eight patient-centered outcome measures, three nursing-centered intervention measures, and four system-centered measures. These standards for nursing care are aggregated measures that characterize the hospital or patient care unit rather than individual patients, precluding the analysis of the effectiveness of nursing care for individual patients.

Patient outcomes used to evaluate nursing practice are at varied levels of abstraction. A number of broad outcome categories without specific measures have been identified. At the other extreme, a multitude of specific outcome measures are used in clinical practice and clinical studies to evaluate patient outcomes for a particular nursing diagnosis or intervention. There also are increasing numbers of outcomes at a middle level of abstraction in nursing care plans, critical paths, quality assurance programs, and nursing information systems. Unfortunately, many of the specific and intermediate level outcomes used in clinical practice are developed for a particular setting with little or no evaluation or relevancy to other settings. Thus there is a pressing need for nursing to continue to identify, standardize, and test outcomes that are sensitive to nursing practice.

A CONCEPTUAL MODEL OF OUTCOMES

Political interest in patient outcomes and health care costs initiated a revolution in health care in the late 1980s that has been labeled the "era of assessment and accountability."[67,151] This has put pressure on health care providers to justify their practice and its effects on patients and national health and has created a distinct area of study. Wennberg has identified unwarrented variations in health care delivery by physicians.[183] Basic questions being raised are: Is the care provided by one organization or agency worth the cost relative to the care provided by other organizations or agencies? What are the benefits patients receive from health care? What is the quality, and is it adequate in light of what is being paid?[159] What are the benefits to the health of the general population and individuals?[67] What outcomes can be expected, given various patient characteristics and states of health? If outcomes are not adequate, what changes are needed for improvement? If outcomes are adequate, can improvements still be achieved?[24] A variety of outcome measures, illustrated in Figure 1-1, have been developed in the last decade to answer these questions.

Patient, system, and provider factors in Figure 1-1 are the health care delivery and individual patient factors that influence outcome achievement. Although much has been written about the effect of these factors on outcomes, only recently has the influence of these factors been empirically investigated in a systematic manner. The nursing literature emphasizes the need to consider these factors when evaluating patient outcomes and when determining quality.[72,110,124] The core of the model represents the global or end outcomes, such as health status. Global, multidisciplinary outcomes measure general health status and patient satisfaction with their health and health care provided. These measures offer useful information for payers evaluating alternative health plans but are not specific enough to determine accountability for changes to improve outcomes and are not suitable for monitoring the health and treatment status of individual patients, particularly those with chronic diseases.[120]

The outer circle represents intermediate outcome measures currently available: outcomes specific to a particular medical diagnosis, system, or type of provider. The outcomes in each of these areas are often intermediate outcomes that must be realized to achieve the more global, long-term outcomes related to health status and satisfaction with care. Intermediate outcomes may include measures that evaluate the effect of interventions on current knowledge, attitudes, and behaviors that affect health status and satisfaction.[173]

1. *System-specific outcomes* include adverse factors such as medication errors, infection rates, and patient falls and measures of organizational effectiveness such as cost and productivity. These measures are commonly found in benchmarking or total quality management systems and emphasize multidisciplinary, system-wide outcomes.
2. *Diagnosis-specific outcomes* are utilized in critical paths and standardized evaluation instruments such as those developed by the Health Outcomes Institute.[59] Outcomes in critical

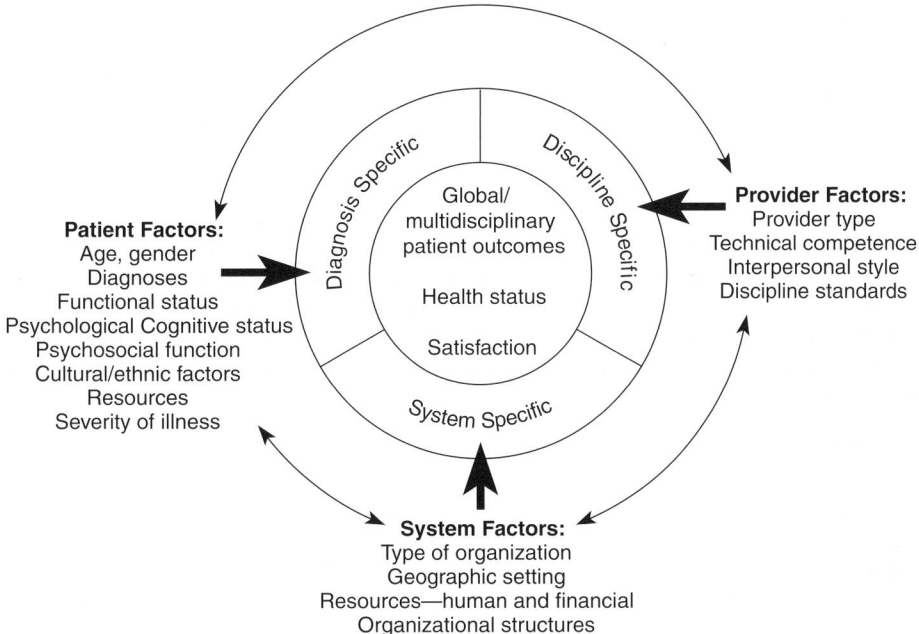

Fig. 1-1 Conceptual Model of Outcomes Research. *(From Iowa Outcomes Project [1997]. Nursing Outcomes Classification [NOC], p. 6, St. Louis: Mosby.)*

paths are often organization-specific and stated as multidisciplinary patient goals that are met or not met. Standardized instruments have primarily captured indicators of physician practice; some may include multidisciplinary outcomes.

3. *Discipline-specific outcomes* reflect the practice and standards of a health care discipline and are important for evaluating the performance and quality of that practice. To date, the focus of effectiveness research using discipline-specific outcomes primarily has been on physician practices or processes of care.[146] Each health care discipline must identify and measure patient outcomes most influenced by its practice to foster the development of knowledge and ensure that standards of care evolve as knowledge increases. Nursing must have validated outcome measures for use in clinical settings, as well as for research, to ensure that outcome data necessary for the elaboration of nursing knowledge and maintenance of the highest standards are available.

Reasons for Standardized Outcomes for Nursing

For the nursing profession to become a full participant in clinical evaluation research, policy development, and interdisciplinary work, it is essential that patient outcomes influenced by nursing care be identified and measured.[73,83,101,103,105,109] While it is recognized that the majority of patient outcomes, including those traditionally used to evaluate physician practice, are not influenced by any one discipline alone, it is essential for each discipline to identify the patient outcomes influenced by its practice to ensure that these discipline-specific outcomes are included in the evaluation of health care effectiveness. If nursing relies on physician-centered information only, the impact of nursing care will remain largely unmeasured and therefore invisible.[108] For nurses to work effectively with managed care organizations to improve quality and reduce costs, nurses must be able to measure and document patient outcomes influenced by nursing care.[143]

For example, the costs of decubitus ulcers are well documented, and prevention is largely a function of nursing[119]; however, information about tissue integrity is not readily available in most clinical evaluation systems. The challenge facing the nursing profession is to create a common language that can be used to organize the phenomena of nursing practice without depersonalizing the patient.[90]

CREATION OF A COMMON NURSING LANGUAGE

Creation of a common language for the nursing profession requires the identification, testing, and application of common terms and measures for nursing diagnoses, nursing interventions, nursing care delivery structures and processes, and patient outcomes. Standardized nursing diagnoses have been under development since 1973, when the first invitational meeting of the National Conference Group for the Classification of Nursing Diagnoses was convened in St. Louis.[160] Development of nursing diagnoses was formalized by the North American Nursing Diagnosis Association (NANDA) in 1992.[37] In addition to the development of new diagnoses, NANDA diagnoses were revised by a research team at The University of Iowa, the Nursing Diagnosis Extension and Classification research team, in conjunction with NANDA members.[131] A comprehensive classification of nursing interventions, Nursing Interventions Classification (NIC), was developed by a research team at The University of Iowa.[69,70] This classification is coded for use in nursing information systems and is being included in the reimbursement system by Alternative Link.[5] This system provides codes for interventions used by multiple health care disciplines as a means for reimbursing complementary and holistic care. Work to standardize administrative data, including information about nursing care delivery systems, has been conducted under the auspices of a research team at The University of Iowa and the American Organization of Nurse Executives.[49] This work, the Nursing Management Minimum Data Set, provides the information necessary to study the effects of nursing administrative and structural variables on patient outcomes.[36]

The outcomes in this text represent the work of a research team at The University of Iowa committed to creating outcomes and related measures at the individual, family, and community level that can be used to evaluate nursing care across the patient care continuum. Individual patient outcome data can be aggregated in a number of ways to assess nursing care effectiveness within an organization and across various settings. The classification is not specific to a patient diagnosis or clinical setting, although some outcomes and related indicators will be used more frequently with a particular patient population or in a particular setting.

Preliminary work to develop and classify nursing interventions laid the foundation for the NOC research, specifically, the conceptualization of outcomes responsive to nursing interventions and the qualitative and quantitative methods used to develop the outcomes and to assess the content validity of the outcomes and indicators. In Phase I of the research, conceptual and methodological issues were identified and resolved, and outcome statements used by nurses were gathered, organized in common referent clusters, and given conceptual outcome labels. Phase II included the refinement and content validation of each outcome through concept analysis and surveys of nurse experts. Preliminary field testing of the nursing-sensitive patient outcomes was accomplished and the outcomes and indicators were organized in a classification structure, supported by hierarchical analysis, with defined rules and principles determining the structure. Phase III focused on testing the psychometric integrity and practicality of measurement scales and procedures with clinical data from 10 field sites representing the continuum of care settings. The validity of the NOC classification structure was evaluated and clinical field data were used to describe the use of the outcomes and linkages among nursing diagnoses, interventions, and outcomes in specific populations and health care settings. Four years of funding for this phase of the research was provided by the National Institute of Nursing Research (RO1-NR03437). This edition of the classification includes refinements identified through this phase of the research and continuing studies. Detailed descriptions of Phases I, II, and III of this research are discussed in the previous edition of NOC.[76,78,120]

Professional practice languages and classification systems are the fundamental vocabularies and categories of thought that define the profession and its scope of practice. The nursing profession has made considerable progress in the last decades in labeling and categorizing the phenomena of nursing. The languages and categories discussed previously attest to the efforts expended toward development of a professional practice language that facilitates the efforts of nursing in the areas described in the following paragraphs.

Computerized Nursing Information Systems

The growth of electronic nursing information systems creates a compelling need for a standardized language for nursing that includes, but is not limited to, patient outcomes influenced by nursing care. Nursing information systems have the potential for improving nursing performance, increasing nursing knowledge, and providing data and information necessary for nursing to participate in the formulation of health care policy.[66] Realization of the potential of such information systems, however, requires turning currently invisible nursing data into visible, productive data[161] that are standardized and can be aggregated and used to answer the pressing questions faced by the nursing profession. Unfortunately, few attempts were initially made to standardize nursing data in clinical information systems. Rather, in many settings, locally specific terminologies and documentation systems have been automated.[69,117] As a consequence, software companies have tended to develop shells that can be individualized for each organization rather than producing software that creates comparable data across organizations.

To move nursing forward, the American Nurses Association (ANA) developed a set of standards for nursing data sets in information systems. The Nursing Information and Data Set Evaluation Center (NIDSEC) is charged with reviewing and evaluating information systems that support nursing practice.[7,12,162,163] Standards used to review the systems include standards related to the nomenclatures, the clinical content linkages, the clinical data repository, and general system requirements. In relation to the nomenclatures, terms from ANA-recognized languages are to be used as the core nursing vocabulary.[7,12] Through this process, the ANA hopes that NIDSEC approval of information system data sets will provide large, retrievable pools of patient data (uniform nursing data sets) that can be used to determine the nature, costs, and effects of nursing practice.[12]

Uniform Nursing Data Sets

A uniform data set "defines the central core of data needed on a routine basis by the majority of decision-makers about a given facet or dimension of the health care delivery system, and it establishes standard measurements, definitions, and classifications for this core."[129] Database development requires a common language and a standard way to organize data.[73] The essential first step in organizing and standardizing nursing information is to develop meaningful categories of data and establish uniform terminology. This can be accomplished with the use of one standard terminology, the use of synonyms linked to current terminologies, and the mapping of current terminologies to each other.[54]

A core set of data, referred to as the Nursing Minimum Data Set (NMDS) was identified in the 1980s under the leadership of Harriet Werley.[184] Consensus was reached on 16 core elements, which were grouped under the categories of nursing care, patient demographics, and service characteristics.[35] Patient demographics and service characteristics are not unique to nursing and can be obtained from other health care databases. The four elements in the nursing care category—nursing diagnosis, nursing intervention, nursing outcome, and intensity of nursing care—are not available in a standardized data set because of the lack of agreement on a standardized language for each nursing care element.[37,111] Recent efforts have focused on creating an interventional nursing minimum data set (i-NMDS).[53]

The National Association for Home Care has developed a uniform data set for home care and hospice. The data set is structured around organizational- and individual-level data items.

Items at the organizational level include service type and use, financial resources and personnel resources. Items at the individual level include patient demographics, medical diagnoses, surgical procedures, and patient use of services. The data set does not contain nursing diagnoses, interventions, or outcomes because these are areas without national consensus[143] and thus represent items that need to be developed.

A number of nursing minimum data sets have been or are being developed in countries other than the United States, including Australia, Canada, and Belgium and other European countries, [140] as well as some South American and Asian countries. The European TELENURSE project included the development of a nursing vocabulary and minimum data set among its objectives.[54] In some instances, nursing data sets are included in multidisciplinary databases and health information systems.

Standardized data sets facilitate the linkage of information in one data set to other data sets. This allows data in clinical information systems to be linked with administrative and other data sets for analysis. The use of logically linked data sets also decreases documentation work by reducing the need for repetitive documentation of information used for multiple purposes in an organization.[185]

National Data Sets

Physicians, health care organizations, and policy makers are extracting and analyzing data from national data sets to compare effectiveness and costs of care by provider and geographic area. "Results of such analyses increasingly form the basis of institutional, regulatory, and reimbursement policy decisions."[142] However, the majority of these data sets contain little information that reflects nursing practice, resulting in a lack of data supporting the effectiveness of nursing practice and its contributions to patient outcomes. The absence of nursing data is the result of medical dominance in health care and the nursing profession's failure to agree on and offer a set of clearly defined, valid, reliable, and standardized nursing data elements for inclusion in national data sets.[141] Therefore the establishment of a set of standardized nursing data elements would allow data collected at the individual patient level to be coded and included in national data sets. This requires agreement on the data elements that are important and relevant for nursing; the terms, measures, or indicators to be used; a uniform coding system; and a cost-effective way to gather the data and input it into a computerized system.[138] The electronic clinical record allows for data input at the point of service.[26,61] There is increasing agreement among health care administrators and policy makers, including those at the federal level, that information technology plays a key role in providing solutions to these challenges.[68,140] A goal of the federal government is to establish an electronic health record for every person in the United States by 2014.[140] As events progress toward this goal, more health care data will be readily available for research and quality assurance. Data will also be available for nursing effectiveness research and quality studies as nursing nomenclatures are included in electronic health records throughout the country. The NOC outcomes presented in Part Three of this edition are coded for use in the electronic record and clinical information systems.

Evaluation of Nursing Care Quality and Effectiveness

Quality patient care requires the collaboration of all health care providers and is measured at the organizational level using outcomes that reflect an interdisciplinary approach to patient care. Illness-related measures have been the traditional measures of quality but are now being expanded to include wellness-related measures and patient satisfaction. The addition of nursing-sensitive patient outcomes related to wellness and satisfaction will contribute to organizational data used to evaluate health care quality. Additionally, knowledge of intermediate outcomes that may be influenced primarily by one discipline is necessary to identify and change structures and processes that inhibit the achievement of quality patient care. For example, functional status may be hindered by decubitus ulcers or inadequate patient knowledge—intermediate outcomes of concern primarily to nurses that will not be available for outcome analysis if not measured and documented by nurses.

Effectiveness research relies on information obtained from large data sets to evaluate the effects of interventions provided by multiple providers in noncontrolled practice situations in which patients are receiving routine care. Because of the multiple factors that influence patient outcomes, large data sets are needed to identify the nursing contribution and to determine patient outcomes sensitive to nursing interventions.[110] Effectiveness research also requires the ability to quantify data, including patient outcomes. Although nursing effectiveness research is still in its infancy, the extent to which nursing is moving forward in effectiveness research is illustrated by the inclusion of the topic in nursing literature.

The need for information about patient outcomes influenced by nursing has increased as organizations have restructured to achieve greater efficiency and concerns have mounted about the cost of health care, the quality of care, and patient safety. Without these data, organizations have little information on which to base decisions about adjusting staff mix, determining cost-effectiveness of various structural or process changes in the nursing care delivery system, or providing information about the quality of nursing care available in the organization.

Although quality of care can be examined from the perspectives of structure, process, and outcome, outcomes are essential components of any quality assurance or quality improvement program. "Outcomes are the changes, either favorable or adverse, in the actual or potential health status of persons, groups, or communities that can be attributed to prior or concurrent care."[44] Outcomes are the trigger for quality assurance programs since they answer the question, "Did the patient benefit or not benefit from the care provided?"[159] Information about patient outcomes should identify not only inadequate outcomes, but also those that are marginal, adequate, and superior to facilitate continual quality improvement. Given that nursing care represents a majority of the hours of care provided in most settings,[4,48] it is essential that health care organizations and nursing practice settings be able to evaluate the quality of care provided by nursing staff. For this to be accomplished, the identification and documentation of patient outcomes influenced by nursing practice are necessary, as well as the application of outcomes influenced by multiple health care providers. However, in a 1996 report, the Institute of Medicine[186] found in a review of nurse staffing and quality of care that existing work in outcome measurement typically has not focused on isolating the contribution of nursing to overall hospital quality.

Concerns about the cost of health care and subsequent methods of cost control raised parallel concerns that quality may be sacrificed. This renewed interest in patient outcomes and their linkage with interventions in studies of health care effectiveness.[33,74,75,77,127] The use of large clinical data sets to assess the effectiveness of health care is now of particular interest. Correspondingly, there is greater recognition of the need to evaluate the effectiveness of nursing interventions. Unfortunately, uniform languages describing nursing practice are often not used for documentation in clinical information systems, and nursing data are too seldom stored in retrievable data repositories that are uniform among settings. This means that nursing data are largely not available for quality analyses in health care organizations and nursing process and outcomes are essentially not represented in national data sets that are routinely analyzed for health policy decisions. It should be clear that the quality of health care cannot be adequately determined to inform health policy if the effectiveness of the practice of the largest group of providers (nurses) in achieving patient outcomes is not evaluated.

Although clinical nursing data sets are now being formed in an increasing number of health care settings, research studies using these data sets are barely beginning. Nurse researchers have been slow to use large data sets to answer questions about nursing quality, and few have analyzed the effectiveness of nursing interventions using large data sets.[180] Yet large data set analyses are very important for nursing quality and effectiveness research in order to detect small outcome effects, to investigate changes in outcomes over time, and to isolate the contribution of nursing from other influences on outcomes. Most large data set studies, to date, have focused on nursing staff and organization level outcomes because of the availability of some large data sets describing nursing structure in organizations, such as staffing, nursing personnel demographics, and characteristics of authority relationships. Studies of nursing process and outcome are rare because nursing process is often difficult to measure and data are typically not collected and stored in data repositories by organizations. At the individual level of analysis, data sets are largely nonexistent because nursing process data are often not directly linked with specific outcomes for individual patients. Studies examining the linkages among nursing structure, process, and outcomes of organizations are few, but slowly increasing, especially some examining the relationship of structure and process.[107,125] Several large data set studies have shown that structural variables, such as the type of nursing care delivery system, nurse authority for decisions, and registered nurse staffing in hospitals and nursing homes, affect mortality rates and other patient outcomes.[2-4,8,20,21,30,31,41,46,89,96,98,99,128,164] A number of studies also have examined the relationship of different aspects of organizational context and a variety of patient outcomes.[9,11,25,55,57,88,91,128,147,155,165] Rantz and colleagues have published several reports of large data set studies using the Long Term Care Minimum Data Set (LTC MDS) to examine nursing home contextual and outcome variable linkages.[56,147-150]

It is clear that more rapid increase in nursing effectiveness and quality studies is dependent on the availability of large clinical nursing data repositories or warehouses. One of the largest local data warehouses (more than 1 million patient records), including discharge data as well as the NMDS, NANDA, NIC, and NOC, was constructed and studied by Delaney and colleagues.[38,39] Findings provided evidence that changes in level of nursing staff expertise (e.g., addition of master's-prepared clinical nurse specialists), practice protocols (e.g., instituting skin care protocol), and national policy (e.g., HCFA length of stay before transfer to skilled care) are reflected in the NMDS nursing care elements' data.[39] A recent study at The University of Iowa, using electronic data from the University of Iowa Hospitals and Clinics, is an analysis of the effectiveness of nursing interventions for patients with hip fracture, congestive heart failure, and risk of falling. This research illustrates the gains that nursing will make in analyzing the quality of care and the effectiveness of nursing interventions.[42,80,160,168,169,170,171] Additional effectiveness research proposals are under development by members of the NOC team using electronic, uniform, nursing clinical data sets from several community hospitals in Nebraska, New York, and Iowa.

Of increasing importance for nursing effectiveness research is the recent work to develop methods for using Knowledge Discovery in Databases (KDD) and data mining in nursing process outcome linkage studies.[1,19,28,39,51,52,102] For example, Autoclass, a KDD tool developed by the National Aerospace Space Administration (NASA) that performs unsupervised classification based on the classical mixture model and supplemented by a Bayesian method for determining optimal classes, was used to find relationships among the NMDS demographic, service, and nursing care variables.[40] Moreover, additional KDD studies based on rough sets have been used to determine decision support rules applicable at the individual patient level.[40,92] Nursing diagnosis, intervention, and outcome linkages are also being analyzed with data collected for the Nursing Outcomes Classification (NOC) study from 10 clinical sites. These analyses describe nursing process outcome linkages for the total sample and within each site. As more health care settings implement nursing clinical information systems that include uniform nursing languages and nursing organization and contextual data, the number of data repositories that can be used for nursing effectiveness and quality studies will undoubtedly increase. SNOMED RT/CT is a reference terminology consisting of a set of concepts and relationships that provides a common reference point for comparison and aggregation of data. SNOMED RT/CT optimizes recording, storage, retrieval, and analysis of data relating to the causes of disease, treatments of patients, and outcomes of the overall health care process in a meaningful way.[16,17,32] Although several issues remain to be resolved for nursing effectiveness research using large clinical data sets to substantially increase, the continuing work with nursing classifications, the development of uniform language systems and reference models, the progress being made with electronic health records, and the development of new methods for analysis of nursing data are hopeful signs.

Advantages of NOC Outcomes for Quality and Effectiveness Research

The Nursing Outcomes Classification described in this book is a comprehensive list of standardized outcomes, definitions, and measures to describe patient outcomes influenced by nursing practice. The outcomes are presented as variable concepts that reflect patient states (e.g., mobility, hydration, coping) that can be measured on a continuum rather than as discrete goals that are met or not met. This variability of concepts will facilitate the identification and analysis of outcome status for specific patient populations and also facilitate the identification of realistic standards of care for specific populations.[105] For example, patients can be aggregated in a number of ways, such as by nursing or medical diagnoses, by service unit, or by severity of illness; and differences in outcome achievement can be analyzed by patient characteristics, such as age, gender, or functional status, as well as by the interventions employed. This type of information will assist nurses in developing realistic standards that reflect currently achieved outcomes if the outcomes are satisfactory or can reflect desired, higher standards of achievement.[105] Such standards reflect variations in outcomes that occur within a patient population because of patient characteristics that cannot be changed. This is quite different from the usual practice of setting one standard or selecting one goal for all patients, regardless of individual patient characteristics that may constitute considerable risk in relation to outcome achievement. "From a quality improvement perspective, it is important to be able to identify a realistic outcome to be achieved. Unrealistic outcome expectations are inefficient in that resources may be expended to no good effect."[122] For comparison of quality across organizations, it is necessary to ensure that the effects of structure and process on patient outcomes are being measured and not the effects of patient characteristics that differ among the organizations.[175]

Outcomes management and effectiveness research has become an imperative in nursing practice in this era of managed care and integrated health care systems,[139] but the evaluation of nursing effectiveness is hindered by a number of factors, including the inability to quantify nursing outcomes in most clinical settings. Outcomes used to evaluate nursing care commonly appear as goal statements designed for use with either a particular patient or specific patient populations and frequently developed for use in one organization. Because they serve different purposes, goal statements vary in their degree of specificity. Statements may be quite specific and designed to reflect a discrete patient status or population (e.g., walks 10 feet without assistance; lists three expected effects of digitalis; systolic blood pressure is between 100 and 150). Goal statements also may be more generic, applicable to a wide range of patients, and require a nursing judgment to determine whether a goal has been met (e.g., anxiety level is decreased; understands activity limitations; blood pressure in desired range).

One problem created by goal statements is that if the goal is not met, the health care professional has no way of knowing how close or how far the patient was from achieving the goal. Another problem is that information about patient status may be lost since patients may move from one health care setting to another over time, and goal accomplishment is often not transferred. However, the major deficit is that goal statements developed in each organization create nonstandardized data that cannot be easily aggregated with data from other settings and populations. The use of a standardized language and classification system with accepted coding enables the aggregation of data internally for organization reports and externally to add more comprehensive data to community and national databases.[45]

Models for the aggregation of data for evaluating effectiveness of nursing interventions have also been developed. One model provides an example of how atomic-level or patient-specific data can be collected once and then aggregated to provide agency, community, national, and worldwide data for decision makers ranging from facility administrators to world health officials.[187] A more recent model illustrates how patient data collected at the individual level can be aggregated and correlated with other data sets to provide information about cost and quality at the unit or organizational level.[71] This model also illustrates aggregation of individual-level data for use in networks, regional, and national data sets.

In the current health care climate, nurses do not have the luxury of waiting for the future, because it is here. The nursing profession must be able to analyze the effectiveness of its interventions and practice and provide information about its role in patient welfare to ensure its role in health care and to influence health care policy. As the electronic health record develops, it is essential that nursing languages be included in the efforts to capture heath care data. If nursing's data needs are not addressed, the efforts of nurses and the outcomes of nursing care for patients will remain invisible and unknown.

Evaluation of Nursing Innovations

Innovations are new ideas or techniques used to solve a problem.[82] They are necessary for the development and refinement of basic and applied knowledge. Nursing innovations can consist of new interventions, revised interventions, or interventions used in a new way to solve clinical problems. They also can be strategies, structures, or processes used to solve management problems.[116] In each instance, patient outcomes are desirable criteria for evaluating innovation effectiveness. In the case of clinical innovations, improved patient outcomes may be the only evaluation criterion. In the case of management innovations, patient outcomes need to be evaluated in conjunction with other outcomes, such as cost reduction or staff mix, to ensure the management innovation did not adversely affect patient outcomes.

Clinical innovations initially are evaluated through controlled clinical studies, with attention given to the measurement of desired or expected outcomes. Many clinical studies in nursing are conducted in one or a few sites and with relatively small samples. Generalizability of such studies can be increased using meta-analysis if study variables are similar. The use of standardized patient outcomes as one of the study variables would increase the ease with which findings can be compared across settings.

Management innovations may be initiated without an evaluation plan, and when such a plan is used, it may not include patient outcomes. The result is a paucity of empirical data about the relationships between structural measures, such as nurse staffing ratios, and quality of care in terms of patient outcomes[186] and the relationship between processes, such as the type of nursing care delivery system, and quality of care. This is particularly bothersome in an era of restructuring and rapid change in health care organizations. Although managers may be forced to make decisions about structural and process changes without empirical data, potential problems can be alleviated if adequate outcome data, including patient outcome data, are identified and routinely collected. The use of standardized outcomes will allow for the comparison of patient outcomes across sites and increase understanding of the effects of structural and process changes on patient outcomes and quality of care.

Participation in Interdisciplinary Care

The use of interdisciplinary teams and collaborative strategies is being promoted as a means of maintaining quality and controlling costs in an increasingly complex health care system. Interdisciplinary teams function when the different disciplines pool their knowledge to jointly evaluate or develop a plan of care to accomplish something that is too complex for one discipline.[115,182] For interdisciplinary teams to be effective, each discipline must contribute their unique perspective and knowledge.[103,115] This requires that nurses have information about their interventions and outcomes to share with other disciplines. Professional languages supply the vocabulary for communication and systematic data collection and analysis, research, and professional literature supply information about the effectiveness of nursing interventions.

Collaboration is the hallmark of interdisciplinary practice and differentiates it from multidisciplinary practice, in which various disciplines contribute to patient care but do not necessarily plan together. Collaboration requires the sharing of each discipline's unique perspective and is characterized by mutual trust and respect for the contribution of each discipline.[182] To be colleagues with members of other disciplines, nurses need a language that allows them to articulate their unique perspective[145] and continue the advancement of nursing knowledge.[115] Without the continual advancement of professional knowledge, the unique contributions of the nursing discipline to interdisciplinary practice will be minimal and decrease the individual member's ability to function in a collegial capacity.

The NOC provides one professional language that nurses can use to identify and evaluate the effects of nursing interventions. Outcome data facilitates nurses participation in collegial relationship as members of an interdisciplinary team and supports development of the knowledge base of nursing necessary for advancing nursing practice.

CONTRIBUTION TO KNOWLEDGE DEVELOPMENT

The development of nursing knowledge requires the use of patient outcome measures. Expanding this knowledge beyond the individual patient to patient populations requires massive amounts of clinical data that describe linkages between and among diagnoses, patient characteristics, interventions, and outcomes.[69] Use of standardized databases with common languages is the most feasible method of obtaining information necessary for analysis of these linkages. Large databases can provide information to a discipline about the effectiveness of current practices and assist in the development of performance goals and practice parameters. Practice parameters, such as the guidelines developed by the Agency for Health Care Policy and Research, provide strategies for patient management and assist clinicians in clinical decision making.[63]

Classifications of nursing diagnoses, nursing interventions, and patient outcomes contain lexical elements for the development of middle-range theories that delineate the substantive structure or the aspects of health care that nurses address,[172] as illustrated in Figure 1-2. Classifications that define the pattern of nursing diagnoses, interventions, and outcomes provide the vertical shafts for the development of middle-range theories used to create the substantive structure of nursing.[172] Using these classifications enables middle-range theory development to build on elements unique to nursing, as well as the "borrowed knowledge" and theories from other disciplines.[152,172] The usefulness of each classification relies on research that links the processes of care to outcomes and the development of explanatory theory.[22,84] Lexical and taxonomic development that provides standardized terms in a constructed classification fosters inductive theory formulation and the empirical testing of deductive theories. It is by accumulating the results of research supporting the effects of interventions on patient outcomes for specific diagnoses and other patient characteristics that evidence-based practice protocols are developed for the discipline. Although the classifications provide the basic elements that are important for the development of substantive nursing theory, they will be expanded or complemented with other knowledge and theories as nursing knowledge develops.

A classification of nursing-sensitive patient outcomes may be the first, but not the only, step for the use of outcomes in the study of nursing practice. Issues related to outcome measurement have been well documented in the literature,[22,58,62,79,85,100] but some of these issues will be best resolved with the use of standardized languages and clinical databases that can be used to study relationships between outcomes, between outcomes and patient characteristics, and between outcomes and nursing interventions. For example, attributing a change in health status to nursing practice requires an understanding of factors that influence patient outcomes and the appropriate timing for data collection. The identification of patient characteristics or risk factors that influence outcome achievement has been used in the study of physician outcomes, but its use has been rare in nursing research. Identification of such factors is a prerequisite in the study of nursing care effectiveness when the controls used in efficacy research are not in place.

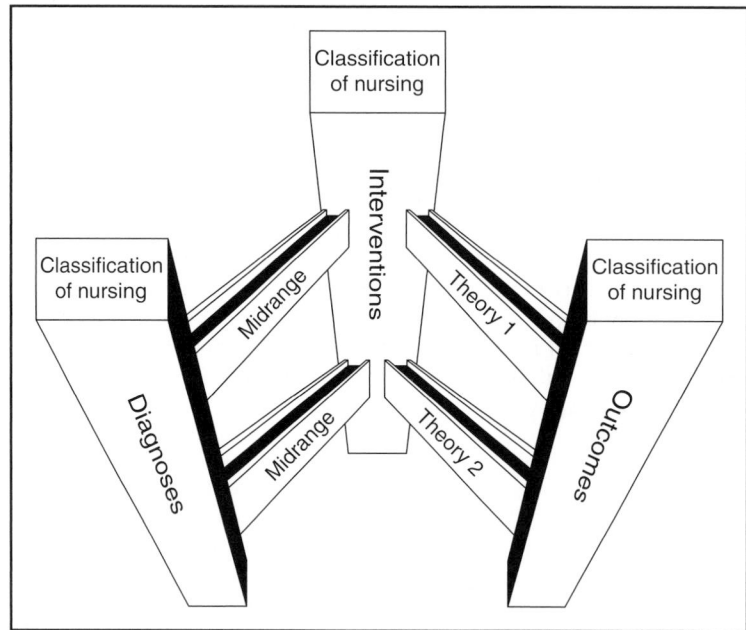

Fig. 1-2 Relationships of nursing diagnoses, interventions, and outcomes of mid-range theories. *(From Tripp-Reimer, T., Woodworth, G., McCloskey, J., & Bulecheck, G.M. [1996]. The dimensional structure of nursing interventions.* Nurs Res, 45, *1.)*

Identification of risk factors also is necessary when comparing outcomes across settings. Recently, Kerr[86] studied risk factors associated with four NOC outcomes. This is beginning work of identifying risk in the area of nursing. While it is recognized that the anticipated change in patient health status may not occur immediately following a nursing intervention, the ideal time for evaluation of clinical outcomes—that is, when treatment outcomes are sufficiently robust to be significant[69]—often is not known. These are only two examples of the questions that must be addressed for nursing to participate fully in outcomes research that focuses on the effectiveness, rather than the efficacy, of health care processes.

ISSUES AND IMPLICATIONS OF RESEARCH WITH NOC OUTCOMES

Understandably, the effectiveness of nursing interventions is less likely to be evaluated if nurses are not confident of the usefulness, reliability, and validity of standardized nursing interventions and patient outcomes that are responsive to nursing, such as the Nursing Interventions Classification (NIC) and the Nursing Outcomes Classification (NOC). Without this confidence, standardized nursing languages are not apt to be widely implemented in electronic clinical documentation systems and hence, will not be available for inclusion in large national data sets. This is one of the main reasons why the research team tested the NOC outcomes with actual clinical data and continues to encourage and plan studies to evaluate the outcomes. The results of the Phase III research in 10 field sites were reported in the third edition of this book.[126] The following is a brief summary of the results and a discussion of the issues and implications for revision of the NOC outcomes.

Summary of Phase III Research Results

Phase III research was enabled by 4 years of National Institute of Nursing funding (RO1-N03437). The research tested the psychometric integrity and practicality of the 190 outcome measures and procedures with the exception of 16 outcomes that pertained to children, published in the first edition of the NOC book.[78] For the evaluation of the NOC outcomes and measures, interrater reliability, construct- or criterion-related validity, change in rating scores (sensitivity), and usefulness of the outcomes and measures were tested in 10 field sites representing the continuum of care. The field settings included two academic, tertiary hospitals; three private, community (intermediate) hospitals; one long-term care nursing home; one community-based parish nursing practice; one ambulatory, academic nursing center staffed by nurse practitioners; and two community health nursing agencies providing home care (Visiting Nurse Associations) in four Midwestern states.[126]

Interrater reliability criteria of 0.80 for near agreement and 0.60 for absolute agreement were considered acceptable evidence of nurse rater. Near agreement is defined as the numerical ratings that do not differ by more than 1 value on the 5-point Likert-type scale for both the label and its indicators. Absolute agreement is defined as two nurses selecting the same numerical rating on the 5-point Likert-type scale. Intraclass correlation was chosen for the final analysis of interrater reliability with an ICC of 0.70 or better considered acceptable evidence of concordance stability.[126]

For most of the outcomes, standardized tools that measure the same or a similar concept were identified and used to estimate the validity of the corresponding NOC outcome. The criterion estimate for validity was set at $r \leq 0.50$ or higher, coupled with statistical significance $p < 0.05$. Sensitivity, the extent that a measure captures change in a phenomenon,[178] was examined for the NOC outcomes by comparing two measurements of the same outcome over time for the same patient. To assess clinical usefulness, nurses were asked to comment on data collection forms about any difficulties using the outcomes to and provide suggestions for revision.[126]

Two thousand three hundred thirty-three (2333) persons for whom the NOC outcomes were rated were distributed among the 10 field sites. Seven hundred and forty-five (745) were in tertiary care settings; 710 were in intermediate care hospitals; 165 were in a nursing home; 646 were cared for in their homes by visiting nurses or were patients who visited a nursing primary care clinic; and 67 were clients of parish nurses. The age of patients ranged from 49 to 87 years. More female patients were rated in each setting except in the tertiary hospitals. Caucasian patients outnumbered other ethnic and minority patients by more than 4 to 1, although there were nearly equal numbers of African American and Caucasian patients rated in the home care and primary nursing clinic sites. More than three fourths of the patients had a high school education or higher degree.[126]

Reliability. For the 109 outcomes with more than 25 ratings, near agreement ranged from 76% to 100%, and agreement was 88% or higher for the majority of these outcomes. Absolute agreement on the outcome labels ranged from 38% to 100%. Absolute agreement on the label was 60% or higher for 75 outcomes. Intraclass correlations ranged from 0.11 to 1.00 and were ≥ 0.70 for 63 of the 109 outcomes. Fifty-three (53) outcomes with at least 25 patient ratings (49%) had near agreement $\geq 80\%$, absolute label agreement $\geq 60\%$, and intraclass correlation coefficients ≥ 0.70.[118]

There were 60 outcomes with fewer than 25 patient ratings. Near agreement scores ranged from 55% to 100% with the majority 90% or higher (n=33) for these outcomes. Absolute agreement ranged from 33% to 100%. The majority of absolute agreements were 60% or higher (n = 42). The range of ICC coefficients was 0.02 to 1.00 and were > 0.70 for 29 of the 60 outcomes. Twenty-five (25) of the outcomes with fewer than 25 ratings (42%) had near agreement $\geq 80\%$, absolute agreement $\geq 60\%$ and ICC ≥ 0.70. Twenty-five of the 52 ICCs computed for the NOC outcomes with fewer than 25 patient ratings were between 0.50 and 0.79 with 18 coefficients 0.80 or higher. For the 169 outcomes that had intraclass coefficients computed, 60% (n = 102) of the coefficients were 0.68 or higher. Each of the NOC core outcomes achieved or exceeded 80% reliability for near agreement.[126]

Validity. For validity, 72 of the outcomes met or exceeded $r = 0.50$ with all but four correlations statistically significant. Eighteen (18) additional outcomes had validity estimates between

0.40 and 0.49 with all but three statistically significant. An additional 32 outcomes achieved estimates of validity between 0.25 and 0.39, and 19 of these correlations were not statistically significant; this may be partly due to the small number of patient ratings. The magnitude of the correlations for 30 outcomes was less than 0.25, and validity was not assessed for 17 of the outcomes. Correlations between the outcome and the criterion measure were ≥ 0.50 for 10 of the 24 core outcomes. Only five outcomes were correlated less than 0.30 with a criterion: Mobility Level; Tissue Integrity: Skin & Mucous Membranes; Safety Behavior: Fall Prevention; Participation: Health Care Decisions; and Comfort Level. Only the Self-Care: Hygiene outcome had no measure of validity.[126]

Sensitivity. Change scores ranged from –3 to +4 with standard deviation (SD) scores ranging from 0.00 to 1.45. Most outcomes (n = 130) showed improvement, 20 indicated regression of the outcome, and 15 showed no change.[126]

Usefulness. Most clinical field nurses reported that the outcomes were clinically useful. The nurses also provided a great deal of feedback about how the outcomes, indicators, and scales might be revised to increase usefulness, including suggestions for revisions of definitions, changes in the indicators, and changes in the scales. The most frequent comments had to do with how to use the indicator rating to arrive at a rating of the outcome label and concerns about indicators that were stated awkwardly for the nurses to rate. The results of the study indicated that nurses must be oriented to the NOC outcomes to use them effectively in their practice and illustrated the importance of training of nurses prior to implementing their use in clinical documentation, as well as the importance of regular monitoring of nurse inter-rater reliability throughout the use of the outcomes.[126]

According to comments, the nurses found most of the outcomes and measures easy to use and were positive about the advantages of the outcomes, whether documented manually or electronically. Nurses who had electronic documentation systems, however, were more positive about use of the outcomes because computerized documentation required less time. Nonetheless, the nurses offered a number of suggestions to make the outcomes more useful. Some were easily accomplished, such as simple editorial changes. Others, however, are more difficult to resolve, such as questions about whether or not to rate each indicator and how ratings of individual indicators should be used to rate the overall outcome. For example, should the indicator ratings only be used as a guide to decide the outcome rating, or should the indicator scores be averaged and that score used as the outcome score? In the study, the nurses used an average of 1.69 to 23 indicators in determining the score on the outcome scales. The average percentage of indicators used for the measurement of each outcome ranged from 16.9% to 100%.[126]

The Phase III study results indicate that many NOC outcomes are sufficiently reliable and valid for use in documenting the efficacy and effectiveness of nursing interventions. Additional testing continues to be needed to refine some measures and to evaluate the outcomes and measures that are developed. Although the findings are not conclusive for all of the 169 outcomes that were tested, they are very encouraging. The findings indicate that nurses rate most outcomes with a high degree of agreement and that the development of valid measures of all patient outcomes is highly probable. The Phase III results also provided evidence that many of the NOC standardized patient outcomes are adequate and useful for evaluating the effectiveness of nursing interventions and for comparisons among patient populations, care settings, and providers. Finally, there are preliminary findings that support the potential that outcome labels alone are reliably rated by nurses in hospitals.[118]

SUMMARY

Outcomes that are reliable, valid, and responsive to nursing interventions are needed for several reasons. Clinicians must have confidence in the integrity of outcome measures to monitor the progress, or lack of progress, of their patients. Administrators and clinician peers need dependable outcome data to evaluate competency and to hold individuals and groups of nurses accountable for a certain standard of practice. Standards of practice, quality and outcome management programs, and the selection of areas of needed knowledge development and dissemination among clinicians are dependent on reliable and valid measurement of patient outcomes that are responsive to nursing interventions. Reliable and valid outcomes are needed for nursing efficacy and effectiveness research to further develop evidence-based practice and to influence health policy. Policy decision makers will not be responsive to a discipline that cannot provide data supporting its effectiveness. Nursing-sensitive patient outcomes provide one of the data elements for the Nursing Minimum Data Set. Development and use of such a data set will provide nurses the information needed for the determination of nursing practice effectiveness.

References

1. Abbott, P. A. (2000). The challenges of data mining in large nursing home datasets. *Information Technology in Nursing, 12*(3), 9-14.
2. Aiken, L. A., Smith, H. L., & Lake, E. T. (1994). Lower Medicare mortality among a set of hospitals known for good nursing care. *Medical Care, 32*, 771-787.
3. Aiken, L. H., Sloane, D., & Sochalski, J. (1998). Hospital organization and outcomes. *Journal of Quality Health Care, 7*, 222-226.
4. Aiken, L., & Sloane, D. (1998). Advances in hospital outcomes research. *Journal of Health Services & Research Policy, 3*(4), 249-250.
5. Alternative Link ABC codes to include NIC. (1998). *NIC/NOC Newsletter, 6*(3), 1.
6. American Nurses Association. (1995). *Nursing care report card for acute care.* Washington, DC: Author.
7. American Nurses Association. (1997). *Nursing informatics & data set evaluation center (NIDSEC) standards and scoring guidelines.* Washington, DC: Author.
8. Anderson, R. A., Hsieh, P.-C., & Su, H.-F. (1998). Resource allocation and resident outcomes in nursing homes: Comparison between the best and worst. *Research in Nursing and Health, 21*(4), 297-313.
9. Anderson, R., & Lawhorne, L. (1999). Variations in staffing and resident care patterns in Michigan nursing homes. *Annals of Long-Term Care, 7*(11), 399-404.
10. Anonymous. (2004). CMS and JCAHO quality measures now are the same: Will that save you time? *Hospital Peer Review, 29*(11), 149-152.
11. Aud, M.A., Zwygart-Stauffacher, M., & Flesner, M. (2007). Measuring quality of care in assisted living: A new tool for providers, consumers, and researchers. *Journal of Nursing Care Quality, 22* (1), 4-7.
12. Averill, C. B., Marek, K. D., Zielstorff, R., Kneedler, J., Delaney, C., & Milholland, D. K. (1998). ANA standards for nursing data sets in information systems. *Computers in Nursing, 16*(3), 157-161.
13. Aydelotte, M. (1962). The use of patient welfare as a criterion measure. *Nursing Research, 11*, 10-14.
14. Badger, K. A. (1998). Patient care report cards: An analysis. *Outcomes Management for Nursing Practice, 2*(1), 29-36.
15. Baernholdt, M., & Lang, N.M. (2003). Why an ICNP? Links among quality information and policy. *International Nursing Review, 50*, 73-78.
16. Bakken, S. (2001). Interactive health communication technology: Where do clinical nursing interventions fit into the picture? *Applied Nursing Research, 14*(3), 173-175.
17. Bakken, S., Warren, J. J., Lundberg, C., Casey, A., Correia, C., Konicek, D., & Zingo, C. (2002). An evaluation of the usefulness of two terminology models for integrating nursing diagnosis concepts into SNOMED Clinical Terms. *International Journal of Medical Informatics, 68*(1-3), 71-77.
18. Benner, P., Sheets, V., Uris, P., Malloch, K., Schwed, K., & Jamison, D. (2002). Individual, practice and system causes of errors in nursing: A taxonomy. *JONA, 32*(10), 509-523.
19. Berger, A. M., & Berger, C. R. (2004). Data mining as a tool for research and knowledge development in nursing. *Computers, Informatics, Nursing (CIN), 22*(3), 123-131.
20. Blegen, M., Goode, C. J., & Reed, L. (1998). Nurse staffing and patient outcomes. *Nursing Research, 47*(1), 43-50.
21. Blegen, M. A., & Vaughn, T. (1998). A multisite study of nurse staffing and patient occurrences. *Nursing Economic$, 16*(4), 196-203.
22. Bond, S., & Thomas, L. H. (1991). Issues in measuring outcomes of nursing. *Journal of Advanced Nursing, 16*, 1492-1502.
23. Brown, D. S. (1992). A conceptual framework for the evaluation of service quality. *Journal of Nursing Care Quality, 6*, 66-74.

24. Carey, R. G., & Lloyd, R. C. (1995). *Measuring quality improvement in healthcare: A guide to statistical process control applications.* New York: Quality Resources, Division of the Kraus Organization Limited.
25. Castle, N. G. (2000). Differences in nursing homes with increasing and decreasing use of physical restraints. *Medical Care, 38*(12), 1154-1163.
26. Center for Health Workforce Planning. (2004). *Status of nursing supply and demand in Iowa: A presentation to the government oversight committee: Iowa department of public health.* Des Moines, IA: Author.
27. Centers for Medicare and Medicaid Services (CMS). (2006). Quality Initiatives. Washington, DC. Retrieved from http://www.cms.hhs.gov/QualityInitiativesGenInfo/
28. Cheung, R., Moody, L., & Cockram, C. (2002). Data mining strategies for shaping nursing and health policy agenda. *Policy, Politics, & Nursing Practice, 3*(3), 248-260.
29. Clark, L. C. (1998). Incorporating OASIS into the Visiting Nurses Association. *Outcomes Management for Nursing Practice, 2*(1), 24-28.
30. Clarke, S. P., & Aiken, L. H. (2003a). Failure to rescue. *American Journal of Nursing, 103*, 42-47.
31. Clarke, S. P., & Aiken, L. H. (2003b). Registered nurse staffing and patient and nurse outcomes in hospitals: A commentary. *Policy, Politics, & Nursing Practice, 4*(2), 104-111.
32. Coenen, A., Marin, H. F., Park, H. A., & Bakken, S. (2001). Collaborative efforts for representing nursing concepts in computer-based systems: International perspectives. *Journal of the American Medical Informatics Association, 8*(3), 289-290.
33. Cox, R. (1998). Implementing nurse sensitive outcomes into care planning at a long-term care facility. *Journal of Nursing Care Quality, 12* (5), 41-51.
34. Daubert, E. A. (1979). Patient classification and outcome criteria. *Nursing Outlook, 27*, 450-454.
35. Delaney, C. (2006). Nursing Minimum Data Set (NMDS) Systems. In V. Saba & K. McCormick (Eds.), *Essentials of nursing informatics* (4th ed., pp. 249-261). New York: McGraw-Hill.
36. Delaney, C., & Huber, D. (1996). *A nursing management minimum data set (NMMDS): A report of an invitational conference.* Chicago, IL: The American Organization of Nurse Executives.
37. Delaney, C., Mehmert, P. A., Prophet, C., Bellinger, S. L., Huber, D. H., & Ellerbe, S. (1992). Standardized nursing language for healthcare information systems. *Journal of Medical Systems, 16*(4), 145-159.
38. Delaney, C., Mehmert, P., Prophet, C., & Crossley, J. (1998). Establishment of the research value of nursing minimum data sets. [Reprint]. In V. Saba, *Nursing and Computers: An Anthology, 1987-1996.* New York: Springer.
39. Delaney, C., Reed, D., & Clarke, M. (2000). Describing patient problems & nursing treatment patterns using Nursing Minimum Data Sets (NMDS & NMMDS) and UHDDS repositories. In J. M. Overhage (Ed.), *AMIA 2000 converging information, technology, & healthcare* (pp. 176-179). Philadelphia: Hanley and Belfus.
40. Delaney, C., Ruiz, M., Clarke, M., & Srinivasan, P. (2000). Knowledge discovery in databases: Data mining the NMDS. In V. Saba, R. Carr, W. Sermeus, & P. Rocha (Eds.), *One step beyond: The evolution of technology & nursing, Proceedings of the 7th International Congress on Nursing Informatics* (pp. 61-65). Aukland, New Zealand: Adis International.
41. Dellefield, M. W. (2000). The relationship between nurse staffing in nursing homes and quality indicators. *Journal of Gerontological Nursing, 26*(6), 14-28.
42. Dochterman, J., Titler, M., Wang, J., Reed, D., Pettit, D., Mathew-Wilson, M., Budreau, G., Bulechek, G., Kraus, V., & Kanak, M. (2005). Describing use of nursing interventions for three groups of patients. *Journal of Nursing Scholarship, 37*(1), 57-66.
43. Donabedian, A. (1966). Evaluating the quality of medical care. *Milbank Memorial Fund Quarterly, 44*(3), 166-206.
44. Donabedian, A. (1985). *The methods and findings of quality assessment and monitoring: An illustrated analysis* (Vol. 3). Ann Arbor, MI: Health Administration Press.
45. Donaldson, M. S., & Lohr, K. N. (Eds.). (1994). *Health data in the information age: Use, disclosure, and privacy.* Washington, DC: National Academy Press.
46. Dyck, M. J. (2007). Nursing staffing and resident outcomes in nursing homes: Weight loss and dehydration. *Journal of Nursing Care Quality, 22*(1), 59-65.
47. Evanoff, B., Potter, P., Wolf, L., Grayson, D., Dunagan, C., & Boxerman, S. (2005). Can we talk? Priorities for patient care differed among health care providers. In K. Henriksen, J. B. Battles, E. Marks, & D. I. Lewin (Eds.), *Advances in patient safety: From research to implementation* (Vol. 1, Research Findings, pp. 5-14). AHRQ Publication No. 05-0021-1. Rockville, MD: Agency for Healthcare Research and Quality.
48. Flarey, D. L., & Blancett, S. S. (1995). Management and organizational restructuring: Reforming the corporate system. In S. S. Blancett & D. Flarey (Eds.), *Reengineering nursing and health care.* Gaithersburg, MD: Aspen.
49. Gardner, D. L., Delaney, C., Crossley, J., Mehmert, P., & Ellerbe, S. (1992). A nursing management minimum data set: Significance and development. *Journal of Nursing Administration, 22*(7), 35-40.
50. Gillette, B., & Jenko, M. (1991). Major clinical functions: A unifying framework for measuring outcomes. *Journal of Nursing Care Quality, 6*, 20-24.
51. Goodwin, L. K., Iannacchione, M. A., Hammond, W. E., Crockett, P., Maher, S., & Schlitz, K. (2001). Data mining methods find demographic predictors of preterm birth. *Nursing Research, 50*(6), 340-345.

52. Goodwin, L., VanDyne, M., Simon, L., & Talbert, S. (2003). Data mining issues and opportunities for building nursing knowledge. *Journal of Biomedical Informatics, 36*(4-5), 379-388.

53. Goossen, W., Delaney, C., Coenen, A., Saba, V., Sermeus, W., Warren, J., Marin, H., Park, H., Junger, A., Hovenga, E., Oyri, K., & Casey, A. (2006). The international nursing minimum data set (i-NMDS). In C. Weaver, C. Delaney, P. Weber, & Carr, R., *Nursing and informatics for the 21st century* (pp. 305-322). Chicago, IL: Healthcare Information and Management Systems Society.

54. Goossen, W., Epping, P., Feuth, T., Dassen, T., Hasman, A. & van den Heuvel, W. (1998). A comparison of nursing minimal data sets. *Journal of the American Medical Informatics Association: JAMIA, 5*(2), 152-163.

55. Gould, M. T. (1992). Nursing home elderly: Social-environmental factors. *Journal of Gerontological Nursing, 18*(8), 13-20.

56. Grando, V. T., Rantz, M. J., Petroski, G. F., Maas, M., Popejoy, L., Conn, V., & Wipke-Tevis, D. (2005). Prevalence and characteristics of nursing homes residents requiring light-care. *Research in Nursing & Health, 28*(3), 210-219.

57. Harrington, C., Woolhandler, S., Mullan, J., Carillo, H., & Himmelstein, D. U. (2002). Does investor-ownership on nursing homes compromise the quality of care? *International Journal of Health Services, 32*(2), 315-325.

58. Harris, M. R., & Warren, J. J. (1995). Patient outcomes: Assessment issues for the CNS. *Clinical Nurse Specialist, 9*(2), 82-86.

59. Health Outcomes Institute. (1993). *Condition-specific type specifications.* Bloomington, MN: Author.

60. Heater, B. S., Becker, A. M., & Olson, R. K. (1988). Nursing interventions and patient outcomes: A meta-analysis of studies. *Nursing Research, 37*, 303-307.

61. Heffler, S., Smith, S., Keehan, S., Borger, C., Clemens, M., & Truffer, C. (2005). U.S. health spending projections for 2004-2014. *Health Affairs, 24*(Suppl 1), 74-85.

62. Hegyvary, S. (1991). Issues in outcomes research. *Journal of Nursing Quality Assurance, 5*(2), 1-6.

63. Hirshfeld, E. B. (1994). Practice parameters versus outcome measurements: How will prospective and retrospective approaches to quality management fit together? *Nutrition in Clinical Practice, 9*(6), 207-215.

64. Horn, B. J., & Swain, M. A. (1978). *Criterion measures of nursing care.* (DHEW Pub. No. PHS 78-3187). Hyattsville, MD: National Center for Health Services Research.

65. Hover, J., & Zimmer, M. (1978). Nursing quality assurance: The Wisconsin system. *Nursing Outlook, 26*, 242-248.

66. Huber, D., Schumacher, L., & Delaney, C. (1997). Nursing Management Minimum Data Set (NMMDS). *Journal of Nursing Administration, 27*, 42-48.

67. Iezzoni, L. I. (1994). Risk and outcomes. In L. I. Iezzoni (Ed.), *Risk adjustment for measuring health care outcomes* (pp. 1-28). Ann Arbor, MI: Health Administration Press.

68. Institute of Medicine. (2001). *Crossing the quality chasm: A new health system for the 21st century.* Washington, DC: National Academy Press.

69. Iowa Intervention Project. (1992). *Nursing interventions classification (NIC).* St. Louis: Mosby.

70. Iowa Intervention Project. (1996). *Nursing interventions classification (NIC)* (2nd ed.). St. Louis: Mosby.

71. Iowa Intervention Project. (1997). Proposal to bring nursing into the information age. *Image, 29*(3), 275-281.

72. Irvine, D., Sidani, S., & Hall, L. M. (1998). Linking outcomes to nurses' roles in health care. *Nursing Economics$, 16*(2), 58-64.

73. Jennings, B. M. (1991). Patient outcomes research: Seizing the opportunity. *Advances in Nursing Science, 14*(2), 59-72.

74. Johnson, M., Bulechek, G., Butcher, H., Maas, M., McCloskey Dochterman, J., Moorhead, S., & Swanson, L. (2006). *NANDA, NOC, and NIC linkages: Nursing diagnoses, outcomes and interventions.* St. Louis: Mosby.

75. Johnson, M., & Maas, M. (1994). Nursing-focused patient outcomes: Challenge for the nineties. In J. McCloskey & H. Grace (Eds.), *Current issues in nursing* (4th ed., pp. 643-649). St. Louis: Mosby.

76 Johnson, M., & Mass, M., (Eds.). (1997). *Nursing outcomes classification (NOC)* (1st ed.). St. Louis, MO: Mosby.

77. Johnson, M., & Maas, M. (1998). The nursing outcomes classification (NOC). *Journal of Nursing Care Quality, 12*(5), 9-20.

78 Johnson, M., Mass, M., & Moorhead, S. (Eds.). (2000). *Nursing outcomes classification (NOC)* (2nd ed.). St. Louis, MO: Mosby.

79. Jones, K. R. (1993). Outcomes analysis: Methods and issues. *Nursing Economics, 11*, 145-152.

80 Kanak, M., Titler, M., Shever, L., Fei, Q., Dochterman, J., & Picone, D. (in press). The effects of hospitalization on multiple units. *Applied Nursing Research.*

81. Kane, R. L., Garrard, J., Skay, C. L., Radosevich, D. M., Buchanan, J. L., McDermott, S. M., Arnold, S. B., & Kepferle, L. (1989). Effects of a geriatric nurse practitioner on process and outcome of nursing home care. *American Journal of Public Health, 79*(9), 1271-1277.

82. Kanter, R. M. (1983). *The change masters: Innovation for productivity in the American corporation.* New York: Simon & Schuster.

83. Keenan, G., & Aquilino, M. L. (1998). Standardized nomenclatures: Keys to continuity of care, nursing accountability and nursing effectiveness. *Outcomes Management for Nursing Practice, 2*(2), 81-85.

84. Keith, R. A. (1995). Conceptual basis of outcome measures. *American Journal of Physical Medicine & Rehabilitation, 74*(1), 73-80.

85. Kelsey, A. (1995). Outcome measures: Problems and opportunities for public health nursing. *Journal of Nursing Management, 3*, 183-187.

86 Kerr, P. (2005). *Nursing interventions & risk adjustment of selected patient outcomes.* Unpublished doctoral dissertation, University of Iowa, Iowa City, Iowa.

87. Kohn, L. T., Corrigan, J. M., & Donaldson, M. S. (2000). *To err is human: Building a safer health system.* Washington, DC: National Academy Press.

88. Kolanowski, A., Hurwitz, S. L., Taylor, L. A., Evans, L., & Strumpf, N. (1994). Contextual factors associated with disturbing behaviors in institutional elders. *Nursing Research, 43*(2), 73-79.

89. Kovner, C., & Gergen, P. J. (1998). Nurse staffing levels and adverse events following surgery in U.S. hospitals. *Image: Journal of Nursing Scholarship, 30*(4), 315-321.

90. Kritek, P. V. (1989). An introduction to the science and art of taxonomy. In American Nurses Association (Ed.), *Classification systems for describing nursing practice: Working papers* (pp. 6-12). Kansas City, KS: American Nurses Association.

91. Kruzich, J. M., Clinton, J. F., & Kelber, S. T. (1992). Personal and environmental influences on nursing home satisfaction. *Gerontologist, 32*(3), 342-350.

92. Kusiak, A., Kern, J. A., Kernstine, K. H., & Tseng, B. T. (2000). Autonomous decision-making: A data mining approach. *IEEE Transaction on Information Technology in Biomedicine, 4*(4), 274-284.

93. Lalonde, B. (1988). Assuring the quality of home care via the assessment of client outcomes. *Caring, 12*(1), 20-24.

94. Lang, N. M., & Clinton, J. F. (1984). Assessment of quality of nursing care. *Annual Review of Nursing Research, 2*, 135-163.

95. Lang, N. M., & Marek, K. D. (1990). The classification of patient outcomes. *Journal of Professional Nursing, 6*, 153-163.

96. Lee, C.-L., Liu, T.-L., Wu, L.-J., Chung, U.-L., & Lee, L.-C. (2002). Cost and care quality between licensed nursing homes under different types of ownership. *Journal of Nursing Research, 10*(2), 151-160.

97 Lee, J. (2006). Reimbursement for alternative providers. In P.S. Cowen & S. Moorhead, Current issues in nursing (pp. 455-468). St. Louis, MO: Mosby.

98. Lee, J. L., Chang, B. L., Pearson, A. L., Kahn, K. L., & Rubenstein, L. V. (1999). Does what nurses do affect clinical outcomes for hospitalized patients? *Health Services Research, 34*(5 pt 1), 1011-1032.

99. Lichtig, L. K., Knauf, R. A., Milholland, D. K. (1999). Some impacts of nursing on acute care hospital outcomes. *Journal of Nursing Administration, 29*(2), 25-33.

100. Lohr, K. N. (1988). Outcome measurement: Concepts and questions. *Inquiry, 25*(1), 37-50.

101. Lower, M. S., & Burton, S. (1989). Measuring the impact of nursing interventions on patient outcomes: The challenge of the 1990s. *Journal of Nursing Quality Assurance, 4*(1), 27-34.

102. Lu, D., Street, W., & Delaney, C. (2006). *Knowledge discovery: Detecting elderly patients with impaired mobility.* Paper presented at The 9th International Congress on Nursing Informatics, Seoul, South Korea, June 11-14, 2006.

103. Maas, M. (1998). Nursing's role in interdisciplinary accountability for patient outcomes. *Outcomes Management for Nursing Practice, 2*(3), 92-94.

104. Maas, M. L., & Delaney, C. (2004). Nursing process outcome linkage research: Issues, current status, and health policy implications. *Medical Care, 42*(2 Suppl), 1140-1148.

105. Maas, M. L., Johnson, M. R., & Kraus, V. L. (1996). In K. Kelly (Ed.), *Outcomes of effective management practice, SONA 8* (pp. 20-35). Thousand Oaks, CA: Sage.

106. Maas, M., Johnson, M., Moorhead, S., Reed, D., & Sweeney, S. (2003). Evaluation of the reliability and validity of nursing outcomes classification patient outcomes and measures. *Journal of Nursing Measurement, 11*(2), 97-117.

107. Maas, M. L., & Specht, J. P. (1999). Quality outcomes and contextual variables in nursing homes. In A. S. Hinshaw, S. L. Feetham, & J. L. F. Shaver (Eds.), *Handbook of clinical nursing research* (pp. 655-663). Thousand Oaks, CA: Sage.

108. Mallison, M. B. (1990). Editorial: Access to invisible expressways. *American Journal of Nursing, 90*(9), 7.

109. Marek, K. D. (1989). Outcomes measurement in nursing. *Journal of Nursing Quality Assurance, 4*(1), 1-9.

110. Marek, K. D. (1997). Measuring the effectiveness of nursing care. *Outcomes Management for Nursing Practice, 1*(1), 8-12.

111. Mark, B.A., & Burleson, D. L. (1995). Measurement of patient outcomes: Data availability and consistency across hospitals. *Journal of Nursing Administration, 25*(4), 52-59.

112. Martin, K.S. (2005). *The Omaha system: A key to practice documentation, and information management.* St. Louis, MO: Saunders.

113. Martin, K. S., Norris, J., & Leak, G. K. (1999). Psychometric analysis of the problem rating scale for outcomes. *Outcomes Management for Nursing Practice, 3*(1), 20-25.
114. Martin, K. S., & Scheet, N. J. (1992). *The Omaha System: Applications for community health nursing.* Philadelphia: W.B. Saunders.
115. McCloskey, J. C., & Maas, M. (1998). Interdisciplinary team: The nursing perspective is essential. *Nursing Outlook, 46*(4), 157-163.
116. McCloskey, J. C., Maas, M. L., Huber, D. G., Kasparek, A., Specht, J. P., Ramler, C. L., Watson, C., Blegen, M., Delaney, C., Ellerbe, S., Etscheidt, C., Gongaware, C., Johnson, M. R., Kelly, K. C., Mehmert, P., & Clougherty, J. (1996). Nursing management innovations: A need for systematic evaluation. In K. Kelly (Ed.), *Outcomes of effective management practice, SONA 8* (pp. 3-19). Thousand Oaks, CA: Sage.
117. McCormick, K. (1991). Future data needs for quality care monitoring, DRG considerations, reimbursement and outcome measurement. *Image, 23*(1), 29-32.
118. McCormick, K. A., Cummings, M. A., & Kovner, C. (1997). The role of the Agency for Health Care Policy and Research (AHCPR) in improving outcomes of care. *The Nursing Clinics of North America, 32*(3), 521-542.
119. McFarland, G. K., & McFarlane, E. A. (1993). *Nursing diagnosis and intervention: A model for clinical practice.* St. Louis: Mosby.
120. McHorney, C. A., & Tarlov, A. R. (1995). Individual-patient monitoring in clinical practice: Are available health status surveys adequate? *Quality of Life Research, 4,* 293-307.
121. Merck Institute of Aging & Health. (2004). *The state of aging and health in America 2004.* Washington, DC: Merck Institute of Aging & Health.
122. Mills, W. C. (1994). Tacking through troubled waters: Toward desired outcomes. In R. M. Carroll-Johnson & M. Paquette (Eds.), *Classification of nursing diagnosis: Proceedings of the tenth conference* (pp. 126-130). Philadelphia: J. B. Lippincott.
123. Mitchell, P. H., Ferketich, S., & Jennings, B. M. (1998). Quality health outcomes model. *Image, 30*(1), 43-46.
124. Mitchell, P. H., Heinrich, J., Moritz, P., & Hinshaw, A. S. (Eds.). (1997). Outcome measures and care delivery systems conference. *Medical Care, 35*(11 Supp.), N51-55.
125. Moorhead, S., Clarke, M. Willits, M., & Tomsha, K.A. (1998). Nursing outcomes classification implementation projects across the care continuum. *Journal of Nursing Care Quality, 12* (5), 52-63.
126. Moorhead, S., Johnson, M., & Maas, M. (Eds.). (2004). *Nursing outcomes classification* (NOC) (3rd ed.). St. Louis: Mosby.
127. Moorhead, S., Johnson, M., Maas, M., & Reed, D. (2003). Testing the nursing outcomes classification in three clinical unites in a community hospital. *Journal of Nursing Measurement, 11*(2), 171-181.
128. Munroe, D. J. (1990). The influence of registered nurse staffing on the quality of nursing home care. *Research in Nursing and Health, 13*(4), 263-270.
129. Murnaghan, H. (1978). Uniform basic data sets for health statistical systems. *International Journal of Epidemiology, 7,* 263-269.
130. Nadzam, D. M., & Nelson, M. (1997). The benefits of continuous performance measurement. *The Nursing Clinics of North America, 32*(3), 543-559.
131. NANDA International. (2003). *Nursing diagnoses: Definitions and classification 2003-2004.* Philadelphia: Author.
132. National Committee for Quality Assurance. (1993). *Health plan employer data and information set 2.0 (HEDIS 2.0).* Washington, DC: Author.
133. National Committee for Quality Assurance. (1995). *Health plan employer data and information set 2.1 (HEDIS 2.1).* Washington, DC: Author.
134. National Committee for Quality Assurance. (2006). *Quality compass.* Washington, DC: Author.
135. National Quality Forum. (2006). *Nursing Quality Measures. National Quality Forum.* Retrieved January 10, 2007 from http://www.qualityforum.org
136. Naylor, M. D., Munro, B. H., & Brooten, D. A. (1991). Measuring the effectiveness of nursing practice. *Clinical Nurse Specialist, 5,* 210-215.
137. Nielsen, G. H., & Mortensen, R. A. (1998). The architecture of ICNP: Time for outcomes—Part II. *International Nursing Review, 45*(1), 27-31.
138. Niemeyer, L. O., & Foto, M. (1995). Using outcomes data. *REHAB Management,* April/May, 105-106.
139. Oermann, M., & Huber, D. (1997). New horizons. *Outcomes Management for Nursing Practice, 1*(1), 1-2.
140. Office of the National Coordinator for Health Information Technology. (2004). Office of the National Coordinator for Health Information Technology: Goals of Strategic Framework Retrieved September 19, 2005, from http://www.os.dhhs.gov/healthit/goals.html
141. Ozbolt, J. (1991). *Strategies for building nursing databases for effectiveness research.* Invited paper presented to National Center for Nursing Research, September 11-13, Rockville, MD.
142. Ozbolt, J. G., Fruchtnight, J. N., & Hayden, J. R. (1994). Toward data standards for clinical nursing information. *Journal of the American Medical Informatics Association: JAMIA, 1*(2), 175-185.

143. Pace, K. B. (1995). Data sets for home care organizations. *Caring, 14*(3), 38-42.

144. Phoon, J., Corder, K., & Barter, M. (1996). Managed care and total quality management: A necessary integration. *Journal of Nursing Care Quality, 10*(2), 25-32.

145. Pike, A. W. (1994). Entering collegial relationships: The demise of nurse as victim. In J. C. McCloskey & H. K. Grace (Eds.), *Current issues in nursing* (4th ed., pp. 643-649). St. Louis: Mosby.

146. Prescott, P. A. (1993). Nursing: An important component of hospital survival under a reformed health care system. *Nursing Economics$, 11*, 192-199.

147. Rantz, M. J., Hicks, L., Grando, V., Petroski, G. F., Madsen, R. W., Mehr, D. R., Conn, V., Zwygart-Staffacher, M., Scott, J., Flesner, M., Bostick, J., Porter, R., & Maas, M. (2004). Nursing home quality, cost, staffing, and staff mix. *The Gerontologist, 44*(1), 24-38.

148. Rantz, M. J., Hicks, L., Petroski, G. F., Madsen, R. W., Mehr, D. R., Conn, V., Zwygard-Staffacher, M., & Maas. M. (2005). Stability and sensitivity of nursing home quality indicators. *Journal of Gerontology: MEDICAL SCIENCES, 59A*(1), 79-82.

149. Rantz, M., Petroski, G., Madsen, R., Scott, J., Conn, V., Popejoy, L., Hicks, L., Porter, R., Zwygart-Stauffacher, M. & Maas, M. (In press). Developing thresholds of quality indicators for nursing homes to use in continuing quality improvement programs. *Journal of Nursing Care Quality.*

150. Rantz, M. J., Zwygart-Stauffacher, M., Popejoy, L. L., Mehr, D. R., Grando, V. T., Wipke-Tevis, D. D., Hicks, L. L., Conn, V. S., Porter, R., & Maas, M. (In press). MDS quality indicators: A useful tool for improving clinical practice and outcomes of care. *Annals of Long Term Care.*

151. Relman, A. S. (1988). Assessment and accountability: The third revolution in medical care. *New England Journal of Medicine, 319*, 1220-1222.

152. Retsas, A. (1995). Knowledge and practice development: Toward an ontology of nursing. *The Australian Journal of Advanced Nursing, 12*(2), 20-25.

153. Reverby, S. (1981). Stealing the golden eggs: Ernest Amory Codman and the science and management of medicine. *Bulletin of the History of Medicine, 55*, 156-171.

154. Ryan, P., & Delaney, C. (1995). Nursing minimum data set. In J. J. Fitzpatrick & J. S. Stevenson (Eds.). *Annual Review of Nursing Research, 13*, 169-194.

155. Ryden, M. B. (1985). Environmental support for autonomy in the institutionalized elderly. *Research in Nursing and Health, 8*(4), 363-371.

156. Saba, V. (1992). The classification of home health care nursing: Diagnoses and interventions. *Caring, 11*(3), 50-57.

157. Saba, V. (2006). *Clinical care classification (CCC) system manual: A guide to nursing documentation.* New York: Springer.

158. Salive, M. E., Mayfield, J. A., & Weissman, N. W. (1990). Patient outcomes research teams and the Agency for Health Care Policy and Research. *Health Services Research, 25*, 697-708.

159. Shaughnessy, P. W., & Crisler, K. S. (1995). *Outcome-based quality improvement: A manual for home care agencies on how to use outcomes.* Washington, DC: National Association for Home Care.

160. Shever, L., Titler, M., Dochterman, J., Fei, Q., & Picone, D.M. (2007). Patterns of nursing intervention use across six days of acute care hospitalization for three older patient populations. *The international Journal of Nursing Terminologies and Classification, 18*(1), 18-29.

161. Simpson, R. (1991). Adopting a nursing minimum data set. *Nursing Management, 22*(2), 20-21.

162. Simpson, R. (1998). A NIDSEC primer. Part 1: Setting the standards. *Nursing Management, 29*(1), 49-50.

163. Simpson, R. (1998). A NIDSEC primer. Part 2: Setting the standards. *Nursing Management, 29*(2), 26-27, 29.

164. Sochalski, J. (2001). Quality of care, nurse staffing and patient outcomes. *Policy, Politics, & Nursing Practice, 2*(1), 9-18.

165. Sochalski, J., & Aiken, L. H. (1999). Accounting for variation in hospital outcomes: A cross-national study. *Health Affairs (Millwood), 18*(3), 256-259.

166. Sovie, M. D. (1989). Clinical nursing practices and patient outcomes: Evaluation, evolution, and revolution. *Nursing Economics$, 7*, 79-85.

167. Tarlov, A. R., Ware, J. E., Greenfield, S., Nelson, E. C., Perrin, E, & Zubkoff, M. (1989). The medical outcomes study: An application of methods for monitoring the results of medical care. *Journal of the American Medical Association, 262*, 925-930.

168. Titler, M., Dochterman, J., Kim, T., Kanak, M., Shever, L., Picone D., Everett, L., & Budreau, G. (2007). Costs of care for seniors hospitalized for hip fractures and related procedures. *Nursing Outlook, 55*(1), 5-14.

169. Titler, M., Dochterman, J., Pettit, D., Everett, L., Xie, X., Kanak, M., & Fei, Q. (2005). Cost of hospital care for elderly at risk fo falling. *Nursing Economics, 23*(6), 290-306.

170. Titler, M., Dochterman, J., Xie, X., Kanak, M., Fei, Q., Picone, D., & Shever, L. (2006). Nursing interventions and other factors associated with discharge disposition in older patients after hip fractures. *Nursing Research, 55*(4), 231-242.

171. Titler, M., Jensen, G.A., Dochterman, J., Xie, X., Kanak, M., & Reed, D. (under review). Cost of hospital care for older adults with heart failure: medical, pharmaceutical, and nursing costs.

172. Tripp-Reimer, T., Woodworth, G., McCloskey, J. C., & Bulechek, G. M. (1996). The dimensional structure of nursing interventions. *Nursing Research, 45*, 10-17.

173. U.S. Department of Health an Human Services. (1992). *The planned approach to community health: A guide for the local PATCH coordinator.* Atlanta, GA: Author.

174. U.S Department of Health and Human Services. (2005). *2005 National healthcare quality report.* Rockville, MD: Author.

175. United States General Accounting Office. (1994). *Health care reform "report cards" are useful but significant issues need to be addressed* (Pub. No. GAO/HEHS 94-219). Gaithersburg, MD: Author.

176. Verran, J. (1996). *Nursing staff in hospitals and nursing homes. Is it adequate?* Washington, DC: Institute of Medicine.

177. Ware, J.E., Kosinski, M., & Keller, S.D. (1995). *How to score the SF-12 physical and mental health summary scales* (2nd ed.). Boston, MA: The Health Institute New England Medical Center.

178. Ware, J. E., & Sherbourne, C. D. (1992). The MOS 36-item short-form health survey (SF-36). I. Conceptual framework and item selection. *Medical Care, 30,* 473-481.

179. Warren, A. (1997). JCAHO's measurement mandate. *The IHS Primary Care Provider, 22*(6), 1-3.

180. Warren, J.J., & Bakken, S. (2002). Update on standardized nursing data sets and terminologies. *Journal of Ahima, 73*(7), 78-83.

181. Warren, J.J., & Hoskins, L. M. (1991). The development of NANDA's nursing diagnosis taxonomy. *Nursing Diagnosis, 1,* 162-168.

182. Warren, M. L., Houston, S., & Luquire, R. (1998). Collaborative practice teams: From multidisciplinary to interdisciplinary. *Outcomes Management for Nursing Practice, 2*(3), 95-98.

183. Wennberg, J.E. (2000). Unwarranted variations in healthcare delivery: Implications for academic medical centres. *British Medical Journal, 325,* 961-964.

184. Werley, H., & Lang, N. (1988). *Identification of the nursing minimum data set.* New York: Springer.

185. Westra, B., & Raup, G. (1995). Computerized charting: An essential tool for survival. *Caring, 14*(8), 57-61.

186. Wunderlich, G.S., Sloan, F.A., & Davis, C.K. (Eds.). (1996). *Nursing staff in hospitals and nursing homes: Is it adequate?* Washington, DC: National Academy Press.

187. Zielstorff, R., Hudgings, C., & Grobe, S. (1993). *Next-generation nursing information systems: Essential characteristics for professional practice.* Washington, DC: American Nurses Association.

CHAPTER TWO

The Current Classification

Identifying outcomes responsive to nursing care is critical work for nursing as we face the challenge of implementing an electronic health record and continue to focus on cost and effectiveness in the health care system. Evidence-based practice is an essential requirement for our professional practice. Efforts by nurses to measure outcomes and capture changes in the status of patients over time provides a way to improve the quality of patient care and add to the knowledge base of nursing. In the past we have been dependent on the use of interdisciplinary outcomes developed mostly for physician practice. Consensus among nurses on standardized nursing-sensitive patient outcomes allows nurses to study the effects of nursing interventions over time and across care settings. This is a very important component of outcomes measurement as the patients move quickly across a variety of care settings. Measurement of outcomes validates whether patients are responding to the nursing interventions provided and helps determine whether changes in care need to be made. The use of standardized outcomes provides the data needed to (1) elucidate nursing knowledge, (2) advance theory development, and (3) determine the effectiveness of nursing care for health care policy formulation. Nurses have been documenting the outcomes of their interventions for decades, but the lack of a common language and associated measures for outcomes has impeded data aggregation, analysis, and synthesis of information about the effects of nursing interventions and practice.

Outcome evaluation in health care has expanded to include not only the efficacy of health care interventions, but also the effectiveness of interventions. In efficacy research, the outcomes of interventions are studied under controlled conditions,[10] whereas in effectiveness research, outcomes are studied in an uncontrolled practice situation. In a sense, efficacy research illustrates what outcomes are possible, given ideal conditions and without consideration of cost, while effectiveness research demonstrates what outcomes are achieved in practice and at what cost. An important result of the emphasis put on the evaluation of health care effectiveness has been the recognition that all initiatives to evaluate effectiveness require the identification, standardization, and the use of valid measurement tools for patient outcomes.[15]

The Nursing Outcomes Classification (NOC) is complementary to taxonomies of the North American Nursing Diagnosis Association (NANDA)[15,17] and the Nursing Interventions Classification (NIC).[6] The NOC provides the language for the outcome identification and evaluation steps of the nursing process and the content for the outcomes element of the Nursing Minimum Data Set (NMDS). NOC can also be used with the OPT Model for clinical reasoning developed by Pesut and Herman.[16] In addition the documentation of the outcomes has been encouraged by the work of NANDA International,[15] the advancement of the Nursing Minimum Data Set,[21,22] the Nursing Interventions Classification work,[6,13,18] the development of computerized information systems in health care and the associated large uniform databases, and the emphasis on demonstrating health care effectiveness. However, the definition and classification of clinically useful nursing-sensitive patient outcomes was not accomplished before the NOC was first published in 1997. Further, there are few conceptual frameworks of nursing-sensitive patient outcomes, and existing ones tend to describe broad categories of outcomes that are not validated. The NOC is especially significant because standardized languages for computerized nursing diagnoses, interventions, and outcomes are needed for the study of linkages among these patient phenomena using actual patient data. Further, the standardized languages represent concepts that describe the basic phenomena for which the nursing discipline is accountable and together with the linkages among the concepts represent an important stage of nursing theory development.

THE CLASSIFICATION

This book presents one way to standardize terminology for nursing-sensitive outcomes for use by nurses and other health care providers interested in changes in patient status after intervention. Each outcome presented in Part Three represents a concept that can be used to assess the state of a patient, caregiver, family, or community/population prior to and after intervention. The outcomes in this classification have been developed for use by nurses, but other disciplines may find them helpful for evaluating the effectiveness of the interventions they provide independently or in interdisciplinary teams with nurses. Each outcome has a definition, a measurement scale or combination of scales, a list of associated indicators for the concept, and supporting references. The NOC taxonomy, described and presented in Part Two facilitates the identification of outcomes in the classification for use in practice. The three levels of the taxonomy help users quickly find the outcomes useful for their practice. In addition, this book provides an alphabetical listing of the outcomes and the page numbers of their locations in the table of contents in the beginning of the text.

The Nursing Outcome Classification: What Is it?

The current classification contains a list of 385 outcomes with definitions, indicators, measurement scales, and supporting references. This includes 58 new outcomes that have been developed since the publication of the third edition. Outcomes in the classification are for use at individual, family, and community levels. In some clinical situations outcomes from a variety of these perspectives may be used for a patient. The term *patient* or *client* is used in the classification to denote an individual who is the recipient of nursing care. It is recognized that the term *client* or *consumer* is used in many community and health-maintenance settings and that *resident* is used in many assisted-living or long-term care settings. For purposes of brevity, the term *patient* or *client* is used in this classification since these terms are commonly used in both nursing and the health care literature. Likewise, the term *caregiver* is used to denote a family member, a significant other, a friend, or another person who cares for or acts on behalf of the patient.

A family is a group of two or more people who are related biologically, legally, or by choice that has a societal expectation to socialize, enculturate, and care for its members. A population is generally understood as a collection of individuals who have one or more personal (e.g., gender, age, illness) or environmental (e.g., country, worksite) characteristics in common.[19] A community is an interactive population with relationships that emerge as members develop and use, in common, some agencies and institutions. The American Nurses Association Division on Community Health Nursing[1] defines community health nursing as a synthesis of nursing practice and public health practice applied to promoting and preserving the health of populations, with the dominant responsibility to the population as a whole.

Community and *population* are terms that suffer from lack of conceptual clarity. When individuals speak of communities, they are ordinarily referring to the social context within which persons reside. Interaction among members is inherent in the notion of community but is not so for a population.[8] Sociologists refer to a community as the immediate social context of an individual's life, the natural area or human landscape that is personally experienced or encountered by an individual in everyday life. Thus the community is the natural area into which a child moves as he or she leaves the immediate circle of the family. In the more common vernacular, *community* may refer to a neighborhood, a town (small to very large, rural or urban), a country, or to any interacting population and the relationships that emerge as members develop and use, in common, some agencies and institutions. Thus one may speak of the "international community" or the "community of nurses." For NOC, a community-level outcome characterizes the immediate social context of persons and the relationships that emerge as members (individuals, families, groups) interact, develop, and use, in common, agencies and institutions. Community-level NOC outcomes also characterize populations of individuals who share an attribute or belong to particular groups, families, neighborhoods, and communities but who do not necessarily interact with one another.

We have fine-tuned our definition of an outcome as this classification has evolved and developed. The definition we developed for the third edition has served our work well. A nursing-sensitive patient outcome is an individual, family, or community state, behavior, or perception that is measured along a continuum in response to nursing intervention(s). The outcomes are variable concepts that can be measured along a continuum using a measurement scale. The outcomes are stated as concepts that reflect a patient, caregiver, family, or community actual state, perception, or behavior rather than as expected goals. A five-point Likert type scale is used with all outcomes and indicators. The five-point scoring format provides an adequate number of options to demonstrate variability in the state, behavior, or perception described by the outcome. This scale structure does not demand the degree of precision required for a 10-point scoring format. A target rating can be used to set a goal for the patient's status, perception, or behavior post intervention. This retains the variability of the outcome and allows measurement of the patient condition at any point in time. For example, the outcome Cognition is measured on a five-point scale from "Severely compromised" to "Not compromised" and Caregiver Performance: Direct Care is measured on a five-point scale from "Not adequate" to "Totally adequate." The measurement scales are standardized so a rating of "5" is always the best possible score and a rating of "1" is the worst possible score. Each of the scales provides modifiers for the scores from 1 to 5. There is an option to rate an indicator as "not applicable" for the patient by selecting the NA column.

By measuring the outcome prior to intervening, the nurse establishes a baseline score on the outcome and can then rate the outcome after the intervention. This allows nurses to follow changes in patient status or maintenance of outcome states over time and across settings. For example, if a patient is rated a "2" prior to intervention and a "4" after intervention, the change score is +2. The true outcome is the change seen in the outcome rating after nursing interventions. This change score can be positive (the outcome rating increased), negative (the outcome rating decreased), or there can be no change (the outcome rating stayed the same). In some cases a change score of zero is the goal. This may be the case in situations where the nurse does not expect the patient to improve but wants to maintain the current status of the patient and provides interventions to do this. This is a common goal when working with elderly patients or the terminally ill. Nurses must be able to quantify the success their interventions bring to maintaining the current status of the patient.

When measuring outcomes, we advocate the use of a "reference person" for comparison with the patient the nurse is caring for. The reference person is a healthy person of the same age and gender. For example, the nurse compares her 60-year-old male patient with a healthy 60-year-old male. This implies that nurses use their experience with other patients in this age-group for the comparison. This is important to have the measurement of outcomes comparable across populations. When the patient has a chronic condition such as arthritis and the nurse is trying to improve the patient's mobility, the comparison person is *not* a 60-year-old male with arthritis but a healthy male of the same age. This comparison maintains the rating of "5" on our measurement scales as the healthy rating. We do not want the "5" rating to be undermined by conditions that reflect the normal best state for the population of patients the nurse works with. This is especially true for populations of patients such as those with renal failure, congestive heart failure, or other serious conditions. This means that the highest rating that this type of patient may be able to achieve on an outcome might be a "3." Since nursing is working toward benchmarking outcomes of care, this is an important requirement for measuring outcomes. Nurses have historically only written goal statements they believed their patients could achieve, so the use of the reference person is a new skill that nurses need to develop as they use the outcomes in this classification. As nursing knowledge increases and more effective interventions are selected or new treatments are developed, improvement in the outcomes achieved may be expected. Lack of change in the outcome score after nursing interventions may indicate that another approach to the problem is required. What is important is that outcomes are measured reliably and validly so that the effectiveness of nursing interventions can be examined.

Outcomes in the classification are at a higher level of abstraction than goal statements typically are. In other instances, the indicators used to determine patient condition in relation to an outcome represent the more specific outcomes often reflected in goal statements. For example, a few of the indicators used in the outcome Cognition are "immediate memory," "remote memory," "communication clear for age," and "information processing." While these may serve as intermediate outcomes or indicators of cognition, when used alone, they do not measure the multidimensional aspects of the concept Cognition. The use of midlevel concepts facilitates the use of outcomes in computerized systems and the aggregation of data for effectiveness research and policy formulation, which for individuals tend to focus on patient conditions that influence functional and health status. The midlevel concept also may be useful in efficacy research. For example, a researcher evaluating an intervention to improve memory can use outcome indicators to determine the effects of the intervention not only on memory but also on other factors that determine cognition. Whereas the outcomes currently do not provide tested measures for assessing the effects of an intervention on memory, they do suggest other factors to consider and can be used in conjunction with tested measures to arrive at a determination of how improvement of memory influences cognition. Further, if outcomes are found to be psychometrically sound, there is potential for the use of outcomes to measure impact variables in efficacy research. Development and testing of outcome measures that have practical use in clinical settings and are valid for use in research have important implications for documenting the nursing profession's contributions to health care and providing data to influence health care policy. These advantages also apply for family- and community-level outcomes.

The outcomes, while representative of broad, midlevel concepts, are at varied levels of specificity. For example, Risk Control is a broad outcome defined as "personal actions to prevent, eliminate, or reduce modifiable health threats" that can be used with any nursing intervention directed at assisting patients to identify and control risks. However, more specific outcomes for risks of common concern to nurses (e.g., Risk Control: Alcohol Use and Risk Control: Drug Use) also are in the classification. Community Health Status versus Community Health Status: Immunity is another example of the variability in level of abstraction among the outcomes in the current classification and taxonomy. As additional outcomes are developed and refined, we expect that greater homogeneity of level of abstraction among outcomes will evolve. Decisions regarding the inclusion of outcomes that are relatively broad versus more specific, however, will depend on what is shown to be useful to nurses. Our experience to date is that nurses in different settings may need different levels of abstraction based on their specialty and the setting in which they provide care. The best example of this is that nurses working in intensive care units prefer the more specific outcomes to use in their practice. In the taxonomic structure, level of abstraction also is reflected in domain, class, and outcome categories, which facilitate the ease with which the classification is used.

The language used in the outcomes reflects the language used by nurses in the nursing literature and practice. Language used most consistently by nurses, rather than by those in other disciplines, was selected for the outcomes whenever possible. However, there are exceptions when terminology most familiar to nurses is too specific to reflect a broad patient state or is stated as a negative outcome. For example, *decubitus ulcer*, or skin breakdown, is a common term used by nurses, but the term used in the classification to describe the condition of the skin is Tissue Integrity: Skin & Mucous Membranes. The wording allows the outcome to be stated as a neutral term and as a midlevel concept that is addressed by nursing interventions. In some instances, undesirable or negative patient conditions are used as the outcome when the concept cannot be captured adequately with a neutral term. For example, the classification contains the outcomes

Pain Level and Infection Severity, both undesirable patient states that represent important outcomes that need to be monitored but cannot be adequately described by terms such as *comfort level* or *immune status*. Undesirable patient conditions also are used as outcomes when the language is commonly accepted and used both by health care providers and by policy makers. For example, the Agency for Health Care Policy and Research uses Pain Level in published guidelines, as do researchers and practitioners when evaluating the effects of interventions on pain. As the number of outcomes in the classification increases the use of terms that are common language in nursing, it becomes easier for nurses to find the outcomes they need to use in practice.

The classification structure uses colons to separate broad outcome terms from terms that make the outcomes more specific. As much as possible, the first term in the outcome reflects the term that the practitioner might select when looking for the outcome. For example, recovery from abuse is found under the broad category Abuse Recovery but is further specified by Abuse Recovery: Emotional; Abuse Recovery: Financial; Abuse Recovery: Physical; and Abuse Recovery: Sexual. In the third edition of the classification a more global outcome called Abuse Recovery Status was added. This is a pattern of outcome development that has been helpful to the development of this classification. Nurses can choose between the specific outcomes or use the more global outcome that contains the more specific content as indicators. Nurses have told us that this means they may select fewer outcomes for some patients.

Each concept represents a patient, caregiver, family, or community/population state, sensitive in varying degrees to nursing interventions. Originally, the research team assessed sensitivity to nursing interventions by (1) selecting the concepts from outcomes in nursing literature and clinical information systems, (2) determining that the outcomes have been used to measure the effects of nursing interventions, and (3) surveying expert nurses about the importance of the outcomes as measures of the effects of nursing interventions. We recognize that the ultimate test of sensitivity will be the widespread selection and use of outcomes in practice and research with careful analyses that isolate the effects of interventions on the outcomes. Because the outcomes have been developed for use in all settings where nurses provide care, some of the outcome indicators may be more applicable in one setting than another. For example, blood values and other diagnostic results used as indicators may be pertinent in an intensive or acute care setting, but they may be less useful in a home or nursing home care setting. When in doubt, we have included indicators that we believe are still used in practice globally, such as urine testing for diabetes, even though the standard in the United States has been focused on blood samples. We need to include these indicators so that the outcomes in this classification have value for nurses in other countries. Finally, community-level outcomes are most likely useful in community health settings or for the evaluation of community responses to disasters. This continues to be the least developed area of the classification.

Many of the nursing-sensitive outcomes are not specific for nursing interventions only and thus could be used to evaluate the care provided by other health care disciplines. For example, physical therapists may greatly influence a patient's overall outcome rating for Mobility. In this case this outcome measures the collaborative results of nursing care and physical therapy. While the outcomes may be used by other disciplines, the indicators used to assess patient condition in relation to the outcome may vary from discipline to discipline. For example, physical therapists may use indicators that measure progress with the use of equipment not routinely used by nursing. The classification also contains outcomes most often associated with nursing interventions such as Breastfeeding Establishment: Infant; Bowel Elimination; Health Promoting Behavior; and Knowledge: Treatment Procedure. The number of outcomes developed for use with teaching interventions continues to increase with each edition. The knowledge outcomes can easily be used by other disciplines providing care to patients.

As standardized NOC outcomes are selected and used in practice, more information will be available to determine their frequency of use and conditions under which they are selected.

Because most NOC outcomes are shared by several disciplines, large clinical databases will be needed to assess the effectiveness of nursing interventions. Variables indicating the contributions of other disciplines; attributes of the individual, caregiver, family, or community; and variables describing the environmental context of care can be controlled to reveal the effects of nursing. For efficacy research, randomized clinical trials (RCT) are the gold standard. Randomization helps control for factors other than nursing interventions that are competing explanations for outcome effects. This type of research, however, is often very difficult to implement and maintain in nursing clinical practice, underscoring the need to build large nursing databases to enable nursing effectiveness research. The use of a classification such as NOC for measuring nursing-sensitive patient outcomes makes this an important step in building the knowledge base of nursing for the future.

The Nursing Outcomes Classification: What It Is Not

Although the classification of outcomes presented in this text contains outcomes frequently used by nurses, at this stage of development, the text does not include all outcomes that might be important for nursing. As nurses review the outcomes and use them in practice and research, other outcomes will be identified and current outcomes may require modification. We anticipate that any classification of outcomes will undergo modification to reflect changes in nursing practice and health care delivery, and therefore, the classification will be continually evolving. The testing of the outcomes in clinical sites resulted in many revisions to the last edition based on feedback from nurses in practice. Changes in this edition of the classification were made to better position the classification for use in electronic health records to ensure that the contributions of nurses can be accurately represented in the future. Efforts of this type enhance the classification, build nursing knowledge, and improve the care nurses provide to patients, families, and communities.

The outcomes published in this edition do not include all outcomes for individuals, groups, families, and communities for which nurses provide interventions. Family and community outcomes are included in this edition, building on our previous work, but more outcomes are needed in this area. However, many individual-level outcomes can be aggregated to characterize families, communities, and populations (e.g., by a nursing or medical diagnosis, by a diagnostic related group [DRG], by the unit or geographic location in which care is provided, or by the nurse providing the care). Additional family and community outcomes will be developed to assess the effectiveness of nursing interventions aimed at these units. It is possible that some of the individual-level outcomes can be modified for use with aggregates, and feedback about such modifications from users will be extremely helpful for future editions. The outcome classification also does not contain outcomes of organizational performance or the cost of health care. These outcomes are important in effectiveness research but do not reflect the effects of interventions on a patient. Rather, organizational and cost outcomes are more often useful for evaluating the effectiveness of nursing management or health services delivery interventions.

The outcomes are not prescriptive. They are not goals for individual patients or patient populations, although they can be translated into goals by identifying the desired state on the measurement scale and setting a target rating for the patient. Individual-level outcomes are not prescribed for a particular nursing diagnosis or nursing intervention. They can be selected for a diagnosis or intervention based on the clinical judgment of the nurse responsible for the care of an individual patient or based on the collective judgment of the health care providers responsible for developing a critical path for a patient population. Possible linkages to NANDA nursing diagnoses are suggested in this book and are found in Part Four. These linkages are presented in this text to assist the user in the selection of outcomes and to stimulate study of the suggested linkages. Additional linkages among diagnoses, interventions and outcomes can be found in a separate publication.[7]

The outcomes are not nursing diagnoses, although many of them assess the same states addressed by nursing diagnoses. A diagnosis identifies a state that is altered, has the potential to be altered, or has the potential to be improved, whereas an outcome assesses the actual state at a given point in time using a five-point measurement scale. Table 2-1 illustrates some of the differences in diagnostic and outcome language using NANDA diagnoses and NOC outcomes.

The comparisons in Table 2-1 illustrate the difference between the language used to identify a state for which a diagnosis is made and the state that is measured as an outcome. They also illustrate that some outcomes are more specific than a related diagnosis (e.g., knowledge outcomes), while some diagnoses are more specific than the related outcome (e.g., diagnoses of bowel function). There also are some global outcomes for which similar language is not used in the NANDA diagnoses; however, these outcomes might be selected for a number of the diagnoses.

Outcomes are not assessments, although indicators may represent patient states, behaviors, or perceptions evaluated during a patient assessment. No outcome represents the total range of individual, family, or community states that make up a comprehensive assessment. An assessment provides the database for clinical reasoning and decisions, including the selection of nursing diagnoses, outcomes, and interventions. Although the defining assessment data for a diagnosis should correspond with outcome indicators that refer to the same patient state, the validation of nursing diagnoses and nursing-sensitive patient outcomes needed to achieve complete correspondence has not yet been done. NOC outcomes can be used as focused assessment tools when determining the baseline rating. When an outcome is selected, the individual, family, or community state, behavior, or perception needs to be evaluated and rated on the measurement

Table 2-1   COMPARISONS OF NANDA DIAGNOSES AND NOC OUTCOMES

NANDA Diagnosis	NOC Outcome
Impaired Physical Mobility	Mobility
Hopelessness	Hope
Deficient Knowledge	Knowledge: Disease Process Knowledge: Medication Knowledge: Diabetes Management Knowledge: Health Behavior Knowledge: Treatment Regimen
Constipation	Bowel Continence
Diarrhea	Bowel Elimination
Stress Urinary Incontinence	Urinary Elimination
Reflex Urinary Incontinence	Urinary Continence Tissue Integrity: Skin & Mucous Membranes Personal Well-Being
Interrupted Family Processes	Family Functioning Family Coping Family Social Climate
Readiness for Enhanced comfort	Comfort Status Comfort Status: Environment Comfort Status: Physical Comfort Status: Psychospiritual Comfort Status: Sociocultural Discomfort Level

scale to provide a baseline measure for comparison with post-intervention measures. It is the baseline measure of a variable outcome state that should correspond to the diagnosis.

Commonly Asked Questions

Initial work on the NOC identified conceptual questions that have formed the foundation on which this work is built. The original research team reviewed the literature on patient outcomes, information systems, taxonomic classification science, effectiveness research, and relevant qualitative and quantitative methods to address these issues. Team members reviewed multiple sources of patient outcomes used by nurses (textbooks, nursing information systems, critical pathways and care plans, outcome studies, standards of practice, conceptual frameworks, and outcome classifications). As nurses begin to use standardized outcomes rather than goals in their practice, many of these initial issues and other questions arise about the NOC. We have included the most commonly asked questions about the classification here and briefly address each question.

Who Is the Patient?   Patient outcomes focus on the recipient of care; however, the traditional use of the term *patient* is too limiting for evaluation of all nursing practice purposes. *Patient* traditionally is defined as an individual recipient of care; however, because family caregivers and significant others often are integrally involved with patients and their care, they also are recipients of nursing care. The term *patient* is used in many of the outcomes, even though the team recognizes that the care recipient may be called *client* or *resident* in some settings. In the first and second editions we used the term patient consistently. When the satisfaction outcomes were added to the third edition, the term *patient satisfaction* as the label name was considered by the research team to be too limiting, so the term *client satisfaction* is used to describe these outcomes. This issue has continued in nursing with some health care organizations wanting to use the term *consumer* for their patients. Regardless of what they are called, individuals are the focus of most of the outcomes in this classification. Data ordinarily are collected on individuals and aggregated to characterize other units of analysis (e.g., patient groups, organizations, communities), but some outcomes require data to be collected at a group level.[5] The research team decided to use individuals as the focal unit for the initial development of the NOC, with family caregivers included to assess the impact of nursing on the family members as individuals. The development and testing of outcomes for other units, such as family and community, were added as experts developed outcomes from the group perspective. This work focuses on developing outcomes that characterize family and community units as a whole. Additional outcomes need to be developed in these areas.

What Do Patient Outcomes Describe?   Like nursing diagnoses, the phenomena of concern with nursing-sensitive patient outcomes are individual patient or caregiver states or behaviors, including perceptions or subjective states.[3,6] These phenomena are in contrast to nursing interventions that describe nurse behaviors.[6] The phenomena of concern for nursing-sensitive patient outcomes also are in contrast to nursing diagnoses where the phenomena of concern are patient states identified because an improvement is desired. Outcomes, on the other hand, define a patient status at a particular point in time and may indicate improvement or deterioration of the state compared with a previous assessment. The defining data for a diagnosis typically correspond to outcomes and indicators at an undesirable point on the status continuum. Patient states that are assessed but do not follow an intervention are not outcomes as we define them. Outcomes describe patient states that follow and are expected to be influenced by an intervention. For the team's research, a *nursing-sensitive patient outcome* is defined as an individual, family, or community state, behavior, or perception that is measured along a continuum in response to nursing intervention(s). Each outcome has an associated group of indicators that are used to determine patient status in relation to the outcome. *Nursing-sensitive patient outcome indicators* are defined as more concrete individual, family, or community states, behaviors, or perceptions that serve as cues for measuring an outcome. The definitions and indicators acknowledge that nurses, family caregivers, and patients supply outcome data and that both the patient and family caregiver are the focus of outcomes. Some outcomes can be measured only by the patient and others only by the nurse, whereas some require measurement by the patient (or family) and the nurse or other health provider. Definitions of some common terms used in the classification are listed in Box 2-1.

In contrast to The Joint Commission's use of the term *indicator* as a quantitative measure,[14] the developers of NOC use the term *nursing-sensitive outcome indicator* to describe the specific patient state that is most sensitive to nursing interventions and for which measurement procedures can be defined. For the purpose of facilitating measurement of change, outcomes are conceptualized as nonevaluative, variable patient states influenced by nursing intervention. Thus patient outcomes represent patient states that vary and can be measured and compared with a baseline over time. As Bond and Thomas[2] note, the requirement of predetermined outcomes that call for a specific change is unnecessary. Unintended consequences of nursing interventions and maintenance of steady states also are valid and may be desirable outcomes.[4] Therefore nursing-sensitive patient outcomes are not viewed as goals, although the outcomes and indicators can be used to set goals for specific patients with baseline status and change in status being assessed over time.

The testing of the NOC in clinical practice indicated that the change in rating after intervention provides important information for nursing to collect. This creates a *change in rating score* when the baseline measurement score prior to intervention is compared with the measurement post-intervention. This *difference in scores* captures the effects of the intervention on the outcome and is one of the main benefits of using variable outcomes rather than goals. The change score can be positive when the second outcome score increases and negative when the outcome score decreases, or the score can be zero if no change occurred.

At What Levels of Abstraction Should Outcomes Be Developed? The nursing-sensitive patient outcomes classification contains patient outcomes and indicators at four general levels of abstraction with measurement procedures at the empirical level (Table 2-2). At the highest levels, outcome categories and classes were derived from the results of hierarchical clustering and qualitative strategies used in the research. These were compared with the outcome categories promulgated by the Medical Outcomes Study[20] and with current nursing outcome.[9,12] The least abstract level contains indicator statements for each outcome label. Outcomes are at middle levels of abstraction, and in some instances, indicators for more abstract, global outcomes are developed as more specific, less abstract outcomes. For example, an indicator for the outcome Mobility is "joint movement," while "flexion" is an indicator for the outcome Joint Movement: Neck. The empirical level includes measurement activities for each outcome and its indicators.

How Should the Outcomes Be Stated? Because the outcomes and indicators are conceptualized as variable patient, caregiver, family, or community states, behaviors, or perceptions, they are given labels representing concepts that can be measured along a continuum as negative or positive states. Whenever possible, the team avoids labels that describe an undesirable state. However, because of the common use of some labels or difficulty identifying an antonym, some do describe an undesirable state. Examples are Infection Severity, Discomfort Level, Fear Level, and Pain Level. Conceptualization of the outcomes as variables allows measurement of negative or positive changes, as well as no change, resulting from nursing interventions.[3] Box 2-2 summarizes the rules used in the development of the outcomes for this classification.

Why Are the Outcomes Not Stated as Goals? The original research team developed the outcomes as variable concepts for several reasons. First, NOC outcomes are developed as

Box 2-1

Selected Terms and Definitions

Ability
Power or capacity to perform actions.

Adequate
Sufficient in quantity or quality to meet a need or function.

Adherence
To hold fast to a selected action to improve health.

Adolescence
Period of time in a child's life from 12 years through 17 years.

Appropriate
Suitable to meet requirements, demands, or needs.

Avoid
Withdraw from something; keep away from.

Behavior
The observable or reported response of an individual, family, or community to its environment.

Care Recipient
A person receiving services from a professional, such as a patient, caregiver (specify), parent (specify), family (specify), or community (specify).

Change in Rating Score
The difference between a baseline rating of the outcome and the postintervention rating(s) of the outcome. This change in score can be positive (the outcome rating increased), negative (the outcome rating decreased), or no change (the outcome rating stayed the same). This change in rating score represents the outcome achieved following a health care intervention(s).

Child
Overall term for childhood from 1 year through 17 years old.

Childcare Provider
Family caregiver or an individual who is paid to provide childcare.

Community
An interactive population with relationships that emerge as members develop and use, in common, some agencies and institutions.

Compliance
To hold fast to a recommendation from a health professional.

Confidence
Belief that one can act to achieve a desired goal.

Data Source
Documentation of where data are obtained from, such as the patient, family member, caregiver, direct observation by health care provider, clinical record, or other source.

Decreased
Lesser in size, degree, or amount.

Disease
A specific pathological process defined by a set of signs and symptoms that affects a body part or the whole body; the etiology, pathology, and prognosis may be known or unknown.

Early Childhood
Period of time in a child's life from 1 year through 5 years (includes toddler and preschool periods).

Effective
Producing desired health-related results.

Family
A group of two or more people who are related biologically, legally, or by choice that has a societal expectation to socialize, enculturate, and care for its members.

Family Caregiver
A family member, significant other, friend, or another person who cares for or acts on behalf of the patient.

Function
Special action or physiological property of an organ or other part of the body to perform its specific work.

Continued

Box 2-1

Selected Terms and Definitions—cont'd

Functioning
Carrying out a set of actions in the expression or performance of a role.

Health
A state of physical, psychological, social, and spiritual functioning.

Health Professionals
Individuals with advanced education and licensure who are reimbursed for providing health care services.

Health Providers
Professional and assistive personnel who are reimbursed for providing health care services.

Inappropriate
Not suitable for meeting requirements, demands, or needs.

Increased
Greater in amount, degree, or size.

Infant
A baby from birth to first birthday.

Late Adulthood
Period of time in an adult's life from 65 years and older.

Measure
A five-point Likert type scale that quantifies a patient outcome or indicator status on a continuum from least to most desirable and provides a rating at a point in time.

Mental
Pertaining to a person's total emotional and intellectual response.

Middle Adulthood
Period of time in an adult's life from 40 years through 64 years.

Middle Childhood
Period of time in a child's life from 6 years through 11 years.

Newborn
A baby from birth to the first 28 days of life.

NOC Taxonomy
A systematic organization of outcomes into groups or categories based on similarities, dissimilarities, and relationships among the outcomes. The NOC taxonomy structure has five levels: domains, classes, outcomes, indicators, and measures.

Nursing-Sensitive Patient Outcome
An individual, family, or community state, behavior, or perception that is measured along a continuum in response to nursing intervention(s). Each outcome has an associated group of indicators that are used to determine patient status in relation to the outcome.

Obtain
To gain or attain by planned effort or action.

Parent
Mother, father, or other individual assuming the childrearing role.

Outcome Indicator
A more concrete individual, family, or community state, behavior, or perception that serves as a cue for measuring an outcome.

Perception
The conscious mental thought, image, or sensation from a sensory stimulus.

Personal Actions
Actions taken by the individual, caregiver, significant other, or family member.

Population
A collection of individuals who have one or more personal (e.g., gender, age, illness) or environmental (e.g., country, worksite) characteristics in common.

Preschool
Period of time in a child's life from 3 years through 5 years.

Recommended
Presented as worthy of confidence, acceptance, or use.

Reference Person
A healthy person of the same age and gender used for comparison when rating an outcome or indicator.

Box 2-1

Selected Terms and Definitions—cont'd

Refrains
Keeps oneself from following a passing impulse.
Reputable
Recognized as positive by health provides or experts in the field.
Resource
Source of supply, support, or information.
Status
State of health of the focus of the outcome. This may be at the individual, family, or community level or a function of a system or state of the body.
Toddler
Period of time in a child's life from 1 year through 2 years.
Well-Being
Extent of positive perception of one's own health status.
Young Adulthood
Period of time in an adult's life from 18 years through 39 years.

Table 2-2   LEVELS OF ABSTRACTION IN THE TAXONOMY

Most Abstract	Nursing-Sensitive Outcome Domain
High Middle Level Abstraction	Nursing-Sensitive Outcome Classes
Middle Level Abstraction	Nursing-Sensitive Outcome
Low Level Abstraction	Nursing-Sensitive Outcome Indicators
Empirical Level	Measurement Activities for Outcomes

variable concepts so that the response of the patient, caregiver, family, or community to nursing interventions can be documented and monitored over time, across settings, and compared. A goal developed for each patient does not allow for this cross comparison. Second, variable outcomes yield more information than just whether or not a goal is met. For clinical and research purposes, either/or type data provide a very limited amount of information and constrain nurses' abilities to adequately evaluate the effectiveness of their interventions. If goals are not met, it is important to know whether any progress was made or the extent that the outcome status deteriorated, if at all. Third, with current short length of stays in acute care settings, it has become very important to be able to document even slight increases in outcome scores at discharge. Goals for short time frames become meaningless for monitoring progress across time. NOC outcomes can be used to state a goal for a patient, family, or community, but this should be in addition to measurement of status on the variable outcome at baseline and over time. Fourth, in many cases, the goal of nursing care may be to maintain a patient at a particular outcome rating when improvement in status is not possible. For example, the goal for a patient with self-care issues may be to maintain his or her outcome status at a "3" for the outcome Self-Care: Bathing. Finally, the strength of using outcomes rather than goals is that a change in rating score can be determined after nursing care is provided. This change in rating score is not possible with goals and is important for evaluating the effectiveness of nursing treatments and comparing outcomes for specific patient populations over time.

> ### Box 2-2
>
> <hr/>
>
> #### Rules for Standardization of Nursing Sensitive Outcomes
>
> - Outcome labels should be concise (stated in five words or less).
> - Outcome labels should be stated in nonevaluative terms rather than as a decreased, increased, or improved state.
> - Outcome labels should use common nursing terms as much as possible.
> - Outcome labels should *not* describe a nurse behavior or interventions.
> - Outcome labels should *not* be stated as a nursing diagnosis.
> - Outcome labels should describe a state, behavior, or perception that is inherently variable and can be measured and quantified.
> - Outcome labels should be conceptualized and stated at a middle level of abstraction.
> - Outcomes labels may be developed using one or two measurement scales.
> - Definitions for outcomes should be consistent with the measurement scale.
> - Wording of indicators should be standardized as much as possible for outcomes using the same measurement scale.
> - Colons should be used to make broader concept labels more specific; however, the broader label is stated first, with the colon and more specific label following (e.g., Nutritional Status: Nutrient Intake, Self Care: Bathing).

What Are Nursing-Sensitive Patient Outcomes? To be useful for assessing the effectiveness of nursing, outcomes and indicators that are influenced by nursing and comprehensive enough to assess all aspects of nursing practice must be identified. The original research team recognized that the majority of patient outcomes, including those traditionally used to evaluate physician care, are not influenced by any one discipline alone. However, for nursing to monitor and improve its practice, it is important to identify the outcomes that are responsive to nursing care. The more abstract and global the outcome, the more likely its achievement will be the result of interventions from several health care disciplines. Specific disciplines will have more influence on certain intermediate outcomes than others. For example, at different times, nursing, medicine, and physical therapy have the most impact on Mobility, although, overall, all share influence on the outcome. It is the specific indicators of outcomes that are more likely to be sensitive to the interventions of a single discipline. Therefore it is essential to identify the indicators most sensitive to nursing interventions to enable nurses to document the effects of their interventions and to hold them individually and collectively accountable for care delivered to patients. To develop and refine the list of nursing-sensitive outcomes and indicators, the original research team defined a set of criteria for evaluating evidence of nursing sensitivity or responsiveness to nursing intervention. These criteria are listed in Box 2-3.

Are Nursing-Sensitive Patient Outcomes the Resolution of Nursing Diagnoses? The majority of nursing-sensitive patient outcomes represent the resolution of nursing diagnoses, although some outcomes are more generic and not necessarily related to specific diagnoses. Clearly, client satisfaction and the financial charges that are attributable to nursing care are not diagnosis specific and cannot be conceived as the resolution of a diagnosis. At this time, it appears that the more general (abstract) the outcome, such as Quality of Life, the less likely it will be diagnosis specific, and conversely, the less abstract the outcome concept, such as Self-Care: Toileting, the more likely it will be nursing diagnosis specific.

How Are the Outcomes Different From Nursing Diagnoses? NOC outcomes describe a variable state, behavior, or perception. The outcome state at a particular time can be at any point on a negative to positive continuum. The outcomes can be used to measure nursing diagnoses stated as problems, risk states, or potential for enhancement diagnoses with the same measure. Nursing diagnoses, on the other hand, for the most part describe states that are in some way less

---

Box 2-3

Criteria for Evaluating Nursing Sensitivity

- A nursing intervention produced a positive outcome.
- A nursing intervention influenced a positive outcome.
- A nursing intervention was carried out with the intent to produce or influence the outcome.
- A nursing intervention produced improvement or maintenance of the outcome or prevented deterioration or occurrence of a negative outcome.
- The nursing intervention occurred before observation of the outcome.
- A failure to provide nursing intervention resulted in failure to achieve a positive outcome or to prevent a negative outcome.
- The interventions that produced or influenced the outcome are within nursing's scope of practice.

---

positive than what is desired. Nursing diagnoses describe problems, actual or potential, that the nurse seeks to resolve through intervention. More recently, nursing diagnoses focused on wellness have been developed. The relationship of these diagnoses and outcomes needs further discussion and evaluation.

When Should Patient Outcomes Be Measured? The appropriate time to measure patient outcomes will vary. This is because some outcomes respond very quickly to intervention, and others respond over a longer period of time. The outcomes of health promotion interventions, for example, are likely to occur over a considerable time period, while the response to interventions to improve nutritional intake could be immediate. There also are outcomes such as Transfer Performance where the full response may take several weeks. One problem is selecting a time for measurement close enough to the intervention to be assured that change is due to the intervention but far enough removed to be able to measure a change. This is why medicine has begun to place more emphasis on intermediate outcomes. In nursing we need to be able to follow the patient across settings to evaluate the effectiveness of interventions for some outcomes.

At What Intervals Should the Outcomes Be Assessed and Documented? More research is needed to definitively answer this question. At present, the nurse determines the intervals for measurement and documentation of the outcome based on clinical judgment as to when the effects of interventions need to be assessed. This is greatly influenced by the setting and characteristics of the patient. Organizational policies also determine the intervals for measurement and documentation in some situations. Overrating of outcomes can become a work load burden for the nurse, so the decision of how often to measure an outcome is a critical one. However, at minimum, the outcomes selected should be rated and documented when (1) the patient or family is admitted to a care setting or makes an initial visit to a nurse for care, (2) the patient or family is discharged, transferred, or referred to another setting or clinician for care, or (3) there is a significant change in status for an outcome. Time intervals for measurement of outcomes should vary based on the characteristics of the concept. For example, the nurse might want to measure Pain Level at least every 4 hours but would not measure the patient's Quality of Life on the same time frames. The nurse and/or interdisciplinary health care team should determine the measurement time frames for outcomes of interest.

How Are the Outcomes Used in Standardized Care Plans/Critical Paths? NOC outcomes are very useful in clinical pathways because they allow quantification of the patient state, behavior, or perception that is expected to occur as specific points in time for a desired pathway of an episode of care. A discussion of the use of the NOC in care plans is found in Chapter 3. Major advantages of their use are (1) the ability to monitor variance from the pathway and

(2) the ability to compare the achievement of specific patient states across settings and providers. Use of the standardized outcomes will greatly facilitate the development of large databases across settings and providers, rather than the more limited, unique setting or provider databases that result when setting- or provider-specific outcomes are used in critical pathways and care planning.

Why Is It Necessary for Nurses to Have Their Own List of Outcomes? The NOC includes patient, caregiver, family, and community outcomes that are responsive to nursing interventions. These outcomes are not intended to be unique to nursing. Clearly, most, if not all, patient outcomes are influenced by multiple health care providers, as well as by other patient, caregiver, family, and community/population characteristics and by environmental factors. However, it is critically important for nurses to measure the effects of their interventions on patient outcomes. The NOC provides a set of indicators for each outcome that is considered to be sensitive to nursing interventions. When used with interdisciplinary teams, different indicators may be the focus of interventions for various disciplines. Without discipline-specific indicators for shared outcomes, it will be impossible to monitor the accountability of each discipline for its contribution to outcome improvement or deterioration. To ensure that the contributions of nursing interventions to patient, caregiver, family, and community outcomes are not credited to other health care providers, standardized nursing data elements must be included in clinical databases. Large data sets that include these data, along with other salient system, patient, caregiver, family, or community characteristics and provider characteristics, are necessary to isolate the independent effects of nursing interventions on patient outcomes.[11]

Why Is It Important to Assess Outcomes Across Care Settings? Continuity of care always is an important value for the nursing profession. Yet communication among settings and nurse providers is constrained. A major obstacle is the lack of standardized nomenclatures to describe the problems that nurses treat, the interventions used, and the resulting outcome states. The inability to optimize continuity of care is costly to patients, families, and the health care system. In the current resource-constrained environment, more emphasis is placed on continuity of care to reduce costs. Further, networks that include providers and settings across the continuum of care are being developed to enhance continuity and optimize care in the most cost-efficient environment. The effort to reduce costs has prompted a corresponding emphasis on the demonstration of outcomes effectiveness. The NOC provides a standardized language for outcomes that can be measured across the entire continuum of care, providing essential information that clinicians need to achieve continuity, and to assess the cost-effectiveness of care.

Why Is It Necessary to Use the Outcome Labels When the Indicators May Be More Useful? Along with medicine, the nursing profession is a key member of the interdisciplinary health care team. The profession's contribution to interdisciplinary outcomes must be documented and the effectiveness of nursing interventions must be evaluated. Large, standardized databases contain outcomes such as those provided by NOC, but likely not discipline-specific indicators in all cases because of space limitations. Therefore it is essential that the nursing profession use standardized outcome labels and that these are included in large databases so that the profession's influence on outcomes will be assessed to determine nursing effectiveness and to influence health policy.

Why Is the Standardization of Outcomes Advocated When Each Patient, Caregiver, Family, or Community/Population Is Unique? Standardizing the language used to describe outcomes in no way interferes with assessing the unique response of each patient, caregiver family, or community/population. Rather, use of the NOC outcomes enables nurses to measure each outcome state for each individual, caregiver, family, and community and provides more information for monitoring the progress of each. Further, specific quantified goals can be set for each and the extent that the goals are or are not met can be documented over time and across settings and compared. In other words, standardized nursing diagnoses, interventions, and outcomes actually *increase* the ability of nurses to identify and document the diagnoses that are unique for each patient, prescribe interventions that are specific for the patient, and document the patient outcomes in response to the interventions for each individual across time and settings.

How Do I Identify Outcomes for Use in My Practice?   With 385 outcomes in the fourth edition of NOC, this task may seem difficult at first. The scope of the classification is to identify all outcomes needed by nurses to evaluate the outcomes of nursing interventions, while most nurses will focus on a limited set of outcomes based on their specialty and practice setting. Beginning efforts to identify core outcomes for specialty practice has supported this belief that nurses can identify a list of outcomes they use daily with their patients. The easiest way to begin to identify outcomes for use in clinical practice is to review the NOC Taxonomy where similar outcomes are grouped under key concepts in nursing. A second way to identify outcomes is to review the list of outcomes identified by nursing specialty to see whether the outcomes identified match the outcomes you need to evaluate the effectiveness of your interventions. It is important that specialty practice is adequately reflected in this classification. A third way to identify NOC outcomes is to examine the linkages provided to Gordon's Health Patterns and NANDA diagnoses and Linkages to the International Classification of Functioning in Part Four.

When Is a New Outcome Developed and How Is It Done?   New outcomes are identified by the developers, by nurses from clinical practice, and through the linkage with other classifications. The NOC team maintains a list of potential concepts for development, and these are addressed as we work on new outcomes. A nurse or group of nurses conducts a concept analysis, defines the outcome, identifies indicators, and chooses a measurement scale(s) for use with the outcome. The NOC focus groups have been primarily responsible for the development of new outcomes. The entire research team reviews the potential outcomes, and revisions are made based on this expert review. Part of this review process involves ensuring that the outcome is useful and clinically accurate for patients across the life span. If it is not, then a target population is identified in the concept label. Many of the outcomes are sent to additional experts for further review. Once the outcome is accepted for inclusion in the NOC, the outcome is placed in the taxonomy and coded. We received several submissions from nurses in practice for this edition. Their names can be found in the front of the book. This edition has 58 new outcomes. Instructions on how to submit an outcome can be found in Appendix B.

Why Are There So Many Different Measurement Scales?   Although we have tried to limit the number of measurement scales used in the classification, there are currently 14 scales used in the 385 outcomes in the fourth edition. There are 298 outcomes that use only one scale. As we develop new outcomes, we establish a scale based on the indicators identified in the literature for the outcome. As more outcomes have been developed, we have attempted to measure similar concepts using the same scale. Since the outcomes focus on state, perceptions, and behavior, it is not surprising that different measurement scales are needed to fit the focus of the outcome. After a careful review of our results from field testing in 10 clinical settings, an effort was made to solve some of the problems encountered by nurses using NOC in practice. In the third edition, the measurement scales for each outcome and the corresponding outcome definition were carefully reviewed and resulted in a reduction in the number of scales and a standard format for definitions based on the specific measurement scale. The evaluation of the anchors for each of the scales resulted in modifications, and some outcomes had a change in measurement scale. A more detailed description of this review is available in the previous edition. Tables 2-3 and 2-4 identify the 14 measurement scales with anchors, provides a definition of the focus of each scale, and lists the outcomes by scale that use a single measure or a combination of two scales.

Table 2-3	SINGLE MEASUREMENT SCALES USED IN NOC		

Scale Letter		Scales and Associated Outcomes	

a	*Severely compromised*	*Substantially compromised*	*Moderately compromised*

DEFINITION: Extent of impairment of health or well-being

Activity Tolerance	Concentration
Ambulation	Coordinated Movement
Ambulation: Wheelchair	Decision-Making
Appetite	Information Processing
Body Positioning: Self-Initiated	Memory
Caregiver Physical Health	Mobility
Cognition	Personal Health Status
Cognitive Orientation	Physical Fitness
Comfort Status	Preterm Infant Organization
Comfort Status: Environment	Rest
Comfort Status: Sociocultural	Self-Care: Activities of Daily Living
Communication	(ADL)
Communication: Expressive	Self-Care: Bathing
Communication: Receptive	Self-Care: Dressing

b	*Severe deviation from normal range*	*Substantial deviation from normal range*	*Moderate deviation from normal range*

DEFINITION: Extent of departure from an established norm or standard

Blood Glucose Level	Joint Movement: Knee
Fetal Status: Antepartum	Joint Movement: Neck
Fetal Status: Intrapartum	Joint Movement: Passive
Growth	Joint Movement: Shoulder
Joint Movement	Joint Movement: Spine
Joint Movement: Ankle	Joint Movement: Wrist
Joint Movement: Elbow	Newborn Adaptation
Joint Movement: Fingers	Nutritional Status
Joint Movement: Hip	

f	*Not adequate*	*Slightly adequate*	*Moderately adequate*

DEFINITION: Extent of sufficiency in quantity or quality to achieve a desired state

Abuse Protection	Caregiver Performance: Direct Care
Breastfeeding Establishment: Infant	Caregiver Performance: Indirect Care
Breastfeeding Establishment: Maternal	Caregiver Role Support
Breastfeeding Maintenance	Community Disaster Readiness
Breastfeeding Weaning	Community Disaster Response
Caregiver Home Care Readiness	

g	*10 and over*	*7-9*	*4-6*

DEFINITION: Number of occurrences

Falls Occurrence	Elopement Occurrence

Mildly compromised	*Not compromised*		

Self-Care: Eating
Self-Care: Hygiene
Self-Care: Instrumental Activities of
    Daily Living (IADL)
Self-Care: Non-Parenteral Medication
Self-Care: Oral Hygiene
Self-Care: Parenteral Medication
Self-Care: Toileting
Self-Care Status
Skeletal Function
Spiritual Health
Transfer Performance

N=38

Mild deviation from normal range	*No deviation from normal range*

Nutritional Status: Biochemical
    Measures
Nutritional Status: Energy
Physical Aging
Physical Maturation: Female
Physical Maturation: Male
Sensory Function
Vital Signs
Weight: Body Mass

N=25

Substantially adequate	*Totally adequate*

Nutritional Status: Food & Fluid Intake
Nutritional Status: Nutrient Intake
Pre-Procedure Readiness
Role Performance
Safe Home Environment
Social Support

N=17

1-3	*None*

N=2

Continued

Table 2-3	SINGLE MEASUREMENT SCALES USED IN NOC—cont'd

Scale Letter		Scales and Associated Outcomes	
i	*None*	*Limited*	*Moderate*

DEFINITION: Range over which an entity extends

Abuse Cessation		Abuse Recovery: Financial
Abuse Recovery		Abuse Recovery: Physical

k	*Never positive*	*Rarely positive*	*Sometimes positive*

DEFINITION: Frequency of an affirmative and accepting perception or characteristics

Body Image		Caregiver-Patient Relationship

l	*Very weak*	*Weak*	*Moderate*

DEFINITION: Extent of intensity

Health Beliefs		Health Beliefs: Perceived Control
Health Beliefs: Perceived Ability to Perform		Health Beliefs: Perceived Resources

m	*Never demonstrated*	*Rarely demonstrated*	*Sometimes demonstrated*

DEFINITION: Frequency of making clear by report or behavior

Abusive Behavior Self-Restraint	Energy Conservation
Acceptance: Health Status	Fall Prevention Behavior
Adaptation to Physical Disability	Family Coping
Adherence Behavior	Family Functioning
Adherence Behavior: Healthy Diet	Family Integrity
Aggression Self-Control	Family Normalization
Alcohol Abuse Cessation Behavior	Family Participation in Professional Care
Anxiety Self-Control	Family Resiliency
Aspiration Prevention	Family Social Climate
Body Mechanics Performance	Family Support During Treatment
Cardiac Disease Self-Management	Fear Self-Control
Caregiver Adaptation to Patient	Grief Resolution
Institutionalization	Health Promoting Behavior
Child Development: 1 Month	Health Seeking Behavior
Child Development: 2 Months	Hearing Compensation Behavior
Child Development: 4 Months	Heedfulness of Affected Side
Child Development: 6 Months	Hope
Child Development: 12 Months	Identity
Child Development: 2 Years	Immunization Behavior
Child Development: 3 Years	Impulse Self-Control
Child Development: 4 Years	Leisure Participation
Child Development: 5 Years	Motivation
Child Development: Middle Childhood	Multiple Sclerosis Self-Management
Child Development: Adolescence	Nausea & Vomiting Control
Compliance Behavior	Ostomy Self-Care
Compliance Behavior: Prescribed Diet	Pain Control

Substantial	Extensive	
Neglect Cessation		
		N=5

Often positive	Consistently positive	
Self-Esteem		
		N=3

Strong	Very strong	
Health Beliefs: Perceived Threat Health Orientation		
		N=6

Often demonstrated	Consistently demonstrated	
Personal Safety Behavior Play Participation Postpartum Maternal Health Behavior Prenatal Health Behavior Psychosocial Adjustment: Life Change Risk Control Risk Control: Alcohol Use Risk Control: Cancer Risk Control: Cardiovascular Health Risk Control: Drug Use Risk Control: Hearing Impairment Risk Control: Hyperthermia Risk Control: Hypothermia Risk Control: Infectious Process Risk Control: Sexually Transmitted Diseases (STDs) Risk Control: Sun Exposure Risk Control: Tobacco Use Risk Control: Unintended Pregnancy Risk Control: Visual Impairment Risk Detection Seizure Control Self-Direction of Care Self-Mutilation Restraint Sexual Functioning Sexual Identity		

Continued

Table 2-3 SINGLE MEASUREMENT SCALES USED IN NOC—cont'd

Scale Letter	Scales and Associated Outcomes

Compliance Behavior: Prescribed Medication	Parent-Infant Attachment	
Coping	Parenting: Adolescent Physical Safety	
Depression Self-Control	Parenting: Early/Middle Childhood Physical Safety	
Diabetes Self-Management	Parenting: Infant/Toddler Physical Safety	
Dignified Life Closure	Parenting Performance	
Discharge Readiness: Supported Living	Parenting: Psychosocial Safety	
Distorted Thought Self-Control	Participation in Health Care Decisions	
Drug Abuse Cessation Behavior	Personal Autonomy	
Elopement Propensity Risk	Personal Resiliency	

n	*Severe*	*Substantial*	*Moderate*

DEFINITION: Extent of a negative or adverse state or response

Acute Confusion Level	Fear Level
Agitation Level	Fear Level: Child
Allergic Response: Localized	Fluid Overload Severity
Allergic Response: Systemic	Hyperactivity Level
Anxiety Level	Infection Severity
Blood Loss Severity	Infection Severity: Newborn
Blood Transfusion Reaction	Loneliness Severity
Caregiver Stressors	Nausea & Vomiting: Disruptive Effects
Depression Level	Nausea & Vomiting Severity
Discomfort Level	Pain: Adverse Psychological Response

r	*Poor*	*Fair*	*Good*

DEFINITION: Extent of proximity to a desired state

Community Competence	Community Risk Control: Chronic Disease
Community Health Status	Community Risk Control: Communicable
Community Health Status: Immunity	Disease
	Community Risk Control: Lead Exposure

s	*Not at all satisfied*	*Somewhat satisfied*	*Moderately satisfied*

DEFINITION: Extent of perception of positive expectations

Caregiver Well-Being	Client Satisfaction: Cultural Needs
Client Satisfaction	Fulfillment
Client Satisfaction: Access to Care	Client Satisfaction: Functional Assistance
Resources	Client Satisfaction: Pain Management
Client Satisfaction: Caring	Client Satisfaction: Physical Care
Client Satisfaction: Case Management	Client Satisfaction: Physical Environment
Client Satisfaction: Communication	Client Satisfaction: Protection of Rights
Client Satisfaction: Continuity of Care	Client Satisfaction: Psychological Care

u	*No knowledge*	*Limited knowledge*	*Moderate knowledge*

DEFINITION: Extent of cognitive information that is understood

Knowledge: Arthritis Management	Knowledge: Fall Prevention
Knowledge: Asthma Management	Knowledge: Fertility Promotion

Smoking Cessation Behavior
Social Interaction Skills
Social Involvement
Suicide Self-Restraint
Symptom Control
Treatment Behavior: Illness or Injury
Vision Compensation Behavior
Weight Gain Behavior
Weight Loss Behavior
Weight Maintenance Behavior

N=104

Mild   *None*

Physical Injury Severity
Stress Level
Substance Addiction Consequences
Substance Withdrawal Severity
Suffering Severity
Symptom Severity
Symptom Severity: Perimenopause
Symptom Severity: Premenstrual
   Syndrome (PMS)

N=28

Very good   *Excellent*

Community Risk Control: Violence
Community Violence Level

N=8

Very satisfied   *Completely satisfied*

Client Satisfaction: Safety
Client Satisfaction: Symptom Control
Client Satisfaction: Teaching
Client Satisfaction: Technical Aspects of
   Care
Personal Well-Being
Quality of Life

N=20

Continued

Table 2-3	Single Measurement Scales Used in NOC—cont'd
Scale Letter	**Scales and Associated Outcomes**

u

DEFINITION: Extent of cognitive information that is understood—cont'd

Substantial knowledge	*Extensive knowledge*
Knowledge: Parenting	
Knowledge: Personal Safety	
Knowledge: Body Mechanics	Knowledge: Health Behavior
Knowledge: Breastfeeding	Knowledge: Health Promotion
Knowledge: Cancer Management	Knowledge: Health Resources
Knowledge: Cancer Threat Reduction	Knowledge: Hypertension Management
Knowledge: Cardiac Disease Management	Knowledge: Illness Care
Knowledge: Child Physical Safety	Knowledge: Infant Care
Knowledge: Conception Prevention	Knowledge: Infection Management
Knowledge: Congestive Heart Failure Management	Knowledge: Labor & Delivery
	Knowledge: Medication
Knowledge: Depression Management	Knowledge: Multiple Sclerosis Management
Knowledge: Diabetes Management	Knowledge: Ostomy Care
Knowledge: Diet	Knowledge: Pain Management
Knowledge: Disease Process	
Knowledge: Energy Conservation	

Why Do Some Outcomes Have Two Scales? An issue identified from the testing of the NOC in clinical sites was the problem that some indicators were difficult to use because they contained double negatives to fit the measurement scale. Nurses felt the negative indicators were important to document because they focus on symptoms indicating complications of the patient's condition and are frequently monitored by nurses in practice. As a solution to this problem, a second scale, for measuring the negative states, was added to 72 outcomes in the third edition. For example, the outcome Sensory Function: Vision uses two scales: "Severe deviation from normal range" to "No deviation from normal range," and "Severe" to "None" for the indicators. The overall outcome rating is based on the Deviation scale. We believe this was an important revision to the classification because it allows for better documentation of complications associated with the outcome. A second problem that made the indicators hard to use was wording such as "free of" (e.g., "free of bleeding"). A second scale allows the nurse to rate the severity of bleeding experienced by the patient, rather than whether bleeding is present or absent in the outcome Oral Hygiene. This provides better data and more information on a change in the status of the patient. In the fourth edition, there are 86 outcomes with two scales. This change in format makes these outcomes easier for nurses to use, and we have received positive feedback for this change. Table 2-4 lists the outcomes using two scales in combination.

Has the NOC Format Changed Over Time? Several key changes were made in the format of the outcomes for the previous edition. The addition of a second scale is discussed in the previous section and has had a major impact on the layout of the outcomes. The area devoted to the overall score for the outcome was increased to make it more prominent in the outcome format. A second header was added for the additional scale when needed. As a result of revisions to the indicators, the numerical sequence of the indicators has changed in a number of outcomes because of moving indicators to a second scale within the outcome. Some indicators were moved

Knowledge: Postpartum Maternal Health
Knowledge: Preconception Maternal Health
Knowledge: Pregnancy
Knowledge: Pregnancy & Postpartum
  Sexual Functioning
Knowledge: Prescribed Activity
Knowledge: Preterm Infant Care
Knowledge: Sexual Functioning
Knowledge: Substance Use Control
Knowledge: Treatment Procedure
Knowledge: Treatment Regimen
Knowledge: Weight Management

N=42

to organize the indicators in a more logical way based on feedback from practicing nurses. The codes attached to the indicators were retained if the meaning did not change. In all outcomes the "other" indicator was deleted and the code retired. The use of abbreviations in the indictors was also greatly reduced.

Another major addition to the format of the outcomes is an area for Outcome Target Ratings. Testing of the classification in a variety of settings and populations revealed the need to identify the goal of nursing interventions in terms of the numerical scale. We have added *Maintain at* and *Increase to* so nurses can identify the expected outcome rating they hope to achieve with an individual, family, or community after intervention. As *change in rating scores* were examined in our clinical sites, it was clear that nurses need a way to document that the goal of interventions might be to maintain a rating at the current state. This was especially true for nursing homes personnel working with the elderly and nurses providing care for terminally ill patients. In these cases it may be a major accomplishment to maintain a patient at a chosen rating, thus preventing a decline in that outcome.

Two additional areas for documentation were added to the top of the outcome for the third edition. *Care Recipient* specified as a Patient, Caregiver, Parent, Family, or Community was added to allow for the documentation of who is receiving the care. This is useful when nurses are working with caregivers and parents and may be maintaining a family record with interventions being used with a variety of family members. *Data Source* deals with the source of information used in the rating; for example, the nurse obtained information from the patient, family member, or caregiver; by direct observation; or from a clinical record. Health care agencies can determine if these areas are useful to them. We believe the source of the data may be more than one of these categories and may become important to document in an electronic patient record.

Testing the outcomes in clinical sites also identified the need to document the location of fractures and wounds within the outcomes. Two diagrams have been added to meet this need. One is a skeleton with the bones of the body coded for the outcome Bone Healing. An area called Site of fracture allows the adding of this code to the outcome. If more than one fracture is pres-

Table 2-4	COMBINATION MEASUREMENT SCALES USED IN NOC		

a and n	*Severely compromised*	*Substantially compromised*	*Moderately compromised*
	Severe	*Substantial*	*Moderate*
	Balance		Immune Status
	Bowel Elimination		Kidney Function
	Caregiver Emotional Health		Medication Response
	Comfort Status: Physical		Neurological Status
	Comfort Status: Psychospiritual		Neurological Status: Autonomic
	Comfortable Death		Neurological Status: Central Motor Control
	Endurance		Neurological Status: Consciousness
	Family Health Status		Neurological Status: Cranial Sensory/Motor Function
	Fatigue Level		Neurological Status: Peripheral
	Fluid Balance		Neurological Status: Spinal Sensory/Motor Function
	Gastrointestinal Function		Oral Hygiene
	Hemodialysis Access		
	Hydration		

b and n	*Severe deviation from normal range*	*Substantial deviation from normal range*	*Moderate deviation from normal range*
	Severe	*Substantial*	*Moderate*
	Blood Coagulation		Post-Procedure Recovery
	Cardiac Pump Effectiveness		Respiratory Status
	Cardiopulmonary Status		Respiratory Status: Airway Patency
	Circulation Status		Respiratory Status: Gas Exchange
	Electrolyte & Acid/Base Balance		Respiratory Status: Ventilation
	Maternal Status: Antepartum		Sensory Function: Cutaneous
	Maternal Status: Intrapartum		Sensory Function: Hearing
	Maternal Status: Postpartum		Sensory Function: Proprioception
	Mechanical Ventilation Response: Adult		Sensory Function: Taste & Smell
	Mechanical Ventilation Weaning Response: Adult		

i and h	*None*	*Limited*	*Moderate*
	Extensive	*Substantial*	*Moderate*
	Abuse Recovery: Emotional		Burn Healing
	Abuse Recovery: Sexual		Burn Recovery
	Bone Healing		Neglect Recovery

m and t	*Never demonstrated*	*Rarely demonstrated*	*Sometimes demonstrated*
	Consistently demonstrated	*Often demonstrated*	*Sometimes demonstrated*
	Asthma Self-Management		Development: Middle Adulthood
	Bowel Continence		Development: Young Adulthood
	Child Adaptation to Hospitalization		Discharge Readiness: Independent Living
	Development: Late Adulthood		Mood Equilibrium

Mildly compromised	*Not compromised*
Mild	*None*
Sleep	
Student Health Status	
Swallowing Status	
Swallowing Status: Esophageal Phase	
Swallowing Status: Oral Phase	
Swallowing Status: Pharyngeal Phase	
Thermoregulation	
Thermoregulation: Newborn	
Tissue Integrity: Skin & Mucous Membranes	
Urinary Elimination	
Will to Live	
	N=35

Mild deviation from normal range	*No deviation from normal range*
Mild	*None*
Sensory Function: Vision	
Systemic Toxin Clearance: Dialysis	
Tissue Perfusion: Abdominal Organs	
Tissue Perfusion: Cardiac	
Tissue Perfusion: Cellular	
Tissue Perfusion: Cerebral	
Tissue Perfusion: Peripheral	
Tissue Perfusion: Pulmonary	
	N=27

Substantial	*Extensive*
Limited	*None*
Wound Healing: Primary Intention	
Wound Healing: Secondary Intention	
	N=8

Often demonstrated	*Consistently demonstrated*
Rarely demonstrated	*Never demonstrated*
Psychomotor Energy	
Safe Wandering	
Urinary Continence	
	N=11

Continued

Table 2-4	COMBINATION MEASUREMENT SCALES USED IN NOC—cont'd	

n *and* *a*	*Severe*	*Substantial*	*Moderate*
	Severely compromised	*Substantially compromised*	*Moderately compromised*
	Caregiver Lifestyle Disruption Immobility Consequences: Physiological		Immobility Consequences: Psycho-Cognitive Immune Hypersensitivity Response

n *and* *b*	*Severe*	*Substantial*	*Moderate*
	Severe deviation from normal range	*Substantial deviation from normal range*	*Moderate deviation from normal range*
	Pain Level		

ent, the nurses can create an outcome for each fracture and measure the outcome separately. The second diagram added is a diagram of the body divided into sites for use with the two wound outcomes: Wound Healing: Primary Intention and Wound Healing: Secondary Intention. Again the outcome provides a means to specify the site and follow more than one wound by identifying separate outcomes for each site. In several places the opportunity to specify exact data about an outcome has been added. For example, in the outcome Blood Loss Severity, the estimated blood loss can be included in the outcome.

The final addition to the original format is documentation at the end of each outcome as to when the outcome was first published in the classification and the edition(s) in which revisions were made. Documenting the history of each outcome is important ongoing work. We believe the inclusion of this information will help in our efforts to maintain a very current classification of nursing-sensitive patient outcomes.

Refinement of the Classification: Ongoing and Future Development

The current classification represents the completion of over 16 years of research to develop and test a classification and taxonomy of nursing-sensitive patient outcomes. The classification contains 385 outcomes designed for measuring the impact of nursing treatments on individual, caregiver, family, and community outcomes. The outcomes are classified in the NOC taxonomy under 7 domains and 31 classes with only new outcomes being added for this edition. This structure has served us well. The name and definition for the class Nutrition was altered slightly to better fit the outcomes in this section. The class name is now called Digestion and Nutrition to better align the outcomes within this class. In the last edition, NOC was also placed in the Taxonomy of Nursing Practice and we anticipate further refinement of this work for combining NANDA, NIC and NOC in the future. This edition includes linkages to NANDA diagnoses and Gordon's health patterns and can be found in Part Four.

Outcomes for individual patients are identified for development by members of the team, educators, and practicing nurses. We maintain a potential list of concepts on a list "for future development." A concept analysis is used to develop and evaluate the outcomes to be added to the NOC. As the classification grows, each new outcome must be evaluated to see how it "fits" with the current outcomes in the classification. Sometimes this involves the modification of an existing outcome or outcomes, or the new outcome may focus on a different age group or patient population. This work is ongoing, and continual updating of the classification is needed to keep it relevant for clinical practice. This is crucial to having valid and reliable standardized language for outcome measurement in

Mild	*None*
Mildly compromised	*Not compromised*

Pain: Disruptive Effects

N=5

Mild	*None*
Mild deviation from normal range	*No deviation from normal range*

N=1

nursing. Since the publication of the last edition, several outcomes have been submitted from students, educators, and practicing nurses. These submissions are very helpful to the development of the classification. We recognize contributors to this work in the front of the book. We need experts from a variety of specialties to work with us to maintain and improve this classification.

Additional efforts are needed to develop and validate family and community outcomes. We especially need experts to help in these two areas. A new community outcome, Community Disaster Response, is included in this edition. Domains and classes for family and community outcomes were added to the NOC taxonomy in the second edition. More family and community outcomes need to be developed to make these areas complete. Input from specialty organizations is also helpful in these areas.

New Features and Revisions for This Edition

We have been approached by a variety of individuals advocating that we standardize the indicator level of NOC. This suggestion comes primarily from nurses and others focusing on language for an electronic health record. Leading this charge, of course, are nurses interested in informatics. The investigators for NOC have conducted extensive reviews of the outcomes published in the third edition, including their respective definitions and indicators. We believed it was crucial to increase the standardization and eliminate as much redundancy as possible in the elements of NOC. At first this was an overwhelming thought because we knew we had over 5000 indicators and had little sense of how many of these were unique. After much discussion and consultation, we decided that we would start this process with this edition. One approach we used was to look at indicators by scale and make an attempt to word indicators that were similar in the same way. Our process was to print all indicators for a scale with the code and outcome they were attached to. For each scale this averaged 5 to 10 pages of indicators to examine. Most of the modifications to indicators were not significant and involved standardization of terms. For instance, we selected the term *strategies* over *techniques* or *methods*, so indicators that included the term *techniques* were rewritten using the word *strategies*. An example would be that the indicator "measures to minimize disease progression" became "strategies to minimize disease progression." We also did searches based on key words such as *demonstrates, communicates, service, drug, medication,* and *pain*.

Another approach we used was to identify the words used as verbs, the total count of unique verbs used, and the selected outcomes that use the respective verbs. We concluded that with this background, when new outcomes were developed, the team could use existing verbs within the classification as opposed to introducing "new" verbs or synonyms of the existing verbs. This process involved only the scales that have indicators that start with verbs—for example, the scale "never demonstrated." To arrive at the number of verbs used within the outcomes, one of the investigators reviewed all of the indicators of the outcomes published in the third edition. Each indicator was reviewed and the verb used to introduce the respective indicator was identified and recorded. The final count of the verbs was arrived at by recording each unique verb within the list of indicators for each outcome. For example, if the verb *acknowledges* introduces three indicators of Risk Control: Unintended Pregnancy, the verb count for that outcome is one, the same as if the word *acknowledges* was used once. In addition to recording the verbs, the investigator recorded the outcome label using the verb within at least one indicator. As the process proceeded, all of the outcomes and the respective indicators were reviewed. The review yielded the use of 256 unique verbs used in the indicators of the 330 outcomes.

Overall, 19 verbs were used in 10 or more outcomes. The specific breakdown showed that 9 verbs were used at least once in 10-19 outcomes; 6 verbs were used at least once in 20-29 outcomes; 2 verbs were used at least once in 30-39 outcomes; 1 verb was used at least once in more than 50 outcomes; and 1 verb was used at least once in more than 60 outcomes. The remaining verbs were used at least once in 1-8 of the outcomes. Examples of the verbs used most frequently in the outcomes were: *Uses* (68); *Maintains* (54); *Seeks* (33); *Monitors* (32); *Participates* (24); *Recognizes* (23); *Identifies* (22); *Performs* (19); *Describes* (19); and *Follows* (19). As revisions to the indicators were made, this verb list was refined and used in our attempts at standardizing the indicators. Further work needs to be done on this project for future editions. This process expanded the terms defined in this chapter in Box 2-1.

This review process also prompted a revision in the measurement scale used with the Knowledge outcomes. As we reviewed the indicators for these outcomes, we decided that the lead phrase "description of" could be eliminated if we changed the scale anchors to "No Knowledge" to "Extensive Knowledge." This shortened the indicator phrase and resulted in only slight modifications of the indicators overall. We believe this is an important change for these outcomes and allows for easier standardization in the future. The content of these indicators clearly becomes the focus of the knowledge outcomes with this revision. This is an area of the classification that continues to grow, reinforcing the importance of teaching as a nursing intervention. We believe the knowledge outcomes focused on helping an individual provide his or her own care related to a disease condition will be important as more patients face chronic illness as they age.

Another change we made for this edition was a greater use of the scale "Deviation from normal range." We have used this scale with the outcome Vital Signs in the past but had not used it with the indicators related to vitals signs in other outcomes. Many times the compromised scale was used to measure indicators related to radial pulse, apical heart rate, blood pressure, or respiratory rate. We attempted to solve this issue in as many outcomes as possible that had these types of indicators. In addition, many of these outcomes also had laboratory or test results that were well suited for the deviation scale. We will continue to work in this manner to further standardize the indicators in future editions.

The steps we have taken to increase the standardization of terms and indicators are only the beginning of this process. The next steps will be to develop a coding system that will standardize the outcome indicators across the outcomes. At the present time the outcome indicators are coded based on the outcome they are within, so although we have standardized many of the indicators, they have multiple codes associated with the same indicator. This next step will probably require a major recoding of our classification. We will continue to work toward this goal, but it was beyond the scope of the work we could accomplish for this edition. We will continue to work with nurses in informatics and vendors using NOC to make revisions of our coding system that address the requirements for an electronic health record.

SUMMARY

This chapter provided an overview of the current outcomes classification and changes made to this edition based on our current work. Fifty-eight new outcomes were added to this edition. Common questions about NOC were posed and answered. Current and future work of the NOC team was reviewed, emphasizing the revisions that are needed for using NOC in an electronic health record. A classification of nursing-sensitive patient, family, and community outcomes will never be complete but will continue to expand and improve with further knowledge of the discipline and testing in practice. Readers and users of the classification are encouraged to provide feedback to the research team. Identification of problems, issues, and outcomes for future development also is encouraged. Appendix B contains a review form that can be completed and returned to the team. We encourage feedback from nurses using NOC.

Although there is increasing interest in outcomes management, quality assessment and improvement, and effectiveness research, nursing remains largely invisible in large data sets and little nursing effectiveness research is being conducted. Those nursing studies completed often are done in a single health care system, and most are not reported. The use of NOC provides data so that contributions made by the nursing profession to health care are documented and made visible. The health care organizations that adopt NOC will be able not only to demonstrate nursing's accountability and contributions to health care but also to compare the achievement of outcomes of care across time and settings. Use of NOC over the last 14 years has demonstrated that nurses can make dramatic improvements in outcomes in a short period of time. With shorter lengths of stay in acute care institutions, it is critical that we learn how to best use our time so that the interventions we choose are effective in improving outcomes. We also need to learn what interventions are ineffective or poorly timed in our current practice strategies. We need to learn more about what outcomes are core to nursing practice and identify key outcomes for specialty practice. This will benefit both education and practice. We also need to see that organizations beyond acute care hospitals use outcomes in evaluating the care provided. The ability to evaluate NOC outcomes across settings is one of its strengths.

Classification work of this kind is essential to our future as a profession. We invite all nurses to join in the effort to include standardized nursing languages in all clinical information systems so that nursing data will be available in large local, national, and international data sets. We also invite our colleagues to assist with further testing of the psychometric integrity and clinical usefulness of the NOC outcomes. Research by nurse scientists, clinicians, and graduate students that is published and shared with the NOC research team will greatly advance this work that is so important for the nursing profession and the clients that nurses serve. Armed with data that demonstrate nursing effectiveness, nurses will influence health policy to optimally benefit the individuals, families, and communities to whom they provide care.

References

1. American Nurses Association. (1986). *Standards of community health nursing practice*. Kansas City, MO: Author.
2. Bond, S., & Thomas, L. H. (1991). Issues in measuring outcomes on nursing. *Journal of Advanced Nursing, 16*, 1492-1502.
3. Erben, R., Franzkowiak, P., & Wenzel, E. (1992). Assessment of the outcomes of health intervention. *Social Science Medicine, 35*(4), 359-365.
4. Grobe, S. J. (1990). Nursing intervention lexicon and taxonomy study; language and classification methods. *Advances in Nursing Science, 13*(2), 22-33.
5. Hegyvary, S. T. (1991). Issues in outcomes research. *Journal of Nursing Quality Assurance, 5*(2), 1-6.
6. Iowa Intervention Project. (2004). Nursing Interventions Classification (NIC). (4th ed.). St. Louis: Mosby.
7. Johnson, M., Bulechek, G., Butcher, H., Maas, M., McCloskey Dochterman, J., Moorhead, S., & Swanson, L. (2006). *NANDA, NOC, and NIC linkages: Nursing diagnoses, outcomes and interventions*. St. Louis: Mosby.

8. Kuss, T., Proulx-Girouard, L., Lovitt, S., Katz, C. B., & Kennelly, P. (1997). A public health nursing model. *Public Health Nursing, 14*(2), 81-91.

9. Lang, N. M., & Clinton, J. F. (1984). Assessment of quality of nursing care. In H. H. Werley & J. J. Fitzpatrick (Eds.), *Annual Review of Nursing Research* (Vol. 2, 135-163). New York: Springer.

10. Lohr, K. (1988). Outcome measurement: Concepts and questions. *Inquiry, 25*(1), 37-50.

11. Marek, K. D. (1997). Measuring the effectiveness of nursing care. *Journal of Nursing Outcomes Management, 1*(1), 8-11.

12. Marek, K. D. (1989). Outcome measurement in nursing. *Journal of Nursing Quality Assurance, 4*(1), 1-9.

13. McCloskey, J. C., & Bulechek, G. M. (1994). Standardizing the language for nursing treatments: An overview of the issues. *Nursing Outlook, 42*(2), 56-63.

14. Nadzam, D. M. (1991). The agenda for change: Update on indicator development and possible implications for the nursing profession. *Journal of Nursing Quality Assurance, 5*(2), 18-22.

15. NANDA International. (2007). *Nursing diagnoses: Definitions & classification, 2007-2008.* Philadelphia: Author.

16. Pesut, D. J., & Herman, J. (1999). Clinical reasoning: The art & science of critical & creative thinking. Albany, NY: Delmar Publishers.

17. Rantz, M. J., & LeMone, P. (Eds.). (1995). Classification of nursing diagnoses: Proceedings of the eleventh conference of the North American Nursing Diagnosis Association.

18. Saba, V. K. (1992). The classification of home health care nursing diagnoses and interventions. *Caring, 11*(3), 50-57.

19. Stanhope, M. (2006). *Foundations of Nursing in the Community* (2nd ed.). St. Louis: Mosby.

20. Tarlov, A. R., Ware, J. E., Greenfield, S. Nelson, E. C., Perren, E., & Zubkoff, M. (1989). The Medical Outcomes Study: An application of methods for monitoring the results of medical care. *Journal of the American Medical Assoication, 262,* 925-930.

21. Werley, H. H., & Lang, N. M. (Eds.) (1988). *Identification of the Nursing Minimum Data Set.* New York: Springer.

22. Werley, H. H., & Devine, E. C. (1987). The Nursing Minimum Data Set: Status and implications (pp. 540-551). In K. J. Hanna, M. Reimer, W. C. Mills, & S. Letourneau (Eds.), *Clinical judgment and decision-making: The future of nursing diagnosis.* New York: John Wiley.

CHAPTER THREE

Using NOC in Clinical Settings

Evaluating the effectiveness of nursing care requires indicators of patient status that can measure both short-term changes following an intervention or episode of care and long-term changes over the course of a chronic illness. The Nursing Outcomes Classification (NOC) was developed to measure just such changes in patient status. Although developed for nursing, other health professionals have found the outcomes useful for evaluating effectiveness of their interventions. The authors encourage the use of the classification by others and encourage other disciplines to contribute indicators specific to their practice. The outcomes are used to measure patient, family or community status in the domains and classes identified in the taxonomy in Part Two. Measurement is not limited to functional and physiological status but includes measures of psychosocial, knowledge, and behavioral status. NOC includes outcomes for an individual patient, a caregiver in the home setting, a family, or a community. This chapter will discuss the selection and use of NOC outcomes in clinical practice. Although written from a nursing perspective, the application process can be used by other disciplines.

SELECTING THE OUTCOME

Selecting patient outcomes for a particular patient or a group of patients is one step in the nurse's clinical decision-making process. The use of standard terms and measures to evaluate outcomes does not decrease in any way the responsibility of the nurse to make an informed assessment and engage in clinical reasoning to identify patient diagnoses/problems, potential outcomes, and interventions to move the patient toward desired outcomes. Outcomes, such as those in the NOC, are selected in much the same manner as an outcome goal. The first judgment the nurse makes is to determine the pertinent health concerns, nursing diagnoses, patient resources, and patient capacities for recovery associated with the patient's presenting condition. This judgment is generally based on a patient assessment that includes both data collection and data analysis. A variety of resources outline the steps and data sources used in the assessment process.[20,21,23] Once the health concerns and/or diagnoses have been identified, the nurse is ready to consider the selection of patient outcomes. A number of factors are considered when selecting an outcome, including (1) the type of health concern; (2) the nursing or medical diagnoses and health problems; (3) patient characteristics; (4) patient resources; (5) patient preferences; (6) patient capacities[1]; and (7) treatment potential.[7]

Type of Health Problem

Health concerns can be categorized as (1) problems for referral that are issues addressed primarily by other health providers; (2) interdisciplinary problems that are issues addressed collaboratively with other providers; and (3) nursing diagnoses that are issues for which the nurse has primary responsibility.[23] If the health concern falls in the first category, the primary responsibility for identifying the desired outcome will usually reside with the responsible health provider. Examples of these concerns may be financial concerns referred to a social worker or spiritual concerns referred to a spiritual advisor. However, associated problems, such as anxiety or depression, may accompany these concerns and require the nurse to work collaboratively with the primary health provider when considering outcomes. If the health concern falls in category two, the nurse and other responsible providers should work together with the patient to identify the outcome. This frequently occurs when the nurse and physical therapist or nurse and dietician collaborate about the outcomes that may be achieved in relation to a rehabilitation program or instructions about a new diet. If the health concern is a nursing diagnosis, the nurse should assume primary responsibility for identifying patient outcomes related to the diagnosis.

Diagnosis or Health Problem

A diagnosis is a judgment based on an assessment and analysis of the patient status. It might be a nursing diagnosis, a medical diagnosis, or a diagnosis made by another health care practitioner. Although all health-related diagnoses are considered when the nurse selects an outcome, many of the outcomes of concern to nurses arise out of a nursing diagnosis. The nursing diagnosis might be related to a medical diagnosis or may represent a patient health problem that is independent of other diagnoses. The common standardized language for nursing diagnoses is that of the NANDA International (NANDA-I).[19] They define a nursing diagnosis as a "Clinical judgment about individual, family, or community responses to actual or potential health problems/life processes" (p. 332)[19] that forms the basis for selecting nursing interventions to achieve patient outcomes. Four types of nursing diagnoses are identified: actual, risk, health-promotion, and wellness. The diagnosis consists of a label, a definition, the defining characteristics, and related factors if an actual diagnosis. A risk diagnosis includes the label, definition, and risk factors. The health-promoting and wellness diagnoses include the label, definition, and defining characteristics. Defining characteristics are the cues that cluster together and characterize the diagnosis. Related factors are associated with the diagnosis as antecedent, contributing, or associated factors.[19]

When selecting an outcome for a patient, consideration should be given to the definition, defining characteristics, and related factors or to the risk factors for a risk diagnosis. Activity Intolerance is defined as "Insufficient physiological or psychological energy to endure or complete required or desired daily activities" (p. 3).[19] Based on this definition, the nurse might select Activity Tolerance, Endurance, Psychomotor Energy, or Self-Care Status as an outcome pertinent to the definition. In the NOC outcomes, Activity Tolerance and Endurance are related to insufficient physiological energy, while Psychomotor Energy is related to insufficient psychological energy. The outcome Self-Care Status may be selected when the nurse is more interested in the patient's ability to carry out required activities of daily living. When considering defining characteristics, such as blood pressure, cardiac response to activity, dyspnea, fatigue, and weakness, outcomes such as Vital Signs or Cardiopulmonary Status might be selected as intermediate outcomes that need improvement if the patient is to increase his or her activity tolerance. If a medical diagnosis is used as a basis for selecting an outcome, the signs and symptoms of the diagnosis, as well as the causative and other related factors, should be considered when choosing the outcome. For example, pulmonary edema may be a symptom of the medical diagnosis Congestive Heart Failure and may suggest the selection of Cardiac Pump Effectiveness, Fluid Overload Severity, or Respiratory Status as outcomes.

Based on the definition of the diagnosis Risk for Activity Intolerance (which is the same as Activity Intolerance but preceded by "at risk for developing"), the outcomes selected for the diagnosis Activity Intolerance can be chosen since that is the problem to be prevented. The risk factors will suggest other possible outcomes, such as Cardiac Pump Effectiveness; Knowledge: Prescribed Activity; Physical Fitness; Respiratory Status: Ventilation; Tissue Perfusion: Cardiac; and Tissue Perfusion: Pulmonary. The fact that more than one outcome may be appropriate for a specific nursing diagnosis supports the clinical decision-making process. Each time the nurse selects an outcome for an individual patient, the nurse is making a clinical judgment based on the factors identified previously and discussed in following sections in greater detail.

Outcomes are frequently associated with both a medical and nursing diagnosis. For example, if the medical diagnosis is Diabetes Mellitus, blood glucose control is a specific outcome for which the nurse may select the NOC outcome Blood Glucose Level. Two other outcomes specific to this medical diagnosis and associated with the nursing diagnoses of

Deficient Knowledge and Ineffective or Effective Therapeutic Regimen Management are Diabetes Self-Management and Knowledge: Diabetes Management. Outcomes selected for standardized nursing care plans or critical paths are those pertinent to the medical or nursing diagnoses or those commonly associated with other health problems accompanying the illness. Part Four contains a list of outcomes commonly associated with each NANDA nursing diagnosis based primarily on expert opinion. Data collected during the evaluation of the outcomes in clinical sites were used when available. Further data collection and analysis are needed to substantiate the associations presented in Part Four and to answer questions about the relationship between diagnoses and outcomes. Are some outcomes selected more frequently for particular nursing diagnoses? Do the outcomes selected for a particular nursing diagnosis vary depending on the site of care, for example, in critical care, home care, or long-term care? Do the outcomes selected for a particular nursing diagnosis vary with patient age, gender, education, or social and economic status? This type of information will be invaluable in designing critical care paths for patient populations as well as in assisting beginning practitioners to make informed judgments about the selection of appropriate patient outcomes.

Patient Characteristics

Patient characteristics affect outcome selection and the amount of improvement a patient can achieve; for this reason, patient characteristics may be referred to as risk adjustment factors. Personal characteristics to be considered include demographic factors, psychological/cognitive factors, illness- and health-related factors, and personal health beliefs or values that influence personal preferences. *Demographic factors,* such as *age* and *gender,* may play an important role in the selection of outcomes. Some NOC outcomes, such as the child and adult development outcomes, are specific for certain ages, while others, such as Cardiac Disease Self-Management, are not appropriate for children. Age might also affect the level of outcome achievement possible. For example, improving Physical Fitness may become more difficult as one ages if one has not been active, and Thermoregulation: newborn may be more difficult to achieve in a low-birthweight neonate. A number of outcomes, such as Maternal Status: Postpartum and Breastfeeding Establishment: Maternal, are obviously for females of childbearing age, while the physical maturation outcomes are written for females or males. *Race* and *ethnicity* can provide information important for considering predisposition to and response to illness as well as indicate cultural beliefs that may affect the acceptance of outcomes by the patient or family. *Education level* is easy to collect and quantify and can act as a proxy for reading level, an important consideration in selecting outcomes related to knowledge and participation in health care.

Psychological and cognitive variables can include emotional states such as depression or anxiety and processes such as concentration, memory, information processing, and decision-making. These factors influence the patient's response to illness, ability to learn, and motivation and therefore need to be considered when selecting outcomes for a particular patient. Knowledge outcomes will not be selected for the patient who has no short-term memory or cannot process information while Anxiety Self-Control may be the most important outcome for the severely anxious patient. NOC has a number of outcomes that can be used to evaluate changes in psychological and cognitive function over time.

Illness and health-related variables such as *initial severity of illness* have a strong influence on outcome selection and outcome achievement. Nursing uses a number of patient acuity measures as well as resource use measures to capture severity of illness. Illness severity may dictate the elimination or inclusion of outcomes. For example, Mobility is generally not selected for a patient in a critical care unit and Comfortable Death would be quite appropriate for a terminally ill patient. *Functional status* and ability to perform activities of daily living will also influence outcome selection. While ambulation is not an appropriate outcome for the quadriplegic patient, Transfer Performance may be important and Self-Direction of Care may be appropriate if the patient is mentally alert but unable to carry out physical self-care activities. Functional status can also affect outcome selection and/or achievement for patients with chronic conditions, such as rheumatoid arthritis. Consideration must be given to limitations posed by the condition when the patient enters an acute care setting.

Available Resources

All supportive resources that influence patient recovery and patient outcomes need to be considered. These can be financial, social, family, and health resources that influence lifestyle, living conditions, and access to health care. They need to be considered because they can influence outcome achievement negatively or positively and, in some cases, limit outcomes that can be considered. For example, improvement in Compliance Behavior or Diabetes Self-Management is not likely to occur if the patient does not have the financial resources to purchase the medications, equipment, or food required to manage the disease. *Social factors* include social support, social relationships, and the availability of someone to assist the patient as needed. Loneliness Severity or Caregiver Performance: Direct Care may become important outcomes if social support is absent or if a caregiver needs to learn multiple procedures and activities to provide care in the home.

Patient Preferences

Including the patient and/or family in the decision-making process when selecting outcomes will ensure that patient preferences are considered. Preferences will be influenced by the patient's personal perceptions about health, desired health goals, treatment options, religious beliefs, and cultural beliefs. Each of these factors can affect which outcomes the patient or family find acceptable. If patients believe their health is satisfactory, they may be less inclined to accept outcomes aimed at measuring improvements in overall health, such as Physical Fitness. If patients are unable to accept emotional or psychological diagnoses because of their religious or cultural beliefs, they are not likely to find outcomes such as Mood Equilibrium or Depression Level acceptable. In addition to collaborating in selecting the outcome, patients should participate in determining where they want to be on the outcome scale, that is, how much change they want to accomplish. It may become important for the nurse to assist the patient in accepting a realistic outcome. An example would be a patient with pulmonary emphysema who wants to achieve a 5 (not compromised) on the outcome Respiratory Status: Ventilation when that is physiologically impossible.

Treatment Potential

The availability of interventions and the potential for them to be delivered should be considered when selecting an outcome. A first step is to determine whether an intervention is available to achieve an outcome for a particular patient. If the diagnosis for a patient is Chronic Confusion secondary to Alzheimer's disease, nursing interventions may be able to assist the patient to maintain his or her current cognitive status for a period of time, but with current interventions eventual decline in cognition can be expected. In such a case, the nurse would be unlikely to select Cognition or Cognitive Orientation as outcomes for which improvement is projected, and as cognition declines, other outcomes related to nutrition, safety, and hygiene may become more important. Likewise, if a patient has the diagnosis of Total Urinary Incontinence secondary to quadriplegia, treatments are not currently available to meet the outcome Urinary Continence, but maintaining a patient at a 5 (none) rating on Infection Severity or 5 (not compromised) rating on Tissue Integrity: Skin and Mucous Membranes may be the important outcomes. A second factor to consider is whether the nursing personnel required to carry out an intervention are available. If teaching a patient or family and evaluating their knowledge requires a professional nurse, then a nurse with the appropriate skills must be available to provide these services if a knowledge outcome is selected. The *Nursing Interventions Classification (NIC)*[4] includes nursing interventions and recommendations for the level of nursing personnel to provide the intervention.

Aids When Selecting Outcomes

There are a number of aids available that can assist in selecting outcomes for the individual patient, patient group, or standardized care plan or when teaching staff about the use of the classification and outcomes. One aid is a list of NOC outcomes with behaviors corresponding to the knowledge outcomes in NOC. This list (Table 4-1) can be helpful in identifying NOC outcomes to assess the effect of knowledge on the desired behavior. The book *NANDA, NOC, and NIC Linkages*[8] provides suggested links among the three languages. Other publications that can be helpful are found in Box 3-1. A number of these have been prepared by the authors of NIC and NOC or by users of the

---

Box 3-1

Publications for Use When Implementing NOC

Behrenbeck, J. G., Timm, J. A., Griebenow, L. K., & Demmer, K. A. (2005). Nursing-sensitive outcome reliability testing in a tertiary care setting. *International Journal of Nursing Terminologies and Classifications, 16*(1), 14-20.

Burkhart, L., & Solari-Twadell, A. (2002). *Integration: A documentation system reporting whole person care.* St. Louis: International Parish Nurse Resource Center, Deaconess Foundation. (www.parish-nurses.org)

Carlson, J. (2006). Consensus validation process: A standardized research method to identify and link the relevant NANDA, NIC, and NOC terms for local populations. *International Journal of Nursing Terminologies and Classifications, 17*(1), 23-24.

Cavendish, R. (2003). School nurses use of NANDA, NIC, and NOC to describe children's abdominal pain. *International Journal of Nursing Terminologies and Classifications, 14*(4), 17-18.

Center for Nursing Classification. (2000). *NIC interventions and NOC outcomes linked to the Oasis information set.* Iowa City, IA: Author.

Cox, R. A. (2001). *Standardized nursing language in long-term care.* Iowa City, IA: Center for Nursing Classification.

Denehy, J., & Poulton, S. (1999). The use of standardized language in individualized healthcare plans. *The Journal of School Nursing, 15*(1), 38-45.

Hayewski, C., Maupin, J., Rapp, D., Sitterding, M., & Pappas, J. (1998). Implementation of nursing intervention classification and nursing outcomes classification in a patient education plan. *Journal of Nursing Care Quality, 12*(5), 30-40.

Iowa Outcomes Project. (2005). *NOC Use Survey.* Iowa City, IA: The University of Iowa, College of Nursing, Center for Nursing Classification & Clinical Effectiveness.

Johnson, M., Bulechek, G., Butcher, H., Dochterman, J. M., Maas, M., Moorhead, S., & Swanson, E. (2006). *NANDA, NOC, and NIC Linkages* (2nd ed). St. Louis: Mosby.

Lunney, M. (2006). Helping nurses use NANDA, NOC, and NIC. *Journal of Nursing Administration, 36*(3), 118-125.

Moorhead, S., Clarke, M., Willits, M., & Tomsha, K. (1998). Nursing outcomes classification implementation projects across the care continuum. *Journal of Nursing Care Quality, 12*(5), 52-63.

Parris, K. M., Place, P. J., Orellana, E., Calder, J., Jackson, K., Karolys, A., Meza, M., Middough, C., Nguyen, V., Shim, N. W., & Smith, D. (1999). Integrating nursing diagnoses, interventions, and outcomes in public health nursing practice. *The Journal of Nursing Language and Classification, 10*(2), 49-56.

Scherb, C. A. (2002). Outcomes research: Making a difference. *Outcomes Management, 6*(1), 22-26.

Stone, P. W., Lee, N., Giannini, M., & Bakken, S. (2004). Economic evaluations and usefulness of standardized nursing terminologies. *International Journal of Nursing Terminologies and Classifications, 15*(4), 101-113.

Titler, M., Dochterman, J., & Reed, D. (2004). *Guideline for conducting effectiveness research in nursing and other healthcare services.* Iowa City, IA: The University of Iowa, College of Nursing, Center for Nursing Classification & Clinical Effectiveness.

Von Krogh, G., Dale, C., & Naden, D. (2005). Framework for integrating NANDA, NIC, and NOC terminology in electronic patient records. *Journal of Nursing Scholarship, 37*(3), 275-281.

In addition to the above articles, the reader might want to review the abstracts from the NANDA, NIC, and NOC conference: Electronic Use of Clinical Nursing Data published in the *International Journal of Nursing Terminologies and Classifications*, January-March 2006, *17*(1).

classification and are available through the Center for Nursing Classification and Clinical Effectiveness (Center) at The University of Iowa. Further information about the center can be found on The University of Iowa, College of Nursing website at **www.nursing.uiowa.edu/cnc**.

COMPLETING THE OUTCOME

Once the outcomes for a patient or patient group are selected, information about the outcome is completed. The outcome label, the outcome definition, and the measurement scales are standardized components of the outcome, meaning the terms for these elements should not change. Although minor changes can be made in the indicators, the indicator concept must remain the same if the indicators are rated and the information kept for further analysis. Two items are provided to retain data that are related to but not part of the outcome; they provide information valuable for analysis. The *Care Recipient* can be the patient, caregiver, parent family, or community. The *Data Source* can be the patient, a family member, a caregiver, direct observation by a health care provider, or the clinical record. Providers may wish to identify additional care recipients or data sources or make the list more specific by identifying the type of health care provider. The other pieces of information to be completed include the current patient rating on the outcome scale and the projected outcome target rating. The indicators may assist the nurse and the patient in making accurate judgments about these two items.

Using the Outcome Indicators

Indicators can be considered more specific measures useful for determining the broader concept measured at the outcome level. The indicators are stated as briefly as possible to facilitate their use. To facilitate electronic versions and future data analysis, indicators have been revised and stated in the same way as much as possible. This has not affected the major concept or focus of the indicator but has standardized how the indicator is stated. Abbreviations are generally not used in the indicator statements but can be used in a facility if there is general agreement on the meaning of the abbreviation. While the language of the indicators should remain standardized as much as possible, practitioners may wish to add some indicators that are pertinent to a specialized area of practice or make the indicators more specific. For example, normal ranges for diagnostic tests or blood pressure can be substituted for the terms in the outcome. Practitioners may also wish to delete indicators that aren't pertinent to an individual patient or patient group with a particular diagnosis.

After selecting the outcomes for an individual patient or for a standardized care plan, the nurse selects the indicators that will be used to determine patient status as reflected in the outcome rating on the measurement scale. In general, the staff should agree on the indicators to be used for the most frequently selected outcomes for their patient population. Some users have found they can limit the indicators for each outcome to four or five, while other users wish to select more indicators. Areas for further study are determining which indicators are most important for an outcome when selected for various patient populations as well as determining whether some of the indicators should carry more weight than others. This will eventually be accomplished if users share this information with others, either through the list-serve managed by the Center, through publications and conferences, or by sharing with the authors so future editions can reflect how the indicators are being used in practice settings.

Rating the status of an individual patient on the selected indicators can assist the nurse to determine the patient's overall rating for the outcome. **As discussed previously, the norm against which the patient is evaluated is that of a healthy individual of approximately the same age and gender (reference person).** If an indicator selected for the patient population is not applicable to a particular patient, the NA column can be checked. A computerized form could include both NA and not known (NK) if desired. Recording the indicators the nurse finds NA will provide data to determine whether some indicators are not pertinent for certain populations or whether they could be eliminated entirely. As the nurse becomes familiar with the selected indicators, it may not be necessary to rate patient status on each indicator since the nurse will automatically consider the indicators when determining the patient's outcome rating. However, it must be recognized that data valuable for determining the indicators most predictive of patient status will be lost when indicator ratings are not retained.

The source of data for the indicators and the outcome will vary. Data may be obtained from the patient record (e.g., biochemical measures or vital signs) or from direct observation or physical assessments (e.g., how well a patient can carry out treatments or if certain signs and symptoms are present). Other indicators may require soliciting information or perceptions from the patient or family (e.g., knowledge about the disease process or treatment, perceptions of health, and satisfaction with care). As noted earlier, the outcome format has a space to record the data source. If the outcomes are entered in a computerized database, the organization can provide codes for each of the sources likely to be used in that organization.

The indicators are less abstract than the outcome and may at times serve as intermediate outcomes in a standardized care plan. Indicators to be used in this way can be selected by the task force as they determine which outcomes are used frequently for the patient population served. If an indicator is considered an important measure of patient progress, nurses may choose to aggregate data on a particular indicator as well as on the outcome. This may be particularly true for patients with short episodes of care in which progress in relation to the outcome may not be evident, but progress in relation to significant indicators may be achieved.

Using the Measurement Scales

The current classification contains 14 measurement scales, which are illustrated in Chapter 2. Measurement scales are provided for both the outcome and the indicators. Each scale is constructed so that the fifth, or end, point reflects the most desirable patient condition relative to the outcome. The nurse can make a judgment about the outcome rating for a patient or patient population without using the indicators; however, most nurses find one or more of the indicators helpful for judging the patient rating on the outcome scale.

Although indicator ratings will assist in determining the patient's rating on the outcome scale, they currently are not weighted to provide a mean or summated rating. It is recommended that the practitioner use both the range and the frequency of patient ratings on the indicator scale as an aid in arriving at the overall outcome rating. In general, low ratings of 1 and 2 on important indicators will mean that the patient has a 1 or 2 rating on the outcome scale. For example, in the outcome Activity Tolerance, equally distributed ratings of 1s and 2s on the indicators would suggest that Activity Tolerance should be rated as "severely compromised" since a number of the indicators are rated as severely compromised. However, if the indicator ratings range from "severely compromised" for ability to speak with physical activity to "mildly compromised" and "not compromised" for the remainder of the indicators, the nurse will want to determine (1) whether the rating is correct and (2) the degree to which this is an indicator of compromised activity tolerance. (Does this occur only with intense activity or with minimal activity?) If the patient has always had difficulty speaking with activity or is having difficulty only with intense activity, the nurse may rate the patient as "mildly compromised" on the outcome. If this is a new symptom and occurs with minimal activity, the nurse may adjust the rating to "moderately compromised" or elect to follow patient ratings for the indicator *ability to speak with physical activity* as well as for the outcome Activity Tolerance.

After rating the patient on the selected outcome using the five-point measurement scale, the nurse can select the desired rating to be achieved following interventions or an episode of care. For example, a patient may enter the care situation with the outcome Endurance rated as "substantially compromised," and because the cause of the decreased endurance cannot be eliminated (e.g., myocardial myopathy), the desired goal for this patient may be to maintain a rating of "substantially compromised" for as long as possible. Another patient may have "extremely compromised" Endurance because of a condition that can be eliminated or partially controlled (e.g., congestive heart failure), and the desired outcome status following an episode of care may be "moderately compromised." The opportunity to provide an Outcome Target Rating based on the measurement scale allows the nurse to set a specific level of attainment as the goal rather than maintain or improve relative to a desired outcome. For example, the nurse would indicate that the rating should be maintained at a 2 in the first instance above and increased to a 3 or possibly a 4 in the second instance.

Outcomes stated as variable concepts and measured along a continuum allow outcome target ratings to be individualized for each patient while maintaining standardized outcome language and measures. They also give recognition to what all nurses know (that not all patients will be able to achieve the most desirable outcome despite the most intensive care). Variable outcomes measured along a continuum allow the nurse to evaluate the amount of progress or lack of progress for an individual patient as well as computing the amount of change that takes place in a particular patient population. This information is not available when outcomes represent only the most desirable patient state, and the evaluation at the conclusion of a care episode represents a goal met or not met.

Using the Outcomes in Standardized Care Plans

The outcomes also can be used to identify goals in critical paths or in standardized care plans. In these situations, the outcome is stated with the desired or expected rating on the measurement scale to be achieved at a certain point in time (e.g., the first post-op day, the third home care visit). The desired goal at the end of an acute care episode for stroke patients with "extremely compromised" Cognition at the time of admission might be "substantially compromised" with a goal of "moderately compromised" or "mildly compromised" following rehabilitation. If the acute care episode is extremely short, the goal may be to maintain the patient at the "extremely compromised" level with some improvement in specified indicators—the intermediate outcomes that indicate progress toward improvement in Cognition. The plan can project the expected outcome at the end of 6 months and the patient's progress followed if in a rehabilitation unit, a nursing home, or at their next clinic visit. On the other hand, the desired goal for patients with hepatic encephalopathy and "extremely compromised" Cognition at the time of admission may be to have the patient's progress to "moderately compromised" or "mildly compromised" after an acute care episode.

Concerns When Using the Scales

A concern frequently voiced by users is the *subjectivity of the scales*. The indicators have been provided to assist the nurse in determining the patient's status and consequent rating on the outcome scale, but they do not eliminate the need for a nursing judgment. Because the scale anchors are not specifically defined for each indicator and outcome, the nurse must make a nursing judgment about the patient status for the indicators, if used, and for the outcome. Although the accuracy of this judgment becomes more important when quantifying outcomes, it requires the same judgment used when evaluating whether the patient has met a goal, has improved in relation to a goal, has not met a goal, or has deteriorated in relation to the goal. Some organizations have elected to provide more specific anchors for the outcomes, as seen in the examples in Table 3-1. This approach is especially useful when the number of outcomes to be used with a particular population is limited, when using the outcomes in a standard plan, or when using a limited number of outcomes in a research study. If nurses elect to do this, they need to provide this information when reporting their findings so other nurses can determine whether the rating has the same meaning and can be used to make comparisons across settings. As the outcomes are used in more settings, it is anticipated that more specificity of the scale anchors will be developed.

Table 3-1	EXAMPLES OF SPECIFIC ANCHORS FOR INDICATORS IN THE OUTCOME DIGNIFIED DYING AND THE KNOWLEDGE OUTCOMES	

Indicator Statement	Rating Scale	Operational Definition
Expresses symptom control	1 = Not at all 2 = To a slight extent 3 = To a moderate extent 4 = To a great extent 5 = None	4 or more symptoms 3 symptoms present 2 symptoms present 1 symptom present No symptoms
Expresses pain relief	1 = Not at all 2 = To a slight extent 3 = To a moderate extent 4 = To a great extent 5 = None	Reports no change in pain, states level at 9-10 Reports 1-2 points lower; states rate is 8 or lower Reports 3-4 points lower, states rate is 6 or lower Reports 5-6 points lower, states rate is 4 or lower Reports 7-10 points lower, states pain is 2 or lower
All knowledge outcomes	1 = None 2 = Limited 3 = Moderate 4 = Substantial 5 = Extensive	Dependent for all information Requires assistive person and resources Requires assistive resource(s) Independent with minimal cues Independently verbalizes/demonstrates information without cues

These examples are taken from Johnson, M., Maas, M., & Moorhead (2000). *Nursing Outcomes Classification (NOC)* (2nd Ed). St. Louis: Mosby. They can be found in that edition in Appendix B (pp. 544, 551). The outcome name for Dignified Dying has been changed to Dignified Life Closure. This illustrates how anchors can be made more specific and how measurements from other tools can be used with a NOC outcome.

Another issue is *how to use published measurement scales* that appear in recognized patient assessment tools, for example, those used to assess pain, neurological status, pedal pulses, and edema or to grade pressure ulcers and burns. In general, these scales tend to measure a more specific or limited concept; in other words, the NOC outcome may be at a more abstract level. We recommend that the user determine what they want to measure and the published measurement scale serves their need; they may elect to use that scale instead of a NOC outcome. For example, the ten-point pain scale that measures the patient report of pain can be used rather than the NOC outcome Pain Level if the patient report of pain is the only measure desired or the scale grading pressure ulcers can be used in place of Wound Healing: Secondary Intention if it captures the dimensions of concern. The scales can also be used as assessment factors and decisions made about how they correspond to the NOC outcome. For an example of how the ten-point pain scale has been used with a NOC outcome, see Table 3-1.

Another concern is the *patient rating on discharge* from a care episode. While it is recognized that the most desirable condition will not be achievable for all patients or patient groups, and therefore the expected outcome may be less than a "5" on the measurement scale, this is quite uncomfortable for many nurses who have been used to stating goals are met when a patient is discharged. Part of staff education when introducing the NOC needs to be a discussion of how to use the measurement scales and what will be done when the patient does not achieve the desired outcome. The following example may be helpful in illustrating this.

One of our test sites was an obstetric unit that admitted a number of teenage mothers. Two of the outcomes used were Knowledge: Infant Care and Knowledge: Postpartum Maternal Health. Initially, staff rated all mothers at a 4 or 5 on discharge from a 48-hour stay. When asked whether all mothers met the criteria for that rating, staff acknowledged that many did not but they were concerned about the legal implications if they didn't rate the patient at a 4 or 5. This issue was discussed, and staff decided to rate the mothers accurately on the rating and allow the mother with a 4 or 5 rating to go home without a referral for follow-up unless she chose to have one, to encourage follow-up for the mother with a 3 rating, and to require follow-up visits for the mother with a 1 or 2 rating. The staff believed the mother with a 3 rating or above was competent to care for herself and the baby until the scheduled follow-up visit with the physician or nurse, but that the mother with a 1 or 2 rating required additional teaching and assistance that would be provided by a follow-up nursing visit within the first 48 hours of returning home. It would be reasonable to assume that prior to using a rating scale, every patient left the hospital having met a goal that stated the patient had the necessary knowledge to care for her infant. The nursing care provided to these patients is now of a higher quality because it provides a rationale for the decisions based on patient status and provides a method to help the mother who needs additional help.

The *legal implications* when using a measurement scale are the same as those when using a goal statement. If a goal is not met, a rationale for why the goal was not met (e.g., the patient's physiological status deteriorated, the patient was unable to comprehend the information) and the action taken should be provided. The same is true when a projected outcome rating is not achieved. For example, the respiratory status is expected to continue to decline due to increased involvement of the lungs secondary to lung cancer; therefore the outcome Comfort Level is replacing the outcome Respiratory Status: Ventilation, indicating that the goal now is to keep the patient as comfortable as possible. As outcome data are collected and analyzed, patient and system characteristics that influence outcome achievement can be identified and the expected outcome rating for various diagnoses or patient populations can be based on clinical evidence.

Timing of Data Collection

The times at which outcomes should be evaluated are not specified by the authors, but the minimum requirement is obtaining a rating when the outcome is selected (i.e., the baseline measure) and when care is completed (i.e., the discharge measure). This may be sufficient in acute care settings if the patient has a short stay; however, some acute care settings have chosen to evaluate patient status once a day or once a shift depending on how rapidly changes in the outcome status are expected. Community agencies may elect to evaluate patient status at each visit or at every other visit if the patient is seen frequently. Since measurement times are not standardized, reporting the patient care day when measures were obtained is important for making comparisons between patient populations and across units. Noting the times when outcomes are measured will provide information to recommend time intervals for the various outcomes and for varied patient populations.

At least two outcome (or indicator) ratings are necessary to determine if change occurs and the degree of change. These types of data are among the most valuable for evaluating how nursing interventions, other aspects of the patient's care, and the patient characteristics affect outcome achievement. If the desired change is not occurring in all patients, data allow nurses to determine what, if any, difference exists between those who achieve the outcome target and those who do not. If it is the type of intervention or care program, these can be changed. If it is a patient characteristic that cannot be changed, such as age, gender, initial severity of illness, then the target outcome can be readjusted to be consistent with the findings. Examples of a few findings related to change in the completed outcome evaluation study are shown in Table 3-2; additional examples can be found in the case study by Brokel.

While the process described for using the outcomes in practice is important, of equal importance are the processes associated with preparing to implement NOC in a clinical setting and in an electronic patient record. The next section briefly overviews these aspects of implementation, and the implementation examples that follow provide examples from two clinical settings.

Table 3-2   CHANGES IN OUTCOME RATINGS FROM BASELINE TO FOLLOW-UP MEASUREMENTS

Outcome[1]	N	Baseline[2]	Follow-Up	Change	Setting/Unit
Ambulation: Walking (Ambulation)	4	2.25	2.50	0.25	Nursing Home
	7	2.29	4.57	2.29	Birth Center
	6	3.83	4.50	0.67	VNA
	12	3.17	3.50	0.33	Medical Unit
	59	1.92	2.51	0.50	Ortho Unit
Aggression Control (Aggression Self-Control)	5	3.60	4.60	1.00	Stress Unit
	13	2.23	3.62	1.38	Behavioral Unit
Caregiver Emotional Health	7	4.00	4.29	0.29	Parish Nursing
	5	4.00	4.00	0.00	VNA
Breastfeeding Establishment: Maternal	6	3.50	4.00	0.50	VNA
	40	3.00	3.78	0.78	Birth Center

[1]Data were collected using outcome Ambulation: Walking has been changed to Ambulation; Aggression has been changed to Aggression Self-Control. Terms from the 2nd edition.
[2]The baseline and follow-up measures are averages of all ratings.

IMPLEMENTING NOC IN PRACTICE

There is increased recognition in clinical settings that standardized languages are a necessary component for the implementation of electronic health records. Standardized outcomes also are important for evaluating the effectiveness of nursing interventions, facilitating the continuity of care in integrated health systems, and ensuring nursing accountability.[10] An Institute of Medicine report[2] on health care quality stresses the following six aims to be met by the health care system:
- Safe: avoiding injury
- Effective: avoiding overuse and underuse
- Patient-centered: responding to patient preferences, needs, and values
- Timely: reducing waits and delays
- Efficient: avoiding waste
- Equitable: providing care that does not vary in quality to all recipients

Evaluation of these aims requires measurement and tracking of patient outcomes, as well as measurement and tracking of other aspects of care. Given these factors, the opportunity for nursing to implement measures to assess nursing effectiveness is timely.

Preparing for Clinical Implementation

Implementing NOC in the clinical setting requires organizational commitment and the development of an implementation plan. Advantages of using NOC must be identified and communicated to organizational leaders and nursing staff. Strengths of NOC that can be emphasized include:
1. Comprehensiveness: NOC includes outcomes for individuals, family caregivers, families, and communities that are applicable across clinical settings.
2. Clinical usefulness: NOC can be used in a manual or electronic clinical information system. The outcomes can be used in critical paths and care plans and can be used to set expected patient goals for individual patients or groups of patients.
3. Data measurement and analysis: Data can be collected from the patient record, quantified, and used in outcome analysis.
4. Recognized nursing language: NOC is one of the nursing languages recognized by the American Nurses Association (ANA) Steering Committee on Databases to Support

Clinical Nursing Practice, has been accepted by Healthcare 7 (HL7), an organization setting standards for the computerized record, and is incorporated into the reference language developed by SNOMED CT.

Organizational leaders and staff may need to be educated about the importance of using standardized languages for nursing practice, although this may be less necessary as plans for the electronic health record progress. A key person, one who is committed to the project and able to articulate the advantages of using standardized languages, needs to be responsible for the implementation process. The nurse in charge of nursing informatics or outcome management is often an ideal person to select as project leader for the implementation process.

Staff members who will use NOC need to be identified and educated about the classification. In our research evaluating the use of NOC in clinical sites, we found that staff education is one of the most important factors for the successful implementation of NOC. The process for using NOC outcomes should be covered as well as the issues and concerns that arise as nurses begin to use the outcomes. Staff should not have to become familiar with the use of NOC and a new computer system at the same time. If an organization is going to select a new computer system, the time used for evaluation and selection of the system should be used to orient nurses to the NOC outcome system and to pilot written forms.

Implementation Planning

A task force of representatives from key areas and pilot sites should be established to assist the project leader with the implementation process.[6] The task force can assist with the development of the implementation plan and with staff education during the implementation process. The implementation plan should include the goals to be accomplished, steps for implementation with the responsible individuals and a time line, the evaluation plan, and the costs associated with implementation. Planning should include the identification of other data that need to be collected in conjunction with the outcome data for clinical and administrative analyses. For example, patient characteristics, staff mix, nursing costs, and nursing diagnoses and interventions may need to be linked with outcome data to answer clinical and administrative questions. During this phase, the ability or inability of the electronic information system to link patient outcomes with other data should be evaluated and, if needed, plans to establish the necessary linkages to other databases should be developed. The ability to collect data on the links between nursing diagnoses, interventions, and outcomes should also be evaluated.

The initial planning should result in the development of a paper format that can be tested prior to implementation throughout the organization or placement in an electronic system. The format used for documenting with standardized languages should not be more time-consuming than that previously used in the organization; however, it must be recognized that documentation may take longer until the staff becomes familiar with the new system. A tri-fold paper form was created for initial use in medical critical care units at The University of Iowa Hospitals and Clinics. It includes information recorded on admission to the unit and provides a standardized format that can be used for nursing diagnoses related to the following nine areas of potential patient problems: (1) sensory; (2) pain; (3) neurologic; (4) motor; (5) pulmonary; (6) cardiac; (7) integument and immune; (8) gastrointestinal and urinary; and (9) nutrition. Examples of how these are set up to include standardized languages are provided in Figures 3-1 and 3-2. This format requires the nurse to make a judgment about the nursing diagnosis and the interventions and outcomes to be used with the diagnosis. Space is provided in the tri-fold for additional comments as necessary. Percentages have been applied to the five-point scale to make the scale more explicit; this technique was used by a number of sites in our evaluation study.

It is recommended that the outcomes be implemented on one or more pilot units to assess and correct problems prior to house-wide implementation. The units selected should be ones on which a majority of the staff members are committed to the project. Once the pilot units are identified, the NOC outcomes used most frequently for the patient population on the unit need to be

CARDIAC PATIENT NURSING DIAGNOSIS (NANDA-I)

Date/Time/Initial Initiated	Date/Time/Initial Resolved

☐ **Altered Tissue Perfusion Cardiopulmonary**
☐ **Risk of Fluid Volume Imbalance (Excess/Deficit)**
☐ **Decrease Cardiac Output**

Parameters:

T < ___ > ___
HR < ___ > ___
SBP < ___ > ___
DBP < ___ > ___
RR < ___ > ___
UO ___
SaO2 > ___
Other: ___

Signs & Symptoms

Edema
Oliguria or anuria
Weak or absent pulse
Altered mental status
Dyspnea/changes in respiratory pattern
Elevated pulmonary artery pressure

Arrhythmia
Jugular vein distention
Decrease blood pressure
Increase pulse rate
Thirst
Changes in skin color/temp.

Related Factors

Excess fluid intake
Hypovolemia/Hypervolemia
Mechanical reduction of venous and/or arterial blood flow
Chest pain. Cardiac ischemia/damage
Loss of fluid through abnormal routes (indwelling tubes, wounds/burns, diarrhea)
Impaired transport of the oxygen across alveolar and/or capillary membrane

NURSING INTERVENTIONS (NIC) & ACTIVITIES

Date/Time/Initial Initiated

Blood Products Administration: Administer per policy and protocol.

Cardiac Care: Acute: R/O MI Protocol. Monitor vital signs q 1-2 hr or as needed. CHAMPS MET level ___ Other:

Fluid/Electrolyte Management: Monitor lab values relevant to fluid & electrolyte balance.

Invasive Hemodynamic Monitoring: Cardiac Indices q ___ PCWP q ___

Hemodynamic Regulation: Monitor vital signs and pulses. Administer vasoactive or inotropic medications as ordered.

Shock Management: Specify:

Teaching (Patient/Family): Instruct the patient/family on cardiac monitor, I.V. lines, hemodynamic monitoring, and hemodynamic medications. Encourage realistic expectations for the patient and family. Inform pt/family of any referral made. Other:

PATIENT OUTCOME (NOC)

Tissue Perfusion: Cardiac: Extent to which blood flows through the coronary vasculature and maintains heart function

Definition of Scale	1 (0%)	2 (25%)	3 (50%)	4 (75%)	5 (100%)
Vital signs within normal limits	Extremely compromised	Substantially compromised	Moderately compromised	Mildly compromised	Not compromised

Day (level/initial)

1	2	3	4	5	6	7
8	9	10	11	12	13	14

Fig. 3-1 Plan for a cardiac patient for a medical intensive care unit. (From Greiner, J., Shelsky, C., Stenger, K., & Crom, E. (2002). Alblo Nursing Diagnoses Standards Form Critical Care. University of Iowa Hospitals and Clinics.)

PAIN PATIENT NURSING DIAGNOSIS (NANDA-I)

Date/Time/Initial Initiated	Date/Time/Initial Resolved	❑ Pain	❑ Chronic Pain	Acceptable pain level:

Possible Signs & Symptoms

		Related Factors

States pain is present
States pain is present > 6 month
Restless
Diaphoresis
Pressure

Muscle guarding
Facial expression of pain
Moaning crying
Autonomic responses

Injuring agents (biological, chemical, physical, psychological)
Chronic physical/psychosocial disability
Surgery/invasive procedure
Cancer
Cardiac

NURSING INTERVENTIONS (NIC) & ACTIVITIES

Date/Time/Initial Initiated

Pain Management: Assess for pain every 2 hr & document on A-1c ICU Flowsheet. Look for nonverbal clues. Consider cultural influences. Consider type & source of pain when selecting pain relief strategy. Other:

Analgesic Administration: Administer analgesia per order. Reassess 10-20 min for parenteral & 30 min to 1 hr for oral medications. Titrate dosage based on intensity. Other:

Analgesic Administration: epidural: NARCAN at bedside. **DO NOT MANIPULATE, CHANGE DRESSING OR ADMINISTER ANYTHING VIA EPIDURAL CATHETER.** For emergencies, if RR 8 or less or undue somnolence call anesthesiology (391) physician. Other:

Teaching (Patient/Family): Instruct the patient/family about pain management & the effects of pain. Review with patient/family medication taken in the past. Provide comfort and reassurance. Instruct to ask for PRN before pain is to severe. Other:

PATIENT OUTCOME

Pain Level: Amount of reported or demonstrated pain.

Day (level/initial)						
1	2	3	4	5	6	7
8	9	10	11	12	13	14

Definition of Scale	1 (0%)	2 (25%)	3 (50%)	4 (75%)	5 (100%)
Reported Pain (0-10)	Severe (8-10)	Substantial (6-7)	Moderate (5-4)	Slight (3-1)	None (0)

Fig. 3-2 Plan for patient with pain for a medical intensive care unit. (From Greiner, J., Shelsky, C., Stenger, K., & Crom, E. (2002). Alblo Nursing Diagnoses Standards Form Critical Care. University of Iowa Hospitals and Clinics.)

identified; this can be done by using the *NOC Use Survey* listed in Box 3-1. The survey tool is an efficient method for identifying outcomes for patient populations and can be completed by all staff. Creating a task force of clinical staff to select the most frequently used outcomes is another way to identify outcomes. The article by Carlson listed in Box 3-1 discusses a method for arriving at a consensus in the selection of NANDA, NOC, and NIC terms. If the unit has a list of the outcome goals used most frequently, the appropriate NOC outcomes can be substituted for the goals. If a needed outcome is not available, the task force can develop the outcome using the guidelines in Appendix B and submit the outcome to the NOC research team or inform the team of the need for a specific outcome.

As noted earlier, a number of articles that users might find helpful in planning for and carrying out implementation can be found in Box 3-1. Some of the articles are specific to a particular area of practice, such as parish nursing or long-term care. Other articles discuss aspects of implementation related to education of staff, testing of outcomes, or processes used in implementation. A couple of articles address issues related to implementation of NOC in electronic patient records.

IMPLEMENTING NOC IN ELECTRONIC SYSTEMS

A primary value of an electronic clinical information system is the ability to collect and analyze large amounts of data. Analyzing data requires that the system be developed in such a way that the information and linkages are available to answer the questions posed. Unfortunately, many current systems do not allow for the types of analyses that nurses need to do. Creating systems that will provide the information nurses need for clinical and administrative decision making requires planning for the type of data sets that will be used and for the linkages among the sets. One way to begin is by determining what such a system should do. It should provide a way to unify data from many information sources, provide a means of detecting trends and possible oversights in care, and provide a basis for outcomes management and a database for epidemiological studies.[15] An important step for nursing is to determine the data sets that are needed, the elements of the data sets, and the types of linkages wanted between the data sets. The book by Titler and colleagues listed in Box 3-1 describes data elements that should be considered and the questions that should be possible to answer.

Identifying Data Sets and Links

Data sets that are of interest to nursing include clinical data sets, provider data sets, fiscal data sets, and utilization data sets. Nurses involved in the development of the electronic nursing system should know the data sets available in the organization and whether the sets can be linked with nursing data. One data set available in all hospital settings is the Uniform Hospital Discharge Data Set (UHDDS).[17] This set includes the 14 items found in Box 3-2, many of which are relevant for nursing. Clinical data sets are generally the largest number of data sets, and in most cases, few of them are coded and organized in a similar fashion. They include data on

---

Box 3-2

Elements in the Uniform Data Set

Personal identification	Admission date	Diagnoses
Date of birth	Discharge date	Procedures and dates
Gender	Physician identification—	Discharge disposition of
Race and ethnicity	attending	patient
Residence (zip code)	Physician identification—	Expected principal source
Hospital identification	operating	of payment

patient medications, laboratory findings, surgical procedures, and radiology results, as well as diagnoses, treatments and interventions, and patient outcomes, to name a few. The electronic clinical nursing sets should contain information about the patient necessary for nursing practice that is not contained elsewhere and about the nursing diagnoses, interventions, and outcomes. In addition to the patient information contained in the UHDDS, nurses will want information discussed in the section on selecting an outcome. Nurses need to give careful consideration to the type of information they want retained about the diagnoses and outcomes. If NANDA diagnoses are used, retaining information about the defining characteristics and related factors or risk factors will increase the types of analyses that can be done. Likewise, obtaining as much information about the outcomes, such as indicators selected and the data source, will facilitate analysis. For the intervention, adequate information to capture important variance in the activities should be maintained.[23] The dose and frequency of the treatment will provide information about the strength of the treatment. The time of day the treatment is administered and the staff providing the treatment can be important information when analyzing the effectiveness of interventions. Perhaps one of the most important factors to consider in the nursing data sets is how linkages between the diagnoses, interventions, and outcomes will be provided. The linkage identifies the problem the intervention is to address and the outcome expected as a result of the intervention.

Provider data sets include information about the nurse, such as age, education, and skill level, and information about the setting, such as unit size, staffing, and type of care delivery system in addition to the type of organization. Fiscal data sets include information about costs and charges that are necessary to compute the cost of nursing and the income generated. The Nursing Management Minimum Data Set[3] includes methods for measuring many of these elements. Utilization data sets are available in most organizations that provide health care services; they are measures of the care provided[11] and will vary with the type of organization. In hospital settings, they will include patient days, hospital admissions, and discharges. In community settings, they will include number of visits, number of admissions, and discharges from the service.

While many of the questions about patient care that clinical nurses want answered will require links among clinical databases, many of the questions that nurse administrators want answered will require links among the clinical, provider, fiscal, and utilization data bases. Nurses have a major opportunity to plan for data sets with the required links when new electronic systems are being put in place. Because electronic systems are costly, mistakes made with the introduction of new systems may be both difficult and costly to rectify at a later date.

Placing NOC in Electronic Systems

In addition to planning for implementation, a number of questions arise about the actual implementation of the NOC outcomes in an electronic system. One of the major problems that nurses have encountered is the amount of space available in the software. There must be adequate space to include the outcome, the definition, and the inclusion of indicators and measurement scales. Eliminating the definition and using indicators as separate outcomes is one way in which nursing addressed these problems in the past. However, this eliminates the opportunity to analyze the indicators that might be most effective or useful for the outcome and may limit analyses that can be done with the data. Overall ratings of each outcome are essential at all measurement points. The development of software programs that will accommodate the information that nurses need to record and evaluate in conjunction with other data are essential. All software providers need to consider the input, collection, and output of nursing data when developing software programs for clinical information systems. We have found that software providers listen to users, and if nurses know what they want their systems to do and demand what is needed for their data collection, changes come about, especially as more emphasis is placed on designing systems for an electronic health record. Software vendors must listen to nurses and include standardized terminology in their clinical information systems to meet the needs of the nursing profession.

LICENSING THE OUTCOMES

A license is needed to use NOC on an electronic information system or in a product for commercial gain. Mosby, Inc., now a part of Elsevier Science, holds the copyright on NOC. The inside front cover of this book contains information about who to contact to use NOC or to obtain a license. The research team elected to publish the classification through a book publisher for a number of reasons. The team had no way to produce and market the product, to provide funding for continued development, or to protect the standardization of the language by protecting the copyright.

Copyright does not restrict fair use. The American Library Association recognizes fair use when the following guidelines are followed: (1) the portion copied is selective and not more than 10% of the work; (2) the materials are not used repeatedly; (3) no more than one copy is made for each person; (4) the source and copyright are included on each copy; and (5) persons are not assessed a fee for the copy beyond the cost of reproduction. Putting NOC on an electronic system requires a license because significant portions of the book will be available for use by multiple users. The use of significant portions of the classification in a book or product that is being sold also requires a license. Fees for the use of NOC in an electronic system to be used in one organization depend on the number of users and average about $5.00 per user per year, an extremely reasonable fee when compared with fees for many other software products. If the user purchases a software product that uses NOC, the license fees will often be included as part of the product cost. Paying licensing fees for the use of nomenclatures or software is familiar to hospital administrators; often it is nurses who are unaware that the organization is paying these fees for other information sets such as those for the pharmacy or laboratory.

Many requests are consistent with fair use and do not require fees. Fees are not required if the organization uses the outcomes in a paper format. However, the organization should purchase enough books so that they do not have to make multiple copies of the classification. Fees are generally not required for schools of nursing that want to use NOC in educational products for their own students; however, if the school is using a significant portion of NOC, it is expected that students will have the books to use with the products produced by the schools. Fees are generally not required for research using NOC. Fees for use in another publication will depend on the number of outcomes used; if only a few are provided as examples, no fee will be assessed for use.

A significant portion of the fees generated through license agreements and use are returned to the Center to fund the upkeep of both NIC and NOC and Center operations. To continue to evaluate NOC in clinical settings, provide a means to update the language, and keep the languages current with changes in federal requirements requires personnel and other resources. The American Nurses Association does not have the resources to fund the continued development of the languages they recognize, so development must be done by the authors. Thus the Center for Nursing Classification and Clinical Effectiveness was created at The University of Iowa for this purpose; however, long-term funding was not provided for the Center. The viability of the Center and its work is dependent on monies earned through publications, licenses, and other products and on donations made to an endowment fund whose purpose is to provide long-term funding for the continued support of the development, refinement, and implementation of NIC and NOC.

CASE STUDIES

The following examples illustrate how two facilities have handled the implementation of NOC in electronic systems. The first example discusses how nursing was able to modify a software product to enable the use of NANDA, NOC, and NIC in their clinical information system. Methods used to assist education of staff are also discussed.

CASE STUDY I

Implementing Standardized Nursing Languages Into an Electronic Medical Record

Jennifer Hafner, BSN, RN, PCCN

Aspirus Wausau Hospital is a 312-bed, multispecialty facility. It is a regional health care facility that provides care to central and northern Wisconsin. In 2005, Aspirus was Magnet-certified and recognized by *U.S. News & World Report* as one of the nation's 50 centers for heart care and digestive care. *U.S. News & World Report* recognized Aspirus as one of the top 100 cardiovascular hospitals again in 2006. Aspirus also received the 2006 Health Grades Distinguished Hospital Award for Clinical Excellence (the only hospital in Wisconsin to receive this award in three consecutive years), the 2007 Health Grades Cardiac Care and Cardiac Surgery Excellence Awards (the only hospital to receive these awards in four consecutive years), the 2007 Health Grades General Surgery Excellence Award, and the 2007 Health Grades Critical Care Excellence Award.[5] Aspirus cares for a large variety of patients in the central and northern Wisconsin area. Aspirus admitted 16,089 patients in 2005; performed 639 open-heart, 498 spine, and 5825 outpatient surgeries; had 26,169 emergency room visits; and delivered 1408 babies. In 2002, it also implemented collaborative practice into its nursing model.

Aspirus implemented NANDA International (NANDA-I),[18] Nursing Interventions Classification (NIC),[4] and Nursing Outcomes Classification (NOC)[16] into its care plan documentation in 2003. At the same time, Aspirus changed its computer system from The Precision Alternative (Gerber Alley) to Epic Systems. Epic Systems uses a graphic user interface similar to windows to manage an electronic medical record (EMR). Epic Systems develops health care software modules for ambulatory care, inpatient, clinical, admission, transfer, discharge functions, financial services, and health information management.

Care plans are a component of the Epic Care inpatient documentation module. There were limitations to the Epic care plan product during the implementation of NANDA, NIC, and NOC into the computerized documentation system. Epic did not have readily available fields for utilizing the NOC rating scales. A workaround was created to allow use of the rating scales. Epic's care plan design also has limitations in that it does not support cross encounters for care path guides. Epic creates a different encounter for each hospital admission or patient visit, and the floor admission is seen as a new encounter. For example, if a patient with heart disease is admitted to the Ambulatory Care Unit for a scheduled cardiac procedure and then admitted to the floor after an intervention, the care plan does not follow the patient when the patient comes back to the hospital for a follow-up schedule surgery. When a patient follows up with cardiac rehabilitation after a myocardial infarction, the care plan cannot follow the patient through the continuum because that is also a new encounter.

Epic also was unable to display an alert to flag that a care plan was required based on assessment data in the documentation flow sheet. Epic functionality did allow programming to suggest a plan of care based on an admission diagnosis or based on the problem list. Epic was able to provide a direct link to an electronic publication of a text. However, there was not an electronic publication for easy reference for the end-user of NANDA, NIC, or NOC. To provide a sound understanding of each NANDA and NOC, definitions of each were displayed in every care plan template.

Smart lists (picklists), and ellipses (wildcards) were compiled and hand-built by the information technology (IT) staff at Aspirus for every single care plan. For care plans that would be built from scratch, the IT staff created a "smart phrase" to give end-users "fields" to complete. A smart phrase was also developed for nursing documentation. The smart phrase "NOC" displays as "Current NOC Outcome Rating (WH-NOC-Current 103447)." The nurse then selects a number from 1 to 5 from the smart list to rate the patient's progress toward the selected outcome. Next, the nurse documents a synopsis of the patient's condition in relation to the indicators chosen, using the Data Action Response (DAR) method of documentation. Selecting a rating on the appropriate scale and then documenting helps ensure inter-rater reliability. Figures 3-3 and 3-4 illustrate how the screens are set up to capture the information necessary to make informed decisions for individual patients and to collect and analyze group data.

In 2003, staff from every nursing unit (subject matter experts) created care plans, based on their experience, for frequent diagnoses or surgeries. These care plans were categorized in Epic under nursing unit and template name (i.e., MSIMC-Carotid Endarectomy {Medical-Surgical Intermediate Care}). Multiple care plans existed for the same diagnosis, based on the inpatient unit, and did not follow across the continuum of the patient's stay.

The outcomes could have been measured at any time; however, it was required that they be measured "at discharge," thus setting outcome or goal attainment at discharge for all outcomes. Aspirus Wausau Hospital was cited by TJC (The Joint Commission) for not individualizing the care plans by setting a specific time to measure each outcome (goal) for each patient. At that time, "expected end dates" were implemented into Epic to make the care plans time-measurable for each patient. The house-wide practice council also created a subcommittee, the care plan task force. The task force was charged to make the care plans more patient specific and measurable to be in compliance with TJC.

The task force recruited Cynthia Finesilver, RN, MSN, CNRN, as a consultant to assist with the revision of the care plans. She is a nationally known expert in NANDA, NIC, and NOC and is currently an adjunct nursing instructor at Northeast Wisconsin Technical College in Green Bay.

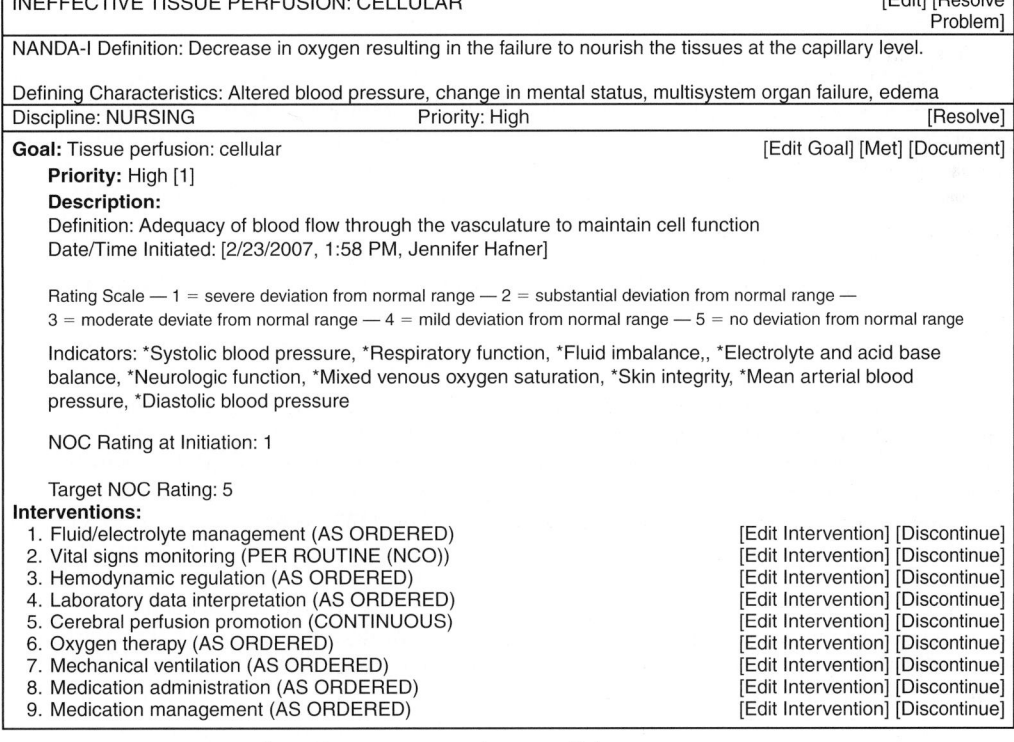

Fig. 3-3 Plan for patient with ineffective tissue perfusion: cellular.

IMPAIRED PHYSICAL MOBILITY	[Edit] [Resolve Problem]
NANDA-I Definition: Limitation in independent, purposeful physical movement of the body or of one or more extemities.	
Defining Characteristics: limited range of motion; limited ability to perform gross and fine motor skills; postural instability	
Discipline: NURSING Priority: High	[Resolve]

Goal: Body positioning: self-initiated   [Edit Goal] [Met] [Document]
Priority: High [1]
Description:
Definition: Ability to change own body position independently, with or without assistive device.
Date/Time Initiated: [2/23/2007, 2:00 PM, Jennifer Hafner]

Rating Scale — 1 = severely compromised — 2 = substantially compromised — 3 = moderately compromised — 4 = mildly compromised — 5 = not compromised

Indicators: Moves from side to side while lying, Moves from lying to sitting and Moves from sitting to standing

NOC Rating at Initiation: 1

Target NOC Rating: 5
Interventions:

1. Exercise therapy: joint mobility (PER ROUTINE (NCO))	[Edit Intervention] [Discontinue]
2. Bedrest care (PER ROUTINE (NCO))	[Edit Intervention] [Discontinue]
3. Skin surveillance (PER ROUTINE (NCO))	[Edit Intervention] [Discontinue]
4. Positioning (PER ROUTINE (NCO))	[Edit Intervention] [Discontinue]
5. Bowel management (AS ORDERED)	[Edit Intervention] [Discontinue]
6. Circulatory precautions (AS ORDERED)	[Edit Intervention] [Discontinue]
7. Pressure management (PER ROUTINE (NCO))	[Edit Intervention] [Discontinue]

Fig. 3-4 Plan for patient with impaired physical mobility.

The president of NANDA-I, T. Heather Herdmann, RN, PhD, who has a degree in nursing informatics, was also consulted to contribute to the design integration into Epic. The revisions of the care plans included implementing the NOC scales and indicators, displaying definitions of each NANDA and NOC, and revising the content of each care plan.

The care plan task force also hosted a 1-day workshop to educate staff about NANDA, NIC, and NOC. The staff then created care plans requested by each unit during the afternoon session. Workdays were then conducted with content experts from each nursing unit and with the author, who was the chair of the care plan task force. The content experts used the workdays to create care plans that were not created at the workshop.

The majority of nurses at Aspirus had not been exposed to NIC and NOC. House-wide education was conducted to educate staff about NIC and NOC and about care plan documentation changes that were implemented at the triannual nursing in-service. Finesilver presented NANDA, NIC, and NOC theory and engaged the staff in case studies to increase the inter-rater reliability. The author presented information specifically related to the NOC scales and Epic implementation. Staff gained an understanding of how to use the NOC scales and how to edit the care plan in Epic.

Staff have to edit the care plan outcome (goal) and choose the indicators (signs or symptoms) that are specific to the patient from a picklist. Staff will reference the indicators and scale specific to that care plan to give a "NOC Rating at Initiation" and a "Target NOC Rating." The "Target NOC Rating" is the patient-specific goal. The "expected end date" is the time frame in which the goal will be achieved. Only short-term goals are used for inpatients, with the exception of hospice, in which short-term and long-term goals are used. NANDA, NIC, and NOC were not used with the home health division of Aspirus.

Staff at Aspirus Wausau Hospital worked very hard to achieve a care plan documentation system that is user-friendly and in compliance and in compliance with TJC. Almost every situation was considered when creating care plans. Multiple care plan templates were devised so that it would be a rare occurrence when an end-user would have to create a care plan from scratch. The care plan revisions were implemented on December 19, 2006.

CASE STUDY II

Acknowledgment: Joan Klehr, for contributions to this case study.

The second case study discusses how a software system was developed using standardized languages to meet the specific needs of the facility. The case also describes how data were handled to produce findings that were used in clinical and administrative decision making.

Selecting and Measuring Nursing Outcomes and Indicators for Use in Case Management

Jane M. Brokel, PhD, RN

This case study illustrates how nursing outcomes were collected over time for a cohort of patients that qualified for case management services. The outcomes used in the study were from the Nursing Outcomes Classification (NOC). The case study will focus on the selection of the NOC outcomes, the workflow process that established the frequency and procedures to measure the nursing-sensitive patient outcome indicators over time, and finally, how the programming of the data set provided rapid extraction of the information on outcomes for the various time periods in an organized manner. This careful up-front preparation provided the information needed to analyze the benefit for patients who received the case management services. This case shows how outcome data were helpful to measure change in patient status in a case management service. The study is presented here to contribute to dialog about the workflow steps to use interface terminologies within practice and research.

Background

In 1992, a Midwest rural referral medical center began providing community case management services to a small group of people at risk for recidivism.[22] The home visits and nursing interventions at the time proved to decrease visits to the emergency room and hospitalization as well as the costs of providing services. Often costs associated with longer lengths of stay and frequent services were denied reimbursement by payers. Hence the patient received services at the provider's loss. The initial patient outcomes were focused on the number of encounters per year and dollars saved to the providers by decreasing losses. In some occurrences, reimbursement could be lost by not hospitalizing the patient when reimbursement was possible. The early case management services were helpful in reducing the losses from nonreimbursed services.[25] The patients benefiting from case management services were people with chronic illnesses and often had two or more chronic diseases to manage.

For this case study, case management services were defined as a nurse, nurse practitioner, or social worker working with the patient and patient's doctor to manage health care needs. Furthermore, the case manager identified the patient's health care needs early on to avoid serious complications and to address the problems or barriers that keep the patient from getting the care needed, thereby avoiding unnecessary hospitalizations. The definition guiding this description was the case management definition from the Nursing Interventions Classification,[14] which is defined as "coordinating care and advocating for specified individuals and patient populations across settings to reduce cost, reduce resource use, improve quality of health care, and achieve desired outcomes" (p. 230).[14] The "desired outcomes" are those the patient was hoping for and were often discussed with the case.

Selection of Nursing Outcomes

In 2000, the case managers submitted an application to participate in a funded research project. In the process of submitting the application, the case managers and Brokel searched for the patient outcomes in Nursing Outcomes Classification (NOC)[9] that best described what the patients were asking for. Some of Brokel's previous work with individual nurse practitioners helped to quickly identify expected outcomes desired by patients. Symptom Control and Quality of Life were two NOC outcomes already used in nurse practitioners' assessments. The synthesizing of case manager's experiences and background literature written about case management[12,13,26] quickly led the case managers to identify the first four NOC outcomes listed below as measures. The number of indicators selected for use with each outcome appears in parentheses following the outcome. The study question for the case managers was, Do the services improve clinical outcomes, quality of life, and self-care management? The burden of adding more outcomes to measure would add to workload. The later three were added later when the collection process was outlined and the case managers were comfortable with time and frequency to collect measurements.

   Symptom Control (2 clinical indicators)
   Quality of Life (6 perception indicators)
   Well-Being (7 perception indicators)
   Self-Care: Instrumental Activities of Daily Living (17 indicators)
   Self-Care: Activities of Daily Living (8 self-care indicators)
   Bowel Continence (2 clinical indicators)
   Urinary Continence (3 clinical indicators)

Collection of Nursing Outcome Indicators

The acknowledgment to participate led to the need to design and develop a data set of key patient variables, nursing variables, and service variables like a Nursing Minimum Data Set[24] for community case management. In 2000, unlike today, the number of programs suited for collection of key nursing variables with service variables was isolated to one possible vendor who had minimal experience. The case managers and Brokel aligned with local programmers to develop a case management program that could ensure the extraction and use of the data in a variety of ways. The technology was designed using Visual Basic proprietary software with a license to use the Nursing Interventions Classification (NIC) and NOC interface terminologies in the design. The case managers identified the subset of indicators for each NOC outcome that they thought pertained to their nursing interventions and activities with the patient. All case managers approved the subset to ensure that everyone was collecting the same indicators for each outcome. The next concern was how frequently the outcomes were going to be measured and the method that would be used to collect the information. The case managers agreed on baseline assessments and agreed that during the first year there would be greater interaction and therefore subsequent assessments of the outcome indicators would be taken at 6 months of service and 1 year. Thereafter, the need for contact was expected to decline and outcomes would be checked annually to see whether the patient stabilized or continued to improve or decline.

Once the NOC indicators were identified, the team described who collected data, when the data were collected, where the data were collected (often in the client's home), and how the case managers were reminded to collect the data. This process generated a workflow showing how to measure outcomes over time. Brokel developed the report format that was used to analyze the data for each of the outcomes. At this time the lead case manager and Brokel provided the report format to the programmers. The programmers could then design the case management program to collect, display, and extract the outcomes indicators of the outcomes. The program was designed to retrieve other variables needed for the study at hand, for example, the NIC interventions. This programming ensured that each of the measurements of NOC indicators (which could be collected at a patient's home, by telephone, or during a visit to a primary care clinic) could be downloaded from the remote sites on a routine basis to facilitate aggregating the information. All aspects of the program were tested with two patients prior to initiating the formal start with a larger cohort of patients to ensure the data set organized, presented, and reported the data as projected.

Measurement of NOC Patient Outcomes

The technology and processes were started in April of 2002 and continue at this time. The new cohort of patients was limited to patients with primary diagnoses of chronic diseases. Those diagnoses included the following: Congestive Heart Failure; Chronic Obstructive Pulmonary Disease; Renal Failure; Arteriosclerosis Vascular Disease Stroke/Cerebral Vascular Disease; Respiratory Failure; and Liver Disease. Those qualified to participate signed informed consents about the larger study and were randomized to receive case management services. During initial planning for the study, the anticipated attrition due to death for the group was expected to be around 14% to 18%.

The local Institutional Review Board approved the study in 2002 and ensures the continued protection of subjects' data. During the first 4 years, 514 people were identified in the randomized group for receiving services. Attrition from this group included 64 due to death and another 79 discontinued services because they moved or for other reasons. Three hundred seventy-one remained in the study and had assessments at 6 months and 1 year. Data were de-identified before analysis and sharing of findings with case managers.

Method of Analysis

The established process required the case manager to request extraction of NOC data from the office manager. Data extraction required the professional version of Microsoft Excel 2000 to pull the extracted data from the case management program database. This software facilitated extracted data into organized files for each NOC outcome and separated the data by time period. In August 2005, the extraction pulled 473 baseline assessments for the Symptom Control indicators; 387 for 6-month assessments; 352 for 1-year assessments; 228 for 2-year assessments; and 47 for 3-year assessments. In June 2006, the number of assessments increased to 170 for a 3-year assessment, and the collection of data began to include 4-year assessments.

The steps to analyze the August 2005 extraction are presented here. The data were examined for assessment of all indicators. A very small number of indicators had missing data and therefore loaded in the data extraction as zeros. All zeros were removed. The data were imported into SSPS version 11 with each indicator as a field of data, and the patient de-identified code and coded time period were two associated fields of data with each indicator for analysis. A first step in analysis was to generate a new column to calculate a mean from the NOC indicators associated with the label. The Case Management program had also calculated an average, but these steps were taken to validate the accuracy of the program's calculation. This process was repeated for each set of NOC indicators and labels. The baseline assessment was considered the patient's control level, and subsequent assessments were compared with the baseline assessment. One-way analysis of variance (ANOVA) was used to analyze changes in scores. Post hoc tests comparing each of the follow-ups to the baseline were used to determine if there were statistically significant changes over time.

Findings

The analysis revealed significant changes indicating improvement in helping patients with chronic disease control symptoms at 6 months, and over time the measurement continued to show improvement from *sometimes demonstrating to often demonstrating* Symptom Control (p = 0.000). The two indicators selected to measure Symptom Control are displayed in Table 3-3 with the average patient outcome scores for each time period. The patients were receiving a variety of nursing interventions, but seven NICs were more frequently performed: Vital Sign

Table 3-3 Symptom Control, NOC Outcome Label and Two Indicators

NOC Outcome	Baseline	6 month	1 year	2 year
Symptom Control	3.87	4.12 (0.001)	4.13 (0.001)	4.30 (0.000)
Monitor symptom variation—indicator	3.91	4.16 (0.01)	4.16 (0.02)	4.38 (0.000)
Uses preventive measures—indicator	3.84	4.08 (0.04)	4.10 (0.04)	4.12 (0.000)

Table 3-4 Quality of Life, NOC Outcome Label, and Six Indicators

NOC Outcome	Baseline	6 month	1 year	2 year
Quality of Life	3.84	4.00 (0.002)	3.95 (0.076)	4.05 (0.000)
Self-concept	3.50	4.06 (0.043)	4.02 (0.216)	4.14 (0.006)
Health status	3.13	3.44 (0.000)	3.36 (0.006)	3.40 (0.004)
Pervasive mood	3.87	3.99 (0.191)	3.99 (0.221)	4.09 (0.008)
Economic status	3.82	3.99 (0.094)	3.91 (0.659)	4.09 (0.010)
Achievement of life goals	3.96	4.13 (0.027)	4.05 (0.468)	4.16 (0.021)
Close relationships	4.36	4.40 (0.943)	4.39 (0.987)	4.44 (0.709)

Monitoring, Teaching: Disease Process, Medication Management, Health Care Information Exchange, Health System Guidance, Decision-Making Support, and Teaching: Prescribed Medications.

The overall average baseline scores for Bowel Continence at 4.81 and Urinary Continence at 4.71 were less of a problem with this cohort. Two indicators were selected to measure Bowel Continence: (1) Recognizes urge to defecate and (2) Maintains predictable pattern. Three indicators were selected to measure Urinary Continence: (1) Recognizes urge to void; (2) Response to urge in timely manner; and (3) Starts and stops stream. The indicators that did change over time were recognizing urges to defecate and void. The overall changes were not significant because most patients did not see this as a problem.

The analysis revealed significant change in the perceptions patients had about their quality of life. The six indicators used to measure the patients' perceptions are presented in Table 3-4. The indicators for perceived health status, self-concept, and achievement of life goals contributed the most to improvements early in care, and over time other perceptions also improved. The indicator for close relationships was rated high at baseline and did not contribute to the change.

The analysis showed some change in patient well-being, but the perceptions were not significant (p = 0.062) as with quality of life perceptions that started out lower. The seven indicators used to measure the patients' perceptions are presented in Table 3-5. The indicators for perceived spiritual life, ability to cope, and ability to relax contributed to improvements over time. Again, most indicators were rated high at baseline and did not contribute to the change.

The analysis revealed independence for the outcome Self-Care: Activities of Daily Living (ALD) with an average baseline of 4.72 that improved to 4.83. The indicators for eating and walking contributed to the improvement and were noticed after 2 years with the case management services.

Table 3-5	PERSONAL WELL-BEING, NOC OUTCOME LABEL WITH SEVEN INDICATORS			
NOC Outcome	**Baseline**	**6 month**	**1 year**	**2 year**
Well-Being	4.02	4.09 (0.400)	4.07 (0.637)	4.13 (0.124)
Social relationships	3.95	4.06 (0.327)	3.94 (1.00)	4.03 (0.777)
Spiritual life	4.19	4.29 (0.269)	4.29 (0.293)	4.38 (0.029)
Cognitive function	3.97	4.04 (0.785)	4.02 (0.931)	4.07 (0.634)
Ability to cope	4.00	4.14 (0.080)	4.07 (0.636)	4.16 (0.090)
Ability to relax	4.01	4.04 (0.977)	4.08 (0.70)	4.17 (0.155)
Level of happiness	4.04	4.06 (0.99)	4.13 (0.357)	4.15 (0.330)
Ability to express emotions	3.96	3.97 (1.00)	3.96 (1.00)	3.96 (1.00)

For example, walking improved from 4.52 to 4.72. Seventeen indicators were measured for the NOC outcome Self-Care: Instrumental Activities of Daily Living (IADL). The average baseline was 3.87. The self-care indicators varied from ability to use a phone (4.8) demonstrated with ease to substantial decline in performing yard work (2.49) and for performing household repairs (2.62). Over time, the ability to perform the yard and household repairs continued to decline within 2 years to 2.37 and 2.47. The case managers were interested in the self-care indicator for managing medications. The baseline was 4.23, which improved to 4.37 in 2 years.

Conclusion

This demonstrates a process and methods that can use NIC and NOC to provide valuable information about patient care with case management services. In addition to the change in outcomes illustrated above, the case managers also had valuable data about the NIC interventions used with these patients. Analyzing the data from the interventions and outcomes together can provide information about the most effective outcomes for selected patient populations. In conclusion, the use of standardized nursing data for individual case use and aggregate patient population use drove the decisions for this design of the computerized application and workflow processes for the nurse working with this patient population.

Acknowledgments: To those who were in the early efforts to establish community case management services for clients and those identifying NIC interventions and NOC outcomes and indicators for use in practice: Larry Schumacher, Kim Larsen, Joan Zenner, Brenda Kern, Marie Cole, Frances Hoffman, Marsha Neff, Christy Wyborny, Marc Anderson, Linda Halsne and Sheila Allison.

SUMMARY

Successful implementation of NOC in a practice setting requires strong leadership and administrative commitment during both the planning and implementation phases. An area of paramount importance that must receive adequate attention in both phases is staff education. Without adequate education and sufficient opportunity to practice the use of a scaled outcome rather than an outcome goal, the implementation process will be faced with more problems than necessary. Questions that staff frequently raise when using NOC have been discussed in the section on issues. In addition to planning for staff education, the plan must address the resources required to implement a new documentation method and the software requirements if an electronic system is used. The examples in this chapter represent early efforts to use NOC in clinical settings. Many issues still need to be investigated related to use of indicators and how to measure the overall outcomes as adoption by agencies occurs.

References

1. Benner, P. (2004). Designing formal classification systems to better articulate knowledge, skills, and meanings in nursing practice. *American Journal of Critical Care, 13*(3), 426-430.
2. Committee on Quality Health Care in America, Institute of Medicine. (2001). *Crossing the quality chasm: A new heath system for the 21st century.* Washington, DC: National Academy Press.
3. Delaney, C., & Huber, D. (1996). *A nursing management minimum data set (NMMDS): A report of an invitational conference.* Chicago: American Organization of Nurse Executives, 1996.
4. Dochterman, J. M., & Bulechek, G. M. (Eds.). (2004). *Nursing interventions classification (NIC)* (4th ed.). St. Louis: Mosby.
5. HealthGrades. (2006). *Clinical excellence-DHA; Patient safety-DHA, Specialty excellence.* Retrieved November 15, 2006, from www.healthgrades.com
6. Iowa Intervention Project. (1997). *NIC implementation manual.* Iowa City, IA: The University of Iowa.
7. Johnson, M. R. (2002). Variables for outcome analysis. *Outcomes Management, 6*(3), 95-98.
8. Johnson, M., Bulechek, G., Butcher, H., Dochterman, J. M., Maas, M., Moorhead, S., & Swanson, E. (2006). *NANDA, NOC, and NIC Linkages.* St. Louis: Mosby.
9. Johnson, M., Maas, M., & Moorhead, S. (2000). *Nursing Outcomes Classification (NOC).* St. Louis: Mosby.
10. Keenan, G., & Aquilino, M. L. (1998). Standardized nomenclatures: Keys to continuity of care, nursing accountability and nursing effectiveness. *Outcomes Management for Nursing, 2*(2), 81-86.
11. Lagoe, R. J., Kurtzig, B. S., & Hohner, V. K. (1999). Health care data and their sources. *Journal of Nursing Care Quality, Special issue 1,* 7-24.
12. Lamb, G. S. (1993). Case management. In J. J. Fitzpatrick & J. S. Stevenson (Eds.), *Annual review of nursing research* (Vol. 13, pp. 117-136). New York: Springer.
13. Leville, S. G., Wagner, E. H., Davis, C., Grothaus, L., Wallace, J., Logerto, M., & Kent, D. (1998). Preventing disability and managing chronic illness in frail older adults. *Journal of American Geriatrics Society, 46*(10), 1191-1198.
14. McCloskey, J., & Bulechek, G. (Eds.). (2000). *Nursing interventions classification (NIC)* (3rd ed.). St. Louis: Mosby.
15. McDonald, C. J., Overhage, J. M., Dexter, P. R., Blevins, L., Meeks-Johnson, J., Suico, J. G., Tucker, M. C., & Schadow, G. (1998). Canopy computing: Using the Web in clinical practice. *Journal of the American Medical Association, 280,* 1325-1329.
16. Moorhead, S., Johnson, M., & Maas, M. (Eds.). (2004). *Nursing outcomes classification* (3rd ed.) (pp. 402, 407, 408). St. Louis: Mosby.
17. National Center for Health Statistics. (1980). *Uniform hospital discharge minimum data set* (Department of Health Education and Welfare Publication No. PHS 80-1157). Washington, DC: Department of Health Education and Welfare.
18. NANDA International. (2003). *Nursing diagnoses: Definitions and classification 2003-2004.* Philadelphia: Author.
19. NANDA International. (2007). *Nursing diagnoses: Definitions and classification 2007-2008.* Philadelphia: Author.
20. Pesut, D. J., & Herman, J. (1999). *Clinical reasoning: The art and science of critical and creative thinking.* Boston: Delmar.
21. Rubenfeld, M. G., & Scheffer, B. K. (1999). *Critical thinking in nursing: An interactive approach* (2nd ed.). Philadelphia: Lippincott Williams & Wilkins.
22. Schumacher, L. P., & Larson, K. A. (1993). Thriving and striving on the turbulence of rural health care. *Nursing Administration Quarterly, 18*(1), 11-15.
23. Sidani, S., & Braden, C. J. (1998). *Evaluating nursing interventions: A theory-driven approach.* Thousand Oaks, CA: Sage.
24. Werley, H. H., & Lang, N. M. (1989). *Identification of the nursing minimum data set.* New York: Springer.
25. White, K. (2003). Case management: Optimizing quality of life. In J. R. Giffith, K. R. White, & P. A. Cahill (Eds.), *Thinking forward: Six strategies for highly successful organizations.* Chicago: Health Administration Press.
26. Zenner, J. (1996). *Use of guarding in adults with chronic illness participating in nursing case management.* Published master's thesis, Mankato, MN: University of Minnesota.

CHAPTER FOUR

Using NOC in Education and Research

For standardized nursing languages such as NOC to become consistently used in nursing, the incorporation of the languages in nursing education and research is necessary. The use of standardized languages in education is becoming more prevalent as nursing textbooks are beginning to use the languages and faculty members are becoming more familiar with the languages. The validation of standardized languages and their use in nursing research is in its infancy, but the implementation of evidence-based practice and the electronic health record will offer more opportunities to test the use of standardized languages in practice settings.

IMPLEMENTING NOC IN EDUCATIONAL PROGRAMS

Implementation of standardized languages, including NOC, throughout a curriculum requires a high level of commitment on the part of faculty and academic administration. All facets of the curriculum—the philosophy, program goals, and individual course objectives—need to reflect this commitment. Frequently, one or more faculty members become interested in piloting a standardized language in a course, use the language in the course, and then encourage its adoption throughout the curriculum. They can act as the project leaders in educating other faculty and demonstrating how course content can be adapted to include NOC and other standardized languages.

Selecting the Standardized Language(s)

Seldom is NOC the only standardized language introduced in a curriculum. Many programs have been using NANDA diagnoses and are moving toward the implementation of NOC and NIC to complete the process of identifying the diagnoses, outcomes, and interventions that students use as they learn the nursing process and plan care for their patients. The fact that the three languages have not been presented together has made implementation throughout the curriculum more difficult. However, movement toward bringing the languages closer together bodes well for expediting their use in curricula. One of the results of the cooperation between NANDA and the authors of NIC and NOC has been the development of a taxonomy structure that can encompass all three languages.[8] The NOC outcomes were placed in the taxonomy and provided in Appendix B in the third edition of the NOC classification.[21] That was the first attempt at using the taxonomy for NOC outcomes, and changes in the taxonomy and the placement of the languages within the taxonomy are likely to occur as a result of feedback from users. The taxonomy is not included in this edition since potential changes are not complete. Another development has been the second edition of a book that links the three languages.[13] The linkages in the book use the terminology from the third edition of NOC[21] and are based on expert opinion and some clinical data. Additionally, publications studying the links among the three languages are beginning to appear in the literature.

Many programs have been using NANDA diagnoses, thereby making it easier to incorporate NIC and NOC, two languages that can be used in conjunction with NANDA. Use of NANDA, NIC, and NOC as the standardized languages in a curriculum has a number of advantages. The languages can be used across all clinical settings in which students have their learning experiences. The languages can be used throughout the curriculum and can serve as an organizing thread. The use of standardized languages better prepare students for the future as electronic records become routine. The languages can increase the student's critical thinking skills if implemented in a manner to do so. Students and nurses who don't have to break other habits often find the languages easier to use than nurses who have not been exposed to standardized languages in their nursing program.

Implementation Strategies

A number of strategies can be used when planning how NOC will be implemented throughout the undergraduate curriculum. One strategy assumes the implementation of NANDA diagnoses, NIC, and NOC and includes the following steps.[6]

1. Determine which diagnoses are used in each course and clinical area. This can be done by individual faculty, by faculty in each course, or by the faculty as a whole.
2. Identify diagnoses used in more than one course and those not used in any of the courses. Determine how these will be handled—taught in more than one course, assigned to one course, not used in the curriculum. This task can be accomplished with a group representing all clinical courses or the faculty as a whole.
3. Select the NOC outcomes that are frequently selected for each of the diagnoses. This can be done by using some of the linkage work or selecting the outcomes that can be used in place of previously used goal statements.
4. Identify the NIC interventions taught in each course. This can be done with a survey that lists all of the courses on the horizontal axis and the interventions on the vertical axis. It can also be accomplished by substituting the appropriate NIC intervention label for the interventions currently taught in each course.
5. As a group, delete all interventions that will not be taught in the undergraduate curriculum.
6. Match all of the interventions that will be used to one of the diagnoses and the associated outcomes. You may find some disparity, most likely some interventions that do not fit a diagnosis. Decide how these interventions will be handled—remain in the curriculum or be deleted.

The end result should be a curriculum that includes a list of diagnoses matched to outcomes and interventions that reflects the goals of the program. The last step is to decide in which course each of the diagnoses and associated interventions and outcomes will be taught. Although time consuming, this strategy preserves critical thinking and allows patient problems, nursing diagnoses, and nursing interventions appropriate for the student level to drive the system.

Another strategy that can be used is to begin with the core interventions used by 43 clinical specialties[7] and determine which of these are appropriate for the undergraduate program. These interventions can be mapped to the interventions currently taught in the course, an exercise that can help faculty decide whether they want to eliminate some of the interventions previously taught or add to the interventions previously taught. Steps similar to those identified above can then be used to link the selected interventions with the appropriate nursing diagnoses and patient outcomes.

Aids for Curriculum Development and Teaching

Detailed suggestions for implementing the languages in a curriculum are provided in a manual by Finesilver and Metzler[10] that can be obtained through the Center for Nursing Classification and Clinical Effectiveness. The manual describes courses in one undergraduate program and includes methods, forms, and teaching aids used in the classes. This and other publications and abstracts that the educator might find helpful are listed in Box 4-1.

The linkages provided in this book, in the Nursing Interventions Classification book,[7] and in the NANDA, NOC, NIC linkage book[13] can assist with the process. These linkages can be used as a teaching tool when students are learning to become familiar with the languages and beginning to plan care. The article by Dr. Yom and associates provides a set of linkages developed for patients undergoing abdominal surgery in Korea.[24] It can provide an opportunity to discuss similarities and differences in the outcomes for patients in Korea and the United States as well as

Box 4-1

Publications Useful for Educators

Burkhart, L. (2006). Integrating NNN into nursing education: A case study. *International Journal of Nursing Terminologies & Classifications, 17*(1), 22.

Denehy, J. (1998). Integrating nursing outcomes classification in nursing education. *Journal of Nursing Care Quality, 12*(5), 73-84.

Finesilver, C., & Metzler, D. (Eds.). (2002). *Curriculum guide for implementation of NANDA, NIC, and NOC into an undergraduate nursing curriculum.* Iowa City, IA: College of Nursing, Center for Nursing Classification and Clinical Effectiveness.

Flatt, M. (2003). Teaching systems transformation. *International Journal of Nursing Terminologies & Classifications, 14*(4), 35.

Kautz, D. D., Kuiper, R., Pesut, D. J., & Williams, R. L. (2006). Using NANDA, NIC, and NOC (NNN) language for clinical reasoning with the outcome-present state-test (OPT) model. *International Journal of Nursing Terminologies and Classifications, 17*(3), 129-138.

Krenz, M. (2003). The use of NOC to direct a competency-based curriculum. *International Journal of Nursing Terminologies & Classifications, 14*(4), 59.

Maas, M. L., Buckwalter, K. C., Hardy, M. D., Tripp-Reimer, T., Titler, M., & Specht, J. P. (Eds.). (2001). *Nursing care of older adults: Diagnoses, outcomes, and interventions.* St. Louis: Mosby. (An example of a text using NANDA, NOC, NIC)

information to use when identifying the NNN linkages for use in the curriculum. (It should be noted that the column on page 85 is mislabeled: the terms in one of the nursing intervention columns are actually the nursing outcome terms.) Another resource is the list-serve available through the Center for Nursing Classification and Clinical Effectiveness at The University of Iowa (to be added to this list-serve send an email to classification-center@uiowa.edu). The members are a diverse group that includes educators as well as practitioners, and they discuss issues related to the use of NIC and NOC in education as well as in practice.

The authors recognize that the knowledge outcomes, while important in their own right, are generally precursors to altering selected patient behaviors. For this reason, we have identified NOC outcomes that can be used to measure behaviors related to the NOC knowledge outcomes; these are provided in Table 4-1. The primary behavioral outcomes are those directly related to the knowledge outcome, for example, Body Mechanics Performance for Knowledge: Body Mechanics. In general, the primary behavioral outcomes reflect both the knowledge definition and indicators found in the knowledge outcome. Secondary behavioral outcomes are those that are related less directly to the knowledge outcome; the relationship can be more directly tied to specific indicators than the overall concept, for example, Transfer Performance for Knowledge: Body Mechanics. The behavioral outcome in the secondary column can also be more specific than the knowledge outcome, for example, Asthma Self-Management for Knowledge: Disease Process, a more generic outcome.

Once decisions about the placement of the standardized languages in the curriculum are made, the next step is the implementation in the curriculum and in course work. The description of the use of NOC in the previous chapter can be helpful in the educational setting. A major difference is the emphasis on teaching students clinical decision making. The following case study presents the implementation of NOC in one academic setting. The Outcome-Present State Test (OPT) model[22] was introduced along with standardized languages throughout the curriculum to teach clinical decision making and critical thinking skills. An additional reference using the OPT model can be found in Box 4-1.

Table 4-1	NOC PERFORMANCE OUTCOMES RELATED TO NOC KNOWLEDGE OUTCOMES	
Knowledge Outcomes	**Primary Behavioral Outcomes**	**Secondary Behavioral Outcomes**
All Knowledge Outcomes	1600 Adherence Behavior 1601 Compliance Behavior 1606 Participation in Health Care Decisions	1705 Health Orientation 1209 Motivation 1614 Personal Autonomy
1831 Knowledge: Arthritis Management	1308 Adaptation to Physical Disability 0200 Ambulation 0206 Joint Movement 0213 & 0221 Joint Movement: Specific Joint 1605 Pain Control 0300 Self-Care: Activities of Daily Living (ADL)	0002 Energy Conservation 1909 Fall Prevention Behavior 0208 Mobility 1309 Personal Resiliency 1305 Psychosocial Adjustment: Life Change 0313 Self-Care Status
1832 Knowledge: Asthma Management	0704 Asthma Self-Management 0002 Energy Conservation 1603 Health Seeking Behavior 1608 Symptom Control 1924 Risk Control: Infectious Process	1300 Acceptance: Health Status 2605 Family Participation in Professional Care 1702 Health Beliefs: Perceived Control 0308 Self-Care: Oral Hygiene 1625 Smoking Cessation Behavior 1609 Treatment Behavior: Illness or Injury
1827 Knowledge: Body Mechanics	1616 Body Mechanics Performance	0200 Ambulation 0201 Ambulation: Wheelchair 0203 Body Positioning: Self-Initiated 0210 Transfer Performance
1800 Knowledge: Breastfeeding	1000 Breastfeeding Establishment: Infant 1001 Breastfeeding Establishment: Maternal 1002 Breastfeeding Maintenance 1003 Breastfeeding Weaning	0110 Growth 1008 Nutritional Status: Food & Fluid Intake 1500 Parent-Infant Attachment
1833 Knowledge: Cancer Management	1603 Health Seeking Behavior 1618 Nausea & Vomiting Control 1605 Pain Control 1606 Participation in Health-Care Decisions 1608 Symptom Control	1302 Coping 1409 Depression Self-Control 2609 Family Support During Treatment 1309 Personal Resiliency 1305 Psychosocial Adjustment: Life Change 1924 Risk Control: Infectious Process
1834 Knowledge: Cancer Threat Reduction	1602 Health Promoting Behavior 1917 Risk Control: Cancer 1906 Risk Control: Tobacco Use 1908 Risk Detection	1704 Health Beliefs: Perceived Threat 1625 Smoking Cessation Behavior
1830 Knowledge: Cardiac Disease Management	1617 Cardiac Disease Self-Management 1622 Compliance Behavior: Prescribed Diet 1603 Health Seeking Behavior 1914 Risk Control: Cardiovascular Health 1608 Symptom Control	1308 Adaptation to Physical Disability 0002 Energy Conservation 2605 Family Participation in Professional Care 2609 Family Support During Treatment 1305 Psychosocial Adjustment: Life Change 1902 Risk Control 1625 Smoking Cessation Behavior 1609 Treatment Behavior: Illness or Injury

Table 4-1	NOC PERFORMANCE OUTCOMES RELATED TO NOC KNOWLEDGE OUTCOMES—cont'd	
Knowledge Outcomes	**Primary Behavioral Outcomes**	**Secondary Behavioral Outcomes**
1801 Knowledge: Child Physical Safety	2902 Parenting: Adolescent Physical Safety 2900 Parenting: Infant/Toddler Physical Safety 2901 Parenting: Early/Middle Childhood Physical Safety 1901 Parenting: Psychosocial Safety 2211 Parenting Performance	2501 Abuse Protection 1910 Safe Home Environment
1821 Knowledge: Conception Prevention	1907 Risk Control: Unintended Pregnancy	1902 Risk Control 1905 Risk Control: Sexually Transmitted Diseases (STD)
1835 Knowledge: Congestive Heart Failure Management	1617 Cardiac Disease Self-Management 1622 Compliance Behavior: Prescribed Diet 0002 Energy Conservation 1603 Health Seeking Behavior 1608 Symptom Control	1308 Adaptation to Physical Disability 2605 Family Participation in Professional Care 1305 Psychosocial Adjustment: Life Change 1902 Risk Control 1914 Risk Control: Cardiovascular Health 1625 Smoking Cessation Behavior 1609 Treatment Behavior: Illness or Injury 1628 Weight Maintenance Behavior
1836 Knowledge: Depression Management	1623 Compliance Behavior: Prescribed Medication 1409 Depression Self-Control 1408 Suicide Self-Restraint	1606 Participation in Health Care Decisions 1503 Social Involvement 1608 Symptom Control
1820 Knowledge: Diabetes Management	1622 Compliance Behavior: Prescribed Diet 1623 Compliance Behavior: Prescribed Medication 1619 Diabetes Self-Management 1603 Health Seeking Behavior 1608 Symptom Control 1628 Weight Maintenance Behavior	1008 Nutritional Status: Food & Fluid Intake 1902 Risk Control 1916 Risk Control: Visual Impairment 0119 Sexual Functioning 1609 Treatment Behavior: Illness or Injury 1611 Vision Compensation Behavior 1627 Weight Loss Behavior
1802 Knowledge: Diet	1621 Adherence Behavior: Healthy Diet 1622 Compliance Behavior: Prescribed Diet 1008 Nutritional Status: Food & Fluid Intake 1626 Weight Gain Behavior 1627 Weight Loss Behavior 1628 Weight Maintenance Behavior	1603 Health Seeking Behavior 1607 Prenatal Health Behavior 1609 Treatment Behavior: Illness or Injury
1803 Knowledge: Disease Process	1603 Health Seeking Behavior 1608 Symptom Control 1609 Treatment Behavior: Illness or Injury	1402 Anxiety Self-Control 1918 Aspiration Prevention 0704 Asthma Self-Management 1616 Body Mechanics Performance 1617 Cardiac Disease Self-Management 1409 Depression Self-Control 1619 Diabetes Self-Management

Continued

Table 4-1 NOC PERFORMANCE OUTCOMES RELATED TO NOC KNOWLEDGE OUTCOMES—cont'd

Knowledge Outcomes	Primary Behavioral Outcomes	Secondary Behavioral Outcomes
		1403 Distorted Thought Self-Control
		1610 Hearing Compensation Behavior
		0918 Heedfulness of Affected Side
		1405 Impulse Self-Control
		1631 Multiple Sclerosis Self-Management
		1618 Nauseas & Vomiting Control
		1615 Ostomy Self-Care
		1605 Pain Control
		1911 Personal Safety Behavior
		1620 Seizure Control
		1406 Self-Mutilation Restraint
		1408 Suicide Self-Restraint
		1611 Vision Compensation Behavior
1804 Knowledge: Energy Conservation	0002 Energy Conservation 1602 Health Promoting Behavior	0200 Ambulation 1616 Body Mechanics Performance
1828 Knowledge: Fall Prevention	1909 Fall Prevention Behavior	0200 Ambulation 0201 Ambulation: Wheelchair 0918 Heedfulness of Affected Side 1910 Safe Home Environment 0210 Transfer Performance
1816 Knowledge: Fertility Promotion	1607 Prenatal Health Behavior 0119 Sexual Functioning	1905 Risk Control: Sexually Transmitted Diseases (STD) 1908 Risk Detection

1805 Knowledge: Health Behavior	1602 Health Promoting Behavior
	1900 Immunization Behavior
	1911 Personal Safety Behavior
	1902 Risk Control
	1903 Risk Control: Alcohol Use
	1917 Risk Control: Cancer
	1914 Risk Control: Cardiovascular
	    Health
	1904 Risk Control: Drug Use
	1915 Risk Control: Hearing Impairment
	
	1922 Risk Control: Hyperthermia
	1923 Risk Control: Hypothermia
	1924 Risk Control: Infectious Process
	1905 Risk Control: Sexually
	    Transmitted Diseases (STD)
	1906 Risk Control: Tobacco Use
	1907 Risk Control: Unintended
	    Pregnancy
	1916 Risk Control: Visual Impairment
	1908 Risk Detection
		1621 Adherence Behavior: Healthy Diet
		1402 Anxiety Self-Control
		1616 Body Mechanics Performance
		2801 Community Risk Control:
		    Chronic Disease
		2802 Community Risk Control:
		    Communicable Disease
		2803 Community Risk Control:
		    Lead Exposure
		2805 Community Risk Control:
		    Violence
		1302 Coping
		0002 Energy Conservation
		1909 Fall Prevention Behavior
		1405 Impulse Self-Control
		1604 Leisure Participation
		1008 Nutritional Status: Food &
		    Fluid Intake
		1607 Prenatal Health Behavior
		1625 Smoking Cessation Behavior
		1628 Weight Maintenance Behavior

1823 Knowledge: Health Promotion	1602 Health Promoting Behavior 1900 Immunization Behavior 1911 Personal Safety Behavior	1903 Risk Control: Alcohol Use 1904 Risk Control: Drug Use 1905 Risk Control: Sexually Transmitted Diseases (STD)

Table 4-1   NOC Performance Outcomes Related to NOC Knowledge Outcomes—cont'd

Knowledge Outcomes	Primary Behavioral Outcomes	Secondary Behavioral Outcomes
	1908 Risk Detection	1906 Risk Control: Tobacco Use 1628 Weight Maintenance Behavior
1806 Knowledge: Health Resources	2206 Caregiver Performance: Indirect Care	1308 Adaptation to Physical Disability 2700 Community Competence 2602 Family Functioning
1837 Knowledge: Hypertension Management	1622 Compliance Behavior: Prescribed Diet 1603 Health Seeking Behavior 1608 Symptom Control	1625 Smoking Cessation Behavior 1609 Treatment Behavior: Illness or Injury 1628 Weight Maintenance Behavior
1824 Knowledge: Illness Care	2205 Caregiver Performance: Direct Care 1603 Health Seeking Behavior 1618 Nausea & Vomiting Control 1605 Pain Control 1613 Self-Direction of Care 1608 Symptom Control 1609 Treatment Behavior: Illness or Injury	1308 Adaptation to Physical Disability 1918 Aspiration Prevention 2206 Caregiver Performance: Indirect Care 1301 Child Adaptation to Hospitalization 0002 Energy Conservation 1909 Fall Prevention Behavior 2605 Family Participation in Professional Care 2609 Family Support During Treatment 1008 Nutritional Status: Food & Fluid Intake 1615 Ostomy Self-Care 1921 Pre-Procedure Readiness 1902 Risk Control 1628 Weight Maintenance Behavior
1819 Knowledge: Infant Care	1500 Parent-Infant Attachment 2900 Parenting: Infant/Toddler Physical Safety 2211 Parenting Performance 1901 Parenting: Psychosocial Safety	2501 Abuse Protection 1400 Abusive Behavior Self-Restraint 1001 Breastfeeding Establishment: Maternal 2608 Family Resiliency 1900 Immunization Behavior
1842 Knowledge: Infection Management	1900 Immunization Behavior 1905 Risk Control: Sexually Transmitted Diseases (STD) 1924 Risk Control: Infectious Process	2800 Community Health Status: Immunity 2802 Community Risk Control: Communicable Disease 1607 Prenatal Health Behavior 1902 Risk Control 1908 Risk Detection
1817 Knowledge: Labor & Delivery		1302 Coping 0002 Energy Conservation 2605 Family Participation in Professional Care 1605 Pain Control
1808 Knowledge: Medication	2205 Caregiver Performance: Direct Care 1623 Compliance Behavior: Prescribed Medication 0307 Self-Care: Non-Parenteral Medication 0309 Self-Care: Parenteral Medication	1911 Personal Safety Behavior 1613 Self-Direction of Care
1838 Knowledge: Multiple Sclerosis Management	1603 Health Seeking Behavior 1631 Multiple Sclerosis Self-Management 1608 Symptom Control	1622 Compliance Behavior: Prescribed Diet 1606 Participation in Health Care Decisions

Continued

Table 4-1	NOC PERFORMANCE OUTCOMES RELATED TO NOC KNOWLEDGE OUTCOMES—cont'd

Knowledge Outcomes	Primary Behavioral Outcomes	Secondary Behavioral Outcomes
1829 Knowledge: Ostomy Care	1615 Ostomy Self-Care 1609 Treatment Behavior: Illness or Injury	0305 Self-Care: Hygiene
1843 Knowledge: Pain Management	1623 Compliance Behavior: Prescribed Medication 1605 Pain Control 1608 Symptom Control	1616 Body Mechanics Performance 1617 Cardiac Disease Self-Management 1601 Compliance Behavior 1302 Coping 0002 Energy Conservation 1618 Nausea and Vomiting Control 1606 Participation in Health Care Decisions 0307 Self-Care: Non-Parenteral Medication 0309 Self-Care: Parenteral Medication
1826 Knowledge: Parenting	2902 Parenting: Adolescent Physical Safety 2901 Parenting: Early/Middle Childhood Physical Safety 2900 Parenting: Infant/Toddler Physical Safety 2211 Parenting Performance 1901 Parenting: Psychosocial Safety	2501 Abuse Protection 2602 Family Functioning 2608 Family Resiliency 1500 Parent-Infant Attachment 0116 Play Participation 1501 Role Performance
1809 Knowledge: Personal Safety	1909 Fall Prevention Behavior 1911 Personal Safety Behavior 1910 Safe Home Environment	1616 Body Mechanics Performance 1405 Impulse Self-Control 1902 Risk Control 1903 Risk Control: Alcohol Use 1904 Risk Control: Drug Use 1922 Risk Control: Hyperthermia 1923 Risk Control: Hypothermia 1908 Risk Detection 0210 Transfer Performance
1818 Knowledge: Postpartum Maternal Health	1302 Coping 1624 Postpartum Maternal Health Behavior 1305 Psychosocial Adjustment: Life Change	1001 Breastfeeding Establishment: Maternal 0002 Energy Conservation 2605 Family Participation in Professional Care 1008 Nutritional Status: Food & Fluid Intake 1907 Risk Control: Unintended Pregnancy
1822 Knowledge: Preconception Maternal Health	1602 Health Promoting Behavior 1607 Prenatal Health Behavior	1911 Personal Safety Behavior 1905 Risk Control: Sexually Transmitted Diseases (STD) 1908 Risk Detection 1910 Safe Home Environment
1810 Knowledge: Pregnancy	1602 Health Promoting Behavior 1607 Prenatal Health Behavior	2501 Abuse Protection 1616 Body Mechanics Performance 0002 Energy Conservation 1618 Nausea & Vomiting Control 1008 Nutritional Status: Food & Fluid Intake 1902 Risk Control 1908 Risk Detection 1910 Safe Home Environment 1628 Weight Maintenance Behavior

Table 4-1	NOC Performance Outcomes Related to NOC Knowledge Outcomes—cont'd	

Knowledge Outcomes	Primary Behavioral Outcomes	Secondary Behavioral Outcomes
1839 Knowledge: Pregnancy & Postpartum Sexual Functioning	1624 Postpartum Maternal Health Behavior 1907 Risk Control: Unintended Pregnancy 0119 Sexual Functioning	2501 Abuse Protection 1607 Prenatal Health Behavior 1905 Risk Control: Sexually Transmitted Diseases (STD)
1811 Knowledge: Prescribed Activity	0200 Ambulation 1609 Treatment Behavior: Illness or Injury	1308 Adaptation to Physical Disability 0201 Ambulation: Wheelchair 1616 Body Mechanics Performance 0203 Body Positioning: Self-Initiated 1607 Prenatal Health Behavior 0210 Transfer Performance
1840 Knowledge: Preterm Infant Care	1500 Parent-Infant Attachment 2211 Parenting Performance	2202 Caregiver Home Care Readiness 2205 Caregiver Performance: Direct Care 2206 Caregiver Performance: Indirect Care 1305 Psychosocial Adjustment: Life Change
1815 Knowledge: Sexual Functioning	0119 Sexual Functioning	1905 Risk Control: Sexually Transmitted Diseases (STD) 1907 Risk Control: Unintended Pregnancy
1812 Knowledge: Substance Use Control	1903 Risk Control: Alcohol Use 1904 Risk Control: Drug Use 1906 Risk Control: Tobacco Use	1405 Impulse Self-Control 1911 Personal Safety Behavior
1814 Knowledge: Treatment Procedure	2205 Caregiver Performance: Direct Care 1921 Pre-Procedure Readiness 1613 Self-Direction of Care 1609 Treatment Behavior: Illness or Injury	1918 Aspiration Prevention 2609 Family Support During Treatment 1615 Ostomy Self-Care 0210 Transfer Performance
1813 Knowledge: Treatment Regimen	2205 Caregiver Performance: Direct Care 1613 Self-Direction of Care 1608 Symptom Control 1609 Treatment Behavior: Illness or Injury	1308 Adaptation to Physical Disability 0704 Asthma Self-Management 1617 Cardiac Disease Self-Management 2206 Caregiver Performance: Indirect Care 1619 Diabetes Self-Management
1841 Knowledge: Weight Management	1626 Weight Gain Behavior 1627 Weight Loss Behavior 1628 Weight Maintenance Behavior	1008 Nutritional Status: Food & Fluid Intake 1622 Compliance Behavior: Prescribed Diet

CASE STUDY

Implementing Languages in an OPT Model Curriculum

Carme Espinosa i Fresnedo

The School of Nursing of the University of Andorra was created in 1988. This is a School of Nursing with some special characteristics. It is the only nursing school in the country of Andorra, and the number of students per course is limited to a maximum of 25. These features are a consequence of the special characteristics of Andorra.

Andorra is a small country located in Europe, between Spain and France in the middle of the Pyrenees. The average elevation is between 838 m and 2942 m above sea level. The country is 468 square kilometers in area, and the current population is around 77,000 inhabitants.

The health system facilities in Andorra consist of one hospital (with around 200 beds, an ICU, an OB unit, etc.), a primary health care network, and some residences for elderly people. The health care system follows a mixed model in which both the people and a welfare system share the accountability for the payment of health care. In the mid-1980s, there was a severe shortage of nurses, and the Andorran government created the School of Nursing in an attempt to solve the problem. From the very beginning, the education of nurses was at the university level. The students obtained the degree of University Diploma in Nursing once they completed the education program. The education program consists of 3 years of full-time education with half of the content in practice and half of the content in theory, which is a total of approximately 4600 education hours.

Currently, the education program of the School of Nursing has finished a review process required to adapt the educational contents to the process of Harmonization of the European Higher Education Area (EHEA). It was at the beginning of the process when the NOC taxonomy was introduced as a part of the educational curriculum in the school.

Rational for Using NOC

In the year 2000, the director of the School of Nursing and two nursing teachers were invited to visit the Center for Nursing Classification and Clinical Effectiveness (CNC) at The University of Iowa. There we had the opportunity to speak with the principal researchers of both the NOC project and the NIC project, along with other researchers and teachers. That experience made us think about the advantages of using Standardized Nursing Languages (SNL) within the curriculum of nursing. Thanks to the people in the CNC, we came back home with the textbooks of NOC and NIC and a textbook that would help us identify a methodology to implement the languages at the basic curriculum of nursing education.

The Situation Before the Use of NOC and NIC

From the very beginning of the School of Nursing, the teachers were very concerned about teaching "nursing," but without a proper language, we were constantly using medical terminology to designate nursing elements. At that time, there was a great effort to implement NANDA diagnoses as a way of describing nursing problems, but the lack of an adequate methodology to teach and learn the diagnostic process made it extremely difficult. The nursing care plan process has been a part of the nursing curriculum from the very beginning of the School, but both the teachers and the students have faced enormous difficulties.

Once a student was able to identify an adequate nursing diagnosis (using NANDA taxonomy), the next challenge was to be able to identify an adequate outcome for the diagnosis. Most of the time, the outcome expressed only the lack of the problem, and each student was using his or her own language to describe that outcome. That made it quite difficult to assess whether the outcome was the most adequate for that situation.

Regarding the identification of nursing interventions, at that time, we were independently using the words *intervention*, *action*, or *type of care* to describe nursing care. Once more, the students identified the nursing interventions using their natural language. Some of them wrote very detailed nursing actions, while others tended to be more general and used wider descriptions for the same activities.

To provide a general picture of the situation, the nursing care plan that we were using at that time was the traditional linear method, which was extremely difficult to understand by the students. That kind of nursing care plan was not used in practice settings by the nurses. The result of that situation was that our students considered the nursing care plan as a "theoretical exercise that they needed to do in order to pass the subject, and then forget about it."

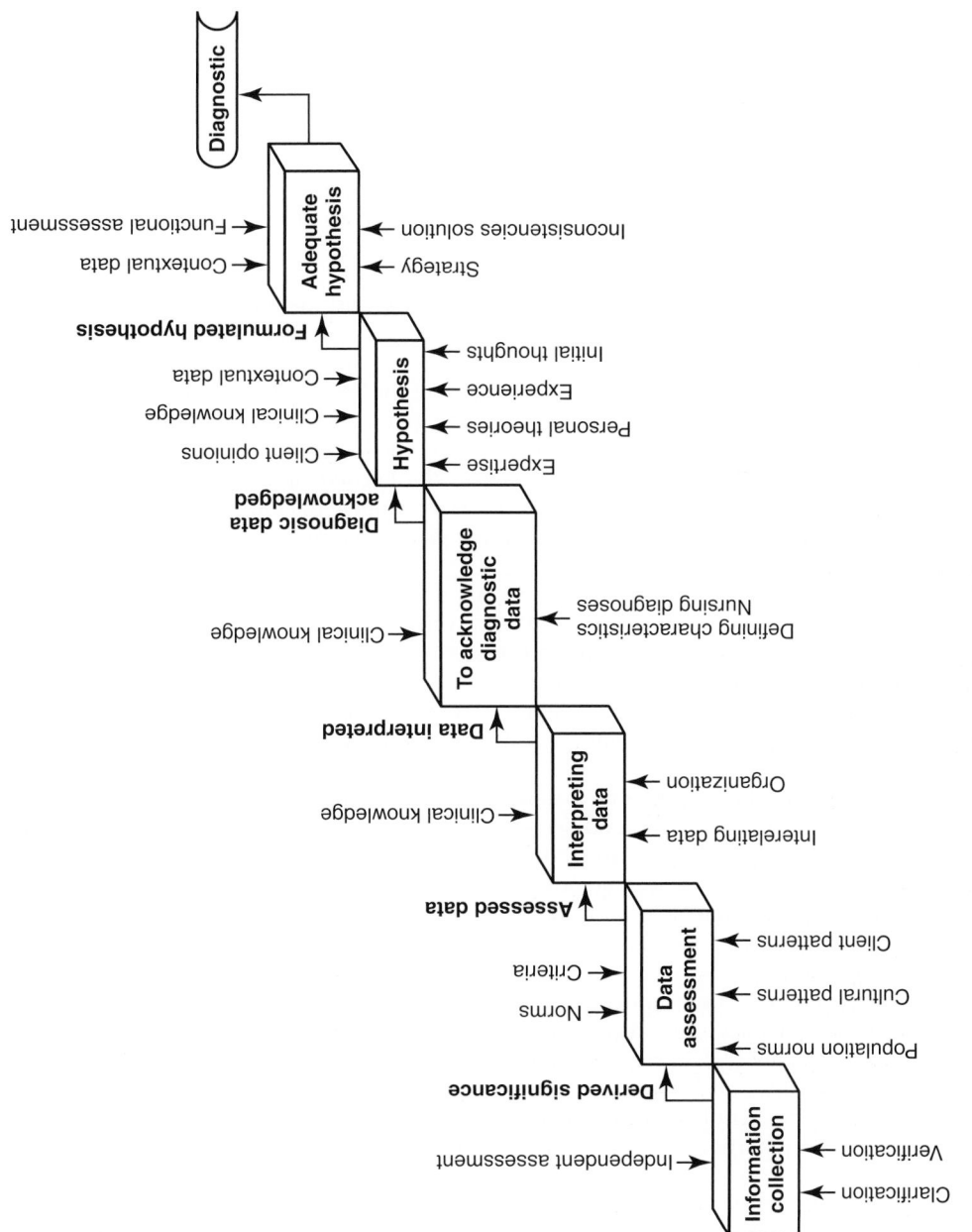

Fig. 4-1 Diagnostic process.

The Change

The first change implemented was the use of Marjory Gordon's Functional Patterns as a guide to collect information. To learn the diagnostic process, we used Gordon's methodology in correlation with the theory of process, resulting in the scheme in Figure 4-1. Later we abandoned the traditional nursing care plan process, and adopted Pesut's Model of Critical Thinking. Together with Pesut's Model, we decided to implement standardized nursing languages (NANDA, NOC, and NIC).

With all of those changes, we expected to solve most of the difficulties that we were facing at that moment. The students should be able to use a model of thinking that was similar to real life, and then be able to describe nursing diagnoses, outcomes, and interventions using SNL. The process was long and complex. But today, nursing languages are now used by all our nursing teachers and all our students as the current and only languages to speak about nursing.

The Implementation Process

We cannot differentiate between the implementation of NOC and the other languages, because we implemented all of them together.

First Things First

The first step was to achieve the support of the Director of the School. Then a person was nominated to be in charge of the implementation process. This person was given all the resources, the books, and the time to think about how to best implement the languages. Then a working group was created with four full-time nurses. Access to all the needed materials was given to the members of the group. The first thing the team did was to evaluate the implications of the implementation of the languages in the curriculum. At that stage, communication with the principal researchers of NOC and NIC was fundamental.

Making a Plan

A plan was made, the targets of the implementation were established, and a study was carried out to assess the factors that could make the process of implementation easier or more difficult. The decision was made that the three languages had to be implemented from the beginning of the curriculum and in all nursing subjects. The next challenge was to decide which NANDA diagnoses, NOC outcomes, and NIC interventions were to be implemented at each level and within which subject.

NOC was revealed to be the keystone to define the level of competency ideally developed by the students in each course. We asked ourselves, "What should a freshman student be able to achieve in relation to different nursing diagnoses? And a second-year student? And a third-year student? Are there outcomes that need an advanced education?" By answering these questions, we were able to determine what NOC outcomes, NIC interventions and NANDA diagnoses were to be taught at each level, and the skeleton of our nursing curriculum began to take shape.

Implementing the Plan

The implementation of the plan included the following main actions:

Revision of the programs for each course and subject. Apart from the revision that was needed to adapt our curriculum to the new EHEA, we tried to establish how nursing content would relate to the content of other disciplines, such as pathophysiology, pharmacology, etc. The pedagogical model to be used needed to be identified because it was vital to the implementation process. The final step was to decide what portion of the existing content needed to be discarded and what needed to be added.

Progressive implementation of the languages. The implementation began in the academic year between 2000 and 2001. We carried out a pilot test on the methodology. After establishing that it worked, we began the implementation of some NANDA nursing diagnoses and some NIC interventions in 2001 and 2002. But the nursing teachers said that it would be very difficult to implement those languages in an adequate way, unless NOC outcomes were added. For this reason, in 2002 and 2003, we introduced some of the NOC outcomes. That was the academic year in which nearly all of the languages were implemented in the three courses and the new curriculum was fully implemented for the freshman year students. The first students fully educated using NANDA, NOC, and NIC graduated in 2005.

Continuous participant information. During the entire implementation process, communication among participants was a key issue. Nurses using the languages have always had someone to help with doubts, problems, questions, etc. The other crucial point of information has been the practice settings. All nurses responsible for students during practice have been informed about the changes, and when needed, special sessions of information and education have been provided. The last action put in place was a postgraduate course on SNL that has been running in our school for the last 3 years, in order to facilitate SNL learning by nurses already working in the health care system.

General Structure of the Curriculum

Once the implementation process was completed, the general structure of our curriculum was as follows:

Freshman year. The students learn about SNL. What are Standardized Nursing Languages, what is their utility, why must nurses use SNL? They also learn the basis of the nursing process to be used along with the languages. In the subject of Adult Nursing, during the second and third term, they begin to use SNL (NANDA, NOC, and NIC) at a very basic level.

Second year. The students use SNL on a daily basis to solve current situations in practice settings and to prepare all Nursing Care Plans. The students learn how to use SNL and combine the autonomous role of the nurse (nursing diagnoses) together with a more collaborative role, relating interdependent problems linked to medical problems.

Third year. The students use SNL to solve case scenarios in critical care settings and specific areas such as Mental Health, Mother and Child Nursing, Gerontological Nursing, etc.

The following examples show how the students of the School of Nursing of Andorra use the OPT model and SNL in the curriculum.

Figure 4-2 illustrates the OPT clinical reasoning model used in the curriculum. Figure 4-3 illustrates the reasoning used to identify the keystone nursing diagnosis for a patient admitted with a cerebrovascular accident (CVA). The outer circles are the nursing diagnoses identified for the patient. The clinical reasoning process used with this model creates the web connecting the diagnoses with the majority of lines converging on the diagnosis: Ineffective Tissue Perfusion: Cerebral, the keystone diagnosis. A similar process is used to identify the outcome (Figure 4-4) and the interventions (Figure 4-5). Figure 4-6 illustrates the outcome indicators selected for this particular patient and the defining characteristics for the diagnosis. Information about the patient taken from the admission history, physical examination, and orders appears on the right side of the figure; the information the nurse would have prior to beginning the reasoning process is used here.

Conclusion

Nursing and the nursing profession existed long before SNL. As a professional activity, modern nursing began with Florence Nightingale in the nineteenth century. Since then, nursing has made great advances both from a humanistic and technological point of view. We need to be aware, though, that nursing is not yet fully considered a science. One of the reasons for this might be the lack of a proper language to communicate what nursing is and what part of science is developed by the nursing discipline. By implementing SNL in basic education, it becomes the natural professional language that allows nurses to communicate within their discipline, as well as with other professionals and the community.

Nursing was defined by Jenkins as "the profession which does what is not measurable, finite, packaged and accountable, in an increasingly IT-dominated world" (p. 90).[12] Without a language that allows nursing to be included in electronic information systems, the profession and its science will stay out of the health system. Nursing will stay as an invisible profession, although nurses are the most numerous professionals in the health system.

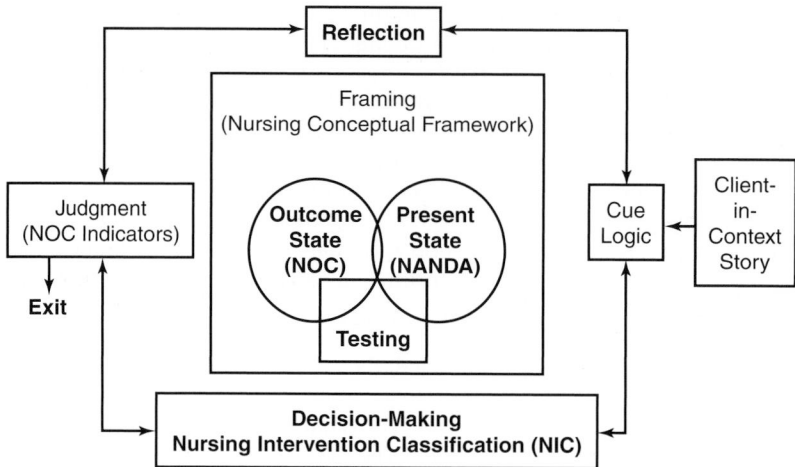

Fig. 4-2 Integrating Outcome Present State Test (OPT) Model with NANDA, NIC, and NOC. (Modified from Pesut and Herman.)

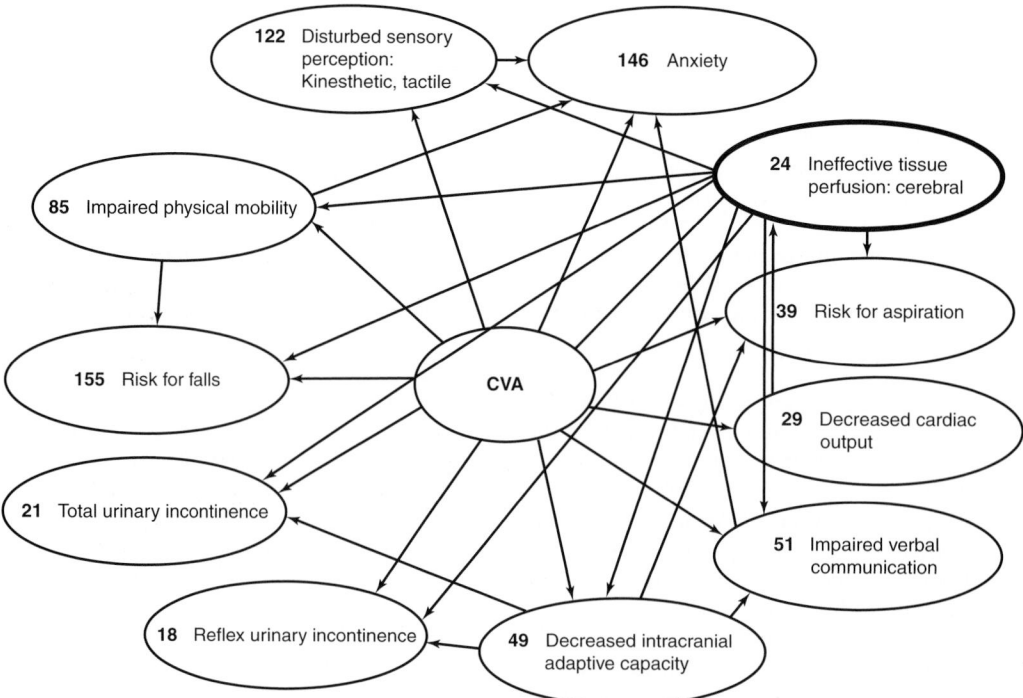

Fig. 4-3 Clinical reasoning web for patient with CVA depicting selection of keystone NANDA diagnosis.

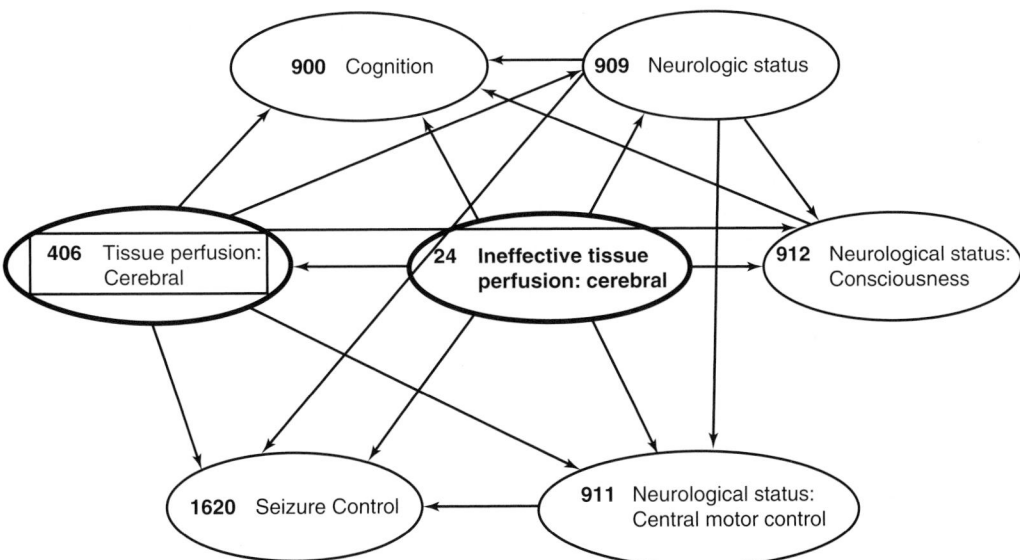

Fig. 4-4 Clinical reasoning web depicting selection of keystone NOC.

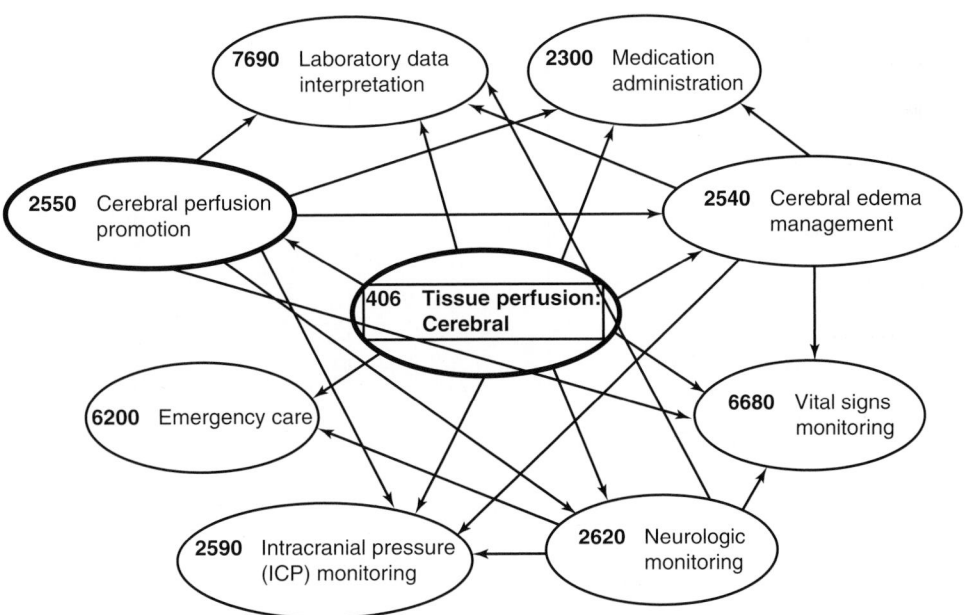

Fig. 4-5 Clinical reasoning web depicting selection of keystone NIC.

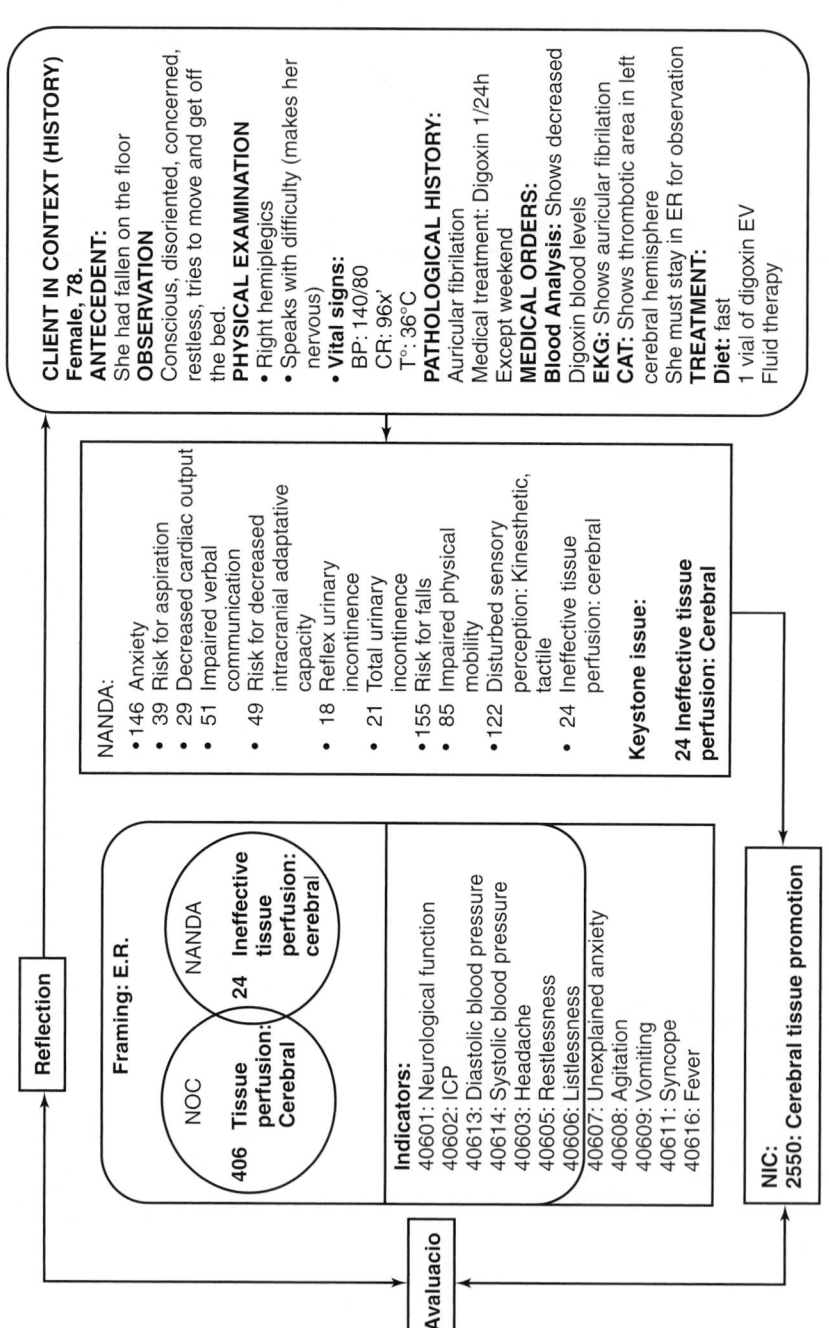

CLIENT IN CONTEXT (HISTORY)
Female, 78.
ANTECEDENT:
She had fallen on the floor
OBSERVATION
Conscious, disoriented, concerned, restless, tries to move and get off the bed.
PHYSICAL EXAMINATION
• Right hemiplegics
• Speaks with difficulty (makes her nervous)
• **Vital signs:**
   BP: 140/80
   CR: 96x'
   T°: 36°C
PATHOLOGICAL HISTORY:
Auricular fibrilation
Medical treatment: Digoxin 1/24h
Except weekend
MEDICAL ORDERS:
Blood Analysis: Shows decreased Digoxin blood levels
EKG: Shows auricular fibrilation
CAT: Shows thrombotic area in left cerebral hemisphere
She must stay in ER for observation
TREATMENT:
Diet: fast
1 vial of digoxin EV
Fluid therapy

NANDA:
• 146 Anxiety
• 39 Risk for aspiration
• 29 Decreased cardiac output
• 51 Impaired verbal communication
• 49 Risk for decreased intracranial adaptative capacity
• 18 Reflex urinary incontinence
• 21 Total urinary incontinence
• 155 Risk for falls
• 85 Impaired physical mobility
• 122 Disturbed sensory perception: Kinesthetic, tactile
• 24 Ineffective tissue perfusion: cerebral

Keystone issue:

24 Ineffective tissue perfusion: Cerebral

Framing: E.R.

NOC · NANDA

406 Tissue perfusion: Cerebral · **24 Ineffective tissue perfusion: cerebral**

Indicators:
40601: Neurological function
40602: ICP
40613: Diastolic blood pressure
40614: Systolic blood pressure
40603: Headache
40605: Restlessness
40606: Listlessness
40607: Unexplained anxiety
40608: Agitation
40609: Vomiting
40611: Syncope
40616: Fever

Reflection

Avaluacio

NIC:
2550: Cerebral tissue promotion

Fig. 4-6 OPT decision-making model applied to patient with CVA.

Currently, more than 50% of the total number of nurses in Andorra can use SNL. Nursing information will be the axis of the electronic system, and the remaining information will be connected. SNL is about the nursing profession and nurses. The nursing profession risks disappearing unless professionals are able to communicate who they are and how nursing care influences the health level of the populations. From our experience, we can say that it is relatively easy to use SNL as natural language if it is learned from the beginning of basic education.

USING NOC IN RESEARCH

The classification and individual outcomes can be used in evaluation research, effectiveness research, and traditional clinical or efficacy research. There is also a pressing need to continue research on the classification itself, particularly attention to the reliability of the measures across populations and settings. These areas cannot be thoroughly addressed in this chapter; rather, this section will discuss the needs for further research on the classification and touch on some of the other research areas and questions that need to be addressed.

Evaluating the Classification

A priority for future research is to continue to evaluate the consistency or stability with which the outcomes are rated. Examination of the reliability and validity of the 169 NOC outcomes that were evaluated in the Phase III study in a more comprehensive sample of settings, types of patient care units, and patient diagnoses is also warranted. Further, 70 outcomes were added to the second edition of NOC, 76 to the third edition, and 46 to this edition, for a total of 376 outcomes in the NOC. These additional outcomes should be tested with clinical data, along with those of the 190 published in the first edition of the NOC book that were not tested in the Phase III study (n = 22). Nurses who choose to use these outcomes in their practice should be aware that reliability and validity data are not available for the additional outcomes, and they should plan to emphasize reliability testing of these outcomes as they are implemented. In sites where the NOC outcomes are implemented in clinical information system, it would be helpful to all if the results of reliability assessment of the outcomes were shared with the Center for Nursing Classification and Effectiveness Research so that a database of results could be maintained and shared with users.

It is also necessary to systematically evaluate the responsiveness of the NOC outcomes to nursing interventions. Responsiveness of the outcomes to nursing interventions is critical for nursing effectiveness and efficacy studies.[18] Responsiveness was assessed using concept analyses and by evaluating change scores with the Phase III data but awaits further empirical verification. A few studies using the NOC outcomes and measures to evaluate the effectiveness of nursing interventions are in process or completed, but more are needed. Now that a comprehensive classification of patient outcomes is available with evidence of the reliability and validity of a large number of the outcomes, nurse researchers can more easily examine the unique contributions of nursing interventions to changes in the status of these outcomes and complete results obtained with standardized evaluation tools.

There are other questions that also should be answered. Among these are the effects of the health care setting, including how different structural variables in different settings influence outcomes with patients. The separate effects of the level of education of the nurse rater, years of experience, staffing, or how well the nurse raters knew the patient on interrater reliability of NOC outcomes need further study. The results will better inform health care organizations about the training and experience needed for use of the NOC outcomes for clinical documentation and the areas in which nurses need additional training. The results would also be helpful in hiring decisions and in determining the responsibilities that are assigned to nurses with specific amounts and types of nursing preparation.

Overall, the Phase III study data provide support for the validity of most of the outcomes; however, further research to estimate validity is clearly needed. This is especially true for outcomes that had correlations below the criterion of 0.50 and for those outcomes for which limited or no data were available to assess their validity. The complete validity data for the 169 outcomes (for which at least some data were collected) are reported in the third edition of the NOC book.

Several other issues have been raised that need further research. Whether or not anchors are needed for scale values and what the anchors should be are important questions. Some sites have attached percentages to the anchors for the scale values. This strategy and the use of other anchors that may be developed need further evaluation to determine whether reliability of measurement is improved. Whether or not the outcome indicators need to be rated or whether the outcome label alone can be reliably rated is an issue that requires further research. Although the preliminary results reported in Chapter 1 suggest that the reliability of outcome ratings may be as good or better when only the outcome label measure is rated, additional research is needed before such a recommendation can be made.

Greater attention must be given to studies of the relationship between the NOC concept and the concept as measured by another standardized tool to better assess criteria and construct validity. Data mining of clinical nursing field data holds some promise for validation of outcome concepts and for identifying the linkages among nursing diagnoses, interventions, and outcomes in order to develop and validate middle-range nursing theories.[17,18,20]

The research team is continuing to develop, validate, and classify outcomes and outcome measures for individuals, families, and communities. There is a list of outcomes to develop and assess for content validity that will require future clinical testing. Outcomes proposed for addition to the classification are regularly received from clinicians throughout the United States. Proposed outcomes from international colleagues need to be received for inclusion as well. Cross-cultural studies of the reliability and validity of the NOC outcomes with clinical data are needed to evaluate their adequacy for use with ethnic and racial minorities and in international education, research, and practice.

The NOC team encourages the use of the outcomes in education, research, and practice and hopes that nurse educators, researchers, and clinicians will assist in the evaluation of the integrity of the outcomes. Nurses who test any of the outcomes for reliability, validity, sensitivity, and/or usefulness are requested to contact the NOC investigators or the Center for Nursing Classification and Clinical Effectiveness, College of Nursing, The University of Iowa, to share the results of their research. Center staff are eager to inform potential investigators of the outcomes that lack clinical testing. It is only through systematic testing by a large number of nurse users that the psychometric integrity of the outcomes will be established and their clinical usefulness optimized. These goals are important to all nurses, the profession, and the clients that nurses serve because of the importance of reliable and valid outcome data for the development of evidence-based nursing practice and the need for nursing to demonstrate its accountability for quality care.

Often nurses may hesitate to begin research studies, thinking they are not prepared or do not have adequate funding. The following case study illustrates how a group of nurses working at different hospitals were able to work together to develop methods for implementing a study using NOC.

Implementing Nursing Outcome Classification in an Electronic Documentation System for Research

Mary E. Kravutske, PhD, RN; Craig Albers, MSN, RN; Penny Hunt, MHSA, RN; Jodi Pahl, MSN, RN-C; LesLea Pitcher, MS, RN; Patricia Strasser-Thomas, RN; Mary Zugcic, MS, RN-BC

Overview

The purpose of the study is to build on previous research of the Nursing Outcome Classification (NOC) research team by collecting nursing data using the clinical and management software system, EXCELCARE, in three hospitals where nurses wanted to incorporate NOC outcomes into their practice. The current study, ECUIP, combines efforts of the Center for Nursing Classification at The University of Iowa College of Nursing (Center); EXCELCARE, Inc; and selected acute care hospitals already using EXCELCARE software. This example will describe the ECUIP project, the IRB approval process, development and implementation of education for the staff registered nurses (RNs) involved in the study, and lessons learned during the process. The various teaching methods, case studies, results, and lessons learned will be discussed.

Background

The acronym ECUIP represents the combined efforts of EXCELCARE (EC) and The University of Iowa (UI) in a Project (P) that focuses on providing RNs with a means to measure and use standardized outcomes of nursing care. The hospital facilities participating in this nursing research are Henry Ford Hospital (HFH) in Detroit, Michigan; St. Rita's Medical Center (SRMC) in Lima, Ohio; and United Health Services (UHS) in Binghamton, New York. The study is focused on establishing how closely nurses rate an overall outcome for the same patient (inter-rater reliability), the change in patient outcome ratings between baseline and postintervention ratings, the identification of key NOC outcomes for specific patient populations, the influence of patient and nurse demographics on patient outcome ratings, and an evaluation of the usefulness of the NOC outcomes in clinical practice.

Each of the three hospital facilities has several RNs assigned to coordinating the research project. The group had three meetings in which the overall project was developed and delineated. A common understanding of the NOC was established within the group, and it was determined how NOCs could be incorporated into the current nursing documentation system. The group wanted to move from the institutional specific outcome statements that were not necessarily nursing outcomes to the standardized language of the Nursing Outcome Classification. The group divided into two work groups: one to address the practice and educational issues and the other to develop the process to input selected NOCs into the software system.

To initiate the study, the practice group, with representatives from each clinical facility, selected 30 of the 330 NOCs based on available patient populations with an emphasis on NOCs not previously studied. Inclusion and deletion criteria were developed before reviewing the indicators for the selected NOCs. Each indicator was reviewed using the established criteria. A consensus decision was made before excluding an indicator to ensure that all clinical facilities were using the same NOCs and indicators.

The practice group also developed a tool to collect demographic data for both the patient and staff RN and an outline for the education materials. The education materials were developed by the initial facility to "go live" and later modified to meet the needs of the other clinical facilities.

The members of the technical group determined the process to input the selected NOCs, indicators, and five-point scale into the current software system. They developed the system, entered the outcomes, and tested the results. Examples of the screens developed for testing are shown in Figures 4-7, 4-8, 4-9, and 4-10.

Each hospital facility then selected the patient care units that would be the pilot sites for documentation using the selected NOCs. The patient care units selected included intensive care, general medicine, general surgical, telemetry, orthopedic, neurology, and oncology. Each study unit was assigned the study NOCs appropriate for the patient population served.

The staff RN would rate each selected indicator for a NOC at the time the NOC was selected for the patient and give an overall rating for the NOC. This would be documented on a software system used for nursing documentation, but only the overall rating would become part of the patient's permanent record. The frequency for evaluating the NOC was dependent on the documentation policy of the clinical facility, but all NOCs were evaluated prior to or at discharge.

It was determined that each site would seek Institutional Review Board (IRB) approval from its hospital facility. The data would be collected at each site, de-identified, and sent to a data manager at the software company. The data manager would forward the data from all of the

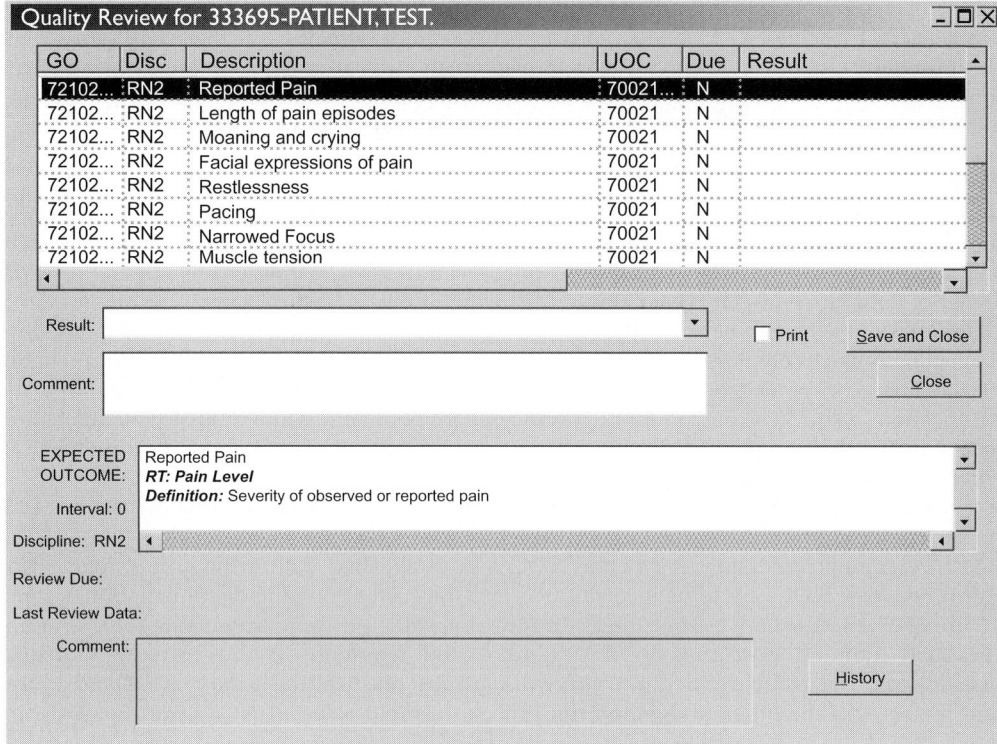

Fig. 4-7 Test screen for reported pain.

clinical facilities to The University of Iowa, College of Nursing Center for Nursing Classification and Clinical Effectiveness. The Center for Nursing Classification and Clinical Effectiveness would seek IRB approval through The University of Iowa, serve as the data repository for the study, and perform data analysis.

Before the study was implemented, the RNs on the study units completed a pre-quiz, a demographic sheet, the educational program, a case study, post-quiz, and evaluation of the education program. After completing all of the above, the RN received continuing education hours (Contact Hours).

The first NOCs selected for this research project were Discharge Readiness: Independent Living; Discharge Readiness: Supported Living; Pain Level; and Cardiac Pump Effectiveness. One research NOC was used at a time, and each unit selected the NOC based on its patient population.

Implementation

Implementation varied slightly at each hospital and from unit to unit based on the research coordinators, the readiness of the staff, and the organization of the hospital. Each hospital identified somewhat different issues, problems, and strengths as it initiated the study. The process is briefly outlined for each hospital.

Henry Ford Hospital

The members of the research team at Henry Ford Hospital (HFH) included a Nurse Scholar, two Clinical Nurse Specialists (CNS), and the RN responsible for maintaining the nursing documentation software system. The Institutional Review Board (IRB) application for HFH was submitted

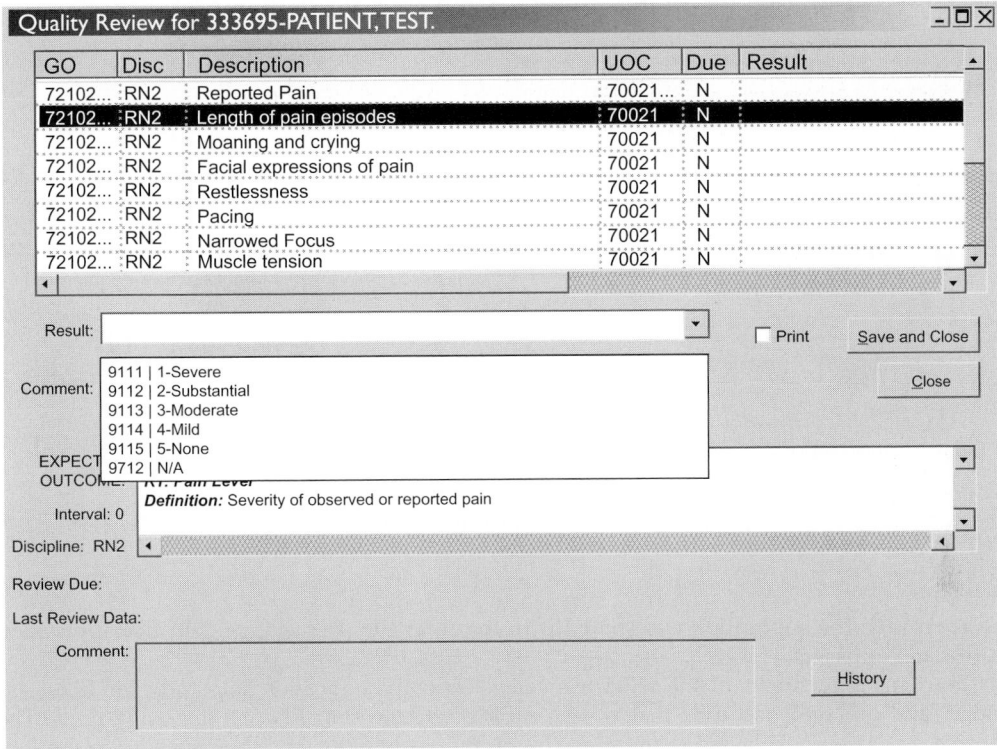

Fig. 4-8 Test screen for length of pain episodes.

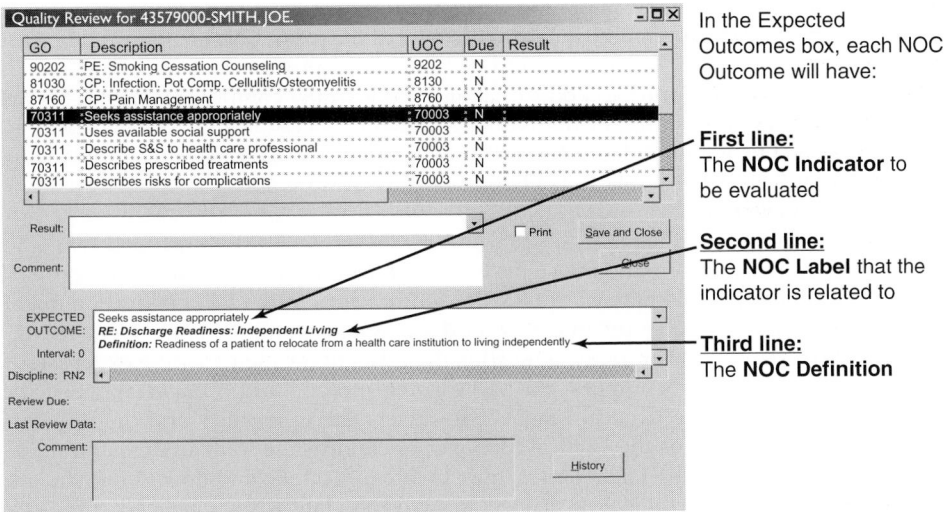

Fig. 4-9 Parts of the documentation screen.

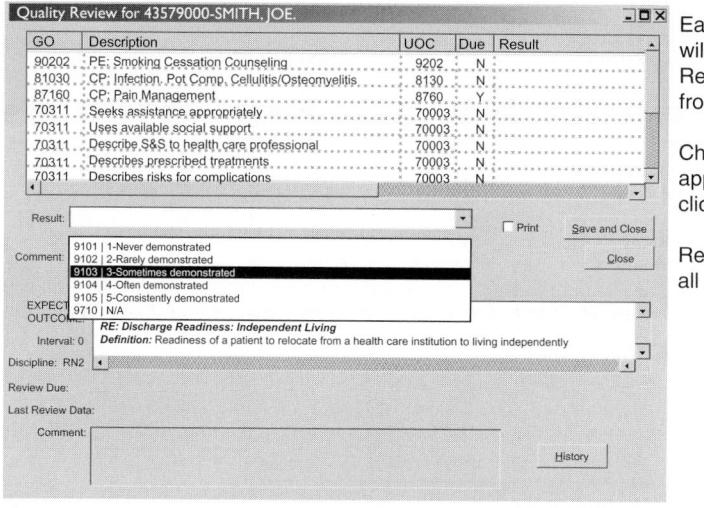

Each NOC Indicator will have a unique Result Set to select from.

Choose the appropriate result and click on it to select it.

Repeat the process for all remaining outcomes.

Fig. 4-10 Using the documentation screen.

and approved. The application was shared with the other sites to facilitate their IRB application process and approval.

The clinical members of the HFH team developed the education self-study module, case studies, and pre- and post-quiz that were completed by the staff RNs on the study units. The research project was explained to the staff RNs on the study units, and they were given the self-study module to complete. A paper and pencil case study was developed so the RN could conceptualize the NOC, indicators, and multiple rating scales prior to documentation using the software system. This was done because the software system does not allow for visualization of more than one indicator at a time. Rating scales for the indicators and overall NOC rating appear one at a time in the software system. The RN would read the case study and rate the patient on each of the indicators for the NOC, then give an overall score (Box 4-2 and Figure 4-11). The CNS would review the case study and the ratings with the RN. The objective was to ensure the RN understood the need to rate each indicator and the overall outcome, and the use of the measurement scales.

The RNs completed a 10-question post-quiz on the e-learning computer system. This was to assess their overall understanding of the Nursing Outcome Classification system. Just-in-time learning was needed to accommodate RNs unable to complete the education prior to initiation of the research study.

St. Rita's Medical Center

The members of the research team at St. Rita's Medical Center (SRMC) included two Clinical Managers and a Clinical Information Systems Specialist. Modifications were made to the HFH IRB application and approval obtained at SRMC. Modifications to the HFH education materials included utilizing the computer for information dissemination and testing, "super users" for training and support, and staff from the education department for their training expertise.

Each nurse completed a Computer Based Learning module and a paper and pencil case study. Each RN met with the Clinical Manager to review the case study and the ratings. The review was an opportunity for the Clinical Manager to confirm the RN's understanding of the research project, how to use the Likert scales, how to rate indicators, and how to rate the overall NOC. Some just-in-time learning was needed to accommodate RNs unable to complete the education prior to initiation of the study.

Box 4-2

Case Study

Discharge Readiness: Independent Living

Day 1: BP 212/98, HR 110, RR 22, T 40° C

Blood glucose 290 mg/dl, pain score 9 (level acceptable to the patient 2)

Mr. K, a 69-year-old with a history of poorly controlled diabetes, was admitted to your unit at 0600 from the emergency department with a diagnosis of cellulites. His right foot is red, tender, and swollen. There is a 2-cm break in the skin on the great toe that is draining purulent fluid.

Mr. K is crying as you enter the room and states, "I'm so tired of these sugar problems. I can't follow the diet and won't take those shots. I'm too sick to do anything. I can't stand this pain any more. Just leave me alone."

Day 3: BP 184/78, HR 90, RR 18, T 38° C

Blood glucose 190 mg/dl, pain score 5 (level acceptable to the patient 2)

Mr. K is up in the chair and using a walker to ambulate in the room. He needs to be reminded to keep his foot elevated when he is sitting up. This morning he drew up his own insulin, but he had trouble seeing the markings on the syringe and couldn't give himself the injection.

His wife has returned from her business trip and is now visiting each evening. She travels frequently and has not been involved in her husband's care prior to this admission. Diabetes education, other than insulin administration, had been put on hold because Mr. K wanted to wait for his wife to participate.

United Health Services

The members of the research team at United Health Services (UHS) included a Nurse Educator and the RN responsible for maintaining the nursing documentation software system. The two participating hospitals in the UHS system were Wilson Memorial Regional Medical Center in Johnson City and Binghamton General Hospital in Binghamton, New York. Modifications were made to the HFH IRB application, and approval was obtained. Modification to the HFH education materials included lunch-and-learn education sessions, resource nurses from each shift on the study units, a list of all the resource nurses, and use of the computer lab to complete the case studies. The resource nurse was used to educate the nurses and to communicate updates.

Lessons Learned

This collaboration provided an excellent opportunity to collaborate with nurses across the three sites and to involve staff nurses in a research process that would impact their practice. The coordinators learned how to modify the research process to meet the needs of each institution while maintaining integrity of the data collected. Additionally, individual lessons were learned at each hospital.

Henry Ford Hospital

Even though the use of the study NOCs was not optional on the study units, the level of participation of the staff RN was increased by providing Contact Hours for the education and encouraging the nurse to view themselves as participants in nursing research.

Support from nursing leadership was increased by selecting initial NOCs to be studied that supported departmental quality goals (pain, discharge planning).

The research team needed to be available to do just-in-time education for those RNs not completing the education prior to the start of the study. Many RNs needed support in becoming comfortable with the use of NOCs.

Nurses see value in standardized nursing language and the use of NOCs but would have preferred the nursing documentation system to utilize more standardized nursing language; they had difficulty using a "mixed" nursing documentation system with existing outcomes and

Definition: Readiness of a patient to relocate from a health care institution to living independently.

Overall Rating: _____

	Never demonstrated 1	Rarely demonstrated 2	Sometimes demonstrated 3	Often demonstrated 4	Consistently demonstrated 5	
Seeks assistance appropriately	1	2	3	4	5	NA
Uses available social support	1	2	3	4	5	NA
Describes signs and symptoms to health care professional	1	2	3	4	5	NA
Describes prescribed treatments	1	2	3	4	5	NA
Describes risks for complications	1	2	3	4	5	NA
Manages own medications	1	2	3	4	5	NA
Performs activities of daily living (ADLs) independently	1	2	3	4	5	NA
Makes appropriate judgments	1	2	3	4	5	NA
	Consistently demonstrated	Often demonstrated	Sometimes demonstrated	Rarely demonstrated	Never demonstrated	
Fever	1	2	3	4	5	NA
Infection	1	2	3	4	5	NA
Confusion	1	2	3	4	5	NA

Fig. 4-11 Discharge readiness: independent living.

the test NOC outcomes. It is conceptually difficult to adopt only a few NOCs without redesigning the existing nursing standards and patient outcomes.

Flexibility was necessary to address unexpected situations. The study NOCs were intended to be used only on the identified study units. It was later discovered that RNs from non-study units found and utilized the study NOCs without any education on their use. Another situation was the normal RN attrition on the study units was not planned for in the development of the study.

St. Rita's Medical Center

The nursing staff participated in the project with minimal resistance and viewed it as a more accurate way to rate patient outcomes. They found the use of the Likert scale to rate indicators a more accurate method than the current method of rating patients as "meeting or not meeting" outcomes.

Use of the Likert scale stimulated interest and increased attention when rating patients because it involved more than just checking a number. The descriptors for each scale involved more thought and evaluation of the patient's condition than would have occurred with a goal statement. For example, rating the indicators increased the nurses' ability to identify pain control issues and motivated them to change the plan of care to achieve more positive outcomes. Rating the indicators helped guide the care of patients by novice nurses.

The preferred educational setting was in the classroom. However, to maximize productive hours of RNs, the education modules were completed during work hours. Meeting with staff prior to the research project "going live" was a challenge and just-in-time learning was necessary. Super user involvement was critical to the success of the project to assist with staff buy-in and off-shift support when the research leads were not on the unit.

The RNs are primarily associate degree–trained nurses with little to no background in nursing taxonomy. However, most nurses at St. Rita's Medical Center saw value in the use of a standardized language after completing the study education. The RNs gained confidence in documenting to standardized outcomes by first using only study NOCs. As the nurses' confidence increased, other study NOCs were added.

United Health Services

Even though it took more coordinating of schedules, the classroom lunch-and-learn instruction and computer lab experience served the nurses well. The RNs were able to ask questions and felt well prepared and confident to begin the project. Using the outcomes from NOC was more time-consuming; however, the nurses could see a real benefit for the patients with the more complete analysis of the patient's condition, and many of the nurses chose to continue using the NOCs when we moved on to study other NOCs.

The Resource Nurses played a major role in supporting the research project and training other nurses on their units. It was important to have adequate resources available for additional training during the initial implementation of this project.

Conclusion

The research project involved multiple clinical facilities with varied documentation policies and resources. All the clinical facilities were strongly supported by their nursing administration. It was possible to introduce standardized nursing outcome language in varied clinical facilities with only minor modifications while maintaining the integrity of the research study. The members from the clinical facility teams brought different perspectives and strengths to the research project and provided support for each other.

Data collection of the indicator and NOC evaluations was simplified using documentation software. The software also made it possible to study the outcome documentation in relation to the individual nurse performing the evaluation. Compared with the original NOC study, resources required to obtain the data were greatly reduced, and it was possible to collect a much greater amount of data in a limited amount of time.

RNs involved in the study were excited to be using standardized nursing outcome language and quickly saw the value of the standardized outcomes. RNs conveyed that the use of both the indicators and overall ratings assisted in evaluating patient progress. Participation in the research study caused individual facilities to evaluate their documentation systems and how nursing outcomes are utilized. RNs were enthusiastic about participating in nursing research and viewed it as an opportunity for professional growth.

Current and Future Research

Although the use of the term "nursing-sensitive patient outcomes" has increased dramatically in the literature, the use of the research-based Nursing Outcomes Classification (NOC) outcomes in reported research is scant. Most reports of studies of nursing-sensitive patient outcomes are either of locally developed outcomes and measures or studies of aggregate quality measures characterizing organizations developed by national groups such as the American Nurses Association and the National Quality Forum. Thus, the advantages of the use of the comprehensive standardized nursing-sensitive patient outcomes that are provided by NOC outcomes are not being optimally realized. We anticipate, however, that the increasing interest in nursing-sensitive patient outcomes and the continued dissemination and adoption of NOC in electronic health records will prompt greater use of the NOC outcomes in all types of research.

In addition to the studies conducted by the NOC research team and reported in previous editions of this book, several other studies have addressed various aspects of the development and testing of the NOC outcomes. These include small studies conducted by faculty, nurse clinicians, and doctoral students and illustrate research that is needed and can be conducted with the NOC outcomes. These investigators can be contacted for more information about their studies.

Doctoral Student Dissertation Research
Validation of Nursing-Sensitive Outcomes for Rural and Urban Community Elderly

Barbara Head, PhD, RN, Assistant Professor, University of Nebraska College of Nursing. Dissertation completed at the University of Iowa College of Nursing, Dissertation publication #AAT 9819945.

A survey research design was used to assess the importance and sensitivity to nursing interventions (nursing contribution), and content validity of six patient outcomes included in the Nursing Outcomes Classification (NOC). The questionnaire was mailed to 368 nurses who were certified as community health nurse specialists by the American Nurses Association Credentialing Center in spring 1997 with a 66% rate of return. The nurse subjects rated indicators of the outcomes (Self-Care: Activities of Daily Living; Self-Care: Instrumental Activities of Daily Living; Treatment Behavior: Illness or Injury; Knowledge: Health Behavior; Caregiver Performance: Direct Care; Caregiver Physical Health) for their importance for determining the outcome rating and for the contribution of nursing to their achievement. Respondents also rated the outcomes for their importance for community health clients and for the community health nurse's contribution to their achievement with community health nursing clients. Results confirmed the importance of the indicators and outcomes for community health nursing and the contribution of community health nursing to achievement of the outcomes. Differences between ratings of importance and contribution were found between rural and urban nurses. Multiple regression techniques were useful for identifying key indicators of the study outcomes. Additional findings are reported in the following articles.

Head, B. J., Aquilino, M. L., Johnson, M., Reed, D., Maas, M., & Moorhead, S. (2000). Content validity and nursing sensitivity of community-level outcomes from the Nursing Outcomes Classification (NOC). *Journal of Nursing Scholarship, 36*(3), 251-255.

Head, B. J., Maas, M., & Johnson, M. (2003). Validity and community-health nursing sensitivity of six outcomes for community health nursing with older clients. *Public Health Nursing, 20*(5), 85-98.

Describing Nursing Effectiveness Through Standardized Nursing Languages and Computerized Clinical Data

Cindy Scherb, PhD, RN, Professor, Winona State University School of Nursing. Dissertation completed at the University of Iowa College of Nursing. Dissertation Abstracts International, 62(12), 5646, #AAT 3034148.

This research was one of the first studies completed using computerized standardized nursing languages to determine the most effective interventions to achieve the best outcomes. NANDA, NIC, and NOC were the standardized nursing languages used in the clinical data repository. Relationships among nursing diagnoses, interventions, and outcomes were investigated for older hospitalized patients with congestive heart failure, pneumonia, and total joint replacement. Linkages among nursing diagnoses, interventions, and outcomes were described and closely approximated linkages recommended by Johnson and colleagues.[14] Two to three nursing interventions were found to be statistically significantly and positively related to NOC outcomes for each of the congestive heart failure, pneumonia, and total joint replacement groups of older patients. Larger samples and inclusion of interventions from other disciplines were recommended for future studies.

A Secondary Analysis of Selected Patient Risk Factors Associated With the Status of Nursing-Sensitive Patient Outcomes

Peggy Kerr, PhD, RN, Post-Doctoral Fellow. The University of Iowa College of Nursing. Dissertation completed at the University of Iowa College of Nursing. Dissertation Abstracts, 2005, 173 pages; #AAT3184722.

This study used secondary data from the NOC Phase III research (R01NR03437) to evaluate patient variables for risk adjustment for four NOC outcomes (Health Promoting Behavior; Self-Care: Activities of Daily Living; Ambulation: Walking; and Vital Signs Status). The purpose was to contribute to the development of risk adjustment methods for nursing effectiveness research. The ability of specific patient characteristics (age, gender, primary medical diagnosis, socioeconomic status, and comorbidities) to explain variation in change in each of the four outcomes was assessed. Contingency table methods and multiple logistic regressions were used to develop a statistical model of risk for each of the four NOC outcomes. Patients with Self Care: Activities of Daily Living and Ambulation: Walking were more likely to experience improvement in these outcomes if they had a musculoskeletal system and connective tissue diagnosis. Those who had an endocrine, nutritional, and metabolic disease or immunity disorder diagnosis or a mental disorder were more likely to have an improved Health Promoting Behavior outcome. Those who had a manually assisted delivery or C-section were more likely to have improved Ambulation: Walking. Those patients in the young-old age-group were almost four times more likely to show no improvement in Self-Care: Activities of Daily Living than those in the youngest age-group. When the youngest age-group, however, was used as the reference group for Vital Signs Status, the patients in the range for 40 to 84 years of age were from 88% to 98% more likely to improve than their younger counterparts. Patients with three or more comorbidities were six times less likely to improve in Self-Care: Activities of Daily Living. Gender was not shown to be significantly related to improvement in any of the four outcomes.

Reliability of Six Outcomes From the Nursing Outcomes Classification (NOC) and the Relationships of Organizational, Patient, and Nurse Characteristics to These Outcomes

Maneewan Sanubol, PhD, RN. Dissertation completed at the University of Iowa College of Nursing. Dissertation publication #AAT 3172437.

This secondary analysis study further investigated the inter-rater reliability of six NOC outcomes by type of health care setting, by nurses' years of experience, and by educational level of nurse raters. The relationships of organizational, nurse, and patient characteristics on the six outcomes were also described. The sample included 2,333 patients for whom clinical data were collected in the NOC Phase III study from ten field sites from 1998 to 2002. Intraclass correlations were used to analyze inter-rater reliability with a criterion of 0.75. The average intraclass (ICC) correlation coefficients of the NOC outcomes rated by paired-nurses by health care setting were 0.75 in community health settings, 0.94 in hospitals, and 0.62 in the nursing home. There were no statistically significant differences in inter-rater reliability coefficients among categories of type of nursing education or years of experience of the nurse raters. Patient age, education, occupation, and medical diagnoses explained a small, but statistically significant amount of the change in outcome scores (R^2 = 0.038, 0.039, 0.013, and 0.042, respectively). Together, patient age, medical diagnoses, and type of health care setting statistically, significantly explained nearly 10% of the variance in outcome change scores (R^2 = 0.098).

Evaluating Home Health Care Nursing Outcomes With OASIS and NOC

Julia Stocker, PhD, RN., University of Michigan, Ann Arbor. Dissertation completed at the University of Michigan School of Nursing.

The sensitivity and responsiveness of the Outcome and Assessment Information Set (OASIS) and the Nursing Outcomes Classification (NOC) to the effects of home health care nursing interventions were measured in this study. Sensitivity refers to the ability of an outcome instrument to detect change attributable to intervention. Alternatively, responsiveness is the ability of an instrument to detect change that is clinically meaningful. Patient outcomes data using the OASIS and the NOC were collected for 106 subjects, referred to home health care for treatment of a cardiac condition, at-home health care admission and discharge. Nursing intervention data were collected at each visit using the Nursing Interventions Classification (NIC). Intervention intensity was calculated by totaling the number of NIC interventions provided over the episode of care. The study findings demonstrated that neither the OASIS nor the NOC were sensitive to the effects of home health care nursing as measured by intervention intensity. However, reliability issues with the measurement of intervention intensity using the NIC could have impacted these findings. Neither measure was sensitive when nursing care was measured using total number of RN visits or total visit time. When effect size and standardized response mean were calculated for the OASIS and the NOC, both measures were sensitive, with the NOC demonstrating greater overall sensitivity. The OASIS was not responsive to clinically discernable change in patient outcomes. However, the NOC was responsive to patient status change in activities of daily living, cardiopulmonary status, coping, and illness management behaviors. The study results demonstrate that outcome measures that are more condition-specific and discipline-specific are more sensitive and responsive to the effects of home health care nursing. Further research is needed to identify and refine outcome measures that are sensitive and responsive to the effects of home health care nursing. While the identification of such measures is a challenge, the ultimate use of sensitive and responsive outcome measures will promote quality and effectiveness in home health care nursing practice.

Pilot Studies
Head, B., PI. Nursing Outcomes Effectiveness: Hospitalized Elders With Pneumonia and Congestive Health Failure; Scherb, C., PI. Hospital Nursing Effectiveness: Elders With Pneumonia/CHF.

Two pilot studies are evaluating the feasibility of a larger multisite nursing effectiveness study and will focus on older persons with pneumonia (DRGs 89 and 90) and congestive health failure (CHF) (DRG 127). The pneumonia and congestive heart failure (CHF) populations are high-cost, high-volume hospitalizations for older persons and health care organizations. The percentage of people over the age of 65 will increase for many years, and it is likely that the elderly population will continue to use the resource intensive services of acute care hospitals. It is necessary to identify the most pertinent nursing interventions to achieve the desired outcomes, so readmissions, complications, and costs can be reduced. Although the use of large data sets is emphasized for health care effectiveness research, data needed to assess nursing effectiveness are lacking. Although steadily increasing, standardized clinical nursing data that are retrievable are rare in single institutions and multiple systems that include services across care settings. As the use of standardized nursing languages increases in hospital information systems, it is important to prepare the nursing research that will be possible using secondary nursing data sets. These pilot studies are using secondary standardized nursing data from two Midwestern urban community hospitals and one Northeastern community hospital to accomplish combined study aims: (1) determine whether the variables that are needed to assess the extent that nursing interventions influence patient outcomes for specific patient populations are available in the hospitals' computerized systems; (2) describe the 10 most frequent North American Nursing Diagnosis Association International (NANDA) diagnoses, Nursing Intervention Classification (NIC) interventions, and Nursing Outcomes Classification (NOC) outcomes documented by nurses for patients 60 to 89 years of age with a primary discharge diagnosis of pneumonia or CHF in the hospitals; (3) describe the intervals of measurement, change, and variation in outcome status throughout the hospital length of stay for the elders with pneumonia and CHF; (4) describe the process of data retrieval for all variables needed to evaluate the clinical and cost effectiveness of nursing interventions for elders with pneumonia in each of the hospitals; and (5) pilot test the development of a data warehouse for a study to evaluate the clinical and cost effectiveness of nursing interventions for elders hospitalized with CHF and pneumonia, using data from all four hospitals. The studies are significant as a preliminary investigation for future studies of the effectiveness of nursing interventions on patient outcomes and will enable subsequent innovative research using standardized clinical data from nurses documenting their practice in integrated information systems across multiple sites.

Scherb, C., PI. Provider Influence on Outcomes for Patients Hospitalized With CHF, TJR, and Pneumonia.

The purpose of the pilot study was to determine whether provider interventions make a difference in patient outcomes. Two rural regional health care organizations (Immanuel St. Joseph's [ISJ-MHS], Albert Lea Medical Center [ALMC-MHS]) and the parent hospital Austin Medical Center (AMC-MHS), which have nursing standardized languages (NANDA, NIC, NOC) in their computerized documentation system, participated in the study. A descriptive design was used to answer this study question: Is there a significant difference in NOC outcome ratings from admission to discharge for CHF, TJR, and pneumonia patients? The study sample included patients who consented to have their medical record used for research and were admitted with the primary DRGs of pneumonia, TJR (hip or knee), or CHF during 1999. The three groups were chosen because of their high volume and high cost to the organization. The nursing staff rated outcomes on the patient at admission and discharge. Data were analyzed for a total of 191 CHF, 220 TJR, and 258 pneumonia patients. A t-test was used to measure for statistically significant differences between admission and discharge ratings. Overall, about half of the outcomes for patients improved significantly from admission to discharge, although a statistically significantly greater percentage of outcomes for CHF and pneumonia patients improved than for TJR patients at discharge. The study results provided important data for the evaluation of their services for these populations and were a beginning for further studies of outcomes with adjustments for risk and the evaluation of the effectiveness and costs of individual disciplines' interventions.

Scherb, C., PI. Outcome Research in Chemical Dependency.

The purpose of this pilot study was to determine whether chemical dependency health care providers' interventions at a Midwestern community hospital made a difference in patient outcomes. A descriptive design was used, and the study questions were (1) is there a significant difference in NOC outcome ratings from admission to discharge for chemical dependency patients; and (2) what are the differences in outcome ratings of nurses and counselors? The study included patients admitted to inpatient and outpatient chemical dependency programs during 1999; a total of 127 patient records were analyzed: 51 inpatients and 76 outpatients. Counselors identified 12 outcomes as pertinent to the population, and 11 of these were significantly improved from admission to discharge. Ten outcomes rated by inpatient nurses were statistically significantly improved, and five were not. This study illustrates how outcomes-based practice can be beneficial for providers and patients by providing standardized outcomes to measure and compare patient progress or decline assessed by interdisciplinary providers.

Keenan, G., PI. Hands-On Automated Nursing Data System (HANDS).

This project that has been under way since the mid-1990s and is focused on creating a viable standardized interdisciplinary plan of care method that provides the patient's current history in "short story form" wherever he or she enters the system, allowing clinicians to access information to assist with immediate and future decisions about care through continuous study and refinement under real time conditions. HANDS contains standardized nursing languages, including NANDA, NOC, and NIC. The mission and vision are to continuously refine the standardized HANDS Plan of Care method, make HANDS gender-neutral and available for widespread and effective use by clinicians, ensure interconnectivity with all electronic health records (EHRs), and enable a consistent approach to evidence-based practice (EBP). The aim is for nurses and interdisciplinary team members to use the HANDS standardized method of documenting and communicating the patient's plan of care and progress toward outcomes in health care settings and during transitions between settings. Wherever and whenever a patient enters the health system, the plan of care history is readily accessible to support future decisions about care. The project is funded by AHRQ (2004-2007) for refinement and revision.

Two proposals that illustrate nursing research made possible by electronic clinical nursing data sets are under review by the Library of Medicine.

Proposed Research
Lu, D-F., PI. Mining Clinical Data Sets for Nursing Dx and Intervention Links and EBP Validation.

This proposed research will use Data Mining Knowledge Discovery methods to describe hospital nurses' use of nursing diagnoses (NANDA) and interventions (NIC). The use of specific nursing interventions to treat specific diagnoses will be compared with recommended linkages published by Johnson and colleagues.[13] Further, the nurses' documented nursing diagnoses and interventions will be compared with evidence-based practice protocols to evaluate the extent that the hospital nurses practices are evidence-based. The study illustrates the use of data mining methods for describing and validating linkages among elements of the nursing process, as well as for answering other research questions. These methods will subsequently be used to describe the linkages among nursing diagnoses, outcomes, and interventions using clinical nursing data sets from multiple settings.

Brokel, J. Testing Reliability and Validity of Decision Support Rules With Electronic Nursing Data.

This research proposes high-risk/high-reward conceptual work and feasibility testing in bioinformatics to test the reliability and validity of clinician expert decision support rules (expert rules) embedded in electronic health records (EHR). The EHR with clinical decision support programming are being deployed in multiple sites. Expert rules are initiated by common events (posted assessment results) for the patient or within clinician's workflow that start (trigger) a programmed evaluation of a pattern of data to find specific content with conditional limits to prompt clinicians to take a specific evidence-based action response. Expert rules are by and large intended to support clinicians in the normal course of their duties, assisting with responsibilities that rely on the processing of data and knowledge. A major problem for nursing is the lack of standards in designing content to operate expert rules within the EHR. The absence of rigorous standards for evaluating reliability and validity in the design and implementation of expert rules leads to inconsistent use of evidence-based nursing practices and safety measures. The conceptual model for expert rules illustrates components to design content for a trigger event in the workflow to start the expert rule, for the conditional limits to evaluate patient data, and for the action response and the clinician performed response. A major component has been how the clinician performs with the expert rule's functions. The study will test methods to estimate the reliability and validity of four expert rules and their use of data from nine hospitals in the Midwest. The specific aims are (1) to describe the expert level of agreement of content congruence (validity) of four expert rules' (newborn jaundice risk assessment, influenza and pneumovax vaccine administrations, and fall risk) trigger events, conditional content and limits, and action response with reported evidence-based practice protocols; (2) to analyze the consistency and reliability of the four expert rules' triggered events over time for specific patient populations across hospitals; and (3) to assess the intrarater reliability of assessment data and interventions documented by nurses in response to triggered events produced for each of the four expert rules for specific patient populations and the interrater reliability across nine hospitals over time. The investigators expect to use the results to propose reliability and validity standards to systematically evaluate more than 100 expert rules in multiple vendor products and to assess the effectiveness of expert rules supporting nursing decisions with extracted clinical data.

These studies will provide the health care industry with validity and reliability standards for the design and use of expert rules across organizations. The research supports a national initiative to certify decision support technology. The results of the proposed and subsequent research will be presented to the American Medical Informatics Association workgroup for consideration of certification standards. This will add to the studies that are available in the literature.

Published Studies

Keenan, G., Yakel, E., & Tschannen, D. (in press). Using evidence to design, test and refine HANDS: The technology supported high reliability nurse handover. In R. Hughes (Ed.), *Advanced in patient safety and quality: An evidence-based handbook for nurse.*

Keenan, G. M., & Tschannen, D. (2006). How has our knowledge of nurse/physician collaboration grown? In J. C. McCloskey Dochterman & H. Grace (Eds.), *Current issues in nursing* (7th ed.). St. Louis: Mosby.

Keenan, G., & Yakel, E. (2004-2007). *HIT support for safe nursing care (7-R01 HS01 5054 02).* Agency for Health Research and Quality (AHRQ).

Keenan, G., Falan, S., Heath, C., & Treder, M. (2003). Establishing competency in the use of NANDA, NOC, and NIC terminology. *Journal of Nursing Measurement, 11*(2), 183-196.

Keenan, G., Stocker, J., Barakauskas, V., Johnson, M., Maas, M., Moorhead, S., & Reed, D. (2003). Establishing the validity, reliability, and sensitivity of NOC in home care settings. *Journal of Nursing Measurement, 11*(2), 135-155.

Keenan, G. M., Barkauskas, V., Stocker, J., Johnson, M., Maas, M., Moorhead, S., et al. (2003). Establishing the validity, reliability, and sensitivity of NOC in an adult care nurse practitioner setting. *Outcomes Management, 7*(2), 74-82.

Keenan, G. M., Falan, S., Heath, C., & Treder, M. (2003). Establishing competency in the use of NANDA, NOC, and NIC terminology. *Journal of Nursing Measurement, 11*(2), 183-196.

Keenan, G. M., Stocker, J., Barkauskas, V., Treder, M., & Heath, C. (2003a). Toward collecting a standardized nursing data set across the continuum: Case of adult care nurse practitioner settings. *Outcomes Management, 7*(3), 113-120.

Keenan, G. M., Stocker, J., Barkauskas, V., Treder, M., & Heath, C. (2003b). Toward integrating a common nursing data set in home care to facilitate monitoring outcomes across settings. *Journal of Nursing Measurement, 11*(2), 157-169.

Macnee, C. L., Edwards, J., Kaplan, A., Reed, S., Bradford, S., Walls, J., & Schaller-Ayers, J. M. (2006). Evaluation of NOC standardized outcome of "Health Seeking Behavior" in nurse-managed clinics. *Journal of Nursing Care Quality, 21*(3), 242-247.

Morrison, R., Burroughs, C., Witt, M., Redden, J., & Leeper, J. D. (2000). Evaluation of NOC instruments with chronically ill patients. *Southern Online Journal of Nursing Research, 1*(1), 1-11. Retrieved from www.snrs.org

Peters, R. M. (2000). Using NOC outcomes of risk control in prevention, early detection, and control of hypertension. *Outcomes Management for Nursing Practice, 4*(1), 39-45.

Scherb, C. A., Stevens, M. S., & Busman, C. (in press). Outcomes related to dehydration in the pediatric population. *Journal of Pediatric Nursing.*

Scherb, C. A. (2002). Outcomes research: Making a difference in practice. *Outcomes Management, 6*(1), 22-26.

Scherb, C. A., Rapp, C. G., Johnson, M., & Maas, M. (1998). The Nursing Outcomes Classification: Validation by rehabilitation nurses. *Rehabilitation Nursing, 23*(4), 174-178.

Tschannen, D., Keenan, G., Yakel, B., & Mandeville, M. (in press). HANDS: A Nursing-oriented standard for documenting and communicating the interdisciplinary plan of care in the EHR to improve safety. *Journal of Healthcare Information Management.*

Williams, J., Skirton, H., Reed, D., Johnson, M., Maas, M., & Daack-Hirsch, S. (2001). Genetic counseling outcomes validation by genetics nurses in the UK and US. *Journal of Nursing Scholarship, 33*(4), 369-374.

Yom, Y., & Yoo, H. S. (2002). Application of nursing diagnoses, interventions, and outcomes to patients undergoing abdominal surgery in Korea. *International Journal of Nursing Terminologies and Classifications, 13*(3), 77-87.

Finally, there are a number of reported studies that define and use nursing-sensitive patient outcomes to assess the adequacy of staffing and effects of other work environment variables, analyze adverse effects of nurses' overtime work, develop quality assessment benchmarks and databases, and measure quality and the effects of nursing interventions in specific patient populations. Selected recent examples are found in the references.[1,2,3,5,9,15,16] These studies and others illustrate intensifying interest in documenting the effects of nursing structures and processes on patient quality outcomes. Because these and future efforts would be strengthened by the use of comprehensive standardized NOC outcomes that could be compared across settings and patient populations, we recommend their use and request investigators assistance in further refinement of the outcomes and measures. We are confident, however, that the several advantages of research using the NOC will become more appealing to investigators as the substantial and sustained adoption and inclusion of NOC in electronic health records continues.

Evaluating Nursing Quality and Effectiveness

Outcomes are the trigger for the evaluation of quality and effectiveness since they answer the question, "Did the patient benefit or not benefit from the care provided?"[23] To facilitate improvement in care quality, information about patient outcomes should identify not only inadequate outcomes, but also those that are marginal, adequate, and superior. The outcomes in NOC are concepts that reflect patient states, are generally neutral (e.g., mobility, hydration, coping), and can be measured on a continuum rather than as a goal that is met or not met. Because of these characteristics, they provide measures that can be aggregated in a number of ways, such as by nursing or medical diagnoses, by service unit, or by severity of illness, to study the effectiveness of nursing interventions. Questions can be addressed about the combination of interventions that is most effective in achieving desired outcomes in a patient group or about the type of nursing care delivery system that produces the best outcomes. They also allow for differences in outcome achievement to be analyzed by patient characteristics, such as age, gender, or functional status. Determining how patient characteristics affect outcome achievement is an important area for further research; data from this type of research will provide information about outcomes that can be realistically achieved with varied patient populations. "From a quality improvement perspective, it is important to be able to identify a realistic outcome to be achieved. Unrealistic outcome expectations are inefficient in that resources may be expended to no good effect" (p. 127)[19] The effect of patient characteristics on outcome achievement is also important when comparing quality across organizations to ensure that the effects of structure and process on patient outcomes are being measured and not the effects of patient characteristics.

Effectiveness research requires the ability to quantify data, including patient outcomes. It generally relies on information obtained from large data sets to evaluate the effects of interventions provided by multiple providers in non-controlled practice situations with patients receiving routine care. New techniques for data mining, data aggregation, and data analysis[11] will foster the expansion of nursing effectiveness research if standardized nursing elements are coded and available in national data sets. At this time, a few studies are beginning to use NOC outcomes to evaluate nursing effectiveness within an organization or patient group.

Clinical innovations initially are evaluated through controlled clinical studies with attention given to the measurement of desired or expected outcomes. Many clinical studies in nursing are conducted in one site and with relatively small samples. The ability to generalize findings can be increased using meta-analysis if study variables are similar. The use of standardized patient outcomes as one of the study variables would increase the ease with which findings could be compared across studies. Because the current outcomes have not been tested as completely as instruments generally selected for controlled studies, the authors would encourage researchers to use the NOC outcomes that correspond to the instrument used in the study, compare results from the two measures, and report these findings when they report their research. The major concern that will need to be considered is whether the research instrument and the NOC outcome are measuring the same concept. If so, this type of testing would facilitate a more rapid evaluation of the outcomes.

For nursing to be a full interdisciplinary participant in health care, to demonstrate accountability to consumers, and to inform policy to optimally benefit patients and families, data must be included in national data sets that can be used to evaluate the effectiveness and cost effectiveness of nursing interventions.[18] It is clear that the quality of health care cannot be adequately determined if the practice of the largest group of providers (nurses) is not evaluated, yet many policy makers, nurses, and consumers appear to remain unconvinced, assuming that nursing care is encompassed by medical care.

The NOC research results and additional studies reported here should encourage and hasten the adoption of NOC outcomes in clinical settings and in computerized clinical information systems and prompt more studies of the NOC outcomes. Many important research questions regarding the reliability, validity, and sensitivity of the outcomes remain unanswered, and the answers are urgently needed. As these research questions continue to be answered and the outcomes are increasingly adopted in electronic nursing clinical information systems, the opportunities for nursing research will increase exponentially. Nursing effectiveness research and effectiveness research of the interventions of other disciplines to inform patients, health care providers, and policy makers are especially needed. The Head and Scherb pilot studies discussed above illustrate important preparations that are required to determine whether or not specific data are available and can be retrieved from hospital data repositories so that nursing studies of effectiveness can be accomplished. Testing methods of retrieval of nursing data and for managing the data are also necessary prior to studies of nursing effectiveness. The use of data mining is an important methodological advance for nursing.[4,11] Many other research studies, such as validation studies of decision support systems that are embedded in nursing information systems, quality assurance studies, and studies of patient safety, will also be enabled by these feasibility and methodological preparations.

SUMMARY

The use of NOC in education is increasing as more textbooks and schools move toward the use of standardized languages. These are important steps for the nursing profession and will ensure that future nurses are better equipped to deal with the changes that will take place with the implementation of electronic records and electronic documentation. Research studies using NOC are beginning to appear in the literature, and it is hoped that research studies and evaluations making use of the classification will increase. Only through research that evaluates patient outcomes related to practice will nurses have the data required to demonstrate the quality and effectiveness of our practice. The potential and importance of the contribution that studies using NOC outcomes will make to quality health care worldwide cannot be overestimated as the electronic health record is implemented containing standardized nursing nomenclatures.

References

1. Aydin, C. E., Bolton, L. B., Donaldson, N., Brown, D. S., Buffrum, M., Elashoff, J. D., & Sandhu, M. (2004). Creating and analyzing a statewide nursing quality measurement database. *Journal of Nursing Scholarship, 36*(4), 371-378.
2. Berney, B., & Needleman, J. (2006). Impact of nursing overtime on nurse-sensitive patient outcomes in New York hospitals. *Policy, Politics, Nursing Practice, 7*(2), 87-100.
3. Capuano, R., Bokovoy, J., Hitchings, K., & Houser, J. (2005). Use of a validated model to evaluate the impact of the work environment on outcomes at a magnet hospital. *Health Care Management Review, 30*(3), 229-236.
4. Cheung, R., Moody, L., & Cockram, C. (2002). Data mining strategies for shaping nursing and health policy agenda. *Policy, Politics, & Nursing Practice, 3*(3), 248-260.
5. Deaton, C., & Grady, K. L. (2004). State of the science for cardiovascular nursing outcomes. *Journal of Cardiovascular Nursing, 19*(5), 329-338.
6. Delaney, C. (April 7, 1998). Personal communication via e-mail.
7. Dochterman, J., & Bulechek, G. (2004). *Nursing interventions classification (NIC)*. St. Louis: Mosby.
8. Dochterman, J., & Jones, D. (2003). *Harmonization in nursing language classification*. Washington, DC: American Nurses Association.
9. Fairley, D., & Closs, S. J. (2006). Evaluation of a nurse consultant's clinical activities and the search for patient outcomes in critical care. *Journal of Clinical Nursing, 15*(9), 1106-1114.
10. Finesilver, C., & Metzler, D. (Eds.). (2002). *Curriculum guide for implementation of NANDA, NIC, and NOC into an undergraduate nursing curriculum*. Iowa City, IA: College of Nursing, Center for Nursing Classification and Clinical Effectiveness.
11. Goodwin, L., VanDyne, M., Simon, L., & Talbert, S. (2003). Data mining issues and opportunities for building nursing knowledge. *Journal of Biomedical Informatics, 36*(2003), 379-388.
12. Jenkins, T. (1988). New roles for nursing professionals. In M. J. Ball, K. J. Hannah, A. Gerdin Telger, & H. Peterson (Eds.), *Nursing informatics: Where caring and technology meet* (pp. 88-95). New York: Springer.
13. Johnson, M., Bulechek, G., Butcher, H., Dochterman, J. M., Maas, M., Moorhead, S., & Swanson, E. (2006). *NANDA, NOC, and NIC Linkages*. St. Louis: Mosby.
14. Johnson, M., Bulechek, G., Dochterman, J., Maas, M., & Moorhead, S. (2001). *Nursing diagnoses, outcomes, & interventions NANDA, NOC, and NIC linkages* (2nd ed.). St. Louis: Mosby.
15. Lacey, S. R., Klaus, S. F., Smith, J. B., Cox, K. S., & Dunton, N. E. (2006). Developing measures of pediatric nursing quality. *Journal of Nursing Care Quality, 21*(3), 210-222.
16. Lake, E. T., & Cheung, R. B. (2006). Are patient falls and pressure ulcers sensitive to nurse staffing? *Western Journal of Nursing Research, 28*(6), 654-657.
17. Lu, D., Street, W., & Delaney, C. (2006, June 11 to 14, 2006). *Knowledge discovery: Detecting elderly patients with impaired mobility*. Paper presented at the 9th International Congress on Nursing Informatics, Seoul, South Korea.
18. Maas, M. L., & Delaney, C. (2004). Nursing process outcome linkage research: Issues, current status, and health policy implications. *Medical Care, 42*(2 Suppl), 1140-1148.
19. Mills, W. C. (1994). Tacking through troubled waters: Toward desired outcomes. In R. M. Carroll-Johnson & M. Paquette (Eds.), *Classification of nursing diagnosis: Proceedings of the tenth conference* (pp. 126-130). Philadelphia: Lippincott.
20. Mitnitski, A. B., Mogilner, A. J., Graham, J. E., & Rockwood, K. (2003). Techniques for knowledge discovery in existing biomedical databases: Estimation of individual aging effects in cognition in relation to dementia. *Journal of Clinical Epidemiology, 56*(2), 116-123.
21. Moorhead, S., Johnson, M., & Maas, M. (Eds.). (2004). *Nursing outcomes classification* (3rd ed.). St. Louis: Mosby.
22. Pesut, D. J., & Herman, J. (1999). *Clinical reasoning: The art and science of critical and creative thinking*. Boston: Delmar.

23. Shaughnessy, P. W. & Crisler, K. S. (1995). *Outcome-based quality improvement: A manual for home care agencies on how to use outcomes.* Washington, DC: National Association for Home Care.
24. Yom, Y., & Yoo, H. S. (2002). Application of nursing diagnoses, interventions, and outcomes to patients undergoing abdominal surgery in Korea. *International Journal of Nursing Terminologies and Classifications, 13*(3), 77-87.

PART TWO

NOC Taxonomy

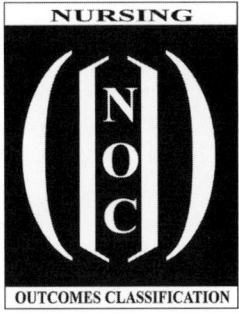

Overview of the NOC Taxonomy

The following section contains the three-level taxonomy for the NOC. This taxonomic structure was developed during the second phase of the research and was first published in the second edition. The NOC taxonomy was created to (1) provide a stable structure for outcome placement over time, (2) allow for the addition of new outcomes as they were developed, (3) allow for the identification of missing outcomes needed for future editions, and (4) assist nurses to identify and select outcomes for the diagnoses they treat for patients, families, and communities. Use of the taxonomy makes identification of possible outcomes for use in practice easier than an alphabetical list of the outcomes. The conceptual grouping of outcomes in the taxonomy has become even more important as the classification has grown over time. Each outcome is listed in only one place in the taxonomy.

DEVELOPMENT OF THE TAXONOMY FOR NOC

The NOC taxonomic structure was developed using strategies refined by the Iowa Intervention Project.[1] The goal was to create a three-level taxonomic structure similar to the one developed for the Nursing Interventions Classification (NIC).[2] This required an inductive approach using qualitative similarity-dissimilarity analysis by many participants sorting outcomes into clusters. Participants assigned a concept label that they felt captured the essence of the cluster. In the first sort, 175 outcomes were grouped in this manner, and the participants were asked to create 15 to 25 clusters based on the sorting process. Hierarchical cluster analysis was then applied to combine the results of each participant's individual sort. This process created the class level of the NOC taxonomy, which when finalized created 24 classes. The classes created using this process are Energy Maintenance, Growth and Development, Mobility, Self-Care, Cardiopulmonary, Elimination, Fluid and Electrolytes, Immune Response, Metabolic Regulation, Neurocognitive, Nutrition, Tissue Integrity, Psychological Well-Being, Psychological Adaptation, Self-Control, Social Interaction, Health Behavior, Health Beliefs, Health Knowledge, Risk Control and Safety, Health and Life Quality, Symptom Status, Family Caregiver Status, and Maltreatment Resolution.

In the second phase of the development of the taxonomy, the 24 classes were sorted by participants to create the top level of the taxonomy. The results of this process identified 6 domains: Functional Health, Physiologic Health, Psychosocial Health, Health Knowledge and Behavior, Perceived Health, and Family Health. A more detailed description of the process used to create the taxonomy is available elsewhere.[3]

REVISIONS MADE IN THE TAXONOMY SINCE ITS CREATION

The third edition has 7 domains and 31 classes in the taxonomic structure. The addition of 2 new classes resulted in some changes in the placement of outcomes within the taxonomy for this edition. Community Health was added as a domain to the taxonomy to allow for inclusion of outcomes focused on the community as the recipient of care. This domain contains outcomes that describe the health, well-being, and functioning of a community or population. Like the Family Domain, the focus of care is on a group rather than an individual. In this case, the population might be an entire community, a neighborhood, or a population of patients with the same health concern.

In addition to the inclusion of two new classes, several other modifications were made in the class level of the taxonomy. The definition of the class Health Knowledge was modified for this edition. The performance aspect of this class was eliminated, so the words "and skills" were removed from the definition. This was done to keep knowledge separate from behavior in the classification. The definition of Domain V, Perceived Health, was modified to describe an individual's health and health care. A new class was added to this domain to include the addition of the client satisfaction outcomes. This class called Satisfaction with Care includes outcomes that describe an individual's perceptions of the quality and adequacy of their health care. Because of this addition, the definition of the class Health and Life Quality was modified. Several changes were made in Domain VI, Family Health. A new class was added called Parenting. This class contains outcomes that describe behaviors of parents that promote growth and development. The class Family Care Status was renamed Family Caregiver Performance to better reflect the outcomes in this class.

CODING OF THE CLASSIFICATION

Once the taxonomic structure was created, coding of the NOC became a high priority for the second edition. Coding is important because it creates a way to (1) represent each of the taxonomic elements, (2) facilitate use of NOC in computer systems, (3) create nursing data sets that can be linked with large regional and national health care databases, and (4) facilitate client outcome evaluation to improve the quality of patient care. The coding structure for NOC includes the domains, classes, outcomes, indicators of each outcome, the measurement scales, and actual scores recorded by users.

Every effort has been made to retain codes used in the second edition in the third edition of this classification. With classification work, it is important to keep coding of the outcomes consistent across editions. When changes were made in this edition, careful consideration of whether the outcome was a new outcome or a revision had to be made. Any outcome that was just updated and revised retained its original code. In a few cases, the outcome revisions resulted in the creation of new outcomes from a previous outcome in the classification. In this case the old outcome was retired (along with its code), and each new outcome was given a new code. Codes for any indicator eliminated from the outcome resulted in the retiring of the code assigned to that indicator. Each outcome had the code for the indicator "Other" retired for that outcome. This indicator was removed because testing in practice demonstrated that data from this indicator was not clinically useful. In many outcomes, the indicators were organized in a new list, but the indicators retained their original codes in spite of placement in the outcome.

Table 2-1 CODING STRUCTURE OF NOC

Domain (1-9)	Class (A-Z) or (a-z)	Outcome (4 numbers)	Indicator (01-99)	Scale (01-99)	Scale Value (1-5)
#	A	####	##	##	###

The addition of a second scale to some outcomes has resulted in the need to modify the coding scheme for the scale data. Scales in the previous addition were coded with a letter of the alphabet. We continue to assign a letter to each scale, but the coding of the scales will need to account for the fact that two scales are in use for some outcomes. The coding will use a number to reflect what scale or scale combinations are used for that outcome, and because there are more than nine scales, the codes for the scales coding will require two spaces in the structure (Table 2-1).

This coding structure allows for expansion of the NOC at every level of the taxonomy and creates a unique identification for each outcome, indicator, and measurement scale. For example, 2 additional domains can be added and the classification can have up to 21 new classes, each containing up to 99 outcomes. This structure allows for substantial additions to the classifications without changing the coding structure. Since the first draft of the taxonomy was created, 155 new outcomes have been developed and placed in the taxonomy. Few changes in the structure have been needed to accomplish this. Changes in the outcomes for this edition are summarized in Appendix A.

The NOC Taxonomy

Level 1 Domains	(1) Domain I	(2) Domain II
	Functional Health Outcomes that describe capacity for and performance of basic tasks of life	**Physiologic Health** Outcomes that describe organic functioning
Level 2 Classes	**A-Energy Maintenance** Outcomes that describe an individual's energy rejuvenation, conservation, and expenditure	**E-Cardiopulmonary** Outcomes that describe an individual's cardiac, pulmonary, circulatory, or tissue perfusion status
	B-Growth & Development Outcomes that describe an individual's physical, emotional, and social maturation	**F-Elimination** Outcomes that describe an individual's waste excretion, elimination patterns, and status
		G-Fluid & Electrolytes Outcomes that describe an individual's fluid and electrolyte status
	C-Mobility Outcomes that describe an individual's physical mobilityand the sequelae of restricted movement	**H-Immune Response** Outcomes that describe an individual's physiological reaction to substances that are foreign or interpreted by the body as foreign
	D-Self-Care Outcomes that describe an individual's ability to accomplish basic and instrumental activities of daily living	**I-Metabolic Regulation** Outcomes that describe an individual's ability to regulate body metabolism
		J-Neurocognitive Outcomes that describe an individual's neurological and cognitive status
		K-Digestion & Nutrition Outcomes that describe an individual's digestion and nutritional patterns
		a-Therapeutic Response Outcomes that describe an individual's systemic reaction to a remedial health treatment, agent, or method
		L-Tissue Integrity Outcomes that describe the condition and function of an individual's body tissues
		Y-Sensory Function Outcomes that describe an individual's perception and use of sensory information

Continued

THE NOC TAXONOMY

Level 1 Domains	(3) Domain III	(4) Domain IV
	Psychosocial Health Outcomes that describe psychological and social functioning	**Health Knowledge & Behavior** Outcomes that describe attitudes, comprehension, and actions with respect to health and illness
Level 2 Classes	**M-Psychological Well-Being** Outcomes that describe an individual's emotional health	**Q-Health Behavior** Outcomes that describe an individual's actions to promote, maintain, or restore health
	N-Psychosocial Adaptation Outcomes that describe an individual's psychological and/or social adaptation to altered health or life circumstances	**R-Health Beliefs** Outcomes that describe an individual's ideas and perceptions that influence health behavior
	O-Self-Control Outcomes that describe an individual's ability to restrain behavior that may be emotionally or physically harmful to self or others	**S-Health Knowledge** Outcomes that describe an individual's understanding in applying information to promote, maintain, and restore health
	P-Social Interaction Outcomes that describe an individual's relationships with others	**T-Risk Control & Safety** Outcomes that describe an action to avoid, limit, or individual's safetystatus and/or actions to avoid, limit, or control identifiable health threats

(5) Domain V	(6) Domain VI	(7) Domain VII
Perceived Health Outcomes that describe impressions of an individual's health and health care	**Family Health** Outcomes that describe health status, behavior, or functioning of the family as a whole or of an individual as a family member	**Community Health** Outcomes that describe the health, well-being, and functioning of a community or population
U-Health & Life Quality Outcomes that describe an individual's perceived health status and related life circumstances	**W-Family Caregiver Performance** Outcomes that describe the adaptation and performance of a family member caring for a dependent child or adult	**b-Community Well-Being** Outcomes that describe the overall health status and social competence of a population or community or population
V-Symptom Status Outcomes that describe an individual's indications of a disease, injury, or loss	**Z-Family Member Health Status** Outcomes that describe the physical, psychological, social, and spiritual health of an individual family member	**c-Community Health Protection** Outcomes that describe the structures and programs of a community to eliminate or reduce health risks and increase community resistance to health threats
e-Satisfaction with Care Outcomes that describe an individual's perceptions of the quality and adequacy of health care provided	**X-Family Well-Being** Outcomes that describe the family environment overall health status and social competence of a family as a unit	
	d-Parenting Outcomes that describe behaviors of parents that promote optimum growth and development of a child	

Continued

Level 1 Domain	**(1) Domain I—Functional Health**	
	Outcomes that describe capacity for and performance of basic tasks of life	
Level 2 Classes	**A-Energy Maintenance** Outcomes that describe an individual's energy rejuvenation, conservation, and expenditure	**B-Growth & Development** Outcomes that describe an individual's physical, emotional, and social maturation
Level 3 Outcomes	0005-Activity Tolerance 0001-Endurance 0002-Energy Conservation 0007-Fatigue Level 0006-Psychomotor Energy 0003-Rest 0004-Sleep	0120-Child Development: 1 Month 0100-Child Development: 2 Months 0101-Child Development: 4 Months 0102-Child Development: 6 Months 0103-Child Development: 12 Months 0104-Child Development: 2 Years 0105-Child Development: 3 Years 0106-Child Development: 4 Years 0107-Child Development: 5 Years 0108-Child Development: Middle Childhood 0109-Child Development: Adolescence 0121-Development: Late Adulthood 0122-Development: Middle Adulthood 0123-Development: Young Adulthood 0111-Fetal Status: Antepartum 0112-Fetal Status: Intrapartum 0110-Growth 0118-Newborn Adaptation 0113-Physical Aging 0114-Physical Maturation: Female 0115-Physical Maturation: Male 0116-Play Participation 0117-Preterm Infant Organization 0119-Sexual Functioning

C-Mobility
Outcomes that describe an individual's physical mobility and the sequelae of restricted movement

0200-Ambulation
0201-Ambulation: Wheelchair
0202-Balance
0203-Body Positioning: Self-Initiated
0212-Coordinated Movement
0204-Immobility Consequences:
    Physiological
0205-Immobility Consequences:
    Psycho-Cognitive
0206-Joint Movement
0213-Joint Movement: Ankle
0214-Joint Movement: Elbow
0215-Joint Movement: Fingers
0216-Joint Movement: Hip
0217-Joint Movement: Knee
0218-Joint Movement: Neck
0207-Joint Movement: Passive
0219-Joint Movement: Shoulder
0220-Joint Movement: Spine
0221-Joint Movement: Wrist
0208-Mobility
0211-Skeletal Function
0210-Transfer Performance

D-Self-Care
Outcomes that describe an individual's ability to accomplish basic and instrumental activities of daily living

0311-Discharge Readiness: Independent
    Living
0312-Discharge Readiness: Supported
    Living
0313-Self-Care Status
0300-Self-Care: Activities of Daily Living (ADL)
0301-Self-Care: Bathing
0302-Self-Care: Dressing
0303-Self-Care: Eating
0305-Self-Care: Hygiene
0306-Self-Care: Instrumental Activities of
    Daily Living (IADL)
0307-Self-Care: Non-Parenteral
    Medication
0308-Self-Care: Oral Hygiene
0309-Self-Care: Parenteral Medication
0310-Self-Care: Toileting

Level 1 Domain	**(2) Domain II—Physiologic Health**	
	Outcomes that describe organic functioning	
Level 2 Classes	**E-Cardiopulmonary** Outcomes that describe an individual's cardiac, pulmonary, circulatory, or tissue perfusion status	**F-Elimination** Outcomes that describe an individual's waste excretion, elimination patterns, and status
Level 3 Outcomes	0409-Blood Coagulation 0413-Blood Loss Severity 0400-Cardiac Pump Effectiveness 0414-Cardiopulmonary Status 0401-Circulation Status 0411-Mechanical Ventilation Response: Adult 0412-Mechanical Ventilation Weaning Response: Adult 0415-Respiratory Status 0410-Respiratory Status: Airway Patency 0402-Respiratory Status: Gas Exchange 0403-Respiratory Status: Ventilation 0404-Tissue Perfusion: Abdominal Organs 0405-Tissue Perfusion: Cardiac 0416-Tissue Perfusion: Cellular 0406-Tissue Perfusion: Cerebral 0407-Tissue Perfusion: Peripheral 0408-Tissue Perfusion: Pulmonary	0500-Bowel Continence 0501-Bowel Elimination 0504-Kidney Function 0502-Urinary Continence 0503-Urinary Elimination

G-Fluid & Electrolytes	**H-Immune Response**	**I-Metabolic Regulation**
Outcomes that describe an individual's fluid and electrolyte status	Outcomes that describe an individual's physiological reaction to substances that are foreign or interpreted by the body as foreign	Outcomes that describe an individual's ability to regulate body metabolism
0600-Electrolyte & Acid/Base Balance 0601-Fluid Balance 0603-Fluid Overload Severity 0602-Hydration	0705-Allergic Response: Localized 0706-Allergic Response: Systemic 0700-Blood Transfusion Reaction 0707-Immune Hypersensitivity Response 0702-Immune Status 0703-Infection Severity 0708-Infection Severity: Newborn	0800-Thermoregulation 0801-Thermoregulation: Newborn 0802-Vital Signs 1006-Weight: Body Mass

Continued

Level 1 Domain	(2) Domain II—Physiologic Health (continued)
	Outcomes that describe organic functioning

Level 2 Classes	**J-Neurocognitive** Outcomes that describe an individual's neurological and cognitive status	**K-Digestion & Nutrition** Outcomes that describe an individual's digestion and nutritional patterns

Level 3 Outcomes	0916-Acute Confusion Level
	0900-Cognition
	0901-Cognitive Orientation
	0902-Communication
	0903-Communication: Expressive
	0904-Communication: Receptive
	0905-Concentration
	0906-Decision-Making
	0918-Heedfulness of Affected Side
	0915-Hyperactivity Level
	0907-Information Processing
	0908-Memory
	0909-Neurological Status
	0910-Neurological Status: Autonomic
	0911-Neurological Status:
	    Central Motor Control
	0912-Neurological Status:
	    Consciousness
	0913-Neurological Status:
	    Cranial Sensory/Motor Function
	0917-Neurological Status:
	    Peripheral
	0914-Neurological Status:
	    Spinal Sensory/Motor Function
		1014-Appetite
		1000-Breastfeeding Establishment:
		    Infant
		1001-Breastfeeding Establishment:
		    Maternal
		1002-Breastfeeding Maintenance
		1003-Breastfeeding Weaning
		1015-Gastrointestinal Function
		1004-Nutritional Status
		1005-Nutritional Status:
		    Biochemical Measures
		1007-Nutritional Status: Energy
		1008-Nutritional Status:
		    Food & Fluid Intake
		1009-Nutritional Status:
		    Nutrient Intake
		1010-Swallowing Status
		1011-Swallowing Status:
		    Esophageal Phase
		1012-Swallowing Status:
		    Oral Phase
		1013-Swallowing Status:
		    Pharyngeal Phase

a-Therapeutic Response	L-Tissue Integrity	Y-Sensory Function
Outcomes that describe an individual's systemic reaction to a remedial health treatment, agent, or method	Outcomes that describe the condition and function of an individual's body tissues	Outcomes that describe an individual's perception and use of sensory information
2300-Blood Glucose Level 2301-Medication Response 2303-Post-Procedure Recovery 2302-Systemic Toxin Clearance: Dialysis	1104-Bone Healing 1106-Burn Healing 1107-Burn Recovery 1105-Hemodialysis Access 1100-Oral Hygiene 1101-Tissue Integrity: Skin & Mucous Membranes 1102-Wound Healing: Primary Intention 1103-Wound Healing: Secondary Intention	2405-Sensory Function 2400-Sensory Function: Cutaneous 2401-Sensory Function: Hearing 2402-Sensory Function: Proprioception 2403-Sensory Function: Taste & Smell 2404-Sensory Function: Vision

Level 1 Domain	**(3) Domain III—Psychosocial Health**
	Outcomes that describe psychological and social functioning

Level 2 Classes	**M-Psychological Well-Being** Outcomes that describe an individual's emotional health	**N-Psychosocial Adaptation** Outcomes that describe an individual's psychological and/or social adaptation to altered health or life circumstances
Level 3 Outcomes	1214-Agitation Level 1211-Anxiety Level 1200-Body Image 1208-Depression Level 1210-Fear Level 1213-Fear Level: Child 1201-Hope 1202-Identity 1203-Loneliness Severity 1204-Mood Equilibrium 1209-Motivation 1205-Self-Esteem 1207-Sexual Identity 1212-Stress Level 1206-Will to Live	1300-Acceptance: Health Status 1308-Adaptation to Physical Disability 1301-Child Adaptation to Hospitalization 1302-Coping 1307-Dignified Life Closure 1304-Grief Resolution 1309-Personal Resiliency 1305-Psychosocial Adjustment: Life Change

O-Self-Control Outcomes that describe an individual's ability to restrain behavior that may be emotionally or physically harmful to self or others	**P-Social Interaction** Outcomes that describe an individual's relationships with others
1400-Abusive Behavior Self-Restraint 1401-Aggression Self-Control 1402-Anxiety Self-Control 1409-Depression Self-Control 1403-Distorted Thought Self-Control 1404-Fear Self-Control 1405-Impulse Self-Control 1406-Self-Mutilation Restraint 1408-Suicide Self-Restraint	1500-Parent-Infant Attachment 1501-Role Performance 1502-Social Interaction Skills 1503-Social Involvement 1504-Social Support

Level 1 Domain	(4) Domain IV—Health Knowledge & Behavior	
	Outcomes that describe attitudes, comprehension, and actions with respect to health and illness	
Level 2 Classes	**Q-Health Behavior** Outcomes that describe an individual's actions to promote, maintain, or restore health	**R-Health Beliefs** Outcomes that describe an individual's ideas and perceptions that influence health behavior
Level 3 Outcomes	1600-Adherence Behavior 1621-Adherence Behavior: Healthy Diet 1629-Alcohol Abuse Cessation Behavior 0704-Asthma Self-Management 1616-Body Mechanics Performance 1617-Cardiac Disease Self-Management 1601-Compliance Behavior 1622-Compliance Behavior: Prescribed Diet 1623-Compliance Behavior: Prescribed Medication 1619-Diabetes Self-Management 1630-Drug Abuse Cessation Behavior 1602-Health Promoting Behavior 1603-Health Seeking Behavior 1610-Hearing Compensation Behavior 1604-Leisure Participation 1631-Multiple Sclerosis Self-Management 1618-Nausea & Vomiting Control 1615-Ostomy Self-Care 1605-Pain Control 1606-Participation in Health Care Decisions 1614-Personal Autonomy 1624-Postpartum Maternal Health Behavior 1607-Prenatal Health Behavior 1620-Seizure Control 1613-Self-Direction of Care 1625-Smoking Cessation Behavior 1608-Symptom Control 1609-Treatment Behavior: Illness or Injury 1611-Vision Compensation Behavior 1626-Weight Gain Behavior 1627-Weight Loss Behavior 1628-Weight Maintenance Behavior	1700-Health Beliefs 1701-Health Beliefs: Perceived Ability to Perform 1702-Health Beliefs: Perceived Control 1703-Health Beliefs: Perceived Resources 1704-Health Beliefs: Perceived Threat 1705-Health Orientation

S-Health Knowledge	T-Risk Control & Safety
Outcomes that describe an individual's understanding in applying information to promote, maintain, and restore health	Outcomes that describe an individual's safety status and/or actions to avoid, limit, or control identifiable health threats

1831-Knowledge: Arthritis Management
1832-Knowledge: Asthma Management
1827-Knowledge: Body Mechanics
1800-Knowledge: Breastfeeding
1833-Knowledge: Cancer Management
1834-Knowledge: Cancer Threat Reduction
1830-Knowledge: Cardiac Disease Management
1835-Knowledge: Congestive Heart Failure
    Management
1801-Knowledge: Child Physical Safety
1821-Knowledge: Conception Prevention
1836-Knowledge: Depression Management
1820-Knowledge: Diabetes Management
1802-Knowledge: Diet
1803-Knowledge: Disease Process
1804-Knowledge: Energy Conservation
1828-Knowledge: Fall Prevention
1816-Knowledge: Fertility Promotion
1805-Knowledge: Health Behavior
1823-Knowledge: Health Promotion
1806-Knowledge: Health Resources
1837-Knowledge: Hypertension Management
1824-Knowledge: Illness Care
1819-Knowledge: Infant Care
1842-Knowledge: Infection Management
1817-Knowledge: Labor & Delivery
1808-Knowledge: Medication
1838-Knowledge: Multiple Sclerosis Management
1829-Knowledge: Ostomy Care
1843-Knowledge: Pain Management
1826-Knowledge: Parenting
1809-Knowledge: Personal Safety
1818-Knowledge: Postpartum Maternal Health
1822-Knowledge: Preconception Maternal Health
1810-Knowledge: Pregnancy
1839-Knowledge: Pregnancy & Postpartum
    Sexual Functioning
1811-Knowledge: Prescribed Activity
1840-Knowledge: Preterm Infant Care
1815-Knowledge: Sexual Functioning
1812-Knowledge: Substance Use Control
1814-Knowledge: Treatment Procedure
1813-Knowledge: Treatment Regimen
1841-Knowledge: Weight Management
	1918-Aspiration Prevention
	1919-Elopement Occurrence
	1920-Elopement Propensity Risk
	1909-Fall Prevention Behavior
	1912-Falls Occurrence
	1900-Immunization Behavior
	1911-Personal Safety Behavior
	1913-Physical Injury Severity
	1921-Pre-Procedure Readiness
	1902-Risk Control
	1903-Risk Control: Alcohol Use
	1917-Risk Control: Cancer
	1914-Risk Control: Cardiovascular Health
	1904-Risk Control: Drug Use
	1915-Risk Control: Hearing Impairment
	1922-Risk Control: Hyperthermia
	1923-Risk Control: Hypothermia
	1924-Risk Control: Infectious Process
	1905-Risk Control: Sexually Transmitted
	    Diseases (STD)
	1925-Risk Control: Sun Exposure
	1906-Risk Control: Tobacco Use
	1907-Risk Control: Unintended Pregnancy
	1916-Risk Control: Visual Impairment
	1908-Risk Detection
	1910-Safe Home Environment
	1926-Safe Wandering

Level 1 Domain	(5) Domain V—Perceived Health	
	Outcomes that describe impressions of an individual's health and health care	
Level 2 Classes	**U-Health & Life Quality** Outcomes that describe an individual's perceived health status and related life circumstances	**V-Symptom Status** Outcomes that describe an individual's indications of a disease, injury, or loss
Level 3 Outcomes	2008-Comfort Status 2009-Comfort Status: Environment 2010-Comfort Status: Physical 2011-Comfort Status: Psychospiritual 2012-Comfort Status: Sociocultural 2007-Comfortable Death 2006-Personal Health Status 2002-Personal Well-Being 2004-Physical Fitness 2000-Quality of Life 2001-Spiritual Health 2005-Student Health Status	2109-Discomfort Level 2106-Nausea & Vomiting: Disruptive Effects 2107-Nausea & Vomiting Severity 1306-Pain: Adverse Psychological Response 2101-Pain: Disruptive Effects 2102-Pain Level 1407-Substance Addiction Consequences 2108-Substance Withdrawal Severity 2003-Suffering Severity 2103-Symptom Severity 2104-Symptom Severity: Perimenopause 2105-Symptom Severity: Premenstrual Syndrome (PMS)

e-Satisfaction with Care
Outcomes that describe an individual's perceptions of the quality and adequacy of their health care provided

3014-Client Satisfaction
3000-Client Satisfaction: Access to Care Resources
3001-Client Satisfaction: Caring
3015-Client Satisfaction: Case Management
3002-Client Satisfaction: Communication
3003-Client Satisfaction: Continuity of Care
3004-Client Satisfaction: Cultural Needs Fulfillment
3005-Client Satisfaction: Functional Assistance
3016-Client Satisfaction: Pain Management
3006-Client Satisfaction: Physical Care
3007-Client Satisfaction: Physical Environment
3008-Client Satisfaction: Protection of Rights
3009-Client Satisfaction: Psychological Care
3010-Client Satisfaction: Safety
3011-Client Satisfaction: Symptom Control
3012-Client Satisfaction: Teaching
3013-Client Satisfaction: Technical Aspects of Care

Level 1 Domain	**(6) Domain VI—Family Health**	
	Outcomes that describe health status, behavior, or functioning of the family as a whole or of an individual as a family member	
Level 2 Classes	**W-Family Caregiver Performance** Outcomes that describe the adaptation and performance of a family member caring for a dependent child or adult	**Z-Family Member Health Status** Outcomes that describe the physical, psychological, social, and spiritual, and emotional health of an individual family member
Level 3 Outcomes	2200-Caregiver Adaptation to Patient Institutionalization 2202-Caregiver Home Care Readiness 2203-Caregiver Lifestyle Disruption 2204-Caregiver-Patient Relationship 2205-Caregiver Performance: Direct Care 2206-Caregiver Performance: Indirect Care 2210-Caregiver Role Support 2208-Caregiver Stressors	2500-Abuse Cessation 2501-Abuse Protection 2514-Abuse Recovery 2502-Abuse Recovery: Emotional 2503-Abuse Recovery: Financial 2504-Abuse Recovery: Physical 2505-Abuse Recovery: Sexual 2506-Caregiver Emotional Health 2507-Caregiver Physical Health 2508-Caregiver Well-Being 2509-Maternal Status: Antepartum 2510-Maternal Status: Intrapartum 2511-Maternal Status: Postpartum 2513-Neglect Cessation 2512-Neglect Recovery

X-Family Well-Being	**d-Parenting**
Outcomes that describe the family environment overall health status and social competence of a family as a unit	Outcomes that describe behaviors of parents that promote optimum growth and development of a child

2600-Family Coping
2602-Family Functioning
2606-Family Health Status
2603-Family Integrity
2604-Family Normalization
2605-Family Participation in
    Professional Care
2608-Family Resiliency
2601-Family Social Climate
2609-Family Support During Treatment
	2902-Parenting: Adolescent Physical Safety
	2901-Parenting: Early/Middle Childhood
	    Physical Safety
	2900-Parenting: Infant/Toddler Physical Safety
	2211-Parenting Performance
	1901-Parenting: Psychosocial Safety

Level 1 Domain	**(7) Domain VII—Community Health** Outcomes that describe the health, well-being, and functioning of a community or population
Level 2 Classes	**b-Community Well-Being** Outcomes that describe the overall health status and social competence of a population or community
Level 3 Outcomes	2700-Community Competence 2701-Community Health Status 2800-Community Health Status: Immunity 2702-Community Violence Level

c-Community Health Protection
Outcomes that describe the structures and programs of a community to eliminate or reduce health risks and increase community resistance to health threats

2804-Community Disaster Readiness
2806-Community Disaster Response
2801-Community Risk Control: Chronic Disease
2802-Community Risk Control: Communicable Disease
2803-Community Risk Control: Lead Exposure
2805-Community Risk Control: Violence

References

1. Iowa Intervention Project. (1993). The NIC taxonomy structure. *Image: Journal of Nursing Scholarship, 25*(3), 187-192.
2. Iowa Intervention Project. J. C. McCloskey, & G. M. Bulechek (Eds.). (1996). *Nursing Interventions Classification (NIC)* (2nd ed.). St. Louis: Mosby Year Book.
3. Moorhead, S., Head, B., Johnson, M. & Maas, M. (1998). The Nursing Outcomes Taxonomy: Development and coding. *Journal of Nursing Care Quality, 12*(6), 56-63.

PART THREE

Outcomes

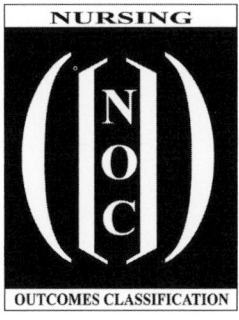

NURSING

NOC

OUTCOMES CLASSIFICATION

Abuse Cessation—2500

Domain-Family Health (VI)

Class-Family Member Health Status (Z)

Scale(s)-None to Extensive (i)

Care Recipient:

Data Source:

Definition: Evidence that the victim is no longer hurt or exploited

OUTCOME TARGET RATING: Maintain at_____   Increase to_____

Abuse Cessation Overall Rating	None 1	Limited 2	Moderate 3	Substantial 4	Extensive 5	
INDICATORS:						
250002 Evidence that physical abuse has ceased	1	2	3	4	5	NA
250003 Evidence that emotional abuse has ceased	1	2	3	4	5	NA
250004 Evidence that sexual abuse has ceased	1	2	3	4	5	NA
250006 Evidence that financial exploitation has ceased	1	2	3	4	5	NA

1st edition 1997; Revised 3rd edition 2004

Outcome Content References:

Amundson, M. J. (1989). Family crisis care: A home based intervention program for child abuse. *Issues in Mental Health Nursing, 10*, 285-296.

Cowen, P. (1991). *The Iowa Crisis Nursery Project as a factor in the prevention of abuse.* Unpublished doctoral dissertation, Iowa City: University of Iowa.

Marshall, E., Buckner, E., Perkins, J., Lowry, J., Hyatt, C., Campbell, C., & Helms, D. (1996). Effects of a child abuse prevention unit in health classes in four schools. *Journal of Community Health Nursing, 13*(2), 107-122.

Olds, D. L., Henderson, C. R., Chamberlin, R., & Tatelbaum, R. (1986). Preventing child abuse and neglect: A randomized trial of nurse home visitation. *Pediatrics, 78*(1), 65-78.

Pressel, D. M. (2000). Evaluation of physical abuse in children. *American Family Physician, 61*(10), 3057-3064.

Reuter, M. M. (1988). Parenting needs of abusing parents: Development of a tool for evaluation of parent education class. *Journal of Community Health Nursing, 5*(2), 129-140.

+Shepard, M., & Campbell, J. A. (1992). The abusive behavior inventory: A measure of psychological and physical abuse. *Journal of Interpersonal Violence, 7*(3), 291-305.

Silverman, J., & Hudson, M. F. (2000). Elder mistreatment: A guide for medical professionals. *North Carolina Medical Journal, 61*(5), 291-296.

Wang, J. J., Lin, J. N., & Lee, F. P. (2006). Psychologically abusive behaviors by those caring for the elderly in a domestic context. *Geriatric Nursing, 27*(5), 284-291.

A

Abuse Protection—2501

Domain-Family Health (VI)

Class-Family Member Health Status (Z)

Scale(s)-Not adequate to Totally adequate (f)

Care Recipient:

Data Source:

Definition: Protection of self and/or dependent others from abuse

OUTCOME TARGET RATING: Maintain at_____   Increase to_____

Abuse Protection Overall Rating	Not adequate 1	Slightly adequate 2	Moderately adequate 3	Substantially adequate 4	Totally adequate 5	
INDICATORS:						
250101 Plan for leaving situation	1	2	3	4	5	NA
250102 Safety of residence	1	2	3	4	5	NA
250103 Plan for avoiding abuse	1	2	3	4	5	NA
250104 Implementation of plan to avoid abuse	1	2	3	4	5	NA
250105 Safety of self	1	2	3	4	5	NA
250106 Safety of children	1	2	3	4	5	NA
250112 Limitation of contact with abuser	1	2	3	4	5	NA
250108 Self-advocacy	1	2	3	4	5	NA
250113 Facilitation of counseling for abused person	1	2	3	4	5	NA
250110 Withdrawal when relationship is unsafe	1	2	3	4	5	NA
250111 Severance of relationship	1	2	3	4	5	NA
250114 Safety of dependent adult	1	2	3	4	5	NA
250115 Use of restraining order	1	2	3	4	5	NA
250116 Social support	1	2	3	4	5	NA

1st edition 1997; Revised 3rd edition 2004; Revised 4th edition

Outcome Content References:

Brendtro, M., & Bowker, L. H. (1989). Battered women: How can nurses help? *Issues in Mental Health Nursing, 10*(2), 169-180.

+Dutton, M. A. (1992). *Empowering and healing the battered women: A model for assessment and intervention.* New York: Springer.

Helton, A., McFarlane, J., & Anderson, E. (1987). Prevention of battering during pregnancy: Focus on nurse behavioral change. *Public Health Nursing, 4*(3), 166-174.

Hoff, L. A. (1992). Battered women: Understanding, identification, and assessment. A psychosocial perspective, Part 1. *Journal of the American Academy of Nurse Practitioners, 4,* 148-155.

Hoff, L. A. (1993). Battered women: Intervention and prevention. A psychosocial cultural perspective, Part 2. *Journal of the American Academy of Nurse Practitioners, 5*(1), 34-39.

Schiamberg, L. B., & Gans, D. (2000). Elder abuse by adult children: An applied ecological framework for understanding contextual risk factors and the intergenerational character of quality of life. *International Aging & Human Development, 50*(4), 329-359.

Theran, S. A., Sullivan, C. M., Bogat, G. A., Stewart, C. S. (2006). Abusive partners and ex-partners: Understanding the effects of relationship to the abuser on women's well-being. *Violence Against Women, 12*(10), 950-969.

Abuse Recovery—2514

Domain-Family Health (VI)

Class-Family Member Health Status (Z)

Scale(s)-None to Extensive (i)

Care Recipient:

Data Source:

Definition: Extent of healing following physical or psychological abuse that may include sexual or financial exploitation

OUTCOME TARGET RATING: Maintain at_____   Increase to_____

Abuse Recovery Overall Rating	None 1	Limited 2	Moderate 3	Substantial 4	Extensive 5	
INDICATORS:						
251401 Recognition of abusive relationship(s)	1	2	3	4	5	NA
251402 Healing of psychological injuries	1	2	3	4	5	NA
251403 Healing of physical injuries	1	2	3	4	5	NA
251404 Healing of physical injuries due to sexual abuse	1	2	3	4	5	NA
251405 Healing of psychological injuries due to sexual abuse	1	2	3	4	5	NA
251406 Control of personal finances following financial exploitation	1	2	3	4	5	NA
251407 Control of legal matters following financial exploitation	1	2	3	4	5	NA
251408 Self-esteem	1	2	3	4	5	NA
251409 Feelings of empowerment	1	2	3	4	5	NA
251410 Positive interpersonal relationships	1	2	3	4	5	NA

3rd edition 2004; Revised 4th edition

Outcome Content References:

Bass, E., & Davis, L. (1994). The courage to heal: A guide for women survivors of child sexual abuse (3rd ed.). New York: Harper & Row.

Campbell, J., McKenna, L. S., Torres, S., Sheridan, D., & Landenburger, K. (1993). Nursing care of abused women. In J. Campbell & J. Humphreys (Eds.), Nursing care of survivors of family violence (pp. 248-289). St. Louis: Mosby.

Hudson, M. F., & Johnson, T. F. (1986). Elder neglect and abuse: A review of the literature. *Annual Review of Nursing Research,* 6(3), 81-134.

Kaplan, S. J., Pelcovitz, D., & Labruna, V. (1999). Child and adolescent abuse and neglect research: A review of the past 10 years. Part I: Physical and emotional abuse and neglect. *Journal of the American Academy of Child & Adolescent Psychiatry,* 38(10), 1214-1222.

Reed, K. (2005). When elders lose their cents: Financial abuse of the elderly. *Clinics in Geriatric Medicine, 21*(2), 365-382.

Smith, M. E., & Kelly, L. M. (2001). The journey of recovery after a rape experience. *Issues in Mental Health Nursing, 22*(4), 337-352.

Taylor, J. Y. (2000). Sisters of the Yam: African American women's healing and self-recovery from intimate male partner violence. *Issues in Mental Health Nursing, 21*(5), 515-531.

Walsh, K., & Bennett, G. (2000). Financial abuse of older people. *Journal of Adult Protection, 2*(1), 21-29.

Wang, J. J., Lin, J. N., & Lee, F. P. (2006). Psychologically abusive behaviors by those caring for the elderly in a domestic context. *Geriatric Nursing, 27*(5), 284-291.

A

Abuse Recovery: Emotional—2502

Domain-Family Health (VI)   *Care Recipient:*

Class-Family Member Health Status (Z)   *Data Source:*

Scale(s)-None to Extensive (i) and Extensive to None (h)

Definition: Extent of healing of psychological injuries due to abuse

OUTCOME TARGET RATING: Maintain at_____   Increase to_____

Abuse Recovery: Emotional Overall Rating	None 1	Limited 2	Moderate 3	Substantial 4	Extensive 5	

INDICATORS:

		None 1	Limited 2	Moderate 3	Substantial 4	Extensive 5	
250202	Self-confidence	1	2	3	4	5	NA
250203	Self-esteem	1	2	3	4	5	NA
250204	Affect appropriate for situation	1	2	3	4	5	NA
250212	Impulse control	1	2	3	4	5	NA
250213	Self-advocacy	1	2	3	4	5	NA
250214	Feelings of empowerment	1	2	3	4	5	NA
250215	Recognition of abusive relationship	1	2	3	4	5	NA
250217	Expressions of comfort with returning home	1	2	3	4	5	NA
250218	Insight into abusive relationship	1	2	3	4	5	NA
250219	Positive social interactions	1	2	3	4	5	NA
250220	Positive interpersonal relationships	1	2	3	4	5	NA
250221	Positive adjustment to change in living arrangements	1	2	3	4	5	NA

		Extensive	Substantial	Moderate	Limited	None	
250201	Depression	1	2	3	4	5	NA
250205	Suicide attempts	1	2	3	4	5	NA
250206	Trauma-induced psychoneurotic behaviors	1	2	3	4	5	NA
250207	Inappropriate attention seeking behaviors	1	2	3	4	5	NA
250208	Trauma-induced conduct disorders	1	2	3	4	5	NA
250209	Trauma-induced learning difficulties	1	2	3	4	5	NA
250210	Self-injurious behaviors	1	2	3	4	5	NA
250211	Neurotic behaviors	1	2	3	4	5	NA

1st edition 1997; Revised 3rd edition 2004

Outcome Content References:

+Briere, J., & Runtz, M. (1989). The trauma symptom checklist (TSC-33): Early data on a new scale. *Journal of Interpersonal Violence, 4*(2), 151-163.

Campbell, J., McKenna, L. S., Torres, S., Sheridan, D., & Landenburger, K. (1993). Nursing care of abused women. In J. Campbell & J. Humphreys (Eds.), *Nursing care of survivors of family violence* (pp. 248-289). St. Louis: Mosby.

Campbell, J., & Fishwick, N. (1993). Abuse of female partners. In J. Campbell & J. Humphreys (Eds.), *Nursing care of survivors of family violence* (pp. 68-104). St. Louis: Mosby.

Humphreys, J., Lee, K., Neylan, T., & Marmar, C. (2001). Psychological and physical distress of sheltered battered women. *Health Care for Women International, 22*(4), 401-414.

Kaplan, S. J., Pelcovitz, D., & Labruna, V. (1999). Child and adolescent abuse and neglect research: A review of the past 10 years. Part I: Physical and emotional abuse and neglect. *Journal of the American Academy of Child & Adolescent Psychiatry, 38*(10), 1214-1222.

Rosen, L. N., & Martin, L. (1998). Long-term effects of childhood maltreatment history on gender-related personality characteristics. *Child Abuse & Neglect, 22*(3), 197-211.

Taylor, J. Y. (2000). Sisters of the Yam: African American women's healing and self-recovery from intimate male partner violence. *Issues in Mental Health Nursing, 21*(5), 515-531.

A

A

Abuse Recovery: Financial—2503

Domain-Family Health (VI)

Class-Family Member Health Status (Z)

Scale(s)-None to Extensive (i)

Care Recipient:

Data Source:

Definition: Extent of control of monetary and legal matters following financial exploitation

OUTCOME TARGET RATING: Maintain at_____   Increase to_____

Abuse Recovery: Financial Overall Rating	None 1	Limited 2	Moderate 3	Substantial 4	Extensive 5	

INDICATORS:

250301	Control of personal possessions	1	2	3	4	5	NA
250303	Control of personal finances	1	2	3	4	5	NA
250306	Control of withdrawal of money from account(s)	1	2	3	4	5	NA
250302	Control of social security and pension income	1	2	3	4	5	NA
250311	Control of earned income	1	2	3	4	5	NA
250313	Control of court-ordered benefits	1	2	3	4	5	NA
250304	Control of legal matters	1	2	3	4	5	NA
250305	Exercise of legal rights	1	2	3	4	5	NA
250315	Knowledge about financial resources	1	2	3	4	5	NA
250308	Knowledge about legal matters	1	2	3	4	5	NA
250309	Participation in financial planning	1	2	3	4	5	NA
250316	Involvement of occupation of choice	1	2	3	4	5	NA
250312	Protection in financial resources	1	2	3	4	5	NA

1st edition 1997; Revised 3rd edition 2004; Revised 4th edition

Outcome Content References:

Anetzberger, G. J. (1987). *The etiology of elder abuse of adult offspring.* Springfield, IL: Charles C. Thomas.

Baumhover, L. A., Beall, S. C., & Pieroni, R. E. (1990). Elder abuse: An overview of social and medical indicators. *Journal of Health and Human Resources Administration, 12*(4), 414-443.

Hudson, M. F., & Johnson, T. F. (1986). Elder neglect and abuse: A review of the literature. *Annual Review of Nursing Research, 6*(3), 81-134.

Lavrisha, M. (1997). What can nurses do about financial exploitation of elders? *Journal of Gerontological Nursing, 23*(7), 49-50.

Reed, K. (2005). When elders lose their cents: Financial abuse of the elderly. *Clinics in Geriatric Medicine, 21*(2), 365-382.

+Sullivan, C., Campbell, R., Angelique, H., Eby, K., & Davidson, W. (1994). An advocacy intervention program for women with abusive partners: Six-month follow-up. *American Journal of Community Psychology, 22*, 101-122.

Walsh, K., & Bennett, G. (2000). Financial abuse of older people. *Journal of Adult Protection, 2*(1), 21-29.

Weiler, K. (1989). Financial abuse of the elderly: Recognizing and acting on it. *Journal of Gerontological Nursing, 15*(8), 10-15.

A

Abuse Recovery: Physical—2504

Domain-Family Health (VI)

Class-Family Member Health Status (Z)

Scale(s)-None to Extensive (i)

Care Recipient:

Data Source:

Definition: Extent of healing of physical injuries due to abuse

OUTCOME TARGET RATING: Maintain at_____   Increase to_____

Abuse Recovery: Physical Overall Rating	None 1	Limited 2	Moderate 3	Substantial 4	Extensive 5	
INDICATORS:						
250403 Timely treatment of injuries	1	2	3	4	5	NA
250401 Healing of physical injuries	1	2	3	4	5	NA
250407 Resolution of physical health problems	1	2	3	4	5	NA
250404 Use of therapeutic health care as needed	1	2	3	4	5	NA
250405 Use of preventive health care	1	2	3	4	5	NA
250411 Evidence of expected response to treatment	1	2	3	4	5	NA
250408 Maintenance of nutritional requirements	1	2	3	4	5	NA
250409 Urinary continence	1	2	3	4	5	NA
250402 Regular bowel elimination	1	2	3	4	5	NA

1st edition 1997; Revised 3rd edition 2004; Revised 4th edition

Outcome Content References:

+Briere, J., & Runtz, M. (1989). The trauma symptom checklist (TSC-33): Early data on a new scale. *Journal of Interpersonal Violence, 4*(2), 151-163.

Campbell, J., McKenna, L. S., Torres, S., Sheridan, D., & Landenburger, K. (1993). Nursing care of abused women. In J. Campbell & J. Humphreys (Eds.), *Nursing care of survivors of family violence* (pp. 248-289). St. Louis: Mosby.

Campbell, J., & Fishwick, N. (1993). Abuse of female partners. In J. Campbell & J. Humphreys (Eds.), *Nursing care of survivors of family violence* (pp. 68-104). St. Louis: Mosby.

Humphreys, J., Lee, K., Neylan, T., & Marmar, C. (2001). Psychological and physical distress of sheltered battered women. *Health Care for Women International, 22*(4), 401-414.

Kaplan, S. J., Pelcovitz, D., & Labruna, V. (1999). Child and adolescent abuse and neglect research: A review of the past 10 years. Part I: Physical and emotional abuse and neglect. *Journal of the American Academy of Child & Adolescent Psychiatry, 38*(10), 1214-1222.

Marshall, C. E., Benton, D., & Brazier, J. M. (2000). Elder abuse. Using clinical tools to identify clues of mistreatment. *Geriatrics, 55*(2), 42-44.

McFarlane, J., Parker, B., & Soeken, K. (1996). Abuse during pregnancy: Associations with maternal health and infant birth weight. *Nursing Research, 45*(1), 37-42.

A

Abuse Recovery: Sexual—2505

Domain-Family Health (VI)

Class-Family Member Health Status (Z)

Scale(s)-None to Extensive (i) and Extensive to None (h)

Care Recipient:

Data Source:

Definition: Extent of healing of physical and psychological injuries due to sexual abuse or exploitation

OUTCOME TARGET RATING: Maintain at_____   Increase to_____

Abuse Recovery: Sexual Overall Rating	None 1	Limited 2	Moderate 3	Substantial 4	Extensive 5	
INDICATORS:						
250502 Acknowledgment of right to disclose abusive situation	1	2	3	4	5	NA
250505 Expressions of right to have been protected from abuse	1	2	3	4	5	NA
250523 Healing of physical injuries	1	2	3	4	5	NA
250509 Relief of anger in non-destructive ways	1	2	3	4	5	NA
250510 Self-advocacy	1	2	3	4	5	NA
250511 Feelings of empowerment	1	2	3	4	5	NA
250512 Expressions of hope	1	2	3	4	5	NA
250513 Consistency of behavior with social norms	1	2	3	4	5	NA
250514 Evidence of non-abusive same-sex relationships	1	2	3	4	5	NA
250515 Evidence of non-abusive opposite-sex relationships	1	2	3	4	5	NA
250524 Expressions of comfort with gender identity	1	2	3	4	5	NA
250525 Expressions of comfort with sexual orientation	1	2	3	4	5	NA
250521 Verbalization of accurate information about sexual functioning	1	2	3	4	5	NA

	Extensive	Substantial	Moderate	Limited	None	
250501 Verbalization of details of abuse	1	2	3	4	5	NA
250503 Verbalization of feelings about the abuse	1	2	3	4	5	NA
250504 Verbalization of feelings of guilt	1	2	3	4	5	NA
250507 Sleep disturbance	1	2	3	4	5	NA
250508 Depression	1	2	3	4	5	NA
250518 Eating disorders	1	2	3	4	5	NA
250519 Self-mutilation	1	2	3	4	5	NA
250520 Suicide attempts	1	2	3	4	5	NA

1st edition 1997; Revised 3rd edition 2004

Outcome Content References:

Bass, E., & Davis, L. (1994). *The courage to heal: A guide for women survivors of child sexual abuse* (3rd ed.). New York: Harper & Row.

+Briere, J., & Runtz, M. (1989). The trauma symptom checklist (TSC-33): Early data on a new scale. *Journal of Interpersonal Violence, 4*(2), 151-163.

DePanfilis, D. (1986). Literature review of sexual abuse (DHHS Publication No. [OHDSA] 87-30530). Washington, DC: USDHHS, National Center on Child Abuse & Neglect.

Gries, L. T., Goh, D. S., Andrews, M. B., Gilbert, J., Praver, F., & Stelzer, D. N. (2000). Positive reaction to disclosure and recovery from child sexual abuse. *Journal of Child Sexual Abuse, 9*(1), 29-51.

Hill, E. L., Gold, S. N., & Bornstein, R. F. (2000). Interpersonal dependency among adult survivors of childhood sexual abuse in therapy. *Journal of Child Sexual Abuse, 9*(2), 71-86.

Sgroi, S. M. (1982). *Handbook of clinical intervention in child sexual abuse.* Lexington, MA: Lexington Books.

Sgroi, S. M. (Ed). (1988). *Vulnerable populations: Evaluation and treatment of sexually abused children and adult survivors* (Vol. 1). Lexington, MA: Lexington Books.

Sgroi, S. M. (Ed). (1988). *Vulnerable populations: Sexual abuse treatment for children, adult survivors, offenders, and persons with mental retardation* (Vol. 2). Lexington, MA: Lexington Books.

Smith, M. E., & Kelly, L. M. (2001). The journey of recovery after a rape experience. *Issues in Mental Health Nursing, 22*(4), 337-352.

Symes, L. (2000). Arriving at readiness to recover emotionally after sexual assault. *Archives of Psychiatric Nursing, 14*(1), 30-38.

Tremblay, C., Hebért, M., & Piché, C. (2000). Type I and type II posttraumatic stress disorder in sexually abused children. *Journal of Child Sexual Abuse, 9*(1), 65-90.

A

Abusive Behavior Self-Restraint—1400

Domain-Psychosocial Health (III)

Class-Self-Control (O)

Scale(s)-Never demonstrated to Consistently demonstrated (m)

Care Recipient:

Data Source:

Definition: Self-restraint of abusive and neglectful behaviors towards others

OUTCOME TARGET RATING: Maintain at_____   Increase to_____

Abusive Behavior Self-Restraint Overall Rating	Never demonstrated 1	Rarely demonstrated 2	Sometimes demonstrated 3	Often demonstrated 4	Consistently demonstrated 5	

INDICATORS:

140022	Obtains needed treatment	1	2	3	4	5	NA
140020	Participates in required treatment regimen	1	2	3	4	5	NA
140006	Discusses the abusive behavior	1	2	3	4	5	NA
140007	Identifies factors contributing to abusive behavior	1	2	3	4	5	NA
140010	Expresses frustrations	1	2	3	4	5	NA
140013	States expectations congruent with developmental level	1	2	3	4	5	NA
140012	Exhibits self-esteem	1	2	3	4	5	NA
140005	Uses alternative coping mechanisms for stress	1	2	3	4	5	NA
140023	Uses personal support system	1	2	3	4	5	NA
140017	Controls impulses	1	2	3	4	5	NA
140018	Uses correct role behaviors	1	2	3	4	5	NA
140024	Uses appropriate caregiving techniques	1	2	3	4	5	NA
140025	Refrains from physically abusive behavior	1	2	3	4	5	NA
140026	Refrains from emotionally abusive behavior	1	2	3	4	5	NA
140027	Refrains from sexually abusive behavior	1	2	3	4	5	NA
140028	Refrains from neglect of dependent's basic needs	1	2	3	4	5	NA
140008	Expresses feelings about victim	1	2	3	4	5	NA
140016	Expresses empathy for victim	1	2	3	4	5	NA
140011	Uses nurturing behavior toward victim	1	2	3	4	5	NA
140009	Identifies available community resources	1	2	3	4	5	NA

1st edition 1997; Revised 2nd edition 2000; Revised 3rd edition 2004; Revised 4th edition

Outcome Content References:

Amundson, M. J. (1989). Family crisis care: A home based intervention program for child abuse. *Issues in Mental Health Nursing, 10,* 285-296.

Anderson, C. L. (1987). Assessing parenting potential for child abuse risk. *Pediatric Nursing, 13*(5), 323-327.

+Buss, A. H., & Perry, M. (1992). The Aggression Questionnaire. *Journal of Personality and Social Psychology, 63*(3), 452-459.

Cowen, P. (1991). *The Iowa Crisis Nursery Project as a factor in the prevention of child abuse.* Unpublished doctoral dissertation, University of Iowa, Iowa City.

Olds, D. L., Henderson, C. R., Chamberlin, R., & Tatelbaum, R. (1986). Preventing child abuse and neglect: A randomized trial of nurse home visitation. *Pediatrics, 78*(1), 65-78.

Marshall, E., Buckner, E., & Powell, K. (1991). Evaluation of a teen parent program designed to reduce child abuse and neglect and to strengthen families. *Journal of Child and Adolescent Psychiatric and Mental Health Nursing, 4*(3), 96-100.

Reuter, M. M. (1988). Parenting needs of abusing parents: Development of a tool for evaluation of parent education class. *Journal of Community Health Nursing, 5*(2), 129-140.

Taylor, D. K., & Beauchamp, C. (1988). Hospital-based primary prevention strategy in child abuse: A multi-level needs assessment. *Child Abuse and Neglect, 12*(3), 343-354.

Tolman, R. M., Edleson, J. L., & Fendrich, M. (1996). The applicability of the theory of planned behavior to abusive men's cessation of violent behavior. *Violence & Victims, 11*(4), 341-354.

A

Acceptance: Health Status—1300

Domain-Psychosocial Health (III)

Class-Psychosocial Adaptation (N)

Scale(s)-Never demonstrated to Consistently demonstrated (m)

Care Recipient:

Data Source:

Definition: Reconciliation to significant change in health circumstances

OUTCOME TARGET RATING: Maintain at_____   Increase to_____

Acceptance: Health Status Overall Rating	Never demonstrated 1	Rarely demonstrated 2	Sometimes demonstrated 3	Often demonstrated 4	Consistently demonstrated 5	
INDICATORS:						
130002 Relinquishes previous concept of personal health	1	2	3	4	5	NA
130008 Recognizes reality of health situation	1	2	3	4	5	NA
130020 Reports positive self-regard	1	2	3	4	5	NA
130016 Maintains relationships	1	2	3	4	5	NA
130007 Reports decreased need to verbalize feelings about health	1	2	3	4	5	NA
130017 Adjusts to change in health status	1	2	3	4	5	NA
130001 Appears peaceful	1	2	3	4	5	NA
130003 Appears calm	1	2	3	4	5	NA
130018 Exhibits resiliency	1	2	3	4	5	NA
130009 Pursues information about health	1	2	3	4	5	NA
130010 Copes with health situation	1	2	3	4	5	NA
130011 Makes decisions about health	1	2	3	4	5	NA
130012 Clarifies personal values	1	2	3	4	5	NA
130019 Clarifies life priorities	1	2	3	4	5	NA
130013 Reports sense of life being worth living	1	2	3	4	5	NA
130014 Performs self-care tasks	1	2	3	4	5	NA

1st edition 1997; Revised 2nd edition 2000; Revised 3rd edition 2004; Revised 4th edition

Outcome Content References:

Clayton, J. W. (1993). Paving the way to acceptance: Psychological adaptation to death and dying in cancer. *Professional Nurse, 8*(4), 206-211.

Kelley, M. P., & Henry, P. (1993). Open discussion can lead to acceptance: The psychosocial effects of stoma surgery. *Professional Nurse, 9*(2), 101-110.

Kübler-Ross, E. (1977). *On death and dying.* London: Tavistock Press.

Lazarus, R. S., & Folkman, S. (1984). *Stress, appraisal and coping.* New York: Springer.

Longo, M. B. (1993). Facilitating acceptance of a patient's decision to stop treatment. *Clinical Nurse Specialist, 7*(3), 233-243.

Melamed, S., Groswasser, Z., & Stern, M. (1992). Acceptance of disability, work involvement and subjective rehabilitation status of traumatic brain-injured (TBI) patients. *Brain Injury, 6*(3), 233-243.

Reynaud, S. N., & Meeker, B. J. (2002). Coping styles of older adults with ostomies. *Journal of Gerontological Nursing, 28*(5), 30-36.

+Wagnild, G. M., & Young, H. M. (1993). Development and psychometric evaluation of the resilience scale. *Journal of Nursing Measurement, 1*(2), 165-178.

Activity Tolerance—0005

A

Domain-Functional Health (I)

Class-Energy Maintenance (A)

Scale(s)-Severely compromised to Not compromised (a)

Care Recipient:

Data Source:

Definition: Physiologic response to energy-consuming movements with daily activities

OUTCOME TARGET RATING: Maintain at_____   Increase to_____

Activity Tolerance Overall Rating	Severely compromised 1	Substantially compromised 2	Moderately compromised 3	Mildly compromised 4	Not compromised 5	
INDICATORS:						
000501 Oxygen saturation with activity	1	2	3	4	5	NA
000502 Pulse rate with activity	1	2	3	4	5	NA
000503 Respiratory rate with activity	1	2	3	4	5	NA
000508 Ease of breathing with activity	1	2	3	4	5	NA
000504 Systolic blood pressure with activity	1	2	3	4	5	NA
000505 Diastolic blood pressure with activity	1	2	3	4	5	NA
000506 Electrocardiogram findings	1	2	3	4	5	NA
000507 Skin color	1	2	3	4	5	NA
000509 Walking pace	1	2	3	4	5	NA
000510 Walking distance	1	2	3	4	5	NA
000511 Stair climbing tolerance	1	2	3	4	5	NA
000516 Upper body strength	1	2	3	4	5	NA
000517 Lower body strength	1	2	3	4	5	NA
000518 Ease of performing activities of daily living (ADL)	1	2	3	4	5	NA
000514 Ability to speak with physical activity	1	2	3	4	5	NA

2nd edition 2000; Revised 3rd edition 2004

Outcome Content References:

Barnett-Damewood, M., & Carlson-Catalano, J. (2000). Physical activity deficit: A proposed nursing diagnosis. *Nursing Diagnosis, 11*(1), 24-31.

Buchner, D. M. (1995). Clinical assessments of physical activity in older adults. In L. Z. Rubenstein, D. Wieland, & R. Bernabei (Eds.), *Geriatric assessment technology: The state of the art* (pp. 147-159). New York: Springer.

Hosking, R., & Hiller, G. (1989). Using nursing diagnosis in a cardiovascular clinical nurse specialist practice. *Journal of Advanced Medical-Surgical Nursing, 1*(3), 33-41.

Larson, J. L., & Leidy, N. K. (1998). Chronic obstructive pulmonary disease: Strategies to improve functional status. *Annual Review of Nursing Research, 16*, 253-286.

Melillo, K. D., Houde, S. C., Williamson, E., & Futrell, M. (2000). Perceptions of nurse practitioners regarding their role in physical activity and exercise prescription for older adults. *Clinical Excellence for Nurse Practitioners, 4*(2), 108-116.

Mol, V. J., & Baker, C. A. (1991). Activity intolerance in the geriatric stroke patient. *Rehabilitation Nursing, 16*(6), 337-344.

Roberts, S. L., & White, B. (1992). Common nursing diagnoses for pulmonary alveolar edema patients. *Dimensions of Critical Care Nursing, 11*(1), 13-27.

Tack, B. B., & Gilliss, C. L. (1990). Nurse-monitored cardiac recovery: A description of the first 8 weeks. *Heart & Lung, 19*(5), 491-499.

Wieseke, A., Twibell, R., Bennett, S., Marine, M., & Schoger, J. (1994). A content validation study of five nursing diagnoses by critical care nurses. *Heart & Lung, 23*(4), 345-351.

A

Acute Confusion Level—0916

Domain-Physiologic Health (II)

Class-Neurocognitive (J)

Scale(s)-Severe to None (n)

Care Recipient:

Data Source:

Definition: Severity of disturbance in consciousness and cognition that develops over a short period of time

OUTCOME TARGET RATING: Maintain at_____   Increase to_____

Acute Confusion Level Overall Rating	Severe 1	Substantial 2	Moderate 3	Mild 4	None 5	
INDICATORS:						
091601 Disorientation of time	1	2	3	4	5	NA
091602 Disorientation of place	1	2	3	4	5	NA
091603 Disorientation of person	1	2	3	4	5	NA
091604 Psychomotor activity	1	2	3	4	5	NA
091605 Impaired cognition	1	2	3	4	5	NA
091606 Impaired memory	1	2	3	4	5	NA
091607 Difficulty following complex commands	1	2	3	4	5	NA
091608 Difficulty interpreting environmental stimuli	1	2	3	4	5	NA
091609 Difficulty maintaining focus	1	2	3	4	5	NA
091610 Difficulty maintaining conversation	1	2	3	4	5	NA
091611 Misinterpretation of cues	1	2	3	4	5	NA
091612 Meaningless verbalizations	1	2	3	4	5	NA
091613 Altered level of consciousness	1	2	3	4	5	NA
091614 Reduction in abstract reasoning	1	2	3	4	5	NA
091615 Restlessness	1	2	3	4	5	NA
091616 Agitation	1	2	3	4	5	NA
091617 Disruption of sleep-wake pattern	1	2	3	4	5	NA
091618 Labile mood	1	2	3	4	5	NA
091619 Sundowning	1	2	3	4	5	NA
091620 Hallucinations	1	2	3	4	5	NA
091620 Delusions	1	2	3	4	5	NA

4th edition

Outcome Content References:

Foreman, M. D., Mion, L. C., Tryostad, L., & Fletcher, K. (1999). Standard of practice protocol: Acute confusion/delirium. *Geriatric Nursing, 20*(3), 147-152.

Johnson, M. (2001). Assessing confused patients. *Journal of Neurology Neurosurgery and Psychiatry, 71*(Suppl. 1), i7-i12.

Miller, J., Neelon, V., Champagne, M., Bailey, D., Ng'andu, N., Belyea, M., Jarrell, E., Montoya, L., & Williams, A. (1997). The assessment of acute confusion as part of nursing care. *Applied Nursing Research, 10*(3), 143-151.

Rapp, C. G., Wakefield, B., Kundrat, M., Mentes, J., Tripp-Reimer, T., Culp, K., Mobiliy, P. Akins, J., & Onega, L. L. (2000). Acute confusion assessment instruments: Clinical versus research usability. *Applied Nursing Research, 13*(1), 37-45.

Trzepacz, P. T. (1999). The delirium rating scale: Its use in consultation-liaison research. *Psychosomatics, 40*(3), 193-204.

Wakefield, B., Mentes, J., Mobily, P., Tripp-Reimer, T., Culp, K. R., Rapp, C. G., Gaspar, P., Kundrat, M., Wadle, K. R., & Akins, J. (2001). Acute confusion. In M. Maas, K. Buckwalter, M. Hardy, T. Tripp-Reimer, M. Titler & J. Specht (Eds.), *Nursing care of older adults: Diagnoses, outcomes & interventions* (pp. 442-454). St. Louis: Mosby.

Adaptation to Physical Disability—1308

Domain-Psychosocial Health (III)   Care Recipient:

Class-Psychosocial Adaptation (N)   Data Source:

Scale(s)-Never demonstrated to Consistently demonstrated (m)

Definition: Adaptive response to a significant functional challenge due to a physical disability

OUTCOME TARGET RATING: Maintain at_____   Increase to_____

Adaptation to Physical Disability Overall Rating	Never demonstrated 1	Rarely demonstrated 2	Sometimes demonstrated 3	Often demonstrated 4	Consistently demonstrated 5	

INDICATORS:

130801	Verbalizes ability to adjust to disability	1	2	3	4	5	NA
130802	Verbalizes reconciliation to disability	1	2	3	4	5	NA
130803	Adapts to functional limitations	1	2	3	4	5	NA
130804	Modifies lifestyle to accommodate disability	1	2	3	4	5	NA
130805	Modifies career goals to accommodate disability	1	2	3	4	5	NA
130806	Uses strategies to reduce stress related to disability	1	2	3	4	5	NA
130807	Identifies ways to increase sense of control	1	2	3	4	5	NA
130808	Identifies ways to cope with life changes	1	2	3	4	5	NA
130809	Identifies risk of complications associated with disability	1	2	3	4	5	NA
130810	Identifies plan to meet activities of daily living	1	2	3	4	5	NA
130811	Identifies plan to meet instrumental activities of daily living	1	2	3	4	5	NA
130812	Accepts need for physical assistance	1	2	3	4	5	NA
130821	Obtains information about disability	1	2	3	4	5	NA
130822	Uses community resources	1	2	3	4	5	NA
130823	Obtains assistance from health professional	1	2	3	4	5	NA
130824	Uses personal support system	1	2	3	4	5	NA
130817	Reports decrease in stress related to disability	1	2	3	4	5	NA
130818	Reports decrease in negative feelings	1	2	3	4	5	NA
130819	Reports decrease in negative body image	1	2	3	4	5	NA
130820	Reports increase in psychological comfort	1	2	3	4	5	NA

Continued

A

3rd edition 2004; Revised 4th edition

Outcome Content References:

Carlsson, E., Berglund, B., & Norgren, S. (2001). Living with an ostomy and short bowel syndrome: Practical aspects and impact on daily life. *Journal of WOCN: Wound, Ostomy, and Continence Nursing, 28*(2), 96-105.

Gignac, M. A., Cott, C., & Badley, E. M. (2000). Adaptation to chronic illness and disability and its relationship to perceptions of independence and dependence. *Journal of Gerontology Series B-Psychological Sciences, 55*(6), P362-P372.

Livneh, H., Antonak, R. F., & Gerhardt, J. (1999). Psychosocial adaptation to amputation: The role of sociodemographic variables, disability-related factors and coping strategies. *International Journal of Rehabilitation Research, 22*(1), 21-31.

Wingate, S. J. (1986). Levels of pacemaker acceptance by patients. *Heart & Lung, 15*(1), 93-100.

Adherence Behavior—1600

Domain-Health Knowledge & Behavior (IV)

Class-Health Behavior (Q)

Scale(s)-Never demonstrated to Consistently demonstrated (m)

Care Recipient:

Data Source:

Definition: Self-initiated actions to promote optimal wellness, recovery, and rehabilitation

OUTCOME TARGET RATING: Maintain at_____   Increase to_____

Adherence Behavior Overall Rating	Never demonstrated 1	Rarely demonstrated 2	Sometimes demonstrated 3	Often demonstrated 4	Consistently demonstrated 5	
INDICATORS:						
160001 Asks health-related questions	1	2	3	4	5	NA
160002 Seeks health information from a variety of sources	1	2	3	4	5	NA
160016 Evaluates accuracy of health information obtained	1	2	3	4	5	NA
160003 Uses reputable health information to develop strategies	1	2	3	4	5	NA
160004 Weighs risks/benefits of health behavior	1	2	3	4	5	NA
160007 Provides rationale for adopting a health behavior	1	2	3	4	5	NA
160008 Uses strategies to eliminate unhealthy behavior	1	2	3	4	5	NA
160009 Uses strategies to optimize health	1	2	3	4	5	NA
160010 Uses health care services congruent with need	1	2	3	4	5	NA
160011 Performs activities of daily living consistent with energy and tolerance	1	2	3	4	5	NA
160012 Performs self-screening	1	2	3	4	5	NA
160013 Describes rationale for deviating from a health regimen	1	2	3	4	5	NA
160014 Performs self-monitoring of health status	1	2	3	4	5	NA

1st edition 1997; Revised 3rd edition 2004, Revised 4th edition

Outcome Content References:

Burkhart, P. V., Dunbar-Jacob, J. M., & Rohay, J. M. (2001). Accuracy of children's self-reported adherence to treatment. *Journal of Nursing Scholarship, 33*(1), 27-32.

Epstein, L., & Cluss, P. A. (1982). A behavioral perspective on adherence to long-term medical regimens. *Journal of Consulting and Clinical Psychology, 50*, 950-971.

Folden, S. L. (1993). Definitions of health and health goals of participants in a community-based pulmonary rehabilitation program. *Public Health Nursing, 10*(1), 31-35.

+Hettler, B. (1982). Wellness promotion and risk reduction on a university campus. In M. Faber & A. Reinhardt (Eds.), *Promoting health through risk reduction*. New York: Macmillan.

Continued

Jensen, L., & Allen, M. (1993). Wellness: The dialect of illness. *Image—The Journal of Nursing Scholarship, 25*(3), 220-224.

Konradi, D. B., & Lyon, B. L. (2000). Measuring adherence to a self-care fitness walking routine. *Journal of Community Health Nursing, 17*(3), 159-169.

Kravits, R., Hays, R. D., Sherbourne, C. D., DiMatteo, M. R., Rogers, W. H., Ordway, L., & Greenfield, S. (1993). Recall of recommendations and adherence to advice among patients with chronic medical conditions. *Archives of Internal Medicine, 153*(16), 1869-1878.

Miller, P., Wikoff, R., & Hiatt, A. (1972). Fishbein's Model of measured behavior of hypertensive patients. *Nursing Research, 41*(2), 104-109.

Pender, N. J. (1990). Expressing health through lifestyle patterns. *Nursing Science Quarterly, 3*(3), 115-122.

Pender, N. J., & Pender, A. R. (1986). Attitudes, subjective norms, and intentions of engagement in health behaviors. *Nursing Research, 35*(1), 15-18.

Shumaker, S. A., Schron, E. B., & Ockene, J. K. (1998). *The handbook of health behavior change* (2nd ed.). New York: Springer.

Toljamo, M., & Hentinen, M. (2001). Adherence to self-care and social support. *Journal of Clinical Nursing, 10*(5), 618-627.

Woods, N. (1989). Conceptualizations of self-care: Toward health-oriented models. *Advances in Nursing Science, 12*(1), 1-13.

A

Adherence Behavior: Healthy Diet—1621

Domain-Health Knowledge & Behavior (IV)

Class-Health Behavior (Q)

Scale(s)-Never demonstrated to Consistently demonstrated (m)

Care Recipient:

Data Source:

Definition: Personal actions to monitor and optimize a healthy and nutritional dietary regimen

OUTCOME TARGET RATING: Maintain at_____   Increase to_____

Adherence Behavior: Healthy Diet Overall Rating	Never demonstrated 1	Rarely demonstrated 2	Sometimes demonstrated 3	Often demonstrated 4	Consistently demonstrated 5	
INDICATORS:						
162101 Sets achievable dietary goals	1	2	3	4	5	NA
162102 Balances caloric intake and caloric requirements	1	2	3	4	5	NA
162103 Seeks information about established nutritional guidelines	1	2	3	4	5	NA
162104 Uses recommended nutritional guidelines to plan meals	1	2	3	4	5	NA
162105 Selects foods consistent with recommended nutritional guidelines	1	2	3	4	5	NA
162106 Selects portions consistent with recommended nutritional guidelines	1	2	3	4	5	NA
162107 Selects foods based on nutritional information on food labels	1	2	3	4	5	NA
162108 Washes fresh fruits and vegetables before eating	1	2	3	4	5	NA
162109 Prepares foods following dietary recommendations for fat, sodium, and carbohydrates	1	2	3	4	5	NA
162110 Cooks meat, poultry, fish, and eggs based on safety recommendations	1	2	3	4	5	NA
162111 Eats recommended servings of fruits per day	1	2	3	4	5	NA
162112 Eats recommended servings of vegetables per day	1	2	3	4	5	NA
162113 Eats more whole grain products than refined grain products	1	2	3	4	5	NA
162114 Minimizes foods with high caloric value and little nutritional value	1	2	3	4	5	NA
162115 Balances fluid intake and fluid loss	1	2	3	4	5	NA
162116 Maintains hydration	1	2	3	4	5	NA

Continued

A

		Never demonstrated	Rarely demonstrated	Sometimes demonstrated	Often demonstrated	Consistently demonstrated	
162117	Selects foods that provide calcium to meet requirements	1	2	3	4	5	NA
162118	Supplements with vitamins/minerals within suggested guidelines	1	2	3	4	5	NA
162119	Chooses foods consistent with cultural religious beliefs	1	2	3	4	5	NA
162120	Discusses use of herbal remedies with health provider						
162121	Avoids foods that interact with medications						
162122	Avoids foods that interact with herbal remedies	1	2	3	4	5	NA
162123	Avoids foods that trigger allergic reactions	1	2	3	4	5	NA

4th edition

Outcome Content References:

Brownell, K. D., & Cohen, L. R. (1995). Adherence to dietary regimen 2: Components of effective intervention. *Behavioral Medicine, 20*(4), 155-164.

Dudek, S. G. (2007). *Nutrition essentials for nursing practice* (5th rev. ed.). Philadelphia: Lippincott Williams & Wilkins.

Marotz, L. R., Rush, J. M., & Cross, M. Z. (2001). Health, safety, and nutrition for the young child. Albany, NY: Thomson Delmar Learning.

Mayo Clinic Staff. (2007). Healthy diet: Do you know what to eat? Retrieved March 9, 2007, from http://www.mayoclinic.com/health/healthy-diet/NU00200

Aggression Self-Control—1401

Domain-Psychosocial Health (III)

Class-Self-Control (O)

Scale(s)-Never demonstrated to Consistently demonstrated (m)

Care Recipient:

Data Source:

Definition: Self-restraint of assaultive, combative, or destructive behaviors toward others

OUTCOME TARGET RATING: Maintain at_____   Increase to_____

Aggression Self-Control Overall Rating	Never demonstrated 1	Rarely demonstrated 2	Sometimes demonstrated 3	Often demonstrated 4	Consistently demonstrated 5	
INDICATORS:						
140110 Identifies when angry	1	2	3	4	5	NA
140111 Identifies when frustrated	1	2	3	4	5	NA
140112 Identifies situations that precipitate hostility	1	2	3	4	5	NA
140113 Identifies responsibility to maintain control	1	2	3	4	5	NA
140114 Identifies when feeling aggressive	1	2	3	4	5	NA
140115 Identifies alternatives to aggression	1	2	3	4	5	NA
140116 Identifies alternatives to verbal outbursts	1	2	3	4	5	NA
140124 Uses effective conflict resolution skills	1	2	3	4	5	NA
140125 Expresses needs in a non-destructive manner	1	2	3	4	5	NA
140117 Vents negative feelings in a non-destructive manor	1	2	3	4	5	NA
140101 Refrains from verbal outbursts	1	2	3	4	5	NA
140126 Avoids violating others' personal space	1	2	3	4	5	NA
140103 Refrains from striking others	1	2	3	4	5	NA
140104 Refrains from harming others	1	2	3	4	5	NA
140105 Refrains from harming animals	1	2	3	4	5	NA
140106 Refrains from destroying property	1	2	3	4	5	NA
140109 Controls impulses	1	2	3	4	5	NA
140121 Uses physical activity to reduce pent-up energy	1	2	3	4	5	NA
140122 Uses techniques to control anger	1	2	3	4	5	NA
140123 Uses techniques to control frustration	1	2	3	4	5	NA
140118 Upholds contract to restrain aggressive behaviors	1	2	3	4	5	NA
140119 Maintains self-control without supervision	1	2	3	4	5	NA

Continued

A

1st edition 1997; Revised 2nd edition 2000; Revised 3rd edition 2004; Revised 4th edition

Outcome Content References:

Berkowitz, L. (1993). *Aggression: Its causes, consequences, and control*. New York: McGraw-Hill.

+Buss, A. H., & Perry, M. (1992). The Aggression Questionnaire. *Journal of Personality and Social Psychology, 63*(3), 452-459.

Crowell, D. H., Evans, I. M., & O'Donnell, C. R. (Eds.). (1987). *Childhood aggression and violence*. New York: Plenum.

Grancola, P. R., & Zeichner, A. (1993). Aggressive behavior in the elderly: A critical review. *Clinical Gerontologist, 13*(2), 3-22.

Ingram, T. N. (2001). Risk for violence: Self-directed or directed at others. In M. Maas, K. Buckwalter, M. Hardy, T. Tripp-Reimer, M. Titler & J. Specht (Eds.), *Nursing care of older adults: Diagnoses, outcomes & interventions* (pp. 696-705). St. Louis: Mosby.

Mason, T., Chandley, M. (1999). *Managing violence and aggression: A manual for nurses and health care workers*. Edinburgh: Churchill Livingstone.

Maxfield, M. C., Lewis, R. E., & Connor, S. (1996). Training staff to prevent aggressive behavior of cognitively impaired elderly patients during bathing and grooming. *Journal of Gerontological Nursing, 22*(1), 37-43.

Pepler, D. J., & Rubin, K. H. (Eds.). (1991). *The development and treatment of childhood aggression*. Hillsdale, NJ: Erlbaum.

Rantz, M. J., & McShane, R. E. (1995). Nursing interventions for chronically confused nursing home residents. *Geriatric Nursing, 16*(1), 22-27.

Ryden, M. B. (1992). Aggressive behavior in persons with dementia who live in the community. *Alzheimer Disease and Associated Disorders, 2*(4), 342-355.

Agitation Level—1214

A

Domain-Psychosocial Health (III)

Class-Psychosocial Well-Being (M)

Scale(s)-Severe to None (n)

Care Recipient:

Data Source:

Definition: Severity of disruptive physiologic and behavioral manifestations of stress or biochemical triggers

OUTCOME TARGET RATING: Maintain at_____   Increase to_____

Agitation Level Overall Rating	Severe 1	Substantial 2	Moderate 3	Mild 4	None 5	
INDICATORS:						
121401 Difficulty processing information	1	2	3	4	5	NA
121402 Restlessness	1	2	3	4	5	NA
121403 Frustration	1	2	3	4	5	NA
121404 Irritability	1	2	3	4	5	NA
121405 Pacing	1	2	3	4	5	NA
121406 Repetitious movements	1	2	3	4	5	NA
121407 Inability to remain seated	1	2	3	4	5	NA
121408 Difficulty staying on tasks	1	2	3	4	5	NA
121409 Resists assistance	1	2	3	4	5	NA
121410 Combativeness	1	2	3	4	5	NA
121411 Thrashing in bed	1	2	3	4	5	NA
121412 Pulling at tubes or restraints	1	2	3	4	5	NA
121413 Repetitious mannerisms	1	2	3	4	5	NA
121414 Grabbing	1	2	3	4	5	NA
121415 Hoarding	1	2	3	4	5	NA
121416 Hitting	1	2	3	4	5	NA
121417 Kicking	1	2	3	4	5	NA
121418 Throwing	1	2	3	4	5	NA
121419 Spitting	1	2	3	4	5	NA
121420 Biting	1	2	3	4	5	NA
121421 Emotional lability	1	2	3	4	5	NA
121422 Verbal outbursts	1	2	3	4	5	NA
121423 Inappropriate verbalizations	1	2	3	4	5	NA
121424 Inappropriate gestures	1	2	3	4	5	NA
121425 Disinhibition	1	2	3	4	5	NA
121426 Interrupted sleep	1	2	3	4	5	NA
121427 Weight loss	1	2	3	4	5	NA
121428 Dehydration	1	2	3	4	5	NA
121429 Increased blood pressure	1	2	3	4	5	NA
121430 Increased radial pulse rate	1	2	3	4	5	NA
121431 Increased respiratory rate	1	2	3	4	5	NA

4th edition

Continued

A

Outcome Content References:

Cohen-Mansfield, J. (1996). Behavioral and mood evaluations: Assessment of Agitation. *International Psychogeriatrics, 8*(2), 233-245.

Gray, K. F. (2004). Managing agitation and difficult behavior in dementia. *Clinics in Geriatric Medicine, 20,* 69-82.

Hamill-Ruth, R. J. (2006). Managing pain and agitation in the critically ill—Are we there yet? *Critical Care Medicine, 34*(6), 1838-1839.

Jaber, S., Chanques, G., Altairac, C., Sebbane, M., Vergne, C., Perrigault, P., Eledjam, J. (2005). A prospective study of agitation in a medical-surgical ICU: Incidence, risk factors, and outcomes. *Chest, 128*(4), 2749-2757.

Nott, M. T., Chapparo, C., & Baguley, I. J. (2006). Agitation following traumatic brain injury: An Australian sample. *Brain Injury, 20*(11), 1175-1182.

Sessler, C. N., Gosnell, M. S., Grap, M. J., Brophy, G. M., O'Neal, P. V., Keane, K. A., Tesoro, E. P., & Elswick, R. K. (2002). The Richmond agitation-sedation scale: Validity and reliability in adult intensive care unit patients. *American Journal of Respiratory Critical Care Medicine, 166,* 1338-1344.

A

Alcohol Abuse Cessation Behavior—1629

Domain-Health Knowledge & Behavior (IV)

Class-Health Behavior (Q)

Scale(s)-Never demonstrated to Consistently demonstrated (m)

Care Recipient:

Data Source:

Definition: Personal actions to eliminate alcohol use that poses a threat to health

OUTCOME TARGET RATING: Maintain at_____   Increase to_____

Alcohol Abuse Cessation Behavior Overall Rating	Never demonstrated 1	Rarely demonstrated 2	Sometimes demonstrated 3	Often demonstrated 4	Consistently demonstrated 5	
INDICATORS:						
162901 Expresses willingness to stop alcohol use	1	2	3	4	5	NA
162902 Expresses belief in the ability to stop alcohol use	1	2	3	4	5	NA
162903 Identifies benefits of eliminating alcohol use	1	2	3	4	5	NA
162904 Identifies negative consequences of alcohol use	1	2	3	4	5	NA
162905 Develops effective strategies to eliminate alcohol use	1	2	3	4	5	NA
162906 Identifies barriers to alcohol elimination	1	2	3	4	5	NA
162907 Identifies emotional states that trigger alcohol use	1	2	3	4	5	NA
162908 Adjusts alcohol elimination strategies as needed	1	2	3	4	5	NA
162909 Commits to alcohol elimination strategies	1	2	3	4	5	NA
162910 Follows selected alcohol elimination strategies	1	2	3	4	5	NA
162911 Participates in screening for associated health problems	1	2	3	4	5	NA
162912 Uses strategies to cope with withdrawal symptoms	1	2	3	4	5	NA
162913 Uses behavior modification strategies	1	2	3	4	5	NA
162914 Uses effective coping strategies	1	2	3	4	5	NA
162915 Obtains assistance from health professional	1	2	3	4	5	NA
162916 Uses personal support system	1	2	3	4	5	NA
162917 Uses reputable sources of information	1	2	3	4	5	NA
162918 Participates in Alcoholics Anonymous	1	2	3	4	5	NA
162919 Contacts sponsor for cessation support	1	2	3	4	5	NA

Continued

A

		Never demonstrated	Rarely demonstrated	Sometimes demonstrated	Often demonstrated	Consistently demonstrated	
162920	Encourages family to participate in Al-Anon	1	2	3	4	5	NA
162921	Uses alternative therapy	1	2	3	4	5	NA
162922	Adjusts lifestyle to promote alcohol elimination	1	2	3	4	5	NA
162923	Uses prescribed medication as recommended	1	2	3	4	5	NA
162924	Uses non-prescription medication as recommended	1	2	3	4	5	NA
162925	Avoids situations that encourage alcohol use	1	2	3	4	5	NA
162926	Uses available support groups	1	2	3	4	5	NA
162927	Uses available community resources	1	2	3	4	5	NA
162928	Participates in counseling	1	2	3	4	5	NA
162929	Monitors for signs of depression	1	2	3	4	5	NA
162930	Eliminates alcohol use	1	2	3	4	5	NA

4th edition

Outcome Content References:

Fox, H. C., Bergquist, K. L., Hong, K., & Sinha, R. (2007). Stress-induced and alcohol cue-induced craving in recently abstinent alcohol-dependent individuals. *Alcoholism: Clinical and Experimental Research*, 31(3), 395-403.

Graham, K., Massak, A., Demers, A., & Rehm, J. (2007). Does the association between alcohol consumption and depression depend on how they are measured? *Alcoholism: Clinical and Experimental Research*, 31(1), 78-88.

Grucza, R. A., & Bierut, L. J. (2006). Cigarette smoking and the risk for alcohol use disorders among adolescent drinkers. *Alcoholism: Clinical and Experimental Research*, 30(12), 2046-2054.

Humphreys, K., & Moos, R. H. (2007). Encouraging posttreatment self-help group involvement to reduce demand for continuing care services: Two-year clinical and utilization outcomes. *Alcoholism: Clinical and Experimental Research*, 31(1), 64-68.

Williams, E. C., Horton, N. J., Samet, J. H., & Saitz, R. (2007). Do brief measures of readiness to change predict alcohol consumption and consequences in primary care patients with unhealthy alcohol use? *Alcoholism: Clinical and Experimental Research*, 31(3), 428-435.

Allergic Response: Localized—0705

Domain-Physiologic Health (II)

Class-Immune Response (H)

Scale(s)-Severe to None (n)

Care Recipient:

Data Source:

A

> **Definition:** Severity of localized hypersensitive immune response to a specific environmental (exogenous) antigen

OUTCOME TARGET RATING: Maintain at_____   Increase to_____

Allergic Response: Localized Overall Rating	Severe 1	Substantial 2	Moderate 3	Mild 4	None 5	

INDICATORS:

070501	Sinus pain	1	2	3	4	5	NA
070502	Headache	1	2	3	4	5	NA
070503	Conjunctivitis	1	2	3	4	5	NA
070504	Lacrimation	1	2	3	4	5	NA
070505	Rhinitis	1	2	3	4	5	NA
070506	Sneezing	1	2	3	4	5	NA
070507	Mucous secretions	1	2	3	4	5	NA
070508	Circumoral edema	1	2	3	4	5	NA
070509	Periorbital edema	1	2	3	4	5	NA
070510	Dark circles under eyes	1	2	3	4	5	NA
070511	Burning sensation of eyes	1	2	3	4	5	NA
070512	Localized itching	1	2	3	4	5	NA
070513	Localized rash	1	2	3	4	5	NA
070514	Localized erythema	1	2	3	4	5	NA
070515	Increased localized skin temperature	1	2	3	4	5	NA
070516	Localized edema	1	2	3	4	5	NA
070517	Localized pain	1	2	3	4	5	NA
070518	Localized granuloma	1	2	3	4	5	NA
070519	Localized necrotizing vasculitis	1	2	3	4	5	NA

3rd edition 2004

Outcome Content References:

Altman, G. B., Buchsel, P., & Coxon, V. (2000). *Delmar's fundamental & advanced nursing skills.* Albany, NY: Thomson Delmar Learning.

Beltrani, V. S. (2004). Dermatologic allergy. *Pediatric Asthma Allergy and Immunology, 17*(1), 97-99.

Huether, S. E., & McCance, K. L. (2000). *Understanding pathophysiology* (2nd ed.). St. Louis: Mosby.

Krause, H. F. (2003). Allergy and chronic rhinosinusitis. *Otolaryngological Head Neck Surgery, 128*(1), 14-16.

Ledgerwood, G. L., & D'Arienzo, P. A. (2004). Allergic eye disorders: identification—and alleviation. *Consultant 44*(6), 781-784, 785-786, 788-789.

Lewis, S., Heitkemper, M., & Dirksen, S. (2000). *Medical-surgical nursing: Assessment and management of clinical problems* (5th ed.). St. Louis: Mosby.

McCance, K. L., & Huether, S. E. (2001). *Pathophysiology: The biological basis for disease in adults and children* (4th ed.). St. Louis: Mosby.

Morris, A. J. (2004). Allergy explained: the new definitive terminology. *Nurse, 4*(2), 40-41.

Mudge-Grout, C., (1992). *Immunologic disorders: Mosby's clinical nursing series.* St. Louis: Mosby.

Opperwall, B. (2003). Asthma, allergy, and upper airway disease. *Nursing Clinics of North America, 38*(4), 697-711.

Scally, R. (2003). Living with latex allergies. *Nursezone 2*(1), 5-7.

Smeltzer, S. C., & Bare, B. G. (Eds.). (2003). *Brunner and Suddarth's textbook of medical-surgical nursing* (10th ed.). Philadelphia: Lippincott Williams & Wilkins.

Thelan, L., Urden, L., Lough, M., & Stacy, K. (1998). *Critical care nursing: Diagnosis and management* (3rd ed.). St. Louis: Mosby.

Tortora, G., & Grabowski, S. (1996). *Principles of anatomy and physiology* (8th ed.). New York, NY: Harper Collins.

A

Allergic Response: Systemic—0706

Domain-Physiologic Health (II)
Class-Immune Response (H)
Scale(s)-Severe to None (n)

Care Recipient:
Data Source:

Definition: Severity of systemic hypersensitive immune response to a specific environmental (exogenous) antigen

OUTCOME TARGET RATING: Maintain at_____ Increase to_____

Allergic Response: Systemic Overall Rating	Severe 1	Substantial 2	Moderate 3	Mild 4	None 5	

INDICATORS:

070601	Laryngeal edema	1	2	3	4	5	NA
070602	Dyspnea at rest	1	2	3	4	5	NA
070603	Wheezing	1	2	3	4	5	NA
070604	Stridor	1	2	3	4	5	NA
070605	Adventitious breath sounds	1	2	3	4	5	NA
070606	Tachycardia	1	2	3	4	5	NA
070607	Decreased blood pressure	1	2	3	4	5	NA
070608	Dysrhythmia(s)	1	2	3	4	5	NA
070609	Pulmonary edema	1	2	3	4	5	NA
070610	Decreased level of consciousness	1	2	3	4	5	NA
070611	Mucous secretions	1	2	3	4	5	NA
070612	Facial edema	1	2	3	4	5	NA
070613	Generalized itching	1	2	3	4	5	NA
070614	Hives	1	2	3	4	5	NA
070615	Body exfoliation	1	2	3	4	5	NA
070616	Petechiae	1	2	3	4	5	NA
070617	Erythema	1	2	3	4	5	NA
070618	Increased skin temperature	1	2	3	4	5	NA
070619	Fever	1	2	3	4	5	NA
070620	Chills	1	2	3	4	5	NA
070621	Nausea	1	2	3	4	5	NA
070622	Vomiting	1	2	3	4	5	NA
070623	Diarrhea	1	2	3	4	5	NA
070624	Abdominal cramping	1	2	3	4	5	NA
070625	Red blood cell hemolysis	1	2	3	4	5	NA
070626	Increased bilirubin	1	2	3	4	5	NA
070627	Enlarged spleen	1	2	3	4	5	NA
070628	Enlarged lymph nodes	1	2	3	4	5	NA
070629	Joint pain	1	2	3	4	5	NA
070630	Muscle pain	1	2	3	4	5	NA
070631	Anaphylactic shock	1	2	3	4	5	NA

3rd edition 2004

Outcome Content References:

Altman, G. B., Buchsel, P., & Coxon, V. (2000). *Delmar's fundamental & advanced nursing skills.* Albany, NY: Thomson Delmar Learning.

Gupta, R., Sheikh, A., Strachan, D., & Anderson H. R. (2003). Increasing hospital admissions for systemic allergic disorders in England: Analysis of national admissions data. *British Medical Journal, 327*(7424), 1142-1143

Huether, S. E., & McCance, K. L. (2000). *Understanding pathophysiology* (2nd ed.). St. Louis: Mosby.

Lewis, S., Heitkemper, M., & Dirksen, S. (2000). *Medical-surgical nursing: Assessment and management of clinical problems* (5th ed.). St. Louis: Mosby.

McCance, K., & Huether, S. (2001). *Pathophysiology: The biological basis for disease in adults and children* (4th ed.). St. Louis: Mosby.

Mudge-Grout, C. (1992). *Immunologic disorders: Mosby's clinical nursing series.* St. Louis: Mosby.

Reading, D. (2004). Managing anaphylaxis. *Practicing Nurse, 28*(3), 28, 30-31.

Ryder, S., & Waldmann, C. (2003). Anaphylaxis. *Care for Critical Illness, 19*(6), 174-176.

Smeltzer, S. C., & Bare, B. G. (Eds.). (2003). *Brunner and Suddarth's textbook of medical-surgical nursing* (10th ed.). Philadelphia: Lippincott Williams & Wilkins.

Thelan, L., Urden, L., Lough, M., & Stacy, K. (1998). *Critical care nursing: Diagnosis and management* (3rd ed.). St. Louis: Mosby.

Tortora, G., & Grabowski, S. (1996). *Principles of anatomy and physiology* (8th ed.). New York, NY: Harper Collins.

A

A

Ambulation—0200

Domain-Functional Health (I)

Class-Mobility (C)

Scale(s)-Severely compromised to Not compromised (a)

Care Recipient:

Data Source:

Definition: Ability to walk from place to place independently with or without assistive device

OUTCOME TARGET RATING: Maintain at_____   Increase to_____

Ambulation Overall Rating	Severely compromised 1	Substantially compromised 2	Moderately compromised 3	Mildly compromised 4	Not compromised 5	
INDICATORS:						
020001 Bears weight	1	2	3	4	5	NA
020002 Walks with effective gait	1	2	3	4	5	NA
020003 Walks at slow pace	1	2	3	4	5	NA
020004 Walks at moderate pace	1	2	3	4	5	NA
020005 Walks at fast pace	1	2	3	4	5	NA
020006 Walks up steps	1	2	3	4	5	NA
020007 Walks down steps	1	2	3	4	5	NA
020008 Walks up inclines	1	2	3	4	5	NA
020009 Walks down inclines	1	2	3	4	5	NA
020010 Walks short distance (< 1 block)	1	2	3	4	5	NA
020011 Walks moderate distance (> 1 block < 5 blocks)	1	2	3	4	5	NA
020012 Walks long distance (5 blocks or >)	1	2	3	4	5	NA
020014 Walks around room	1	2	3	4	5	NA
020015 Walks around dwelling	1	2	3	4	5	NA
020016 Adjusts to different surface textures	1	2	3	4	5	NA
020017 Walks around obstacles	1	2	3	4	5	NA

1st edition 1997; Revised 3rd edition 2004; Revised 4th edition

Outcome Content References:

Green, J., Forster, A., & Young, J. (2002). Reliability of gait speed measured by a timed walking test in patients one year after stroke. *Clinical Rehabilitation, 16*(3), 306-314.

+Uniform Data System for Medical Rehabilitation. (1997). *Guide for the Uniform Data Set for Medical Rehabilitation* (including the FIM™ instrument), (version 5.1). Buffalo, NY: UDSMR.

Hoeman, S. (2002). *Rehabilitation nursing: Process, application, and outcomes* (3rd ed.). St. Louis: Mosby.

Jirovec, M. M. (1991). The impact of daily exercise on the mobility, balance, and urine control of cognitively impaired nursing home residents. *International Journal of Nursing Studies, 28*(2), 145-151.

Lord, S. R., & Menz, H. B. (2002). Physiologic, psychologic, and health predictors of 6-minute walk performance in older people. *Archives of Physical Medicine & Rehabilitation, 83*(7), 907-911.

Mikulic, M. A., Griffith, E. R., & Jebsen, R. H. (1976). Clinical application of a standardized mobility test. *Archives of Physical Medicine and Rehabilitation, 57*(3), 143-146.

Pomeroy, V. (1990). Development of an ADL-oriented assessment-of-mobility scale suitable for use for elderly people with dementia. *Physiotherapy, 76*(8), 446-448.

Tinetti, M. E. (1986). Performance-oriented assessment of mobility problems in elderly patients. *Journal of the American Geriatric Society, 34*(2), 119-126.

Ambulation: Wheelchair—0201

A

Domain-Functional Health (I)

Class-Mobility (C)

Scale(s)-Severely compromised to Not compromised (a)

Care Recipient:

Data Source:

Definition: Ability to move from place to place in a wheelchair

OUTCOME TARGET RATING: Maintain at_____   Increase to_____

Ambulation: Wheelchair Overall Rating	Severely compromised 1	Substantially compromised 2	Moderately compromised 3	Mildly compromised 4	Not compromised 5	
INDICATORS:						
020101 Transfers to and from wheelchair	1	2	3	4	5	NA
020102 Propels wheelchair safely	1	2	3	4	5	NA
020103 Propels wheelchair short distance	1	2	3	4	5	NA
020104 Propels wheelchair moderate distance	1	2	3	4	5	NA
020105 Propels wheelchair long distance	1	2	3	4	5	NA
020106 Maneuvers curbs	1	2	3	4	5	NA
020107 Maneuvers doorways	1	2	3	4	5	NA
020108 Maneuvers ramps	1	2	3	4	5	NA

1st edition 1997; Revised 3rd edition 2004

Outcome Content References:

Hoeman, S. (2002). *Rehabilitation nursing: Process, application, and outcomes* (3rd ed.). St. Louis: Mosby.

Kane, R. L., & Kane, R. A. (2000). *Assessing older persons: Measures, meaning, and practical applications.* New York: Oxford University Press.

Lan, T. Y., Melzer, D., Tom, B. D., & Guralnik, J. M. (2002). Performance tests and disability: Developing an objective index of mobility-related limitation in older populations. *Journals of Gerontology. Series A, Biological Sciences & Medical Sciences, 57*(5), M294-M301.

Mikulic, M. A., Griffith, E. R., & Jebsen, R. H. (1976). Clinical application of a standardized mobility test. *Archives of Physical Medicine and Rehabilitation, 57*(3), 143-146.

+Uniform Data System for Medical Rehabilitation. (1997). *Guide for the Uniform Data Set for Medical Rehabilitation* (including the FIM™ instrument), (version 5.1). Buffalo, NY: UDSMR.

A

Anxiety Level—1211

Domain-Psychosocial Health (III)   *Care Recipient:*

Class-Psychosocial Well-Being (M)   *Data Source:*

Scale(s)-Severe to None (n)

Definition: Severity of manifested apprehension, tension, or uneasiness arising from an unidentifiable source

OUTCOME TARGET RATING: Maintain at_____   Increase to_____

Anxiety Level Overall Rating	Severe 1	Substantial 2	Moderate 3	Mild 4	None 5	
INDICATORS:						
121101 Restlessness	1	2	3	4	5	NA
121102 Pacing	1	2	3	4	5	NA
121103 Hand wringing	1	2	3	4	5	NA
121104 Distress	1	2	3	4	5	NA
121105 Uneasiness	1	2	3	4	5	NA
121106 Muscle tension	1	2	3	4	5	NA
121107 Facial tension	1	2	3	4	5	NA
121108 Irritability	1	2	3	4	5	NA
121109 Indecisiveness	1	2	3	4	5	NA
121110 Outbursts of anger	1	2	3	4	5	NA
121111 Problem behavior	1	2	3	4	5	NA
121112 Difficulty concentrating	1	2	3	4	5	NA
121113 Difficulty learning	1	2	3	4	5	NA
121114 Difficulty problem solving	1	2	3	4	5	NA
121115 Panic attack	1	2	3	4	5	NA
121116 Verbalized apprehension	1	2	3	4	5	NA
121117 Verbalized anxiety	1	2	3	4	5	NA
121118 Exaggerated concern about life events	1	2	3	4	5	NA
121119 Increased blood pressure	1	2	3	4	5	NA
121120 Increased pulse rate	1	2	3	4	5	NA
121121 Increased respiratory rate	1	2	3	4	5	NA
121122 Dilated pupils	1	2	3	4	5	NA
121123 Sweating	1	2	3	4	5	NA
121124 Dizziness	1	2	3	4	5	NA
121125 Fatigue	1	2	3	4	5	NA
121126 Decreased productivity	1	2	3	4	5	NA
121127 Decreased school achievement	1	2	3	4	5	NA
121128 Withdrawal	1	2	3	4	5	NA
121129 Sleep disturbance	1	2	3	4	5	NA
121130 Change in bowel pattern	1	2	3	4	5	NA
121131 Change in eating pattern	1	2	3	4	5	NA

3rd edition 2004

Outcome Content References:

American Psychiatric Association. (2000). *Diagnostic and statistical manual of mental disorders* (4th ed. text revision). Washington DC: Author.

Byrne, B. (2000). Relationships between anxiety, fear, self-esteem, and coping strategies in adolescence. *Adolescence, 35*(137), 201-216.

Charron, H. S. (1998). Anxiety disorders. In E. M. Varcarolis (Ed.), *Foundations of psychiatric mental health nursing* (3rd ed., pp. 443-477). Philadelphia: W.B. Saunders.

Kim, M., Sertella, R., Gulanick, M., Moyer, K., Parsons, E., Scherbel, J., Stafford, M., Suhayada, R., & Yocum, C. (1984). Clinical validation of cardiovascular nursing diagnoses. In M. Kim, G. McFarland, & A. McLane (Eds.), *Classification of nursing diagnoses: Proceedings of the fifth national conference* (pp. 128-137). St. Louis: Mosby.

Shuldham, C. M., Cunningham, G., Hiscock, M., & Luscombe, P. (1995). Assessment of anxiety in hospital patients. *Journal of Advanced Nursing, 22*(1), 87-93.

Taylor-Loughran, A. E., O'Brien, M. E., LaChapelle, R., & Rangel, S. (1989). Defining characteristics of the nursing diagnoses fear and anxiety: A validation study. *Applied Nursing Research, 2*(4), 178-186.

Whitley, G. G., & Tousman, S. A. (1996). A multivariate approach for validation of anxiety and fear. *Nursing Diagnosis, 7*(3), 116-124.

A

Anxiety Self-Control—1402

Domain-Psychosocial Health (III)

Class-Self-Control (O)

Scale(s)-Never demonstrated to Consistently demonstrated (m)

Care Recipient:

Data Source:

Definition: Personal actions to eliminate or reduce feelings of apprehension, tension, or uneasiness from an unidentifiable source

OUTCOME TARGET RATING: Maintain at_____   Increase to_____

Anxiety Self-Control Overall Rating	Never demonstrated 1	Rarely demonstrated 2	Sometimes demonstrated 3	Often demonstrated 4	Consistently demonstrated 5	
INDICATORS:						
140201 Monitors intensity of anxiety	1	2	3	4	5	NA
140202 Eliminates precursors of anxiety	1	2	3	4	5	NA
140203 Decreases environmental stimuli when anxious	1	2	3	4	5	NA
140204 Seeks information to reduce anxiety	1	2	3	4	5	NA
140205 Plans coping strategies for stressful situations	1	2	3	4	5	NA
140206 Uses effective coping strategies	1	2	3	4	5	NA
140207 Uses relaxation techniques to reduce anxiety	1	2	3	4	5	NA
140208 Monitors duration of episodes	1	2	3	4	5	NA
140209 Monitors length of time between episodes	1	2	3	4	5	NA
140210 Maintains role performance	1	2	3	4	5	NA
140211 Maintains social relationships	1	2	3	4	5	NA
140212 Maintains concentration	1	2	3	4	5	NA
140213 Monitors sensory perceptual distortions	1	2	3	4	5	NA
140214 Maintains adequate sleep	1	2	3	4	5	NA
140215 Monitors physical manifestations of anxiety	1	2	3	4	5	NA
140216 Monitors behavioral manifestations of anxiety	1	2	3	4	5	NA
140217 Controls anxiety response	1	2	3	4	5	NA

1st edition 1997; Revised 2nd edition 2000; Revised 3rd edition 2004

Outcome Content References:

+Hudson, W. W. (1992). *The WALMYR assessment scales scoring manual.* Tempe, AZ: WALMYR Publishing Co.

Laraia, M. T., Stuart, G. W., & Best, C. L. (1989). Behavioral treatment of panic-related disorders: A review. *Archives of Psychiatric Nursing, 3*(3), 125-133.

Moorhead, S. A., & Brighton, V. A. (2001). Anxiety and fear. In M. Maas, K. Buckwalter, M. Hardy, T. Tripp-Reimer, M. Titler, & J. Specht (Eds.), *Nursing care of older adults: Diagnoses, outcomes & interventions* (pp. 571-592). St. Louis: Mosby.

Stuart, G. W., & Laraia, M. T. (2001). *Principles and practice of psychiatric nursing* (7th ed.). St. Louis: Mosby.

Tucker, S., Moore, W., & Luedtke, C. (2000). Outcomes of a brief inpatient treatment program for mood and anxiety disorders. *Outcomes Management for Nursing Practice, 4*(3), 117-123.

Waddell, K. L., & Demi, A. S. (1993). Effectiveness of an intensive partial hospitalization program for treatment of anxiety disorders. *Archives of Psychiatric Nursing, 7*(1), 2-10.

Appetite—1014

Domain-Physiologic Health (II)

Class-Digestion & Nutrition (K)

Scale-Severely compromised to Not compromised (a)

Care Recipient:

Data Source:

Definition: Desire to eat when ill or receiving treatment

OUTCOME TARGET RATING: Maintain at_____   Increase to_____

Appetite Overall Rating	Severely compromised 1	Substantially compromised 2	Moderately compromised 3	Mildly compromised 4	Not compromised 5	
INDICATORS:						
101401 Desire to eat	1	2	3	4	5	NA
101402 Craving for food	1	2	3	4	5	NA
101403 Enjoyment of food	1	2	3	4	5	NA
101404 Pleasant taste of food	1	2	3	4	5	NA
101405 Reports energy to eat	1	2	3	4	5	NA
101406 Food intake	1	2	3	4	5	NA
101407 Nutrient intake	1	2	3	4	5	NA
101408 Fluid intake	1	2	3	4	5	NA
101409 Stimulus to eat	1	2	3	4	5	NA

3rd edition 2004

Outcome Content References:

Anderson, K. N., Anderson, L. E., & Glanze, W. D. (2002). *Mosby's medical, nursing, & allied health dictionary* (6th ed.). St. Louis: Mosby.

Dudek, S. G. (2001). *Nutrition essentials for nursing practice*. Philadelphia: Lippincott Williams & Wilkins.

Lewis, S. M., Heitkemper, M. M., & Dirksen, S. R. (2000). *Medical surgical nursing: Assessment and management of clinical problems*. St. Louis: Mosby.

McCanse, K. L., & Huether, S. E. (2002). *Pathophysiology: The biological basis for disease in adults and children*. St. Louis: Mosby.

Potter, P. A., & Perry, A. G. (2001). *Fundamentals of nursing* (5th ed.). St. Louis: Mosby.

Thomas, C. L. (Ed.). (1993). *Taber's cylcopedic medical dictionary* (17th ed.). Philadelphia: F.A. Davis.

A

Aspiration Prevention—1918

Domain-Health Knowledge & Behavior (IV)

Class-Risk Control & Safety (T)

Scale(s)-Never demonstrated to Consistently demonstrated (m)

Care Recipient:

Data Source:

Definition: Personal actions to prevent the passage of fluid and solid particles into the lung

OUTCOME TARGET RATING: Maintain at_____   Increase to_____

Aspiration Prevention Overall Rating	Never demonstrated 1	Rarely demonstrated 2	Sometimes demonstrated 3	Often demonstrated 4	Consistently demonstrated 5	
INDICATORS:						
191801 Identifies risk factors	1	2	3	4	5	NA
191802 Avoids risk factors	1	2	3	4	5	NA
191809 Maintains oral hygiene	1	2	3	4	5	NA
191803 Positions self upright for eating and drinking	1	2	3	4	5	NA
191805 Positions self on side for eating and drinking as needed	1	2	3	4	5	NA
191804 Selects foods according to swallowing ability	1	2	3	4	5	NA
191806 Selects food and fluid of proper consistency	1	2	3	4	5	NA
191808 Uses liquid thickeners as needed	1	2	3	4	5	NA
191810 Remains upright for 30 minutes after eating	1	2	3	4	5	NA

2nd edition 2000; Revised 3rd edition 2004; Revised 4th edition

Outcome Content References:

Fellows, L. S., Miller, E. H., Frederickson, M., Bly, B., & Felt, P. (2000). Evidence-based practice for enteral feedings: Aspiration prevention strategies, bedside detection, and practice change. *Medsurg Nursing, 9*(1), 27-31.

The Joanna Briggs Institute for Evidence Based Nursing and Midwifery. (2000). Identification and nursing management of dysphagia in adults with neurological impairment. *Best Practice, 4*(2), Blackwell Science-Asia, Australia.

Johnson, J. L., & Hirsch, C. S. (2003). Aspiration pneumonia. *Postgraduate Medicine, 113*(3), 99-107.

Lewis, S. M., Collier, I. C., Heitkermper, M. M., & Dirksen, S. R. (2000). *Medical-surgical nursing: Assessment & management of clinical problems* (5th ed.). St. Louis: Mosby.

McCance, K. L., & Huether, S. E. (2002). *Pathophysiology: The biologic basis for disease in adults and children* (4th ed.). St. Louis: Mosby.

Oh, E., Weintraub, N., & Dhanai, S. (2004). Can we prevent aspiration pneumonia in the nursing home? *Journal of the American Medical Directors Association, 6*(3-Suppl. 1), S76-S80.

Smeltzer, S. C., & Bare, B. G. (Eds.). (2003). *Brunner and Suddarth's textbook of medical-surgical nursing* (10th ed.). Philadelphia: Lippincott Williams &Wilkins.

A

Asthma Self-Management—0704

Domain-Health, Knowledge, & Behavior (IV)
Class-Health Behavior (Q)
Scale(s)-Never demonstrated to Consistently demonstrated (m) and Consistently demonstrated to Never demonstrated (t)

Care Recipient:
Data Source:

Definition: Personal actions to prevent or reverse inflammatory condition resulting in bronchial constriction of the airways

OUTCOME TARGET RATING: Maintain at_____   Increase to_____

Asthma Self-Management Overall Rating	Never demonstrated 1	Rarely demonstrated 2	Sometimes demonstrated 3	Often demonstrated 4	Consistently demonstrated 5	
INDICATORS:						
070418 Describes causal factors	1	2	3	4	5	NA
070419 Recognizes onset of asthma	1	2	3	4	5	NA
070401 Initiates action to avoid personal triggers	1	2	3	4	5	NA
070402 Initiates action to manage personal triggers	1	2	3	4	5	NA
070426 Shares acute asthma management with relevant individual(s)	1	2	3	4	5	NA
070427 Shares emergency plan with relevant individual(s)	1	2	3	4	5	NA
070428 Follows emergency plan for acute attacks	1	2	3	4	5	NA
070429 Adjusts life routine for optimal health	1	2	3	4	5	NA
070403 Makes appropriate environmental modifications	1	2	3	4	5	NA
070420 Uses diary to monitor symptoms over time	1	2	3	4	5	NA
070430 Obtains early treatment for infection	1	2	3	4	5	NA
070405 Participates in age-appropriate activities	1	2	3	4	5	NA
070406 Sleeps through the night with no cough or wheeze	1	2	3	4	5	NA
070431 Reports energy restored after rest	1	2	3	4	5	NA
070432 Maintains access to medication	1	2	3	4	5	NA
070433 Monitors medication side effects	1	2	3	4	5	NA
070409 Reports symptom control with minimal medication use	1	2	3	4	5	NA
070410 Monitors peak flow routinely	1	2	3	4	5	NA
070411 Monitors peak flow when symptoms occur	1	2	3	4	5	NA

Continued

A

		Never demonstrated	Rarely demonstrated	Sometimes demonstrated	Often demonstrated	Consistently demonstrated	
070412	Makes appropriate medication choices	1	2	3	4	5	NA
070434	Uses inhalers, spacers, and nebulizers correctly	1	2	3	4	5	NA
070414	Self-manages exacerbations	1	2	3	4	5	NA
070415	Reports uncontrolled symptoms to health professional	1	2	3	4	5	NA
070435	Uses support group	1	2	3	4	5	NA
070421	Reports asthma controlled	1	2	3	4	5	NA

		Consistently demonstrated (4 + occurrences)	Often demonstrated (3 occurrences)	Sometimes demonstrated (2 occurrences)	Rarely demonstrated (1 occurrence)	Never demonstrated (no occurrence)	
070422	Emergency visits related to asthma within the last year	1	2	3	4	5	NA
070423	Hospitalizations related to asthma within the last year	1	2	3	4	5	NA
070424	School absences related to asthma within the school year	1	2	3	4	5	NA
070425	Work absences related to asthma within the last year	1	2	3	4	5	NA

2nd edition 2000; Revised 3rd edition 2004; Revised 4th edition

Outcome Content References:

Cross, S. (1997). Revised guidelines on asthma management. *Professional Nurse, 12*(6), 408-410.

Gallagher, C. (2002). Childhood asthma: Tools that help parents manage it. *American Journal of Nursing, 102*(8), 71-83.

Le, J. T., Pearlman, D. S., Nickals, R., Lowenthal, M., & Rosenthal, R. (1998). Algorithm for the diagnosis and management of asthma: A practice parameter update. *Annals of Allergy, Asthma and Immunology, 81*, 415-420.

National Heart, Lung, and Blood Institute. National Asthma Education Program. (1997). *Expert panel report 2: Guidelines for the diagnosis and management of asthma* (NIH Publication No. 97-4051). Bethesda, MD: U.S. Department of Health and Human Services.

Perry, C. S., & Toole, K. A. (2000). Impact of school nurse case management on asthma control in school-aged children. *Journal of School Health, 70*(7), 303-304.

Tettersell, M. J. (1993). Asthma patients' knowledge in relation to compliance with drug therapy. *Journal of Advanced Nursing, 18*(1), 103-113.

Yawn, B. P. (2005). Asthma. In D. L. Huber (Ed.), *Disease management: A guide for case managers* (pp. 100-131). St. Louis: Saunders.

Yoos, H. L., & McMullen, A. (1999). Symptom perception and evaluation in childhood asthma. *Nursing Research, 48*(1) 2-8.

Yoos, H. L., Philipson, E., McMullen, A. (2003). Asthma management across the life span: The child with asthma. *Nursing Clinics of North America, 38*(4), 635-652.

B

Balance—0202

Domain-Functional Health (I)

Class-Mobility (C)

Scale(s)-Severely compromised to Not compromised (a) and Severe to None (n)

Care Recipient:

Data Source:

Definition: Ability to maintain body equilibrium

OUTCOME TARGET RATING: Maintain at_____   Increase to_____

Balance Overall Rating	Severely compromised 1	Substantially compromised 2	Moderately compromised 3	Mildly compromised 4	Not compromised 5	
INDICATORS:						
020201 Maintains balance while standing	1	2	3	4	5	NA
020202 Maintains balance while sitting without back support	1	2	3	4	5	NA
020203 Maintains balance while walking	1	2	3	4	5	NA
020209 Maintains balance while standing on one foot	1	2	3	4	5	NA
020210 Maintains balance while shifting balance from one foot to another	1	2	3	4	5	NA
020211 Posture	1	2	3	4	5	NA
	Severe	**Substantial**	**Moderate**	**Mild**	**None**	
020205 Weaving	1	2	3	4	5	NA
020206 Dizziness	1	2	3	4	5	NA
020207 Shakiness	1	2	3	4	5	NA
020208 Stumbling	1	2	3	4	5	NA

1st edition 1997; Revised 3rd edition 2004; Revised 4th edition

Outcome Content References:

+Berg, K., Wood-Dauphinee, S., Williams, J. I., & Gayton, D. (1989). Measuring balance in the elderly: Preliminary development of an instrument. *Physiotherapy Canada, 41*, 304-311.

Dittmar, S. (1989). *Rehabilitation nursing: Process and application.* St. Louis: Mosby.

Our balancing act. (2006). *Harvard Health Letter, 31*(10), 1-3.

Pettersson, A. F., Engardt, M., & Wahlund, L. O. (2002). Activity level and balance in subjects with mild Alzheimer's disease. *Dementia & Geriatric Cognitive Disorders, 13*(4), 213-216.

Pomeroy, V. (1990). Development of an ADL-oriented assessment-of-mobility scale suitable for use with elderly people with dementia. *Physiotherapy, 76*(8), 446-448.

Roberts, B. L. (1989). Effects of walking on balance among elders. *Nursing Research, 38*(3), 180-182.

Tinetti, M. E. (1986). Performance-oriented assessment of mobility problems in elderly patients. *Journal of the American Geriatric Society, 34*(2), 119-126.

B

Blood Coagulation—0409

Domain-Physiologic Health (II)

Class-Cardiopulmonary (E)

Scale(s)-Severe deviation from normal range to No deviation from normal range (b) and Severe to None (n)

Care Recipient:

Data Source:

Definition: Extent to which blood clots within normal period of time

OUTCOME TARGET RATING: Maintain at_____   Increase to_____

Blood Coagulation Overall Rating	Severe deviation from normal range 1	Substantial deviation from normal range 2	Moderate deviation from normal range 3	Mild deviation from normal range 4	No deviation from normal range 5	
INDICATORS:						
040901 Clot formation	1	2	3	4	5	NA
040912 Prothrombin time (PT)	1	2	3	4	5	NA
040905 Prothrombin time— international normalized ratio (PT-INR)	1	2	3	4	5	NA
040907 Partial thromboplastin time (PTT)	1	2	3	4	5	NA
040913 Hemoglobin (Hgb)	1	2	3	4	5	NA
040908 Platelet count	1	2	3	4	5	NA
040909 Plasma fibrinogen	1	2	3	4	5	NA
040914 Fibrin split products (FSP)	1	2	3	4	5	NA
040910 Hematocrit (Hct)	1	2	3	4	5	NA
040915 Activated clotting time (ACT)	1	2	3	4	5	NA
	Severe	**Substantial**	**Moderate**	**Mild**	**None**	
040902 Bleeding	1	2	3	4	5	NA
040903 Bruising	1	2	3	4	5	NA
040904 Petechiae	1	2	3	4	5	NA
040916 Ecchymosis	1	2	3	4	5	NA
040917 Purpura	1	2	3	4	5	NA
040918 Hematuria	1	2	3	4	5	NA
040919 Blood in stool	1	2	3	4	5	NA
040920 Hemoptysis	1	2	3	4	5	NA
040921 Hematemesis	1	2	3	4	5	NA
040922 Bleeding gums	1	2	3	4	5	NA

2nd edition 2000; Revised 3rd edition 2004

Outcome Content References:

Arnett, C. (1998). Thrombocytopenia in the newborn. *Neonatal Network—Journal of Neonatal Nursing, 17*(8), 27-37.

Beyth, R. J. (2001). Thromboembolic disease and anticoagulation in the elderly: Hemorrhagic complications of oral anticoagulant therapy (electronic version). *Clinics in Geriatric Medicine, 17*(1), 49-56.

Clochesy, J. M., Brey, C., Cardin, S., Whittaker, A. A., & Rudy, E. B. (1996). *Critical care nursing* (2nd ed.). Philadelphia: W.B. Saunders.

Fahey, V. A. (Ed.). (1999). *Vascular nursing* (3rd ed.). Philadelphia: W.B. Saunders.

Fihn, S. D., Callahan, C. M., Martin, D., McDonell, M. B., Henikoff, J. G., & White, R. H. (1996). The risk for and severity of bleeding complications in elderly patients treated with warfarin. *Annals of Internal Medicine, 124*(11), 970-979.

Lewis, S. M., Collier, I. C., Heitkemper, M. M., & Dirksen, S. R. (2000). *Medical-surgical nursing: Assessment & management of clinical problems* (5th ed.). St. Louis: Mosby.

McCance, K. L., & Huether, S. E. (2002). *Pathophysiology: The biologic basis for disease in adults and children* (4th ed.). St. Louis: Mosby.

Smeltzer, S. C., & Bare, B. G. (Eds.). (2003). *Brunner and Suddarth's textbook of medical-surgical nursing* (10th ed.). Philadelphia: Lippincott Williams & Wilkins.

Blood Glucose Level—2300

Domain Physiologic Health (II)

Class-Therapeutic Response (a)

Scale(s)-Severe deviation from normal range to No deviation from normal range (b)

Care Recipient:

Data Source:

B

Definition: Extent to which glucose levels in plasma and urine are maintained in normal range

OUTCOME TARGET RATING: Maintain at_____   Increase to_____

Blood Glucose Level Overall Rating	Severe deviation from normal range 1	Substantial deviation from normal range 2	Moderate deviation from normal range 3	Mild deviation from normal range 4	No deviation from normal range 5	
INDICATORS:						
230001 Blood glucose	1	2	3	4	5	NA
230004 Glycosylated hemoglobin	1	2	3	4	5	NA
230005 Fructosamine	1	2	3	4	5	NA
230007 Urine glucose	1	2	3	4	5	NA
230008 Urine ketones	1	2	3	4	5	NA

2nd edition 2000; Revised 3rd edition 2004

Outcome Content References:

American Diabetes Association. (1998). Standards of medical care for patients with diabetes mellitus. *Diabetes Care, 21* (Suppl. 1), S23-S31.

American Diabetes Association. (1998). Testing of glycemia in diabetes. *Diabetes Care, 21*(Suppl. 1), S69-S71.

Cryer, P. E. (2001). Hypoglycemia risk reduction in type 1 diabetes. *Experimental & Clinical Endocrinology & Diabetes, 109*(Suppl. 2), S412-S423.

Dalewitz, J., Khan, N., & Hershey, C. (2000). Barriers to control of blood glucose in diabetes mellitus. *American Journal of Medical Quality, 15*(1), 16-25.

Funnell, M. M., Hunt, C., Kulkarni, K., Rubin, R. R., & Yarborough, P. C. (Eds.). (1998). *A core curriculum for Association of Diabetes Educators.* Chicago: American Association of Diabetes Educators.

Kelley, D. B. (Ed.). (1998). *Intensive diabetes management* (2nd ed.). Alexandria, VA: American Diabetes Association.

Lebovitz, H. E. (Ed.). (1998). *Therapy for diabetes mellitus and related disorders* (3rd ed.). Alexandria, VA: American Diabetes Association.

Lewis, S. M., Collier, I. C., Heitkermper, M. M., & Dirksen, S. R. (2000). *Medical-surgical nursing: Assessment & management of clinical problems* (5th ed.). St. Louis: Mosby.

McCance, K. L., & Huether, S. E. (2002). *Pathophysiology: The biologic basis for disease in adults and children* (4th ed.). St. Louis: Mosby.

Zgibor, J. C., & Simmons, D. (2002). Barriers to blood glucose monitoring in a multiethnic community. *Diabetes Care, 25*(10), 1772-1777.

B

Blood Loss Severity—0413

Domain-Physiologic Health (II)

Class-Cardiopulmonary (E)

Scale(s)-Severe to None (n)

Care Recipient:

Data Source:

Definition: Severity of internal or external bleeding/hemorrhage

OUTCOME TARGET RATING: Maintain at_____   Increase to_____

Blood Loss Severity Overall Rating	Severe 1	Substantial 2	Moderate 3	Mild 4	None 5	
INDICATORS:						
041301 Visible blood loss	1	2	3	4	5	NA
041302 Hematuria	1	2	3	4	5	NA
041303 Frank blood from anus	1	2	3	4	5	NA
041304 Hemoptysis	1	2	3	4	5	NA
041305 Hematemesis	1	2	3	4	5	NA
041306 Abdominal distention	1	2	3	4	5	NA
041307 Vaginal bleeding	1	2	3	4	5	NA
041308 Post surgical bleeding	1	2	3	4	5	NA
041309 Decreased systolic blood pressure	1	2	3	4	5	NA
041310 Decreased diastolic blood pressure	1	2	3	4	5	NA
041311 Increased apical heart rate	1	2	3	4	5	NA
041312 Loss of body heat	1	2	3	4	5	NA
041313 Skin and mucous membrane pallor	1	2	3	4	5	NA
041314 Anxiety	1	2	3	4	5	NA
041315 Decreased cognition	1	2	3	4	5	NA
041316 Decreased hemoglobin (Hgb)	1	2	3	4	5	NA
041317 Decreased hematocrit (Hct)	1	2	3	4	5	NA

Estimated blood loss_____(ml)

3rd edition 2004

Outcome Content References:

American College of Surgeons Committee on Trauma. (1997). *Advanced trauma life support for doctors.* Chicago: American College of Surgeons.

Baron, B. J., Sinert, R., Zehtabchi, S., Stavile, K. L., & Scalea, T. M. (2004). Diagnostic utility of sublingual PCO_2 for detecting hemorrhage in penetrating trauma patients. *Journal of Trauma, 57*(1), 69-74.

Blankenship, J. C. (1999). Bleeding complications of glycoprotein IIb-IIIa receptor inhibitors (electronic version). *American Heart Journal, 138*, 287-296.

Bose, P., Regan, F., & Paterson-Brown, S. (2006). Improving the accuracy of estimated blood loss at obstetric haemorrhage using clinical reconstructions. *BJOG: An International Journal of Obstetrics & Gynaecology, 113*(8), 919-924.

deGuzman, E., Shankar, M. N., & Mattox, K. L. (1999). Limited volume resuscitation in penetrating thoracoabdominal trauma. *AACN Clinical Issues, 10*, 61-68.

Fihn, S. D., Callahan, C. M., Martin, D., McDonell, M. B., Henikoff, J. G., & White, R. H. (1996). The risk for and severity of bleeding complications in elderly patients treated with warfarin. *Annals of Internal Medicine, 124*, 970-979.

Maxson, J. H. (2000). Management of disseminated intravascular coagulation. *Critical Care Nursing Clinics of North America, 12*, 341-352.

Sims, C., Seigne, P., Menconi, M., Monarca, J., Barlow, C., Pettit, J., & Puyana, J. C. (2001). Skeletal muscle acidosis correlates with the severity of blood volume loss during shock and resuscitation. *Journal of Trauma, 51*(6), 1137-1146.

Swearington, P. L., & Keen, J. H. (2001). *Manual of critical care nursing: Nursing interventions and collaborative management* (4th ed.). St. Louis: Mosby.

B

Blood Transfusion Reaction—0700

Domain-Physiologic Health (II)

Class-Immune Response (H)

Scale(s)-Severe to None (n)

Care Recipient:

Data Source:

Definition: Severity of complications with blood transfusion reaction

OUTCOME TARGET RATING: Maintain at_____   Increase to_____

Blood Transfusion Reaction Overall Rating	Severe 1	Substantial 2	Moderate 3	Mild 4	None 5	
INDICATORS:						
070020 Shortness of breath	1	2	3	4	5	NA
070003 Decreased urine output	1	2	3	4	5	NA
070004 Increased apical heart rate	1	2	3	4	5	NA
070022 Decreased blood pressure	1	2	3	4	5	NA
070007 Fever	1	2	3	4	5	NA
070008 Chills	1	2	3	4	5	NA
070009 Itching	1	2	3	4	5	NA
070010 Rash	1	2	3	4	5	NA
070011 Restlessness	1	2	3	4	5	NA
070012 Anxiety	1	2	3	4	5	NA
070013 Malaise	1	2	3	4	5	NA
070021 Nausea	1	2	3	4	5	NA
070014 Chest pain	1	2	3	4	5	NA
070015 Lumbar pain	1	2	3	4	5	NA
070017 Hemoglobinuria	1	2	3	4	5	NA
070023 Muscle spasms	1	2	3	4	5	NA
070024 Twitching	1	2	3	4	5	NA

1st edition 1997; Revised 3rd edition 2004; Revised 4th edition

Outcome Content References:

McCance, K. L., & Huether, S. E. (2002). *Pathophysiology: The biologic basis for disease in adults and children* (4th ed.). St. Louis: Mosby.

Raife, T. J. (1997). Adverse effects of transfusions caused by leukocytes. *Journal of Intravenous Nursing, 20*(5), 238-244.

Smeltzer, S. C., & Bare, B. G. (Eds.). (2003). *Brunner and Suddarth's textbook of medical-surgical nursing* (10th ed.). Philadelphia: Lippincott Williams & Wilkins.

B

Body Image—1200

Domain-Psychosocial Health (III)

Class-Psychological Well-Being (M)

Scale(s)-Never positive to Consistently positive (k)

Care Recipient:

Data Source:

Definition: Perception of own appearance and body functions

OUTCOME TARGET RATING: Maintain at_____   Increase to_____

Body Image Overall Rating	Never positive 1	Rarely positive 2	Sometimes positive 3	Often positive 4	Consistently positive 5

INDICATORS:

120001	Internal picture of self	1	2	3	4	5	NA
120002	Congruence between body reality, body ideal, and body presentation	1	2	3	4	5	NA
120003	Description of affected body part	1	2	3	4	5	NA
120016	Attitude toward touching affected body part	1	2	3	4	5	NA
120017	Attitude toward using strategies to enhance appearance	1	2	3	4	5	NA
120005	Satisfaction with body appearance	1	2	3	4	5	NA
120018	Attitude toward using strategies to enhance function	1	2	3	4	5	NA
120006	Satisfaction with body function	1	2	3	4	5	NA
120007	Adjustment to changes in physical appearance	1	2	3	4	5	NA
120008	Adjustment to changes in body function	1	2	3	4	5	NA
120009	Adjustment to changes in health status	1	2	3	4	5	NA
120013	Adjustment to body changes due to injury	1	2	3	4	5	NA
120014	Adjustment to body changes due to surgery	1	2	3	4	5	NA
120015	Adjustment to body changes due to aging	1	2	3	4	5	NA

1st edition 1997; Revised 3rd edition 2004; Revised 4th edition

Outcome Content References:

Fritz, G. K. (Ed). (2004). Body image—tips for parents. *The Brown University Child and Adolescent Behavior Letter*. Providence, RI: Manisses Communications Group.

Comunale, D. L. (1992). Collaborative care planning with the arthritic client at home. *Journal of Home Health Care Practice, 4*(2), 8-15.

Dixon, J. B., Dixon, M. E., & O'Brien, P. E. (2002). Body image: Appearance orientation and evaluation in the severely obese. Changes with weight loss. *Obesity Surgery, 12*(1), 65-71.

Kater, K. J., Rohwer, J., & Londre, K. (2002). Evaluation of an upper elementary school program to prevent body image, eating, and weight concerns. *Journal of School Health, 72*(5), 199-204.

Key, A., George, C. L., Beattie, D., Stammers, K., Lacey, H., & Waller, G. (2002). Body image treatment within an inpatient program for anorexia nervosa: The role of mirror exposure in the desensitization process. *International Journal of Eating Disorders, 31*(2), 185-190.

LeMone, P. (1991). Analysis of human phenomenon: Self-concept. *Nursing Diagnosis, 2*(3), 129-130.

Low, M. B. (1993). Women's body image: The nurse's role in promotion of self-acceptance. *AWONN's Clinical Issues, 4*(2), 213-219.

MacGinley, K. J. (1993). Nursing care of the patient with altered body image. *British Journal of Nursing, 2*(22), 1098-1102.

Martin, H., & Ammerman, S. D. (2002). Adolescents with eating disorders: Primary care screening, identification, and early intervention. *Nursing Clinics of North America, 37*(3), 537-551.

Newell, R. (1991). Body-image disturbance: Cognitive behavioral formulation and intervention. *Journal of Advanced Nursing, 16*(12), 1400-1405.

Price, B. (1990). A model for body image care. *Journal of Advanced Nursing, 15*(5), 585-593.

Price, B. (1992). Living with altered body image: The cancer experience. *British Journal of Nursing, 1*(13), 641-645.

Price, B. (1993). Profiling the high-risk altered body image patient. *Senior Nurse, 13*(4), 17-21.

+Rosen, J. C., Srebnik, D., Saltzberg, E., & Wendt, S. (1991). Development of a body image avoidance questionnaire. *Psychological Assessment: A Journal of Consulting and Clinical Psychology, 3*(1), 32-37.

Van Deusen, J., Harlowe, D., & Baker, L. (1989). Body image perceptions of the community-based elderly. *The Occupational Therapy Journal of Research, 9*(4), 243-248.

Wasson, D., & Anderson, M. A. (1995). Chemical dependency and adolescent self-esteem. *Clinical Nursing Research, 4*(3), 274-289.

B

B

Body Mechanics Performance—1616

Domain-Health Knowledge & Behavior (IV)

Class-Health Behavior (Q)

Scale(s)-Never demonstrated to Consistently demonstrated (m)

Care Recipient:

Data Source:

Definition: Personal actions to maintain proper body alignment and to prevent muscular skeletal strain

OUTCOME TARGET RATING: Maintain at_____   Increase to_____

Body Mechanics Performance Overall Rating	Never demonstrated 1	Rarely demonstrated 2	Sometimes demonstrated 3	Often demonstrated 4	Consistently demonstrated 5	
INDICATORS:						
161601 Uses correct standing posture	1	2	3	4	5	NA
161602 Uses correct sitting posture	1	2	3	4	5	NA
161603 Uses correct lying posture	1	2	3	4	5	NA
161604 Uses correct lifting techniques	1	2	3	4	5	NA
161605 Uses correct carrying techniques	1	2	3	4	5	NA
161612 Uses correct pushing technique	1	2	3	4	5	NA
161607 Uses supportive devices correctly	1	2	3	4	5	NA
161608 Obtains assistance with heavy load	1	2	3	4	5	NA
161613 Maintains muscle strength	1	2	3	4	5	NA
161614 Maintains joint flexibility	1	2	3	4	5	NA
161611 Uses prescribed exercises to prevent injury	1	2	3	4	5	NA
161615 Uses proper body mechanics	1	2	3	4	5	NA

3rd edition 2004; Revised 4th edition

Outcome Content References:

Chan, D., Laporte, D. M., & Sveistrup, H. (1999). Rising from sitting in elderly people, Part 2: Strategies to facilitate rising. *British Journal of Occupational Therapy, 62*(2), 64-68.

Laporte, D. M., Chan, D., & Sveistrup, H. (1999). Rising from sitting in elderly people, Part 1: Implications of biomechanics and physiology. *British Journal of Occupational Therapy, 62*(1), 36-42.

Potter, P. A., & Perry, A. G. (2001). *Fundamentals of nursing* (5th ed.). St. Louis: Mosby.

Body Positioning: Self-Initiated—0203

Domain-Functional Health (I)

Class-Mobility (C)

Scale(s)-Severely compromised to Not compromised (a)

Care Recipient:

Data Source:

B

Definition: Ability to change own body position independently with or without assistive device

OUTCOME TARGET RATING: Maintain at_____   Increase to_____

Body Positioning: Self-Initiated Overall Rating	Severely compromised 1	Substantially compromised 2	Moderately compromised 3	Mildly compromised 4	Not compromised 5	
INDICATORS:						
020302 Moves from lying to sitting	1	2	3	4	5	NA
020303 Moves from sitting to lying	1	2	3	4	5	NA
020304 Moves from sitting to standing	1	2	3	4	5	NA
020305 Moves from standing to sitting	1	2	3	4	5	NA
020306 Moves from standing to kneeling	1	2	3	4	5	NA
020307 Moves from kneeling to standing	1	2	3	4	5	NA
020308 Moves from standing to squatting	1	2	3	4	5	NA
020309 Moves from squatting to standing	1	2	3	4	5	NA
020310 Bends at waist while standing	1	2	3	4	5	NA
020311 Moves from side to side while lying	1	2	3	4	5	NA
020301 Moves from front to back while lying	1	2	3	4	5	NA
020313 Moves from back to front while lying	1	2	3	4	5	NA

1st edition 1997; Revised 2nd edition 2000; Revised 3rd edition 2004

Outcome Content References:

+Berg, K., Wood-Dauphinee, S., Williams, J. I., & Gayton, D. (1989). Measuring balance in the elderly: Preliminary development of an instrument. *Physiotherapy Canada, 41,* 304-311.

Melzer, I., Benjuya, N., & Kaplanski, J. (2000). Age related changes in muscle strength and fatigue. *Isokinetics & Exercise Science, 8*(2), 73-83.

Mikulic, M. A., Griffith, E. R., & Jebsen, R. H. (1976). Clinical application of a standardized mobility test. *Archives of Physical Medicine and Rehabilitation, 57*(3), 143-146.

Bone Healing—1104

Domain-Physiologic Health (II)

Class-Tissue Integrity (L)

Scale(s)-None to Extensive (i) and Extensive to None (h)

Care Recipient:

Data Source:

Definition: Extent of regeneration of cells and tissues following bone injury

OUTCOME TARGET RATING: Maintain at_____   Increase to_____

Bone Healing Overall Rating	None 1	Limited 2	Moderate 3	Substantial 4	Extensive 5	
INDICATORS:						
110402 Cellular proliferation	1	2	3	4	5	NA
110403 Callus formation	1	2	3	4	5	NA
110404 Ossification, consolidation, and remodeling	1	2	3	4	5	NA
110405 Intact peripheral circulation	1	2	3	4	5	NA
110406 Return of skeletal function	1	2	3	4	5	NA
	Extensive	Substantial	Moderate	Limited	None	
110401 Hematoma	1	2	3	4	5	NA
110407 Pain	1	2	3	4	5	NA
110408 Edema	1	2	3	4	5	NA
110410 Infection in surrounding tissue	1	2	3	4	5	NA
110411 Infection in bone	1	2	3	4	5	NA

Site of fracture (# from skeleton) _____

1st edition 1997; Revised 3rd edition 2004

Outcome Content References:

Abdullah, D., Ford, T. R., Papaioannou, S., Nicholson, J., & McDonald, F. (2002). An evaluation of accelerated Portland cement as a restorative material. *Biomaterials, 23*(19), 4001-4010.

Mandracchia, V. J., Nelson, S. C., & Barp, E. A. (2001). Current concepts of bone healing. *Clinics in Podiatric Medicine & Surgery, 18*(1), 55-77.

Porth, C. M. (2002). *Pathophysiology: Concepts of altered health states* (6th ed.). Philadelphia: Lippincott Williams & Wilkins.

Potter, P. A., & Perry, A. G. (2001). *Fundamentals of nursing* (5th ed.). St. Louis: Mosby.

Wade, R., & Richardson, J. (2001). Outcome in fracture healing: A review. *Injury, 32*(2), 109-114.

B

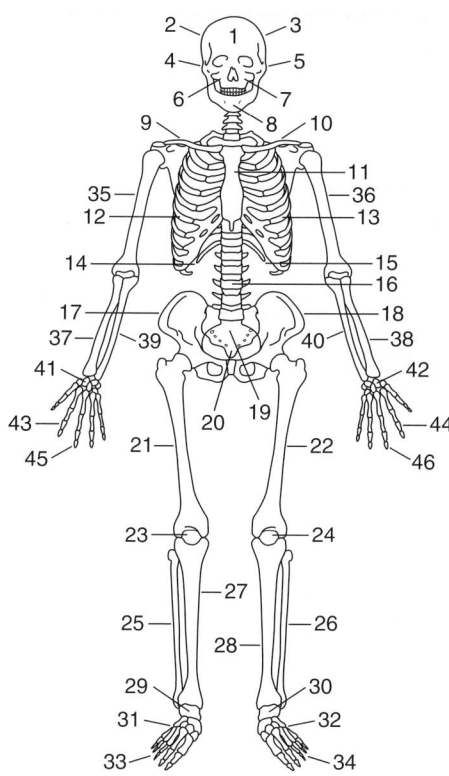

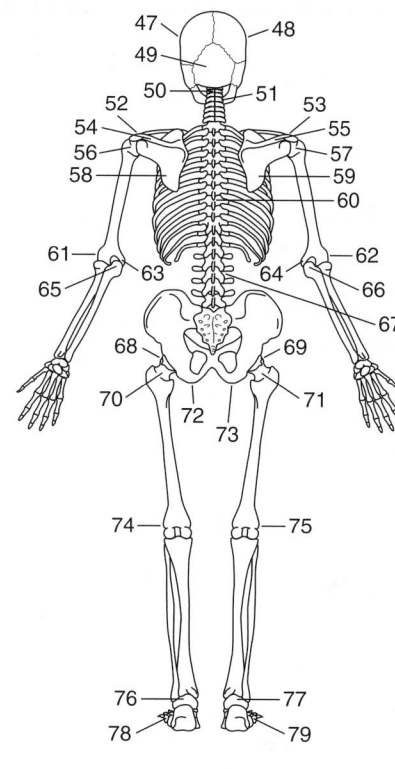

Bones of the head
1. Frontal
2. Right temporal
3. Left temporal
4. Right zygomatic
5. Left zygomatic
6. Right maxilla
7. Left maxilla
8. Mandible
47. Left parietal
48. Right parietal
49. Occipital

Bones of the neck and chest
9. Right clavicle
10. Left clavicle
11. Sternum
12. Right ribs
13. Left ribs
14. Right floating rib
15. Left floating rib
16. Vertebral column
50. Atlas
51. Cervical vertebra(e) specify _____
52. Left acromion
53. Right acromion
54. Left spine of scapula
55. Right spine of scapula
58. Left scapula
59. Right scapula
60. Thoracic vertebra(e) specify _____

Bones of the abdomen
16. Vertebral column
17. Right ilium
18. Left ilium
19. Sacrum
20. Coccyx
72. Left ischium
73. Right ischium
67. Lumbar vertebra(e) specify _____

Bones of the arm
35. Right humerus
36. Left humerus
37. Right radius
38. Left radius
39. Right ulna
40. Left ulna
41. Right carpals
42. Left carpals
43. Right metacarpals
44. Left metacarpals
45. Right phalanges
46. Left phalanges
56. Right head of humerus
57. Left head of humerus
61. Left epicondyle
62. Right epicondyle
63. Left epitrochlea
64. Right epitrochlea
65. Left olecranon
66. Right olecranon

Bones of the leg
21. Right femur
22. Left femur
23. Right patella
24. Left patella
25. Right fibula
26. Left fibula
27. Right tibia
28. Left tibia
29. Right tarsals
30. Left tarsals
31. Right metatarsals
32. Left metatarsals
33. Right phalanges
34. Left phalanges
68. Left head of femur
69. Right head of femur
70. Left neck of femur
71. Right neck of femur
74. Left condyle of femur
75. Right condyle of femur
76. Left talus
77. Right talus
78. Left calcaneus
79. Right calcaneus

B

Bowel Continence—0500

Domain-Physiologic Health (II)

Class-Elimination (F)

Care Recipient:

Data Source:

Scale(s)-Never demonstrated to Consistently demonstrated (m) and Consistently demonstrated to Never demonstrated (t)

Definition: Control of passage of stool from the bowel

OUTCOME TARGET RATING: Maintain at_____   Increase to_____

Bowel Continence Overall Rating	Never demonstrated 1	Rarely demonstrated 2	Sometimes demonstrated 3	Often demonstrated 4	Consistently demonstrated 5	

INDICATORS:

050008	Recognizes urge to defecate	1	2	3	4	5	NA
050001	Maintains predictable pattern of stool evacuation	1	2	3	4	5	NA
050002	Maintains control of stool passage	1	2	3	4	5	NA
050003	Evacuates stool at least every 3 days	1	2	3	4	5	NA
050006	Sphincter tone adequate to control defecation	1	2	3	4	5	NA
050007	Sphincter innervation functional	1	2	3	4	5	NA
050009	Responds to urge in timely manner	1	2	3	4	5	NA
050012	Gets to toilet between urge and evacuation of stool	1	2	3	4	5	NA
050017	Maintains barrier-free environment for independent toileting	1	2	3	4	5	NA
050013	Ingests adequate amount of fluid	1	2	3	4	5	NA
050014	Ingests adequate amount of fiber	1	2	3	4	5	NA
050015	Describes relationship of food intake to stool consistency	1	2	3	4	5	NA
050018	Monitors amount and consistency of stool	1	2	3	4	5	NA
050019	Toilets independently	1	2	3	4	5	NA

		Consistently demonstrated	Often demonstrated	Sometimes demonstrated	Rarely demonstrated	Never demonstrated	
050004	Diarrhea	1	2	3	4	5	NA
050005	Constipation	1	2	3	4	5	NA
050020	Overuse of laxatives	1	2	3	4	5	NA
050021	Overuse of enemas	1	2	3	4	5	NA
050022	Soils clothing during day	1	2	3	4	5	NA
050023	Soils clothing or bedding during night	1	2	3	4	5	NA

1st edition 1997; Revised 3rd edition 2004; Revised 4th edition

Outcome Content References:

Hogstel, M. O., & Nelson, M. (1992). Anticipation and early detection can reduce bowel elimination complications. *Geriatric Nursing, 13*(1), 28-33.

Maas, M. L., & Specht, J. P. (2001). Bowel incontinence. In M. Maas, K. Buckwalter, M. Hardy, T. Tripp-Reimer, M. Titler, & J. Specht (Eds.), *Nursing care of older adults: Diagnoses, outcomes & interventions* (pp. 238-251). St. Louis: Mosby.

McLane, A. (1987). *Classification of nursing diagnoses: Proceedings of the 7th conference*. St. Louis: Mosby.

+Morris, J. N., Hawes, C., Fries, B. E., Phillips, C. D., Mor, V., Katz, S., Murphy, K., Drugovich, M. L., & Friedlob, A. S. (1990). Designing the national resident assessment instrument for nursing homes. *Gerontologist, 30*(3), 293-307.

Bowel Elimination—0501

Domain-Physiologic Health (II)

Class-Elimination (F)

Scale(s)-Severely compromised to Not compromised (a) and Severe to None (n)

Care Recipient:

Data Source:

Definition: Formation and evacuation of stool						

OUTCOME TARGET RATING: Maintain at_____   Increase to_____

Bowel Elimination Overall Rating	Severely compromised 1	Substantially compromised 2	Moderately compromised 3	Mildly compromised 4	Not compromised 5	
INDICATORS:						
050101 Elimination pattern	1	2	3	4	5	NA
050102 Control of bowel movements	1	2	3	4	5	NA
050103 Stool color	1	2	3	4	5	NA
050104 Stool amount for diet	1	2	3	4	5	NA
050105 Stool soft and formed	1	2	3	4	5	NA
050112 Ease of stool passage	1	2	3	4	5	NA
050118 Sphincter tone	1	2	3	4	5	NA
050119 Muscle tone to evacuate stool	1	2	3	4	5	NA
050121 Passage of stool without aids	1	2	3	4	5	NA
050129 Bowel sounds	1	2	3	4	5	NA
	Severe	**Substantial**	**Moderate**	**Mild**	**None**	
050107 Fat in stool	1	2	3	4	5	NA
050108 Blood in stool	1	2	3	4	5	NA
050109 Mucus in stool	1	2	3	4	5	NA
050110 Constipation	1	2	3	4	5	NA
050111 Diarrhea	1	2	3	4	5	NA
050123 Abuse of elimination aids	1	2	3	4	5	NA
050128 Pain with passage of stool	1	2	3	4	5	NA

1st edition 1997; Revised 3rd edition 2004; Revised 4th edition

Outcome Content References:

Heading, C. (1987). Factors affecting bowel functions. *Nursing, 3*(21), 773-783.

Hogstel, M. O., & Nelson, M. (1992). Anticipation and early detection can reduce bowel elimination complications. *Geriatric Nursing, 13*(1), 28-33.

Lepshy, M. S., & Michael, A. (1993). Chronic diarrhea: Evaluation and treatment. *American Family Physician, 48*(8), 1461-1466.

Loening-Baucke, V. (1994). Management of chronic constipation in infants and toddlers. *American Family Physician, 46*(2), 397-406.

McKenna, S., Wallis, M., Brannelly, A., & Cawood, J. (2001). The nursing management of diarrhoea and constipation before and after the implementation of a bowel management protocol. *Australian Critical Care, 14*(1), 10-16.

McLane, A. M., & McShane, R. E. (2001). Constipation. In M. Maas, K. Buckwalter, M. Hardy, T. Tripp-Reimer, M. Titler, & J. Specht (Eds.), *Nursing care of older adults: Diagnoses, outcomes & interventions* (pp. 220-226). St. Louis: Mosby.

McShane, R. E., & McLane, A. M. (1988). Constipation: Impact of etiological factors. *Journal of Gerontological Nursing, 14*(4), 31-34.

Potter, P. A., & Perry, A. G. (2001). *Fundamentals of nursing* (5th ed.). St. Louis: Mosby.

Wadle, K. R. (2001). Diarrhea. In M. Maas, K. Buckwalter, M. Hardy, T. Tripp-Reimer, M. Titler, & J. Specht (Eds.), *Nursing care of older adults: Diagnoses, outcomes & interventions* (pp. 227-237). St. Louis: Mosby.

Breastfeeding Establishment: Infant—1000

Domain-Physiologic Health (II)

Class-Digestion & Nutrition (K)

Scale(s)-Not adequate to Totally adequate (f)

Care Recipient:

Data Source:

B

Definition: Infant attachment to and sucking from the mother's breast for nourishment during the first 3 weeks of breastfeeding

OUTCOME TARGET RATING: Maintain at_____   Increase to_____

Breastfeeding Establishment: Infant Overall Rating	Not adequate 1	Slightly adequate 2	Moderately adequate 3	Substantially adequate 4	Totally adequate 5	

INDICATORS:

100001	Proper alignment and latch on	1	2	3	4	5	NA
100002	Proper areolar grasp	1	2	3	4	5	NA
100003	Proper areolar compression	1	2	3	4	5	NA
100004	Correct suck and tongue placement	1	2	3	4	5	NA
100005	Audible swallow	1	2	3	4	5	NA
100006	Nursing a minimum of 5-10 minutes per breast	1	2	3	4	5	NA
100007	Minimum 8 feedings per day	1	2	3	4	5	NA
100008	Urinations per day appropriate for age	1	2	3	4	5	NA
100009	Loose, yellow, seedy stools per day appropriate for age	1	2	3	4	5	NA
100010	Weight gain appropriate for age	1	2	3	4	5	NA
100011	Infant contentment after feeding	1	2	3	4	5	NA

1st edition 1997; Revised 3rd 2004

Outcome Content References:

Biancuzzo, M. (2003). *Breastfeeding the newborn* (2nd ed.). St. Louis: Mosby.

Cricco-Lizza, R. (2006). Black Non-Hispanic mother's perception about the promotion of infant feeding methods by nurses and physicians. *Journal of Obstetric, Gynecologic, and Neonatal Nursing (JOGNN), 35*(2), 173-180.

Henderson, A. M., Pincombe, J., & Stamp, G. E. (2000). Assisting women to establish breastfeeding: Exploring midwives' practices. *Breastfeeding Review, 8*(3), 11-17.

Lang, S. (2002). *Breastfeeding special care babies* (2nd ed.). London: Bailliere Tindall.

Lawrence, R. A., & Lawrence, R. M. (1999). *Breastfeeding: A guide for the medical profession* (5th ed.). St. Louis: Mosby.

Minchin, M. K. (1989). Positioning for breastfeeding. *Birth, 16*(2), 67-80.

+Muldford, C. (1992). The mother-baby assessment (MBA): An "Apgar Score" for breastfeeding. *Journal of Human Lactation, 8*(2), 79-82.

Neifert, M. R., & Seacat, J. M. (1986). A guide to successful breastfeeding. *Contemporary Pediatrics, 3*, 1-14.

Page-Goertz, S. (1989). Discharge planning for the breastfeeding dyad. *Pediatric Nursing, 15*(5), 543-544.

Righard, L., & Alade, M. O. (1992). Sucking technique and its effect on success of breastfeeding. *Birth, 19*(4), 185-189.

Riordan, J., & Auerbach, K. G. (1999). *Breastfeeding and human lactation* (2nd ed.). Sudbury, MA: Jones and Bartlett.

Shrago, L., & Bocar, D. (1990). The infant's contribution to breastfeeding. *Journal of Obstetric, Gynecologic, & Neonatal Nursing, 19*(3), 209-213.

Walker, M. (1989). Functional assessment of infant breastfeeding patterns. *Birth, 16*(3), 140-147.

Breastfeeding Establishment: Maternal—1001

Domain-Physiologic Health (II)

Class-Digestion & Nutrition (K)

Scale(s)-Not adequate to Totally adequate (f)

Care Recipient:

Data Source:

B

Definition: Maternal establishment of proper attachment of an infant to and sucking from the breast for nourishment during the first 3 weeks of breastfeeding

OUTCOME TARGET RATING: Maintain at_____   Increase to_____

Breastfeeding Establishment: Maternal Overall Rating	Not adequate 1	Slightly adequate 2	Moderately adequate 3	Substantially adequate 4	Totally adequate 5	
INDICATORS:						
100101 Comfort of position during nursing	1	2	3	4	5	NA
100102 Supports breast using "C" hold (cupping)	1	2	3	4	5	NA
100103 Breast fullness prior to feeding	1	2	3	4	5	NA
100104 Milk ejection (let-down) reflex	1	2	3	4	5	NA
100106 Recognition of infant swallowing	1	2	3	4	5	NA
100107 Suction broken before removing infant from breast	1	2	3	4	5	NA
100121 Techniques to prevent nipple tenderness	1	2	3	4	5	NA
100109 Avoidance of artificial nipple use with infant	1	2	3	4	5	NA
100110 Avoidance of giving water to infant	1	2	3	4	5	NA
100122 Supplemental feedings	1	2	3	4	5	NA
100112 Response to infant's temperament	1	2	3	4	5	NA
100113 Recognition of early hunger cues	1	2	3	4	5	NA
100120 Fluid intake of mother	1	2	3	4	5	NA
100123 Pumping of breast	1	2	3	4	5	NA
100115 Safe storage of breastmilk	1	2	3	4	5	NA
100124 Use of family support	1	2	3	4	5	NA
100125 Use of community support	1	2	3	4	5	NA
100118 Satisfaction with breastfeeding process	1	2	3	4	5	NA

1st edition 1997; Revised 3rd edition 2004; Revised 4th edition

Outcome Content References:

Biancuzzo, M. (2003). *Breastfeeding the newborn* (2nd ed.). St. Louis: Mosby.

Cricco-Lizza, R. (2006). Black Non-Hispanic mother's perception about the promotion of infant feeding methods by nurses and physicians. *Journal of Obstetric, Gynecologic, and Neonatal Nursing (JOGNN), 35*(2), 173-180.

Henderson, A. M., Pincombe, J., & Stamp, G. E. (2000). Assisting women to establish breastfeeding: Exploring midwives' practices. *Breastfeeding Review, 8*(3), 11-17.

Hill, P., & Aldag, J. (1991). Potential indicators of insufficient milk supply syndrome. *Research in Nursing and Health, 14(1)*, 11-19.

Lawrence, R. A., & Lawrence, R. M. (1999). Breastfeeding: A guide for the medical profession (5th ed.). St. Louis: Mosby.

Lowdermilk, D. & Perry, S. (2004). Maternity & women's health care (8th ed.). St. Louis: Mosby.

Continued

B

Minchin, M. K. (1989). Positioning for breastfeeding. *Birth*, 16(2), 67-80.

+Muldford, C. (1992). The mother-baby assessment (MBA): An "Apgar Score" for breastfeeding. *Journal of Human Lactation*, 8(2), 79-82.

Neifert, M. R., & Seacat, J. M. (1986). A guide to successful breastfeeding. *Contemporary Pediatrics, 3*, 1-14.

Page-Goertz, S. (1989). Discharge planning for the breastfeeding dyad. *Pediatric Nursing, 15*(5), 543-544.

Righard, L., & Alade, M. O. (1992). Sucking technique and its effect on success of breastfeeding. *Birth, 19*(4), 185-189.

Riordan, J., & Auerbach, K. G. (1999). *Breastfeeding and human lactation* (2nd ed.). Sudbury, MA: Jones and Bartlett.

Shrago, L., & Bocar, D. (1990). The infant's contribution to breastfeeding. *Journal of Obstetric, Gynecologic, & Neonatal Nursing, 19*(3), 209-213.

Walker, M. (1989). Functional assessment of infant breastfeeding patterns. *Birth, 16*(3), 140-147.

Breastfeeding Maintenance—1002

Domain-Physiologic Health (II)

Class-Digestion & Nutrition (K)

Scale(s)-Not adequate to Totally adequate (f)

Care Recipient:

Data Source:

Definition: Continuation of breastfeeding from establishment to weaning for nourishment of an infant/toddler

OUTCOME TARGET RATING: Maintain at_____   Increase to_____

Breastfeeding Maintenance Overall Rating	Not adequate 1	Slightly adequate 2	Moderately adequate 3	Substantially adequate 4	Totally adequate 5	
INDICATORS:						
100201 Infant's growth in normal range	1	2	3	4	5	NA
100202 Infant's development in normal range	1	2	3	4	5	NA
100205 Ability to safely collect and store breastmilk	1	2	3	4	5	NA
100217 Ability to safely thaw and warm stored breastmilk	1	2	3	4	5	NA
100218 Techniques to prevent breast tenderness	1	2	3	4	5	NA
100208 Recognition of signs of decreased milk supply	1	2	3	4	5	NA
100219 Recognition of signs of plugged ducts	1	2	3	4	5	NA
100220 Recognition of signs of mastitis	1	2	3	4	5	NA
100221 Awareness that breastfeeding can continue beyond infancy	1	2	3	4	5	NA
100210 Avoidance of self-medication without checking with health professional	1	2	3	4	5	NA
100222 Perceived family support for breastfeeding	1	2	3	4	5	NA
100223 Perceived support for continuation of lactation on return to work	1	2	3	4	5	NA
100224 Perceived support for continuation of lactation on return to school	1	2	3	4	5	NA
100204 Knowledge of benefits from continued breastfeeding	1	2	3	4	5	NA
100225 Knowledge of resources for support	1	2	3	4	5	NA
100215 Satisfaction with breastfeeding process	1	2	3	4	5	NA

1st edition 1997; Revised 3rd edition 2004; Revised 4th edition

Outcome Content References:

Bear, K., & Tigges, B. B. (1993). Management strategies for promoting successful breastfeeding. *Nurse Practitioner, 18*(6), 50, 53-54, 56-58, 60.

Callahan, S., Sejourne, N., & Denis, A. (2006). Fatigue and breastfeeding—An inevitable relationship. *Journal of Human Lactation, 22*(2), 182-187.

Continued

B

Coreil, J., & Murphy, J. E. (1988). Maternal commitment, lactation practices, and breastfeeding duration. *Journal of Obstetric, Gynecologic, & Neonatal Nursing, 17*(4), 273-278.

Cricco-Lizza, R. (2006). Black Non-Hispanic mother's perception about the promotion of infant feeding methods by nurses and physicians. *Journal of Obstetric, Gynecologic, and Neonatal Nursing (JOGNN), 35*(2), 173-180.

Dick, M. J., Evans, M. L., Arthurs, J. B., Barnes, J. K., Caldwell, R. S., Hutchins, S. S., & Johnson, L. K. (2002). Predicting early breastfeeding attrition. *Journal of Human Lactation, 18*(1), 21-28.

Hauck, Y., & Reinbold, J. (1996). Criteria for successful breastfeeding: Mothers' perceptions. *Journal—Australian College of Midwives, 9*(1), 21-27.

Lawrence, R. A., & Lawrence, R. M. (1999). *Breastfeeding: A guide for the medical profession* (5th ed.). St. Louis: Mosby.

Rentschler, D. D. (1991). Correlates of successful breastfeeding. *Image—The Journal of Nursing Scholarship, 23*(3), 151-154.

Riordan, J., & Auerbach, K. G. (1999). *Breastfeeding and human lactation* (2nd ed.). Sudbury, MA: Jones and Bartlett.

Breastfeeding Weaning—1003

Domain-Physiologic Health (II)

Class-Nutrition (K)

Scale(s)-Not adequate to Totally adequate (f)

Care Recipient:

Data Source:

Definition: Progressive discontinuation of breastfeeding of an infant/toddler

OUTCOME TARGET RATING: Maintain at_____   Increase to_____

Breastfeeding Weaning Overall Rating	Not adequate 1	Slightly adequate 2	Moderately adequate 3	Substantially adequate 4	Totally adequate 5	

INDICATORS:

100302	Recognition of weaning readiness cues	1	2	3	4	5	NA
100318	Recognition of signs of decreased milk supply	1	2	3	4	5	NA
100304	Knowledge of benefits of gradual weaning	1	2	3	4	5	NA
100305	Knowledge of guidelines for rapid "emergency" weaning	1	2	3	4	5	NA
100319	Knowledge of appropriate methods to reduce breast tenderness	1	2	3	4	5	NA
100320	Mother's freedom from plugged ducts	1	2	3	4	5	NA
100321	Mother's freedom from or mastitis	1	2	3	4	5	NA
100322	Introduction of solids as recommended by health professional	1	2	3	4	5	NA
100308	Replacement of one additional breastfeeding with solids every few days	1	2	3	4	5	NA
100323	Replacement of breastmilk with other fluids	1	2	3	4	5	NA
100309	Introduction of solid foods one at a time	1	2	3	4	5	NA
100310	Introduction of solid foods using a spoon	1	2	3	4	5	NA
100311	Additional physical touch during time of weaning	1	2	3	4	5	NA
100313	Knowledge of resources available for support	1	2	3	4	5	NA
100314	Use of available resources	1	2	3	4	5	NA
100316	Satisfaction with weaning process	1	2	3	4	5	NA

1st edition 1997; Revised 3rd edition 2004; Revised 4th edition

Continued

B

Outcome Content References:

Castiglia, P. T. (1992). Weaning. *Journal of Pediatric Health Care, 6*(1), 38-39.

Hendricks, K. M., & Badruddin, S. H. (1992). Weaning recommendations: The scientific basis. *Nutrition Reviews, 50*(5), 125-133.

Hervada, A. R. (1992). Weaning: Historical perspectives, practical recommendations, and current controversies. *Current Problems in Pediatrics, 22*(5), 223-241.

Huggins, K., & Ziedrich, L. (1994). *The nursing mother's guide to weaning.* Boston: The Harvard Common Press.

Kleinman, R. E. (Ed.). (1998). *Pediatric nutrition handbook* (4th ed.). Elk Grove Village, IL: American Academy of Pediatrics.

Lawrence, R. A., & Lawrence, R. M. (1999). *Breastfeeding: A guide for the medical profession* (5th ed.). St. Louis: Mosby.

Lewallen, L. P., Dick, M. J., Flowers, J., Powell, W., Zickefoose, K. T., Wall, Y. G., & Price, Z. M. (2006). Breastfeeding support and early cessation. *Journal of Obstetric, Gynecologic, and Neonatal Nursing (JOGNN), 35*(2), 166-172.

Riordan, J., & Auerbach, K. G. (1999). *Breastfeeding and human lactation* (2nd ed.). Sudbury, MA: Jones and Bartlett.

Rogers, C. S., Morris, S., & Taper, L. J. (1987). Weaning from the breast: Influences on maternal decisions. *Pediatric Nursing, 13*(5), 341-345.

Spangler, A. (1992). *Amy Spangler's breastfeeding: A parent's guide.* Atlanta: Amy Spangler.

Walker, C. (1995). When to wean: Whose advice do mothers find helpful? *Health Visitor, 68*(3), 109-111.

Burn Healing—1106

Domain-Physiologic Health (II)

Class-Tissue Integrity (L)

Scale(s)-None to Extensive (i) and Extensive to None (h)

Care Recipient:

Data Source:

Definition: Extent of healing of a burn site

OUTCOME TARGET RATING: Maintain at_____   Increase to_____

Burn Healing Overall Rating	None 1	Limited 2	Moderate 3	Substantial 4	Extensive 5	
INDICATORS:						
110601	Percent of graft site healed	1	2	3	4	5	NA
110602	Percent of burn site healed	1	2	3	4	5	NA
110603	Tissue granulation	1	2	3	4	5	NA
110604	Joint movement of affected extremity	1	2	3	4	5	NA
110605	Tissue perfusion of burn site	1	2	3	4	5	NA

	Extensive	Substantial	Moderate	Limited	None	
110606	Pain	1	2	3	4	5	NA
110607	Infection	1	2	3	4	5	NA
110608	Blistered skin	1	2	3	4	5	NA
110609	Purulent drainage	1	2	3	4	5	NA
110610	Foul wound odor	1	2	3	4	5	NA
110611	Burn site edema	1	2	3	4	5	NA
110612	Difficulty breathing	1	2	3	4	5	NA
110613	Tissue necrosis	1	2	3	4	5	NA

Grafted Yes / No

Location of burn _____ __

001 Head	007 Right upper arm	013 Right thigh
002 Neck	008 Left upper arm	014 Left thigh
003 Anterior trunk	009 Right lower arm	015 Right leg
004 Posterior trunk	010 Left lower arm	016 Left leg
005 Buttock	011 Right hand	017 Right foot
006 Genitalia	012 Left hand	018 Left foot

4th edition

Outcome Content References:

American Burn Association: Hospital and prehospital resources for optimal care of patients with burn injury: Guidelines for development and operation of burn centers. (1990). *Journal of Burn Care and Rehabilitation, 11*(2), 98-104.

Black, J., & Hawks, J. (2005). *Medical-surgical nursing. Clinical management for positive outcomes* (7th ed.). St. Louis: Saunders.

Mendez-Eastman, S. (2005). Burn injuries. *Plastic Surgical Nursing 25*(3), 133-139.

Nowlin, A. (2006). The delicate business of burn care. *RN, 69*(1), 52-58.

Osborn, K. (2003). Nursing burn injuries (Critical Care). *Nursing Management, 34*(5), 49-56.

Regojo, P. (2003). Burn care basics: How to extinguish problems. *Nursing 2003, 3*(3), 50-53.

B

Burn Recovery—1107

Domain-Physiologic Health (II)

Class-Tissue Integrity (L)

Scale(s)-None to Extensive (i) and Extensive to None (h)

Care Recipient

Data Source

Definition: Extent of overall physical and psychological healing following major burn injury

OUTCOME TARGET RATING: Maintain at_____   Increase to_____

Burn Recovery Overall Rating	None 1	Limited 2	Moderate 3	Substantial 4	Extensive 5	
INDICATORS:						
110701 Tissue granulation	1	2	3	4	5	NA
110702 Tissue perfusion of burn site	1	2	3	4	5	NA
110703 Percent of burn healed	1	2	3	4	5	NA
110704 Temperature stability	1	2	3	4	5	NA
110705 Electrolyte stability	1	2	3	4	5	NA
110706 Fluid balance	1	2	3	4	5	NA
110707 Self-care ability	1	2	3	4	5	NA
110708 Joint movement of extremities	1	2	3	4	5	NA
110709 Ambulation tolerance	1	2	3	4	5	NA
110710 Positive attitude toward touching affected part	1	2	3	4	5	NA
110711 Psychological adjustment to changes in physical appearance	1	2	3	4	5	NA
110712 Psychological adjustment to changes in body function	1	2	3	4	5	NA

	Extensive 1	Substantial 2	Moderate 3	Limited 4	None 5	
110713 Pain	1	2	3	4	5	NA
110714 Decreased cognition	1	2	3	4	5	NA
110715 Pain medication requirements	1	2	3	4	5	NA
110716 Decreased oxygen saturation	1	2	3	4	5	NA
110717 Difficulty breathing	1	2	3	4	5	NA
110718 Weight loss	1	2	3	4	5	NA
110719 Infection	1	2	3	4	5	NA
110720 Blistered skin	1	2	3	4	5	NA
110721 Purulent drainage	1	2	3	4	5	NA
110722 Foul wound odor	1	2	3	4	5	NA
110723 Burn site edema	1	2	3	4	5	NA
110724 Tissue necrosis	1	2	3	4	5	NA
110725 Generalized edema	1	2	3	4	5	NA
110726 Gastrointestinal complications	1	2	3	4	5	NA
110727 Decreased urine output	1	2	3	4	5	NA
110728 Burn site grafting required	1	2	3	4	5	NA

Outcome Content References:

American Burn Association. (1990). Hospital and prehospital resources for optimal care of patients with burn injury: Guidelines for development and operation of burn centers. *Journal of Burn Care and Rehabilitation, 11*(2), 98-104.

Black, J., & Hawks, J. (2005). *Medical-surgical nursing. Clinical management for positive outcomes* (7th ed.). St. Louis: Saunders.

Mendez-Eastman, S. (2005). Burn injuries. *Plastic Surgical Nursing 25*(3), 133-139.

Nowlin, A. (2006). The delicate business of burn care. *RN, 69*(1), 52-58.

Osborn, K. (2003). Nursing burn injuries (Critical Care). *Nursing Management, 34*(5), 49-56.

Regojo, P. (2003). Burn care basics: How to extinguish problems. *Nursing 2003, 3*(3), 50-53.

B

Cardiac Disease Self-Management—1617

Domain-Health Knowledge & Behavior (IV)

Class-Health Behavior (Q)

Scale(s)-Never demonstrated to Consistently demonstrated (m)

Care Recipient:

Data Source:

C

> **Definition:** Personal actions to manage heart disease, its treatment, and prevent disease progression

OUTCOME TARGET RATING: Maintain at_____   Increase to_____

Cardiac Disease Self-Management Overall Rating	Never demonstrated 1	Rarely demonstrated 2	Sometimes demonstrated 3	Often demonstrated 4	Consistently demonstrated 5	

INDICATORS:

161701	Accepts health provider's diagnosis	1	2	3	4	5	NA
161702	Seeks information about methods to maintain cardiovascular health	1	2	3	4	5	NA
161703	Participates in health care decision making process	1	2	3	4	5	NA
161704	Participates in prescribed cardiac rehabilitation program	1	2	3	4	5	NA
161705	Performs treatment regimen as prescribed	1	2	3	4	5	NA
161706	Monitors symptom onset	1	2	3	4	5	NA
161707	Monitors symptom persistence	1	2	3	4	5	NA
161708	Monitors symptom severity	1	2	3	4	5	NA
161709	Monitors symptom frequency	1	2	3	4	5	NA
161710	Reports symptoms of worsening disease	1	2	3	4	5	NA
161711	Reports signs and symptoms of depression	1	2	3	4	5	NA
161712	Uses diary to monitor symptoms over time	1	2	3	4	5	NA
161713	Uses preventive measures to reduce risk of complications	1	2	3	4	5	NA
161714	Uses symptom-relief measures	1	2	3	4	5	NA
161744	Obtains health care when warning signs occur	1	2	3	4	5	NA
161716	Monitors pulse rate and rhythm	1	2	3	4	5	NA
161717	Monitors blood pressure	1	2	3	4	5	NA
161718	Limits sodium intake	1	2	3	4	5	NA
161719	Limits fat and cholesterol intake	1	2	3	4	5	NA
161720	Follows recommended diet	1	2	3	4	5	NA
161721	Follows fluid restriction recommendations	1	2	3	4	5	NA
161722	Monitors effects of stimulants	1	2	3	4	5	NA

		Never demonstrated	Rarely demonstrated	Sometimes demonstrated	Often demonstrated	Consistently demonstrated	
161723	Monitors body weight	1	2	3	4	5	NA
161724	Uses effective weight control strategies	1	2	3	4	5	NA
161725	Maintains optimum weight	1	2	3	4	5	NA
161726	Follows recommendations for alcohol use	1	2	3	4	5	NA
161727	Participates in smoking cessation regimen	1	2	3	4	5	NA
161728	Participates in recommended exercise program	1	2	3	4	5	NA
161729	Uses energy conservation techniques	1	2	3	4	5	NA
161730	Balances activity and rest	1	2	3	4	5	NA
161731	Performs usual life routine	1	2	3	4	5	NA
161732	Follows recommendations for sexual activity	1	2	3	4	5	NA
161733	Obtains required medication	1	2	3	4	5	NA
161734	Uses medication as prescribed	1	2	3	4	5	NA
161735	Monitors prescribed medication therapeutic effects	1	2	3	4	5	NA
161736	Uses only over-the-counter medication approved by health professional	1	2	3	4	5	NA
161737	Uses stress management techniques	1	2	3	4	5	NA
161738	Obtains flu and pneumonia immunizations	1	2	3	4	5	NA
161739	Uses health care services congruent with need	1	2	3	4	5	NA
161740	Participates in screening for cholesterol	1	2	3	4	5	NA
161741	Reports need for financial assistance	1	2	3	4	5	NA
161742	Keeps appointments with health professional	1	2	3	4	5	NA
161743	Maintains plan for medical emergencies	1	2	3	4	5	NA
161745	Adjusts life routine for optimal health	1	2	3	4	5	NA

3rd edition 2004; Revised 4th edition

Outcome Content References:

Cannon, C. P., Battler, A., Brindis, R. G., Cox, J. L., Ellis, S. G., Every, N. R., Flaherty, J. T., Harrington, R. A., Krumholz, H. M., Simoons, M. L., Van De Werf, F. J. J., & Weintraub, W. S. (2001). ACC key data elements and definitions for measuring the clinical management and outcomes of patients with acute coronary syndromes: A report of the American College of Cardiology task force on clinical data standards (acute coronary syndrome writing committee). *Journal of the American College of Cardiology, 38,* 2114-2130.

Continued

Dunbar, S. B., Jacobson, L. H., & Deaton, C. (1998). Heart failure: Strategies to enhance patient self-management. *AACN Clinical Issues: Advanced Practice in Acute & Critical Care, 9,* 244-256.

Dusseldorp, E., Van Elderan, T., Maes, S., Meulman, J., & Kraaij, V. (1999). A meta-analysis of psychoeducational programs for coronary heart disease patients. *Health Psychology, 18,* 506-519.

Hunt, S. A., Baker, D. W., Chin, M. H., Cinquegrani, M. P., Feldman, A. M., Grancis, G. S., Ganiats, T. G., Goldstein, S., Gregoratos, G., Jessup, M. L., Noble, R. J., Packer, M., Silver, M. A., & Steven, L. W. (2001). ACC/AHA guidelines for the evaluation and management of chronic heart failure in the adult: A report of the American College of Cardiology/American Heart Association Task Force on Practice Guidelines (Committee to revise the 1995 Guidelines for the Evaluation and Management of Heart Failure). *Journal of the American College of Cardiology, 38,* 2101-2113.

Johnson, J., & Pearson, V. (2000). The effects of a structured education course on stroke survivors living in the community (including commentary by Phipps, M.). *Rehabilitation Nursing, 25,* 59-65.

National Institutes of Health, National Heart, Lung, and Blood Institute (NHLBI), & National High Blood Pressure Education Program (1997). *The Sixth Report of the Joint National Committee on Prevention, Detection, Evaluation, & Treatment of High Blood Pressure* (NIH Publication No. 98-4080). Bethesda, MD: Author.

Sheps, S. G., Black, H. R., Cohen, J. D., Kaplan, N. M., Ferdinand, K. C., Chobanian, A. V., Dustan, H. P., Gifford, R. W., Moser, M., et al. (1997). *The Sixth Report of the Joint National Committee on Prevention, Detection, Evaluation, & Treatment of High Blood Pressure* (NIH Publication No. 98-4080). Bethesda, MD: National Institutes of Health, National Heart, Lung, and Blood Institute (NHLBI), & National High Blood Pressure Education Program.

Cardiac Pump Effectiveness—0400

Domain-Physiologic Health (II)

Class-Cardiopulmonary (E)

Scale(s)-Severe deviation from normal range to No deviation from normal range (b) and Severe to None (n)

Care Recipient:

Data Source:

C

Definition: Adequacy of blood volume ejected from the left ventricle to support systemic perfusion pressure

OUTCOME TARGET RATING: Maintain at_____   Increase to_____

Cardiac Pump Effectiveness Overall Rating	Severe deviation from normal range 1	Substantial deviation from normal range 2	Moderate deviation from normal range 3	Mild deviation from normal range 4	No deviation from normal range 5	
INDICATORS:						
040001 Systolic blood pressure	1	2	3	4	5	NA
040019 Diastolic blood pressure	1	2	3	4	5	NA
040002 Apical heart rate	1	2	3	4	5	NA
040003 Cardiac index	1	2	3	4	5	NA
040004 Ejection fraction	1	2	3	4	5	NA
040006 Peripheral pulses	1	2	3	4	5	NA
040007 Heart size	1	2	3	4	5	NA
040020 Urine output	1	2	3	4	5	NA
040022 24-hour intake and output balance	1	2	3	4	5	NA
040025 Central venous pressure	1	2	3	4	5	NA
	Severe	Substantial	Moderate	Mild	None	
040009 Neck vein distension	1	2	3	4	5	NA
040010 Dysrhythmia	1	2	3	4	5	NA
040011 Abnormal heart sounds	1	2	3	4	5	NA
040012 Angina	1	2	3	4	5	NA
040013 Peripheral edema	1	2	3	4	5	NA
040014 Pulmonary edema	1	2	3	4	5	NA
040015 Diaphoresis	1	2	3	4	5	NA
040016 Nausea	1	2	3	4	5	NA
040017 Fatigue	1	2	3	4	5	NA
040023 Dyspnea at rest	1	2	3	4	5	NA
040026 Dyspnea with mild exertion	1	2	3	4	5	NA
040024 Weight gain	1	2	3	4	5	NA
040027 Ascites	1	2	3	4	5	NA
040028 Hepatomegaly	1	2	3	4	5	NA
040029 Impaired cognition	1	2	3	4	5	NA
040030 Activity intolerance	1	2	3	4	5	NA
040031 Pallor	1	2	3	4	5	NA
040032 Cyanosis	1	2	3	4	5	NA
040033 Flushed	1	2	3	4	5	NA

Continued

C

1st edition 1997; Revised 3rd edition 2004; Revised 4th edition

Outcome Content References:

Bumann, R., & Speltz, M. (1989). Decreased cardiac output: A nursing diagnosis. *Dimensions of Critical Care Nursing, 8*(1), 6-15.

Dalton, J. (1985). A descriptive study: Defining characteristics of the nursing diagnosis cardiac output, alterations in: Decreased. *Image—The Journal of Nursing Scholarship, 17*(4), 113-117.

Dougherty, C. (1986). Decreased cardiac output: Validation of a nursing diagnosis. *Dimensions of Critical Care Nursing, 5*(3), 182-188.

Dougherty, C. M. (2001). Decreased cardiac output. In M. Maas, K. Buckwalter, M. Hardy, T. Tripp-Reimer, M. Titler, & J. Specht (Eds.), *Nursing care of older adults: Diagnoses, outcomes & interventions* (pp. 285-297). St. Louis: Mosby.

Futrell, A. (1990). Decreased cardiac output: Case for a collaborative diagnosis. *Dimensions of Critical Care Nursing, 9*(4), 202-209.

U.S. Department of Health and Human Services. (1994). *Heart failure: Evaluation and care of patients with left-ventricular systolic dysfunction* (AHCPR Publication No. 94-0612). Rockville, MD: Public Health Service Agency for Health Care Policy and Research.

U.S. Department of Health and Human Services. (1994). *Unstable angina: Diagnosis and management* (AHCPR Publication No 94-0602). Rockville, MD: Public Health Service Agency for Health Care Policy and Research.

Cardiopulmonary Status—0414

Domain-Physiologic Health (II)

Class-Cardiopulmonary (E)

Scale(s)-Severe deviation from normal range to No deviation from normal range (b) and Severe to None (n)

Care Recipient:

Data Source:

C

Definition: Adequacy of blood volume ejected from the ventricles and exchange of carbon dioxide and oxygen at the alveolar level

OUTCOME TARGET RATING: Maintain at_____   Increase to_____

Cardiopulmonary Status Overall Rating	Severe deviation from normal range 1	Substantial deviation from normal range 2	Moderate deviation from normal range 3	Mild deviation from normal range 4	No deviation from normal range 5	
INDICATORS:						
041401 Systolic blood pressure	1	2	3	4	5	NA
041402 Diastolic blood pressure	1	2	3	4	5	NA
041403 Peripheral pulses	1	2	3	4	5	NA
041404 Apical heart rate	1	2	3	4	5	NA
041405 Cardiac rhythm	1	2	3	4	5	NA
041406 Respiratory rate	1	2	3	4	5	NA
041407 Respiratory rhythm	1	2	3	4	5	NA
041408 Depth of inspiration	1	2	3	4	5	NA
041409 Expulsion of air	1	2	3	4	5	NA
041410 Urinary output	1	2	3	4	5	NA
041411 Cardiac index	1	2	3	4	5	NA
041412 Oxygen saturation	1	2	3	4	5	NA
041413 Movement of sputum out of airway	1	2	3	4	5	NA

	Severe	Substantial	Moderate	Mild	None	
041414 Activity intolerance	1	2	3	4	5	NA
041415 Impaired cognition	1	2	3	4	5	NA
041416 Pallor	1	2	3	4	5	NA
041417 Cyanosis	1	2	3	4	5	NA
041418 Flushed	1	2	3	4	5	NA
041419 Neck vein distention	1	2	3	4	5	NA
041420 Chest retraction	1	2	3	4	5	NA
041421 Pursed lip breathing	1	2	3	4	5	NA
041422 Peripheral edema	1	2	3	4	5	NA
041423 Pulmonary edema	1	2	3	4	5	NA
041424 Dyspnea at rest	1	2	3	4	5	NA

Continued

		Severe	Substantial	Moderate	Mild	None	
041425	Dyspnea with mild exertion	1	2	3	4	5	NA
041426	Fatigue	1	2	3	4	5	NA
041427	Restlessness	1	2	3	4	5	NA
041428	Somnolence	1	2	3	4	5	NA
041429	Weight gain	1	2	3	4	5	NA
041430	Weight loss	1	2	3	4	5	NA
041431	Diaphoresis	1	2	3	4	5	NA

Outcome Content References:

Berry, B. E., & Pinard, A. E. (2002). Assessing tissue oxygenation. *Critical Care Nurse, 22*(3), 22-36.

Dougherty, C. M. (2001). Decreased cardiac output. In M. Maas, K. Buckwalter, M. Hardy, T. Tripp-Reimer, M. Titler, & J. Specht (Eds.), *Nursing care of older adults: Diagnoses, outcomes & interventions* (pp. 285-297). St. Louis: Mosby.

Smeltzer, S. C., & Bare, B. G. (2004). *Brunner & Suddarth's textbook of medical surgical nursing* (Vol. 1 & 2) (10th ed.). Philadelphia: Lippincott Williams & Wilkins.

Wakefield, B. (2001). Ineffective breathing pattern. In M. Maas, K. Buckwalter, M. Hardy, T. Tripp-Reimer, M. Titler, & J. Specht (Eds.), *Nursing care of older adults: Diagnoses, outcomes & interventions* (pp. 313-323). St. Louis: Mosby.

Caregiver Adaptation to Patient Institutionalization—2200

Domain-Family Health (VI)

Class-Family Caregiver Performance (W)

Scale(s)-Never demonstrated to Consistently demonstrated (m)

Care Recipient:

Data Source:

C

Definition: Adaptive response of family caregiver when the care recipient is moved to an institution

OUTCOME TARGET RATING: Maintain at_____   Increase to_____

Caregiver Adaptation to Patient Institutionalization Overall Rating	Never demonstrated 1	Rarely demonstrated 2	Sometimes demonstrated 3	Often demonstrated 4	Consistently demonstrated 5	

INDICATORS:

220001	Trusts non-family caregiver	1	2	3	4	5	NA
220002	Maintains desired control over care	1	2	3	4	5	NA
220003	Participates in care as desired	1	2	3	4	5	NA
220004	Maintains caregiver-care recipient relationship	1	2	3	4	5	NA
220016	Collaborates with health provider in determining care	1	2	3	4	5	NA
220006	Reports decreased need to verbalize feelings about change	1	2	3	4	5	NA
220007	Resolves feelings of guilt	1	2	3	4	5	NA
220008	Resolves feelings of anger	1	2	3	4	5	NA
220009	Uses conflict resolution strategies	1	2	3	4	5	NA
220017	Reports comfort with role transition	1	2	3	4	5	NA
220011	Provides consent for treatment	1	2	3	4	5	NA
220012	Provides information about patient's routine	1	2	3	4	5	NA
220013	Provides patient's comfort items	1	2	3	4	5	NA
220014	Communicates needs of nonverbal patient	1	2	3	4	5	NA

1st edition 1997; Revised 3rd edition 2004; Revised 4th edition

Outcome Content References:

Gaugler, J. E., Pearlin, L. I., Leitsch, S. A., & Davey, A. (2001). Relinquishing in-home dementia care: Difficulties and perceived helpfulness during the nursing home transition. *American Journal of Alzheimer's Disease & Other Dementias, 16*(1), 32-42.

Kaus, K. J. (1990). Fostering family integrity. In M. Craft & J. A. Denehy (Eds.), *Nursing Interventions for infants and children* (pp. 181-200). Philadelphia: W.B. Saunders.

Langford, M. (2001). A view from the front lines. Residential treatment: Have I done the right thing? *Premier Outlook, 2*(1), 16,18.

Lindgren, C. L. (1993). The caregiver career. *Image—The Journal of Nursing Scholarship, 25*(3), 214-219.

Lindsay, J. K., Roman, L., DeWys, M., Eager, M., Levick, J., & Quinn, M. (1993). Creative caring in the NICU: Parent to parent support. *Neonatal Network, 12*(4), 37-44.

Maas, M., Buckwalter, K., Swanson, E., Specht, J., Tripp-Reimer, T., & Hardy, M. (1994). The caring partnership: Staff and families of persons institutionalized with Alzheimer's disease. *The American Journal of Alzheimer's Care and Related Disorders & Research, 9*(6), 21-30.

Continued

+Montgomery, R. J. V., Gonyea, J. G., & Hooyman, N. R. (1985). Caregiving and the experience of subjective and objective burden. *Family Relations, 34,* 19-26.

Moyle, W., Edwards, H., & Clinton, M. (2002). Living with loss: Dementia and the family caregiver. *Australian Journal of Advanced Nursing, 19*(3), 25-31.

Olson, R. K., Heater, B. S., & Becker, A. M. (1990). A meta-analysis of the effects of nursing interventions on children and parents. *Maternal-Child Nursing, 15*(2), 104-108.

+Picot, S. J., Youngblut, J., & Zeller, R. (1997). Development and testing of a measure of perceived caregiver rewards in adults. *Journal of Nursing Measurement, 5*(1), 33-52.

Stevenson, J. E. (1990). Family stress related to home care of Alzheimer's disease patients and implications for support. *Journal of Neuroscience Nursing, 22*(3), 179-188.

Swanson, E., Jensen, D. P., Specht, J., Saylor, D., Johnson, M., & Maas, M. (1997). Caregiving: Concept analysis and outcomes. *Scholarly Inquiry for Nursing Practice, 11*(1), 65-79.

Wilson, H. S. (1989). Family caregiving for a relative with Alzheimer's dementia: Coping with negative choices. *Nursing Research, 38*(2), 94-98.

C

Caregiver Emotional Health—2506

Domain-Family Health (VI)

Class-Family Member Health Status (Z)

Scale(s)-Severely compromised to Not compromised (a) and Severe to None (n)

Care Recipient:

Data Source:

C

Definition: Emotional well-being of a family care provider while caring for a family member

OUTCOME TARGET RATING: Maintain at_____   Increase to_____

Caregiver Emotional Health Overall Rating	Severely compromised 1	Substantially compromised 2	Moderately compromised 3	Mildly compromised 4	Not compromised 5	
INDICATORS:						
250601 Satisfaction with life	1	2	3	4	5	NA
250602 Sense of control	1	2	3	4	5	NA
250603 Self-esteem	1	2	3	4	5	NA
250610 Certainty about future	1	2	3	4	5	NA
250611 Perceived social connectedness	1	2	3	4	5	NA
250612 Perceived spiritual well-being	1	2	3	4	5	NA
250614 Perceived adequacy of resources	1	2	3	4	5	NA
	Severe	**Substantial**	**Moderate**	**Mild**	**None**	
250604 Anger	1	2	3	4	5	NA
250605 Resentfulness	1	2	3	4	5	NA
250606 Guilt	1	2	3	4	5	NA
250607 Depression	1	2	3	4	5	NA
250608 Frustration	1	2	3	4	5	NA
250609 Ambivalence about situation	1	2	3	4	5	NA
250613 Perceived burden	1	2	3	4	5	NA
250615 Psychotropic medication use	1	2	3	4	5	NA

1st edition 1997; Revised 3rd edition 2004

Outcome Content References:

Brown, M. A., & Powell-Cope, G. M. (1991). AIDS family caregiving: Transitions through uncertainty. *Nursing Research, 40*(6), 338-345.

Bull, M. J. (1990). Factors influencing family caregiver burden and health. *Western Journal of Nursing Research, 12*(6), 758-776.

Croog, S. H., Sudilovsky, A., Burleson, J. A., & Baume, R. M. (2001). Vulnerability of husband and wife caregivers of Alzheimer disease patients to caregiving stressors. *Alzheimer Disease & Associated Disorders, 15*(4), 201-210.

Ducharme, F., LeVesque, L., Gendron, M., & Legault, A. (2001). Development process and qualitative evaluation of a program to promote the mental health of family caregivers. *Clinical Nursing Research, 10*(2), 182-201.

Fruewirth, S. E. (1989). An application of Johnson's Behavioral Model: A case study. *Journal of Community Health Nursing, 6*(2), 61-71.

Given, B. A., Kozachik, S. L., Collins, C. E., DeVoss, D. N., & Given, C. W. (2001). Caregiver role strain. In M. Maas, K. Buckwalter, M. Hardy, T. Tripp-Reimer, M. Titler, & J. Specht (Eds.), *Nursing care of older adults: Diagnoses, outcomes & interventions* (pp. 679-695). St. Louis: Mosby.

Grant, I., Adler, K. A., Patterson, T. L., Dimsdale, J. E., Ziegler, M. G., & Irwin, M. R. (2002). Health consequences of Alzheimer's caregiving transitions: Effects of placement and bereavement. *Psychosomatic Medicine, 64*(3), 477-486.

Continued

Haley, W. E., LaMonde, L. A., Han, B., Narramore, S., & Schonwetter, R. (2001). Family caregiving in hospice: Effects on psychological and health functioning among spousal caregivers of hospice patients with lung cancer or dementia. *Hospice Journal, 15*(4), 1-18.

Lindgren, C. L. (1990). Burnout and social support in family caregivers. *Western Journal of Nursing Research, 12*(4), 469-487.

Ptok, U., Papassotiropoulos, A., & Heun, R. (2001). Mental health in spouses of patients with gerontopsychiatric disorders. *International Journal of Geriatric Psychiatry, 16*(10), 1014-1016.

Romeis, J. C. (1989). Caregiver strain. *Journal of Aging and Health, 1*(2), 188-208.

+Robinson, B. C. (1983). Validation of a caregiver strain index. *Journal of Gerontology, 38*(3), 344-348.

Thompson, E. H., Futterman, A. M., Gallagher-Thompson, D., Rose, J. M., & Lovett, S. B. (1993). Social support and caregiving burden in family caregivers of frail elders. *Journal of Gerontology, 48*(5), S245-S254.

C

Caregiver Home Care Readiness—2202

Domain-Family Health (VI)

Class-Family Caregiver Performance (W)

Scale(s)-Not adequate to Totally adequate (f)

Care Recipient:

Data Source:

C

Definition: Preparedness of a caregiver to assume responsibility for the health care of a family member in the home

OUTCOME TARGET RATING: Maintain at_____   Increase to_____

Caregiver Home Care Readiness Overall Rating	Not adequate 1	Slightly adequate 2	Moderately adequate 3	Substantially adequate 4	Totally adequate 5	

INDICATORS:

220201	Willingness to assume caregiving role	1	2	3	4	5	NA
220204	Participation in decisions about home care	1	2	3	4	5	NA
220202	Knowledge about caregiving role	1	2	3	4	5	NA
220203	Demonstration of positive regard for care recipient	1	2	3	4	5	NA
220205	Knowledge of care recipient's disease process	1	2	3	4	5	NA
220206	Knowledge of recommended treatment regimen	1	2	3	4	5	NA
220207	Knowledge of recommended procedures	1	2	3	4	5	NA
220219	Knowledge of equipment and supplies required	1	2	3	4	5	NA
220220	Knowledge of equipment operation	1	2	3	4	5	NA
220208	Knowledge of prescribed activity	1	2	3	4	5	NA
220209	Knowledge of follow-up care	1	2	3	4	5	NA
220210	Knowledge of emergency care	1	2	3	4	5	NA
220211	Knowledge of financial resources	1	2	3	4	5	NA
220212	Financial resources for caregiving	1	2	3	4	5	NA
220213	Knowledge of when to contact health professional	1	2	3	4	5	NA
220214	Perceived social support for caregiving	1	2	3	4	5	NA
220215	Confidence in ability to manage care at home	1	2	3	4	5	NA
220217	Willingness to involve care recipient in planning care	1	2	3	4	5	NA
220218	Evidence of plans for caregiver backup	1	2	3	4	5	NA
220222	Participation in discharge planning	1	2	3	4	5	NA

Continued

1st edition 1997; Revised 3rd edition 2004; Revised 4th edition

Outcome Content References:

Axelrod, J., Geismar, L., & Ross, R. (1994). Families of chronically mentally ill patients: Their structure, coping resources, and tolerance for deviant behavior. *Health & Social Work, 19*(4), 271-278.

Baginski, Y. (1994). Roadblocks to home care. *Continuing Care, 13*(8), 16-18, 24, 28-29.

Bull, M. J., Hansen, H. E., & Gross, C. R. (2000). Differences in family caregiver outcomes by their level of involvement in discharge planning. *Applied Nursing Research, 13*(2), 76-82.

Coppa, C., Hepburn, J., Strauss, D., & Yody, B. B. (1999). Return to home after acquired brain injury: Is the family ready? *Brain Injury Source, 3*(2), 18-20, 22.

Gennaro, S., & Bakewell-Sachs, S. (1992). Discharge planning and home care for low-birth weight infants. *NAACOGS Clinical Issues in Perinatal & Womens Health Nursing, 3*(1), 129-145.

Magilvy, J. K., & Lakomy, J. M. (1991). Transitions of older adults to home care. *Home Health Care Services Quarterly, 12*(4), 59-70.

+Picot, S. J., Youngblut, J., & Zeller, R. (1997). Development and testing of a measure of perceived caregiver rewards in adults. *Journal of Nursing Measurement, 5*(1), 33-52.

Scherbring, M. (2002). Effect of caregiver perception of preparedness of burden in an oncology population. *Oncology Nursing Forum, 29*(6), E70-E76.

Titler, M. G., & Pettit, D. M. (1995). Discharge readiness assessment. *Journal of Cardiovascular Nursing, 9*(4), 64-74.

Caregiver Lifestyle Disruption—2203

Domain-Family Health (VI)   Care Recipient:

Class-Family Caregiver Performance (W)   Data Source:

Scale(s)-Severe to None (n) and Severely compromised to Not compromised (a)

C

Definition: Severity of disturbances in the lifestyle of a family member due to caregiving

OUTCOME TARGET RATING: Maintain at_____   Increase to_____

Caregiver Lifestyle Disruption Overall Rating	Severe 1	Substantial 2	Moderate 3	Mild 4	None 5	
INDICATORS:						
220315 Disruption of routine	1	2	3	4	5	NA
220317 Disruption of family dynamics	1	2	3	4	5	NA
220318 Disruption of living environment	1	2	3	4	5	NA
220319 Financial burden from caregiving	1	2	3	4	5	NA

	Severely compromised	Substantially compromised	Moderately compromised	Mildly compromised	Not compromised	
220310 Role responsibilities	1	2	3	4	5	NA
220302 Role performance	1	2	3	4	5	NA
220320 Sleep	1	2	3	4	5	NA
220303 Role flexibility	1	2	3	4	5	NA
220304 Opportunities for privacy	1	2	3	4	5	NA
220305 Relationships with family members	1	2	3	4	5	NA
220306 Social interactions	1	2	3	4	5	NA
220307 Social support	1	2	3	4	5	NA
220308 Diversional activities	1	2	3	4	5	NA
220312 Relationships with friends	1	2	3	4	5	NA
220313 Relationships with pets	1	2	3	4	5	NA
220309 Work productivity	1	2	3	4	5	NA

1st edition 1997; Revised 3rd edition 2004; Revised 4th edition

Outcome Content References:

Baldwin, B. A., Kleeman, K. M., Stevens, G. L., & Rasin, J. (1989). Family caregiver stress: Clinical assessment and management. *International Psychogeriatrics, 1*(2), 183-193.

Gaynor, S. E. (1990). The long haul: The effects of home care on caregivers. *Image—The Journal of Nursing Scholarship, 22*(4), 208-212.

Given, B. A., & Given, C. W. (1991). Family caregiving for the elderly. *Annual Review of Nursing Research, 9*, 77-101.

Hinds, C. (1992). Suffering: A relatively unexplored phenomenon among family caregivers of non-institutionalized patients with cancer. *Journal of Advanced Nursing, 17*(8), 918-925.

Kuhlman, G. J., Wilson, H. S., Hutchison, S. A., & Wallhagen, M. (1991). Alzheimer's disease and family caregiving: Critical syntheses of the literature and research agenda. *Nursing Research, 40*(6), 331-337.

Lindgren, C. L. (1990). Burnout and social support in family caregivers. *Western Journal of Nursing Research, 12*(4), 469-487.

Lindgren, C. L. (1993). The caregiver career. *Image—The Journal of Nursing Scholarship, 25*(3), 214-219.

Continued

Oberst, M. T., Thomas, S. E., Gass, K. A., & Ward, S. E. (1989). Caregiving demands and appraisal of stress among family caregivers. *Cancer Nursing, 12*(4), 209-215.

+Robinson, B. C. (1983). Validation of a caregiver strain index. *Journal of Gerontology, 38*(3), 344-348.

Robinson, K. (1990). The relationships between social skills, social support, self-esteem and burden in adult caregivers. *Journal of Advanced Nursing, 15*(7), 788-795.

Robinson, K. M. (1989). Predictors of depression among wife caregivers. *Nursing Research, 38*(8), 359-363.

Stern, S., Doolan, M., Staples, E., Szmukler, G. L., & Eisler, I. (1999). Disruption and reconstruction: Narrative insights into the experience of family members caring for a relative diagnosed with serious mental illness. *Family Process, 38*(3), 353-369.

Stevenson, J. E. (1990). Family stress related to home care of Alzheimer's disease patients and implications for support. *Journal of Neuroscience Nursing, 22*(3), 179-188.

Thompson, E. H., Futterman, A. M., Gallagher-Thompson, D., Rose, J. M., & Lovette, S. B. (1993). Social support and caregiving burden in family caregivers of frail elders. *Journal of Gerontology, 48*(5), S245-S254.

C

Caregiver-Patient Relationship—2204

Domain-Family Health (VI)

Class-Family Caregiver Performance (W)

Scale(s)-Never positive to Consistently positive (k)

Care Recipient:

Data Source:

C

Definition: Positive interactions and connections between the caregiver and care recipient

OUTCOME TARGET RATING: Maintain at_____   Increase to_____

Caregiver-Patient Relationship Overall Rating	Never positive 1	Rarely positive 2	Sometimes positive 3	Often positive 4	Consistently positive 5	
INDICATORS:						
220401 Effective communication	1	2	3	4	5	NA
220402 Patience	1	2	3	4	5	NA
220404 Calmness	1	2	3	4	5	NA
220405 Nurturance and affirmation	1	2	3	4	5	NA
220406 Companionship	1	2	3	4	5	NA
220407 Caring	1	2	3	4	5	NA
220408 Long-term commitment	1	2	3	4	5	NA
220409 Mutual acceptance	1	2	3	4	5	NA
220410 Mutual respect	1	2	3	4	5	NA
220411 Collaborative problem solving	1	2	3	4	5	NA
220412 Sense of responsibility	1	2	3	4	5	NA
220413 Mutual sense of attachment	1	2	3	4	5	NA

1st edition 1997; Revised 3rd edition 2004; Revised 4th edition

Outcome Content References:

Caldwell, S. M. (1988). Measuring family well-being: Conceptual model, reliability, validity and use. In C. F. Waltz & O. L. Strickland (Eds.), *Measurement of nursing outcomes: Measuring client outcomes* (Vol. 1, pp. 396-422). New York: Springer.

Clemen-Stone, S., McGuire, S., & Eigsti, D. (2002). *Comprehensive community health nursing: Family, aggregate and community practice* (6th ed.). St. Louis: Mosby.

Craft, M. J., & Willadsen, J. A. (1992). Interventions related to family. *Nursing Clinics of North America, 27*(20), 517-540.

+Picot, S. J., Youngblut, J., & Zeller, R. (1997). Development and testing of a measure of perceived caregiver rewards in adults. *Journal of Nursing Measurement, 5*(1), 33-52.

Gaynor, S. E. (1990). The long haul: The effects of home care on caregivers. *Image—The Journal of Nursing Scholarship, 22*(4), 208-212.

Hooyman, M., Gonyea, J., & Montgomery, R. (1985). Impact of in-home services termination on family caregivers. *The Gerontologist, 25*(2), 141-145.

O'Neill, C., & Sorenson, E. S. (1991). Home care of the elderly: A family perspective. *Advances in Nursing Science, 13*(4), 28-37.

Phillips, L. R. (1988). The fit of elder abuse with the family violence paradigm, and the implications of a paradigm shift for clinical practice. *Public Health Nursing, 5*(4), 222-229.

Printz-Feddersen, V. (1990). Group process effect on caregiver burden. *Journal of Neuroscience Nursing, 22*(3), 164-168.

+Vermooij-Dassen, M. J. F. J. (1993). *Dementia and home care: Determinants of the sense of competence of primary caregivers and the effect of professionally guided caregiver support* (in Dutch). Lisse, The Netherlands: Swets & Seitliger.

C

Caregiver Performance: Direct Care—2205

Domain-Family Health (VI)
Class-Family Caregiver Performance (W)
Scale(s)-Not adequate to Totally adequate (f)

Care Recipient:
Data Source:

Definition: Provision by family care provider of appropriate personal and health care for a family member

OUTCOME TARGET RATING: Maintain at_____   Increase to_____

Caregiver Performance: Direct Care Overall Rating	Not adequate 1	Slightly adequate 2	Moderately adequate 3	Substantially adequate 4	Totally adequate 5	

INDICATORS:

220503	Knowledge of disease process	1	2	3	4	5	NA
220504	Knowledge of treatment regimen	1	2	3	4	5	NA
220505	Adherence to treatment regimen	1	2	3	4	5	NA
220516	Performance of procedures	1	2	3	4	5	NA
220502	Assistance with care recipient's activities of daily living needs	1	2	3	4	5	NA
220506	Assistance with care recipient's instrumental activities of daily living needs	1	2	3	4	5	NA
220501	Provision of emotional support to care recipient	1	2	3	4	5	NA
220508	Surveillance of health status of care recipient	1	2	3	4	5	NA
220509	Surveillance of behavior of care recipient	1	2	3	4	5	NA
220510	Anticipation of care recipient's needs	1	2	3	4	5	NA
220517	Unconditional positive regard for care recipient	1	2	3	4	5	NA
220518	Competence monitoring own caregiving skill level	1	2	3	4	5	NA
220513	Confidence performing needed tasks	1	2	3	4	5	NA
220515	Provision of safe environment	1	2	3	4	5	NA

1st edition 1997; Revised 3rd edition 2004; Revised 4th edition

Outcome Content References:
Given, B. A., Kozachik, S. L., Collins, C. E., DeVoss, D. N., & Given, C. W. (2001). Caregiver role strain. In M. Maas, K. Buckwalter, M. Hardy, T. Tripp-Reimer, M. Titler, & J. Specht (Eds.), *Nursing care of older adults: Diagnoses, outcomes & interventions* (pp. 679-695). St. Louis: Mosby.
Given, B. A., & Given, C. W. (1991). Family caregiving for the elderly. *Annual Review of Nursing Research, 9*, 77-101.
Oberst, M. T., Thomas, S. E., Gass, K. A., & Ward, S. E. (1989). Caregiving demands and appraisal of stress among family caregivers. *Cancer Nursing, 12*(4), 209-215.
+Picot, S. J., Youngblut, J., & Zeller, R. (1997). Development and testing of a measure of perceived caregiver rewards in adults. *Journal of Nursing Measurement, 5*(1), 33-52.
Pierson, M. A., & Irons, K. (1992). Identification of a cluster of nursing diagnoses for a caregiver support group. *Nursing Diagnosis, 3*(1), 36-41.
Printz-Feddersen, V. (1990). Group process effect on caregiver burden. *Journal of Neuroscience Nursing, 22*(3), 164-168.
Thomas, V. M., Ellison, K., Howell, E. V., & Winters, K. (1992). Caring for the person receiving ventilatory support at home: Caregivers' needs and involvement. *Heart & Lung, 21*(2), 180-186.
+Vermooij-Dassen, M. J. F. J. (1993). *Dementia and home care: Determinants of the sense of competence of primary caregivers and the effect of professionally guided caregiver support* (in Dutch). Lisse, The Netherlands: Swets & Seitliger.
Wallhagen, M. I., & Kagan, S. H. (1993). Staying within bounds: Perceived control and the experience of elderly caregivers. *Journal of Aging Studies, 7*(2), 197-213.

Caregiver Performance: Indirect Care—2206

Domain-Family Health (VI)

Class-Family Caregiver Performance (W)

Scale(s)-Not adequate to Totally adequate (f)

Care Recipient:

Data Source:

C

Definition: Arrangement and oversight by family care provider of appropriate care for a family member

OUTCOME TARGET RATING:　Maintain at_____　　Increase to_____

Caregiver Performance: Indirect Care Overall Rating	Not adequate 1	Slightly adequate 2	Moderately adequate 3	Substantially adequate 4	Totally adequate 5	
INDICATORS:						
220601 Confidence in problem solving	1	2	3	4	5	NA
220602 Recognition of changes in health status of care recipient	1	2	3	4	5	NA
220603 Recognition of changes in behavior of care recipient	1	2	3	4	5	NA
220614 Anticipation of care recipient's needs	1	2	3	4	5	NA
220605 Procurement of needed health care services for care recipient	1	2	3	4	5	NA
220611 Procurement of needed transportation for care recipient	1	2	3	4	5	NA
220612 Procurement of needed equipment and supplies for care recipient	1	2	3	4	5	NA
220606 Skill in overseeing provision of care	1	2	3	4	5	NA
220615 Unconditional positive regard for care recipient	1	2	3	4	5	NA
220608 Skill in pursuing care problems with direct care providers	1	2	3	4	5	NA
220609 Confidence in performing needed tasks	1	2	3	4	5	NA
220613 Recognition of requirements for safety	1	2	3	4	5	NA

1st edition 1997; Revised 3rd edition 2004; Revised 4th edition

Outcome Content References:

Bowers, B. J. (1987). Intergenerational caregiving: Adult caregivers and their aging parents. *Advances in Nursing Science, 9*(2), 20-31.

Given, B. A., Kozachik, S. L., Collins, C. E., DeVoss, D. N., & Given, C. W. (2001). Caregiver role strain. In M. Maas, K. Buckwalter, M. Hardy, T. Tripp-Reimer, M. Titler, & J. Specht (Eds.), *Nursing care of older adults: Diagnoses, outcomes & interventions* (pp. 679-695). St. Louis: Mosby.

Given, B. A., & Given, C. W. (1991). Family caregiving for the elderly. *Annual Review of Nursing Research, 9*, 77-101.

Oberst, M. T., Thomas, S. E., Gass, K. A., & Ward, S. E. (1989). Caregiving demands and appraisal of stress among family caregivers. *Cancer Nursing, 12*(4), 209-215.

Pierson, M. A., & Irons, K. (1992). Identification of a cluster of nursing diagnoses for a caregiver support group. *Nursing Diagnosis, 3*(1), 36-41.

Printz-Feddersen, V. (1990). Group process effect on caregiver burden. *Journal of Neuroscience Nursing, 22*(3), 164-168.

Thomas, V. M., Ellison, K., Howell, E. V., & Winters, K. (1992). Caring for the person receiving ventilatory support at home: Caregivers' needs and involvement. *Heart & Lung, 21*(2), 180-186.

+Vermooij-Dassen, M. J. F. J. (1993). *Dementia and home care: Determinants of the sense of competence of primary caregivers and the effect of professionally guided caregiver support* (in Dutch). Lisse, The Netherlands: Swets & Seitliger.

Wallhagen, M. I., & Kagan, S. H. (1993). Staying within bounds: Perceived control and the experience of elderly caregivers. *Journal of Aging Studies, 7*(2), 197-213.

Caregiver Physical Health—2507

Domain-Family Health (VI)

Class-Family Member Health Status (Z)

Scale(s)-Severely compromised to Not compromised (a)

Care Recipient:

Data Source:

C

Definition: Physical well-being of a family care provider while caring for a family member

OUTCOME TARGET RATING: Maintain at_____   Increase to_____

Caregiver Physical Health Overall Rating	Severely compromised 1	Substantially compromised 2	Moderately compromised 3	Mildly compromised 4	Not compromised 5	
INDICATORS:						
250715 Physical fitness	1	2	3	4	5	NA
250702 Sleep-rest pattern	1	2	3	4	5	NA
250703 Blood pressure	1	2	3	4	5	NA
250704 Energy level	1	2	3	4	5	NA
250705 Physical comfort	1	2	3	4	5	NA
250706 Mobility level	1	2	3	4	5	NA
250707 Resistance to infection	1	2	3	4	5	NA
250708 Physical function	1	2	3	4	5	NA
250709 Weight	1	2	3	4	5	NA
250710 Gastrointestinal function	1	2	3	4	5	NA
250716 Cardiac function	1	2	3	4	5	NA
250717 Pulmonary function	1	2	3	4	5	NA
250718 Nutritional status	1	2	3	4	5	NA
250719 Cognitive status	1	2	3	4	5	NA
250711 Medication use	1	2	3	4	5	NA
250712 Perceived general health	1	2	3	4	5	NA

1st edition 1997; Revised 3rd edition 2004; Revised 4th edition

Outcome Content References:

Collins, C. E., Given, B. A., & Given, C. W. (1994). Interventions with family caregivers of persons with Alzheimer's disease. *Nursing Clinics of North America, 29*(1), 127-131.

Given, B. A., Kozachik, S. L., Collins, C. E., DeVoss, D. N., & Given, C. W. (2001). Caregiver role strain. In M. Maas, K. Buckwalter, M. Hardy, T. Tripp-Reimer, M. Titler, & J. Specht (Eds.), *Nursing care of older adults: Diagnoses, outcomes & interventions* (pp. 679-695). St. Louis: Mosby.

Given, B. A., & Given, C. W. (1991). Family caregiving for the elderly. *Annual Review of Nursing Research, 9*, 77-101.

Grant, I., Adler, K. A., Patterson, T. L., Dimsdale, J. E., Ziegler, M. G., & Irwin, M. R. (2002). Health consequences of Alzheimer's caregiving transitions: Effects of placement and bereavement. *Psychosomatic Medicine, 64*(3), 477-486.

Grasel, E. (2002). When home care ends—Changes in the physical health of informal caregivers caring for dementia patients: A longitudinal study. *Journal of American Geriatric Society, 50*(5), 843-849.

Haley, W. E., LaMonde, L. A., Han, B., Narramore, S., & Schonwetter, R. (2001). Family caregiving in hospice: Effects on psychological and health functioning among spousal caregivers of hospice patients with lung cancer or dementia. *Hospice Journal, 15*(4), 1-18.

Pepin, J. I. (1992). Family caring and caring in nursing: *Image—The Journal of Nursing Scholarship, 24*(2), 127-131.

+Robinson, B. C. (1983). Validation of a caregiver strain index. *Journal of Gerontology, 38*(3), 344-348.

Springer, D., & Brubaker, T. H. (1984). *Caregiving and the dependent elderly.* Thousand Oaks, CA: Sage.

Winslow, B., & O'Brien, R. (1992). Use of formal community resources by spouse caregivers of chronically ill adults. *Public Health Nursing, 9*(27), 128-132.

Zeisel, J., Hyde, J., & Levkoff, S. (1994). Best practices: An environment-behavior (E-B) model for Alzheimer special care units. *The American Journal of Alzheimer's Care and Related Disorders & Research, 9*(2), 4-21.

Caregiver Role Endurance—2210

Domain-Family Health (VI)

Class-Family Caregiver Performance (W)

Scale(s)-Not adequate to Totally adequate (f)

Care Recipient:

Data Source:

C

Definition: Factors that promote family care provider's capacity to sustain caregiving over an extended period of time

OUTCOME TARGET RATING: Maintain at_____   Increase to_____

Caregiver Role Endurance Overall Rating	Not adequate 1	Slightly adequate 2	Moderately adequate 3	Substantially adequate 4	Totally adequate 5	

INDICATORS:

221001	Mutually satisfying care recipient-caregiver relationship	1	2	3	4	5	NA
221002	Mastery of direct care activities	1	2	3	4	5	NA
221003	Mastery of indirect care activities	1	2	3	4	5	NA
221004	Supplemental services to assist with care	1	2	3	4	5	NA
221012	Health provider support for caregiver	1	2	3	4	5	NA
221013	Supplies for caregiving	1	2	3	4	5	NA
221011	Financial resources for caregiving	1	2	3	4	5	NA
221005	Social support for caregiver	1	2	3	4	5	NA
221008	Respite for caregiver	1	2	3	4	5	NA
221009	Opportunities for caregiver leisure activities	1	2	3	4	5	NA

1st edition 1997; Revised 3rd edition 2004; Revised 4th edition (formerly Caregivimg Endurance Potential)

Outcome Content References:

Czaja, S. J., & Rubert, M. P. (2002). Telecommunications technology as an aid to family caregivers of persons with dementia. *Psychosomatic Medicine, 64*(3), 469-476.

Given, B. A., Stommel, M., Collins, C., King, S., & Given, C. W. (1990). Responses of elderly spouse caregivers. *Research in Nursing & Health, 13,* 77-85.

Oberst, M. T., Thomas, S. E., Gass, K. A., & Ward, S. E. (1989). Caregiving demands and appraisal of stress among family caregivers. *Cancer Nursing, 12*(4), 209-215.

+Picot, S. J., Youngblut, J., & Zeller, R. (1997). Development and testing of a measure of perceived caregiver rewards in adults. *Journal of Nursing Measurement, 5*(1), 33-52.

Rawlins, S. R. (1991). Using the connecting process to meet family caregiver needs. *Journal of Professional Nursing, 7*(4), 213-220.

Romeis, J. C. (1989). Caregiver strain. *Journal of Aging and Health, 1*(2), 188-208.

Stevenson, J. E. (1990). Family stress related to home care of Alzheimer's disease patients and implications for support. *Journal of Neuroscience Nursing, 22*(3), 179-188.

Thompson, E. H., Futterman, A. M., Gallagher-Thompson, D., Rose, J. M., & Lovett, S. B. (1993). Social support and caregiving burden in family caregivers of frail elders. *Journal of Gerontology, 48*(5), S245-S254.

Wallhagen, M. I. (1992). Caregiving demands: Their difficulty and effects on the well-being of elderly caregivers. *Scholarly Inquiry for Nursing Practice: An International Journal, 6*(2), 111-133.

Winslow, B., & O'Brien, R. (1992). Use of formal community resources by spouse caregivers of chronically ill adults. *Public Health Nursing, 9*(27), 128-132.

Caregiver Stressors—2208

Domain-Family Health (VI)

Class-Family Caregiver Performance (W)

Scale(s)-Severe to None (n)

Care Recipient:

Data Source:

C

> **Definition:** Severity of biopsychosocial pressure on a family care provider caring for another over an extended period of time

OUTCOME TARGET RATING: Maintain at_____   Increase to_____

Caregiver Stressors Overall Rating	Severe 1	Substantial 2	Moderate 3	Mild 4	None 5	

INDICATORS:

220801	Reported stressors of caregiving	1	2	3	4	5	NA
220802	Physical limitations for caregiving	1	2	3	4	5	NA
220803	Psychological limitations for caregiving	1	2	3	4	5	NA
220804	Cognitive limitations	1	2	3	4	5	NA
220805	Role conflict	1	2	3	4	5	NA
220815	Sense of isolation	1	2	3	4	5	NA
220807	Perceived lack of social support	1	2	3	4	5	NA
220818	Perceived lack of health professional support	1	2	3	4	5	NA
220816	Loss of personal time	1	2	3	4	5	NA
220819	Conflict between work and caregiver responsibilities	1	2	3	4	5	NA
220820	Perceived burden of care recipient's progressive health problems	1	2	3	4	5	NA
220813	Impairment of caregiver-patient relationship	1	2	3	4	5	NA
220821	Impairment of family relationships	1	2	3	4	5	NA

1st edition 1997; Revised 3rd edition 2004; Revised 4th edition

Outcome Content References:

Andersson, A., Levin, L. A., Emtinger, B. G. (2002). The economic burden of informal care. *International Journal of Technology Assessment in Health Care, 18*(1), 46-54.

Brown, M. A., & Powell-Cope, G. M. (1991). AIDS family caregiving: Transitions through uncertainty. *Nursing Research, 40*(6), 338-345.

Chambers, M., Ryan, A. A., & Connors, S. L. (2001). Exploring the emotional needs and coping strategies of family carers. *Journal of Psychiatric and Mental Health Nursing, 8,* 99-106.

Davis, L. L. (2001). Altered family processes. In M. Maas, K. Buckwalter, M. Hardy, T. Tripp-Reimer, M. Titler, & J. Specht (Eds.), *Nursing care of older adults: Diagnoses, outcomes & interventions* (pp. 719-727). St. Louis: Mosby.

Given, C. W., Given, B., Stommel, M., Collins, C., King, S., & Franklin, S. (1992). The Caregiver Reaction Assessment (CRA) for caregivers to persons with chronic physical and mental impairments. *Research in Nursing & Health, 15*(4), 271-283.

Glasscock, R. (2000). A phenomenological study of the experience of being a mother of a child with cerebral palsy. *Pediatric Nursing, 26*(4), 407-410.

Laidlaw, T. M., Coverdale, J. H., Falloon, I. R., & Kydd, R. R. (2002). Caregivers' stresses when living together or apart from patients with chronic schizophrenia. *Community Mental Health Journal, 38*(4), 303-310.

Levesque, L., Ducharme, F., & Lachance, L. (1999). Is there a difference between family caregiving of institutionalized elders with or without dementia? *Western Journal of Nursing Research, 21*(4), 472-497.

+Robinson, B. C. (1983). Validation of a caregiver strain index. *Journal of Gerontology, 38*(3), 344-348.

Stevenson, J. E. (1990). Family stress related to home care of Alzheimer's disease patients and implications for support. *Journal of Neuroscience Nursing, 22*(3), 179-188.

Thompson, E. H., Futterman, A. M., Gallagher-Thompson, D., Rose, J. M., & Lovett, S. B. (1993). Social support and caregiving burden in family caregivers of frail elders. *Journal of Gerontology, 48*(5), S245-S254.

Wallhagen, M. I. (1992). Caregiving demands: Their difficulty and effects on the well-being of elderly caregivers. *Scholarly Inquiry for Nursing Practice: An International Journal, 6*(2), 111-133.

C

Caregiver Well-Being—2508

Domain-Family Health (VI)

Class-Family Member Health Status (Z)

Scale(s)-Not at all satisfied to Completely satisfied (s)

Care Recipient:

Data Source:

C

Definition: Extent of positive perception of primary care provider's health status

OUTCOME TARGET RATING: Maintain at_____   Increase to_____

Caregiver Well-Being Overall Rating	Not at all satisfied 1	Somewhat satisfied 2	Moderately satisfied 3	Very satisfied 4	Completely satisfied 5	
INDICATORS:						
250801 Physical health	1	2	3	4	5	NA
250802 Psychological health	1	2	3	4	5	NA
250803 Lifestyle	1	2	3	4	5	NA
250804 Performance of usual roles	1	2	3	4	5	NA
250805 Social support	1	2	3	4	5	NA
250806 Support for instrumental activities of daily living	1	2	3	4	5	NA
250807 Health professional support	1	2	3	4	5	NA
250808 Social relationships	1	2	3	4	5	NA
250811 Family sharing of responsibilities for caregiving	1	2	3	4	5	NA
250812 Availability for respite	1	2	3	4	5	NA
250813 Ability to cope	1	2	3	4	5	NA
250809 Caregiver role	1	2	3	4	5	NA
250814 Financial resources for caregiving	1	2	3	4	5	NA

1st edition 1997; Revised 3rd edition 2004; Revised 4th edition

Outcome Content References:

Brown, M. A., & Powell-Cope, G. M. (1991). AIDS family caregiving: Transitions through uncertainty. *Nursing Research, 40*(6), 338-345.

Given, B. A., Kozachik, S. L., Collins, C. E., DeVoss, D. N., & Given, C. W. (2001). Caregiver role strain. In M. Maas, K. Buckwalter, M. Hardy, T. Tripp-Reimer, M. Titler, & J. Specht (Eds.), *Nursing care of older adults: Diagnoses, outcomes & interventions* (pp. 679-695). St. Louis: Mosby.

Given, C. W., Given, B., Stommel, M., Collins, C., King, S., & Franklin, S. (1992). The Caregiver Reaction Assessment (CRA) for caregivers to persons with chronic physical and mental impairments. *Research in Nursing & Health, 15*(4), 271-283.

Jungbauer, J., & Angermeyer, M. C. (2002). Living with a schizophrenic patient: A comparative study of burden as it affects parents and spouses. *Psychiatry, 65*(2), 110-123.

Pender, N., Murdaugh, C., & Parsons, M. A. (2001). *Health promotion in nursing practice* (4th ed.). Upper Saddle River, NJ: Prentice Hall.

+Picot, S. J., Youngblut, J., & Zeller, R. (1997). Development and testing of a measure of perceived caregiver rewards in adults. *Journal of Nursing Measurement, 5*(1), 33-52.

Stevenson, J. E. (1990). Family stress related to home care of Alzheimer's disease patients and implications for support. *Journal of Neuroscience Nursing, 22*(3), 179-188.

Thompson, E. H., Futterman, A. M., Gallagher-Thompson, D., Rose, J. M., & Lovett, S. B. (1993). Social support and caregiving burden in family caregivers of frail elders. *Journal of Gerontology, 48*(5), S245-S254.

Wade, S. L., Taylor, H. G., Drotar, D., Stancin, T., Yeates, K. O., & Minich, N. M. (2002). A prospective study of long-term caregiver and family adaptation following brain injury in children. *Journal of Health Trauma Rehabilitation, 17*(2), 96-111.

Wallhagen, M. I. (1992). Caregiving demands: Their difficulty and effects on the well-being of elderly caregivers. *Scholarly Inquiry for Nursing Practice: An International Journal, 6*(2), 111-133.

Warfield, M. E. (2001). Employment, parenting, and well-being among mothers of children with disabilities. *Mental Retardation, 39*(4), 297-309.

Child Adaptation to Hospitalization—1301

Domain-Psychosocial Health (III)

Class-Psychosocial Adaptation (N)

Scale(s)-Never demonstrated to Consistently demonstrated (m) and Consistently demonstrated to Never demonstrated (t)

Care Recipient:

Data Source:

C

Definition: Adaptive response of a child from 3 years through 17 years of age to hospitalization

OUTCOME TARGET RATING: Maintain at_____   Increase to_____

Child Adaptation to Hospitalization Overall Rating	Never demonstrated 1	Rarely demonstrated 2	Sometimes demonstrated 3	Often demonstrated 4	Consistently demonstrated 5	
INDICATORS:						
130112 Interacts with parent	1	2	3	4	5	NA
130121 Maintains usual routine	1	2	3	4	5	NA
130113 Recognizes reason for hospitalization	1	2	3	4	5	NA
130115 Participates in decision-making	1	2	3	4	5	NA
130123 Asks questions about illness	1	2	3	4	5	NA
130124 Asks questions about treatment	1	2	3	4	5	NA
130125 Describes illness	1	2	3	4	5	NA
130126 Describes prescribed treatment	1	2	3	4	5	NA
130127 Maintains sense of control	1	2	3	4	5	NA
130118 Cooperates with procedures	1	2	3	4	5	NA
130109 Responds to comfort measures	1	2	3	4	5	NA
130110 Responds to diversional therapy	1	2	3	4	5	NA
130111 Participates in social interaction	1	2	3	4	5	NA
130119 Interacts with peers	1	2	3	4	5	NA
130117 Maintains pre-admission self-care behaviors	1	2	3	4	5	NA

	Consistently demonstrated	Often demonstrated	Sometimes demonstrated	Rarely demonstrated	Never demonstrated	
130101 Agitation	1	2	3	4	5	NA
130102 Separation anxiety	1	2	3	4	5	NA
130103 Regressive behaviors	1	2	3	4	5	NA
130104 Anxiety	1	2	3	4	5	NA
130105 Fear	1	2	3	4	5	NA
130106 Anger	1	2	3	4	5	NA
130128 Withdrawal	1	2	3	4	5	NA
130129 Aggressive behaviors	1	2	3	4	5	NA

1st edition 1997; Revised 3rd edition 2004; Revised 4th edition

Continued

C

Outcome Content References:

Coucouvanis, J. A. (1990). Behavior management. In M. Craft & J. A. Denehy (Eds.), *Nursing interventions for infants and children* (pp. 151-165). Philadelphia: W.B. Saunders.

Hockenberry, M. J., Wilson, D., Winkelstein, M. L., & Kline, N. E. (2003). *Wong's nursing care of infants and children* (7th ed.). St. Louis: Mosby.

Manion, J. (1990). Preparing children for hospitalization, procedures, or surgery. In M. Craft & J. A. Denehy (Eds.), *Nursing interventions for infants and children* (pp. 74-90). Philadelphia: W.B. Saunders.

Olson, R. K., Heater, B. S., & Becker, A. M. (1990). A meta-analysis of the effects of nursing interventions on children and parents. *Maternal-Child Nursing, 15*(2), 104-108.

Shields, L. (2001). A review of the literature from developed and developing countries relating to the effects of hospitalization on children and parents. *International Nursing Review, 48*(1), 29-37.

Wolfer, J. A., & Visintainer, M. A. (1975). Pediatric surgical patients' and parents' stress responses and adjustment as a function of psychologic preparation and stress-point nursing care. *Nursing Research, 24*(4), 244-255.

Ziegler, D. B., & Prior, M. M. (1994). Preparation for surgery and adjustment to hospitalization. *Nursing Clinics of North America, 29*(4), 655-669.

Child Development: 1 Month—0120

Domain-Functional Health (I)

Class-Growth & Development (B)

Scale(s)-Never demonstrated to Consistently demonstrated (m)

Care Recipient:

Data Source:

C

Definition: Milestones of physical, cognitive and psychosocial progression by 1 month of age

OUTCOME TARGET RATING: Maintain at_____   Increase to_____

Child Development: 1 Month Overall Rating	Never demonstrated 1	Rarely demonstrated 2	Sometimes demonstrated 3	Often demonstrated 4	Consistently demonstrated 5	

INDICATORS:

012001	Signals hunger	1	2	3	4	5	NA
012002	Signals discomfort	1	2	3	4	5	NA
012003	Responds to sounds	1	2	3	4	5	NA
012004	Responds to voice	1	2	3	4	5	NA
012005	Responds to face	1	2	3	4	5	NA
012006	Coos	1	2	3	4	5	NA
012007	Smiles spontaneously	1	2	3	4	5	NA
012008	Eyes follow to mid-line	1	2	3	4	5	NA
012009	Signals overstimulation	1	2	3	4	5	NA
012010	Exhibits five sleep and alert states	1	2	3	4	5	NA
012011	Flexes extremity	1	2	3	4	5	NA
012012	Holds head erect momentarily	1	2	3	4	5	NA
012013	Turns head side to side when prone	1	2	3	4	5	NA
012014	Holds head in horizontal line with back when prone	1	2	3	4	5	NA
012015	Moro reflex	1	2	3	4	5	NA
012016	Tonic neck reflex	1	2	3	4	5	NA
012017	Dance reflex	1	2	3	4	5	NA
012018	Crawl reflex	1	2	3	4	5	NA
012019	Babinski reflex	1	2	3	4	5	NA
012020	Suck reflex	1	2	3	4	5	NA
012021	Palmer reflex	1	2	3	4	5	NA
012022	Plantar reflex	1	2	3	4	5	NA
012023	Rooting reflex	1	2	3	4	5	NA

3rd edition 2004

Outcome Content References:

Berger, K. S. (2001). *The developing person through the life span* (5th ed.). New York: Worth Publishers.

Broome, M. E., & Rollins, J. A. (Eds.). (1999). *Core curriculum for the nursing care of children and their families.* Pitman, NJ: Anthony J. Jannetti.

Darrah, J., Redfern, L., Maguire, T. O., Beaulne, A. P., & Watt, J. (1998). Intra-individual stability of rate of gross motor development in full-term infants. *Early Human Development, 52*(2), 169-179.

Hockenberry, M. J., Wilson, D., Winkelstein, M. L., & Kline, N. E. (2003). *Wong's nursing care of infants and children* (7th ed.). St. Louis: Mosby.

Kimmel, S. R., Quinn, E. A., & Phelps, K. A. (1994). Assessing child development. *Primary Care, 21*(4), 673-692.

Piper, M. C., Pinnell, L. E., Darrah, J., Maguire, T., & Byrne, P. J. (1992). Construction and validation of the Alberta Infant Motor Scale (AIMS). *Canadian Journal of Public Health, 83*(Suppl. 2), S46-S50.

Trachtenbarg, D. E., & Golemon, T. B. (1998). Care of the premature infant, Part 1: Monitoring growth and development. *American Family Physician, 57*(9), 2123-2131.

Child Development: 2 Months—0100

Domain-Functional Health (I)

Class-Growth & Development (B)

Scale(s)-Never demonstrated to Consistently demonstrated (m)

Care Recipient:

Data Source:

C

Definition: Milestones of physical, cognitive, and psychosocial progression by 2 months of age

OUTCOME TARGET RATING: Maintain at_____   Increase to_____

Child Development: 2 Months Overall Rating	Never demonstrated 1	Rarely demonstrated 2	Sometimes demonstrated 3	Often demonstrated 4	Consistently demonstrated 5	
INDICATORS:						
010002 Crawl reflex disappearance	1	2	3	4	5	NA
010003 Lifts head, neck, and upper chest with support of forearms while in prone position	1	2	3	4	5	NA
010004 Shows some head control in upright position	1	2	3	4	5	NA
010005 Hands frequently open	1	2	3	4	5	NA
010006 Grasp reflex fading	1	2	3	4	5	NA
010007 Coos and vocalizes	1	2	3	4	5	NA
010008 Shows interest in auditory stimuli	1	2	3	4	5	NA
010009 Shows interest in visual stimuli	1	2	3	4	5	NA
010010 Smiles	1	2	3	4	5	NA
010011 Shows pleasure in interactions, especially with primary caregivers	1	2	3	4	5	NA

1st edition 1997; Revised 3rd edition 2004

Outcome Content References:

Berger, K. S. (2001). *The developing person through the life span* (5th ed.). New York: Worth Publishers.

Bricker, D. (Ed.). (2002). *Assessment, evaluation, and programming system for infants and children* (2nd ed.). Baltimore: Paul H. Brookes Publishing.

Cowen, P., & Van Hoozer, H. L. (under submission). *Building blocks for healthy tots.*

Darrah, J., Redfern, L., Maguire, T. O., Beaulne, A. P., & Watt, J. (1998). Intra-individual stability of rate of gross motor development in full-term infants. *Early Human Development*, 52(2), 169-179.

Green, M., & Palfrey, J. S. (Eds.). (2002). *Bright futures: Guidelines for health supervision of infants, children and adolescents.* Arlington, VA: National Center for Education in Maternal and Child Health.

Hockenberry, M. J., Wilson, D., Winkelstein, M. L., & Kline, N. E. (2003). *Wong's nursing care of infants and children* (7th ed.). St. Louis: Mosby.

Child Development: 4 Months—0101

Domain-Functional Health (I)

Class-Growth & Development (B)

Scale(s)-Never demonstrated to Consistently demonstrated (m)

Care Recipient:

Data Source:

C

Definition: Milestones of physical, cognitive, and psychosocial progression by 4 months of age

OUTCOME TARGET RATING: Maintain at_____   Increase to_____

Child Development: 4 Months Overall Rating	Never demonstrated 1	Rarely demonstrated 2	Sometimes demonstrated 3	Often demonstrated 4	Consistently demonstrated 5	
INDICATORS:						
010101 Holds head erect and raises body on hands while in prone position	1	2	3	4	5	NA
010102 Controls head well	1	2	3	4	5	NA
010103 Rolls over from prone to supine	1	2	3	4	5	NA
010104 Holds own hands	1	2	3	4	5	NA
010105 Grasps rattle	1	2	3	4	5	NA
010106 Reaches for objects	1	2	3	4	5	NA
010107 Bats at objects	1	2	3	4	5	NA
010108 Babbles and coos	1	2	3	4	5	NA
010109 Recognizes parents' voices	1	2	3	4	5	NA
010110 Recognizes parents' touch	1	2	3	4	5	NA
010111 Looks at and becomes excited by mobile	1	2	3	4	5	NA
010112 Smiles, laughs, and squeals	1	2	3	4	5	NA
010116 Exhibits a nocturnal sleep pattern	1	2	3	4	5	NA
010114 Comforts self	1	2	3	4	5	NA

1st edition 1997; Revised 3rd edition 2004; Revised 4th edition

Outcome Content References:

Berger, K. S. (2001). *The developing person through the life span* (5th ed.). New York: Worth Publishers.

Cowen, P., & Van Hoozer, H. L. (under submission). *Building blocks for healthy tots.*

Green, M., & Palfrey, J. S. (Eds.). (2002). *Bright futures: Guidelines for health supervision of infants, children and adolescents.* Arlington, VA: National Center for Education in Maternal and Child Health.

Hockenberry, M. J., Wilson, D., Winkelstein, M. L., & Kline, N. E. (2003). *Wong's nursing care of infants and children* (7th ed.). St. Louis: Mosby.

Child Development: 6 Months—0102

Domain-Functional Health (I)

Class-Growth & Development (B)

Scale(s)-Never demonstrated to Consistently demonstrated (m)

Care Recipient:

Data Source:

C

Definition: Milestones of physical, cognitive, and psychosocial progression by 6 months of age

OUTCOME TARGET RATING: Maintain at_____   Increase to_____

Child Development: 6 Months Overall Rating	Never demonstrated 1	Rarely demonstrated 2	Sometimes demonstrated 3	Often demonstrated 4	Consistently demonstrated 5	

INDICATORS:

010201	Supports head when pulled to sit	1	2	3	4	5	NA
010202	Rolls over	1	2	3	4	5	NA
010203	Sits with support	1	2	3	4	5	NA
010204	Stands when placed and bears weight	1	2	3	4	5	NA
010205	Grasps and mouths objects	1	2	3	4	5	NA
010206	Gestures (e.g., points, shakes head)	1	2	3	4	5	NA
010207	Starts to self-feed	1	2	3	4	5	NA
010208	Shows interest in toys	1	2	3	4	5	NA
010209	Transfers small objects from hand to hand	1	2	3	4	5	NA
010210	Vocalizes/sings syllables (dada, baba)	1	2	3	4	5	NA
010211	Babbles reciprocally	1	2	3	4	5	NA
010212	Smiles, laughs, squeals, imitates noise	1	2	3	4	5	NA
010213	Turns to sounds	1	2	3	4	5	NA
010214	Shows beginning signs of stranger anxiety	1	2	3	4	5	NA
010215	Comforts self	1	2	3	4	5	NA

1st edition 1997; Revised 3rd edition 2004

Outcome Content References:

Berger, K. S. (2001). *The developing person through the life span* (5th ed.). New York: Worth Publishers.

Bricker, D. (Ed). (2002). *Assessment, evaluation, and programming system for infants and children* (2nd ed.). Baltimore: Paul H. Brookes Publishing.

Cowen, P., & Van Hoozer, H. L. (under submission). *Building blocks for healthy tots.*

Green, M., & Palfrey, J. S. (Eds.). (2002). *Bright futures: Guidelines for health supervision of infants, children and adolescents.* Arlington, VA: National Center for Education in Maternal and Child Health.

Hockenberry, M. J., Wilson, D., Winkelstein, M. L., & Kline, N. E. (2003). *Wong's nursing care of infants and children* (7th ed.). St. Louis: Mosby.

Rossetti, L. M. (1990). *Infant-toddler assessment: An interdisciplinary approach.* Boston: Little, Brown & Company.

Child Development: 12 Months—0103

Domain-Functional Health (I)

Class-Growth & Development (B)

Scale(s)-Never demonstrated to Consistently demonstrated (m)

Care Recipient:

Data Source:

C

Definition: Milestones of physical, cognitive, and psychosocial progression by 12 months of age

OUTCOME TARGET RATING: Maintain at_____   Increase to_____

Child Development: 12 Months Overall Rating	Never demonstrated 1	Rarely demonstrated 2	Sometimes demonstrated 3	Often demonstrated 4	Consistently demonstrated 5	

INDICATORS:

010301	Pulls to stand	1	2	3	4	5	NA
010302	Cruises around furniture	1	2	3	4	5	NA
010303	Attempts to take steps alone	1	2	3	4	5	NA
010304	Precise pincer grasp	1	2	3	4	5	NA
010305	Points with index fingers	1	2	3	4	5	NA
010306	Bangs blocks together	1	2	3	4	5	NA
010307	Drinks from cup	1	2	3	4	5	NA
010308	Feeds self finger foods	1	2	3	4	5	NA
010309	Feeds self with spoon	1	2	3	4	5	NA
010310	Uses vocabulary of one to three words in addition to mama, dada	1	2	3	4	5	NA
010311	Imitates vocalizations	1	2	3	4	5	NA
010312	Looks for dropped or hidden object	1	2	3	4	5	NA
010313	Plays social games	1	2	3	4	5	NA
010314	Waves bye-bye	1	2	3	4	5	NA

1st edition 1997; Revised 3rd edition 2004

Outcome Content References:

Berger, K. S. (2001). *The developing person through the life span* (5th ed.). New York: Worth Publishers.

Bricker, D. (Ed.). (2002). *Assessment, evaluation, and programming system for infants and children* (2nd ed.). Baltimore: Paul H. Brookes Publishing.

Cowen, P., & Van Hoozer, H. L. (under submission). *Building blocks for healthy tots.*

Green, M., & Palfrey, J. S. (Eds.). (2002). *Bright futures: Guidelines for health supervision of infants, children and adolescents.* Arlington, VA: National Center for Education in Maternal and Child Health.

Hockenberry, M. J., Wilson, D., Winkelstein, M. L., & Kline, N. E. (2003). *Wong's nursing care of infants and children* (7th ed.). St. Louis: Mosby.

Rossetti, L. M. (1990). *Infant-toddler assessment: An interdisciplinary approach.* Boston: Little, Brown & Company.

Santos, D. C., Gabbard, C., & Goncalves, V. M. (2001). Motor development during the first year: A comparative study. *Journal of Genetic Psychology, 162*(2), 143-153.

Vaivre-Douret, L., & Burnod, Y. (2001). Development of a global motor rating scale for young children (0-4 years) including eye-hand grip coordination. *Child Care Health & Development, 27*(6), 515-534.

C

Child Development: 2 Years—0104

Domain-Functional Health (I)

Class-Growth & Development (B)

Scale(s)-Never demonstrated to Consistently demonstrated (m)

Care Recipient:

Data Source:

Definition: Milestones of physical, cognitive, and psychosocial progression by 2 years of age

OUTCOME TARGET RATING: Maintain at_____   Increase to_____

Child Development: 2 Years Overall Rating	Never demonstrated 1	Rarely demonstrated 2	Sometimes demonstrated 3	Often demonstrated 4	Consistently demonstrated 5	

INDICATORS:

010401	Walks quickly	1	2	3	4	5	NA
010402	Stoops well	1	2	3	4	5	NA
010403	Walks up and down stairs one step at a time	1	2	3	4	5	NA
010404	Walks backwards	1	2	3	4	5	NA
010405	Kicks a ball	1	2	3	4	5	NA
010406	Throws a ball	1	2	3	4	5	NA
010407	Makes circular and horizontal strokes with crayon	1	2	3	4	5	NA
010408	Stacks five to six blocks	1	2	3	4	5	NA
010409	Feeds self with spoon and fork	1	2	3	4	5	NA
010410	Follows two-step commands	1	2	3	4	5	NA
010411	Indicates wants verbally	1	2	3	4	5	NA
010412	Uses phrases of two to three words	1	2	3	4	5	NA
010413	Listens to story looking at pictures	1	2	3	4	5	NA
010414	Points to some body parts	1	2	3	4	5	NA
010415	Begins parallel play	1	2	3	4	5	NA
010416	Imitates adults	1	2	3	4	5	NA
010417	Interacts with adults in simple games	1	2	3	4	5	NA

1st edition 1997; Revised 3rd edition 2004

Outcome Content References:

Berger, K. S. (2001). *The developing person through the life span* (5th ed.). New York: Worth Publishers.

Bricker, D. (Ed.). (2002). *Assessment, evaluation, and programming system for infants and children* (2nd ed.). Baltimore: Paul H. Brookes Publishing.

Cowen, P., & Van Hoozer, H. L. (under submission). *Building blocks for healthy tots.*

Green, M., & Palfrey, J. S. (Eds.). (2002). *Bright futures: Guidelines for health supervision of infants, children and adolescents.* Arlington, VA: National Center for Education in Maternal and Child Health.

Hockenberry, M. J., Wilson, D., Winkelstein, M. L., & Kline, N. E. (2003). *Wong's nursing care of infants and children* (7th ed.). St. Louis: Mosby.

Provost, B., Crowe, T. K., & McClain, C. (2000). Concurrent validity of the Bayley Scales of Infant Development II Motor Scale and the Peabody Developmental Motor Scales in two-year-old children. *Physical & Occupational Therapy in Pediatrics, 20*(1), 5-18.

Rossetti, L. M. (1990). *Infant-toddler assessment: An interdisciplinary approach.* Boston: Little, Brown & Company.

Vaivre-Douret, L., & Burnod, Y. (2001). Development of a global motor rating scale for young children (0-4 years) including eye-hand grip coordination. *Child Care Health & Development, 27*(6), 515-534.

Child Development: 3 Years—0105

Domain-Functional Health (I)

Class-Growth & Development (B)

Scale(s)-Never demonstrated to Consistently demonstrated (m)

Care Recipient:

Data Source:

C

Definition: Milestones of physical, cognitive, and psychosocial progression by 3 years of age

OUTCOME TARGET RATING: Maintain at_____   Increase to_____

Child Development: 3 Years Overall Rating	Never demonstrated 1	Rarely demonstrated 2	Sometimes demonstrated 3	Often demonstrated 4	Consistently demonstrated 5	

INDICATORS:

010501	Balances on one foot	1	2	3	4	5	NA
010502	Pedals a riding toy	1	2	3	4	5	NA
010503	Dresses self	1	2	3	4	5	NA
010504	Manipulates writing/coloring instruments	1	2	3	4	5	NA
010505	Copies a circle	1	2	3	4	5	NA
010506	Copies a cross	1	2	3	4	5	NA
010507	Controls bowel in daytime	1	2	3	4	5	NA
010508	Controls bladder in daytime	1	2	3	4	5	NA
010509	Distinguishes gender differences	1	2	3	4	5	NA
010510	Gives own first name	1	2	3	4	5	NA
010511	Gives own age	1	2	3	4	5	NA
010512	Engages in magical thinking/fantasy	1	2	3	4	5	NA
010513	Plays interactive games with peers	1	2	3	4	5	NA
010514	Begins cooperative group play	1	2	3	4	5	NA
010515	Uses sentences of three or four words	1	2	3	4	5	NA
010516	Speech understood by strangers	1	2	3	4	5	NA

1st edition 1997; Revised 3rd edition 2004

Outcome Content References:

Berger, K. S. (2001). *The developing person through the life span* (5th ed.). New York: Worth Publishers.

Bricker, D. (Ed.). (2002). *Assessment, evaluation, and programming system for infants and children* (2nd ed.). Baltimore: Paul H. Brookes Publishing.

Cowen, P., & Van Hoozer, H. L. (under submission). *Building blocks for healthy tots.*

Green, M., & Palfrey, J. S. (Eds.). (2002). *Bright futures: Guidelines for health supervision of infants, children and adolescents.* Arlington, VA: National Center for Education in Maternal and Child Health.

Hemgren, E., & Persson, K. (1999). A model for combined assessment of motor performance and behaviour in 3-year-old children. *Upsala Journal of Medical Sciences, 104*(1), 49-85.

Hockenberry, M. J., Wilson, D., Winkelstein, M. L., & Kline, N. E. (2003). *Wong's nursing care of infants and children* (7th ed.). St. Louis: Mosby.

Vaivre-Douret, L., & Burnod, Y. (2001). Development of a global motor rating scale for young children (0-4 years) including eye-hand grip coordination. *Child Care Health & Development, 27*(6), 515-534.

Child Development: 4 Years—0106

Domain-Functional Health (I)

Class-Growth & Development (B)

Scale(s)-Never demonstrated to Consistently demonstrated (m)

Care Recipient:

Data Source:

C

Definition: Milestones of physical, cognitive, and psychosocial progression by 4 years of age

OUTCOME TARGET RATING: Maintain at_____   Increase to_____

Child Development: 4 Years Overall Rating	Never demonstrated 1	Rarely demonstrated 2	Sometimes demonstrated 3	Often demonstrated 4	Consistently demonstrated 5	
INDICATORS:						
010601 Walks, climbs, runs	1	2	3	4	5	NA
010602 Walks up and down stairs	1	2	3	4	5	NA
010603 Hops and jumps on one foot	1	2	3	4	5	NA
010604 Rides tricycle or bicycle with training wheels	1	2	3	4	5	NA
010605 Throws overhand ball	1	2	3	4	5	NA
010606 Builds tower of 10 blocks	1	2	3	4	5	NA
010607 Draws person with three parts	1	2	3	4	5	NA
010608 Gives first and last name	1	2	3	4	5	NA
010609 Uses sentences of four to five words, short paragraphs	1	2	3	4	5	NA
010610 Uses past tense in vocabulary	1	2	3	4	5	NA
010611 Describes a recent experience	1	2	3	4	5	NA
010612 Sings a song	1	2	3	4	5	NA
010613 Distinguishes fantasy from reality	1	2	3	4	5	NA
010614 Describes use of common items in home	1	2	3	4	5	NA
010616 Engages in creative play	1	2	3	4	5	NA

1st edition 1997; Revised 3rd edition 2004

Outcome Content References:

Berger, K. S. (2001). *The developing person through the life span* (5th ed.). New York: Worth Publishers.

Green, M., & Palfrey, J. S. (Eds.). (2002). *Bright futures: Guidelines for health supervision of infants, children and adolescents.* Arlington, VA: National Center for Education in Maternal and Child Health.

Hockenberry, M. J., Wilson, D., Winkelstein, M. L., & Kline, N. E. (2003). *Wong's nursing care of infants and children* (7th ed.). St. Louis: Mosby.

Vaivre-Douret, L., & Burnod, Y. (2001). Development of a global motor rating scale for young children (0-4 years) including eye-hand grip coordination. *Child Care Health & Development, 27*(6), 515-534.

Child Development: 5 Years—0107

Domain-Functional Health (I)

Class-Growth & Development (B)

Scale(s)-Never demonstrated to Consistently demonstrated (m)

Care Recipient:

Data Source:

C

Definition: Milestones of physical, cognitive, and psychosocial progression by 5 years of age

OUTCOME TARGET RATING: Maintain at_____   Increase to_____

Child Development: 5 Years Overall Rating	Never demonstrated 1	Rarely demonstrated 2	Sometimes demonstrated 3	Often demonstrated 4	Consistently demonstrated 5	
INDICATORS:						
010717 Walks	1	2	3	4	5	NA
010718 Climbs	1	2	3	4	5	NA
010719 Runs	1	2	3	4	5	NA
010702 Skips	1	2	3	4	5	NA
010703 Dresses self without assistance	1	2	3	4	5	NA
010704 Draws a person with head, body, arms, and legs	1	2	3	4	5	NA
010705 Copies a triangle or square	1	2	3	4	5	NA
010706 Counts using fingers	1	2	3	4	5	NA
010707 Recognizes most letters of alphabet	1	2	3	4	5	NA
010708 Prints some letters	1	2	3	4	5	NA
010709 Uses complete sentence of five words	1	2	3	4	5	NA
010710 Uses future tense in vocabulary	1	2	3	4	5	NA
010711 Speaks short paragraphs	1	2	3	4	5	NA
010712 Gives own address	1	2	3	4	5	NA
010713 Gives own phone number	1	2	3	4	5	NA
010714 Follows simple rules of interactive games with peers	1	2	3	4	5	NA
010716 Engages in creative play	1	2	3	4	5	NA

1st edition 1997; Revised 3rd edition 2004; Revised 4th edition

Outcome Content References:

Berger, K. S. (2001). *The developing person through the life span* (5th ed.). New York: Worth Publishers.

Boucher, B. H., Doescher, S. M., & Sugawara, A. I. (1993). Preschool children's motor development and self-concept. *Perceptual & Motor Skills, 76*(1), 11-17.

Green, M., & Palfrey, J. S. (Eds.). (2002). *Bright futures: Guidelines for health supervision of infants, children and adolescents.* Arlington, VA: National Center for Education in Maternal and Child Health.

Hockenberry, M. J., Wilson, D., Winkelstein, M. L., & Kline, N. E. (2003). *Wong's nursing care of infants and children* (7th ed.). St. Louis: Mosby.

Child Development: Middle Childhood—0108

Domain-Functional Health (I)

Class-Growth & Development (B)

Scale(s)-Never demonstrated to Consistently demonstrated (m)

Care Recipient:

Data Source:

C

Definition: Milestones of physical, cognitive, and psychosocial progression from 6 years through 11 years of age

OUTCOME TARGET RATING: Maintain at_____   Increase to_____

Child Development: Middle Childhood Overall Rating	Never demonstrated 1	Rarely demonstrated 2	Sometimes demonstrated 3	Often demonstrated 4	Consistently demonstrated 5	
INDICATORS:						
010801 Practices good health habits	1	2	3	4	5	NA
010802 Plays in groups	1	2	3	4	5	NA
010803 Develops close friendships	1	2	3	4	5	NA
010804 Identifies with same-sex peer group	1	2	3	4	5	NA
010805 Assumes responsibility for selected household tasks	1	2	3	4	5	NA
010806 Follows through with commitments to extracurricular activities	1	2	3	4	5	NA
010807 Expresses feelings constructively	1	2	3	4	5	NA
010808 Displays self-confidence	1	2	3	4	5	NA
010809 Understands right and wrong	1	2	3	4	5	NA
010810 Follows safety rules	1	2	3	4	5	NA
010811 Expresses increasingly complex thoughts	1	2	3	4	5	NA
010812 Shows creativity	1	2	3	4	5	NA
010813 Comprehends increasingly complex ideas	1	2	3	4	5	NA
010814 Assumes responsibility for homework	1	2	3	4	5	NA
010815 Performs in school to level of ability	1	2	3	4	5	NA

1st edition 1997; Revised 3rd edition 2004

Outcome Content References:

Berger, K. S. (2001). *The developing person through the life span* (5th ed.). New York: Worth Publishers.

Green, M., & Palfrey, J. S. (Eds.). (2002). *Bright futures: Guidelines for health supervision of infants, children and adolescents.* Arlington, VA: National Center for Education in Maternal and Child Health.

Hockenberry, M. J., Wilson, D., Winkelstein, M. L., & Kline, N. E. (2003). *Wong's nursing care of infants and children* (7th ed.). St. Louis: Mosby.

Child Development: Adolescence—0109

Domain-Functional Health (I)

Class-Growth & Development (B)

Scale(s)-Never demonstrated to Consistently demonstrated (m)

Care Recipient:

Data Source:

Definition: Milestones of physical, cognitive, and psychosocial progression from 12 years through 17 years of age

OUTCOME TARGET RATING: Maintain at_____   Increase to_____

Child Development: Adolescence Overall Rating	Never demonstrated 1	Rarely demonstrated 2	Sometimes demonstrated 3	Often demonstrated 4	Consistently demonstrated 5	

INDICATORS:

010901	Practices good health habits	1	2	3	4	5	NA
010904	Uses effective social interaction skills	1	2	3	4	5	NA
010905	Uses conflict resolution strategies	1	2	3	4	5	NA
010920	Vents negative feelings in a non-destructive manner	1	2	3	4	5	NA
010906	Maintains good peer relationships with same gender	1	2	3	4	5	NA
010907	Maintains good peer relationships with opposite gender	1	2	3	4	5	NA
010921	Respects others	1	2	3	4	5	NA
010911	Uses effective coping strategies	1	2	3	4	5	NA
010922	Discusses feelings of distress with supportive adult	1	2	3	4	5	NA
010912	Displays increasing levels of autonomy	1	2	3	4	5	NA
010913	Describes personal value system	1	2	3	4	5	NA
010914	Uses formal operational thinking	1	2	3	4	5	NA
010915	Sets academic goals	1	2	3	4	5	NA
010916	Performs in school to level of ability	1	2	3	4	5	NA
010923	Participates in extracurricular school activities	1	2	3	4	5	NA
010924	Performs in work to level of ability	1	2	3	4	5	NA
010925	Identifies occupational goals	1	2	3	4	5	NA
010926	Observes rules	1	2	3	4	5	NA
010927	Obeys laws	1	2	3	4	5	NA
010908	Shows capacity for intimacy	1	2	3	4	5	NA
010902	Describes sexual development	1	2	3	4	5	NA

Continued

		Never demonstrated	Rarely demonstrated	Sometimes demonstrated	Often demonstrated	Consistently demonstrated	
010903	Expresses comfort with own sexual identity	1	2	3	4	5	NA
010928	Postpones sexual activity	1	2	3	4	5	NA
010929	Avoids high-risk sexual activity	1	2	3	4	5	NA
010910	Avoids alcohol use	1	2	3	4	5	NA
010918	Avoids tobacco use	1	2	3	4	5	NA
010919	Avoids recreational drug use	1	2	3	4	5	NA

1st edition 1997; Revised 3rd edition 2004; Revised 4th edition

OUTCOME CONTENT REFERENCES:

Berger, K. S. (2001). *The developing person through the life span* (5th ed.). New York: Worth Publishers.

Hockenberry, M. J., Wilson, D., Winkelstein, M. L., & Kline, N. E. (2003). *Wong's nursing care of infants and children* (7th ed.). St. Louis: Mosby.

Green, M., & Palfrey, J. S. (Eds.). (2002). *Bright futures: Guidelines for health supervision of infants, children and adolescents.* Arlington, VA: National Center for Education in Maternal and Child Health.

Krueger, D. W. (2001). Body self. Development, psychopathologies, and psychoanalytic significance. *Psychoanalytic Study of the Child, 56,* 238-259.

Mitchell, J. J. (1996). *Adolescent vulnerability: A sympathetic look at the frailties and limitations of youth.* Calgary, Alberta, Canada: Detselig Enterprises Ltd.

Circulation Status—0401

Domain-Physiologic Health (II)

Class-Cardiopulmonary (E)

Scale(s)-Severe deviation from normal range to No deviation from normal range (b) and Severe to None (n)

Care Recipient:

Data Source:

C

Definition: Unobstructed, unidirectional blood flow at an appropriate pressure through large vessels of the systemic and pulmonary circuits

OUTCOME TARGET RATING: Maintain at_____   Increase to_____

Circulation Status Overall Rating	Severe deviation from normal range 1	Substantial deviation from normal range 2	Moderate deviation from normal range 3	Mild deviation from normal range 4	No deviation from normal range 5	
INDICATORS:						
040101 Systolic blood pressure	1	2	3	4	5	NA
040102 Diastolic blood pressure	1	2	3	4	5	NA
040103 Pulse pressure	1	2	3	4	5	NA
040104 Mean blood pressure	1	2	3	4	5	NA
040105 Central venous pressure	1	2	3	4	5	NA
040106 Pulmonary wedge pressure	1	2	3	4	5	NA
040141 Right carotid pulse strength	1	2	3	4	5	NA
040142 Left carotid pulse strength	1	2	3	4	5	NA
040143 Right brachial pulse strength	1	2	3	4	5	NA
040144 Left brachial pulse strength	1	2	3	4	5	NA
040145 Right radial pulse strength	1	2	3	4	5	NA
040146 Left radial pulse strength	1	2	3	4	5	NA
040147 Right femoral pulse strength	1	2	3	4	5	NA
040148 Left femoral pulse strength	1	2	3	4	5	NA
040149 Right pedal pulse strength	1	2	3	4	5	NA
040150 Left pedal pulse strength	1	2	3	4	5	NA
040135 PaO_2 (Partial pressure of oxygen in arterial blood)	1	2	3	4	5	NA
040136 $PaCO_2$ (Partial pressure of carbon dioxide in arterial blood)	1	2	3	4	5	NA
040137 Oxygen saturation	1	2	3	4	5	NA
040112 Arterial-venous oxygen difference	1	2	3	4	5	NA
040140 Urine output	1	2	3	4	5	NA
040151 Capillary refill	1	2	3	4	5	NA

	Severe	Substantial	Moderate	Mild	None	
040107 Orthostatic hypotension	1	2	3	4	5	NA
040113 Adventitious breath sounds	1	2	3	4	5	NA

Continued

C

	Severe	Substantial	Moderate	Mild	None	
040118 Large vessel bruits	1	2	3	4	5	NA
040119 Neck vein distention	1	2	3	4	5	NA
040120 Peripheral edema	1	2	3	4	5	NA
040121 Ascites	1	2	3	4	5	NA
040123 Fatigue	1	2	3	4	5	NA
040152 Weight gain	1	2	3	4	5	NA
040153 Impaired cognition	1	2	3	4	5	NA
040154 Pallor	1	2	3	4	5	NA
040155 Dependent rubor	1	2	3	4	5	NA
040156 Intermittent claudication	1	2	3	4	5	NA
040157 Decreased skin temperature	1	2	3	4	5	NA
040158 Paresthesia	1	2	3	4	5	NA
040159 Syncope	1	2	3	4	5	NA
040160 Pitting edema	1	2	3	4	5	NA
040161 Lower extremity ulcers	1	2	3	4	5	NA
040162 Numbness	1	2	3	4	5	NA

1st edition 1997; Revised 3rd edition 2004; Revised 4th edition

Outcome Content References:

Andreoli, K. G., Zipes, D. P., Wallace, A. G., Kinney, M. R., & Fowkes, V. K. (Eds.). (1996). *Comprehensive cardiac care* (8th ed.). St. Louis: Mosby.

Cullen, L. (1992). Interventions related to circulatory care. *Nursing Clinics of North America, 27*(2), 445-477.

Dougherty, C. M. (2001). Decreased cardiac output. In M. Maas, K. Buckwalter, M. Hardy, T. Tripp-Reimer, M. Titler, & J. Specht (Eds.), *Nursing care of older adults: Diagnoses, outcomes & interventions* (pp. 285-297). St. Louis: Mosby.

Fahey, V. A. (Ed.). (1999). *Vascular nursing* (3rd ed.). Philadelphia: W.B. Saunders.

Murphy, T. G., & Bennett, E. J. (1992). Low-tech, high-touch perfusion assessment. *American Journal of Nursing, 92*(5), 36-46.

Reischman, R. R. (2002). Critical care cardiovascular nurse expert and novice diagnostic cue utilization. *Journal of Advanced Nursing, 39*(1), 24-34.

Sheehy, S. B. (1999). *Manual of emergency care* (5th ed.). St. Louis: Mosby.

Smeltzer, S. C., & Bare, B. G. (Eds.). (2003). *Brunner and Suddarth's textbook of medical-surgical nursing* (10th ed.). Philadelphia: Lippincott Williams & Wilkins.

Smith, S. L. (1990). Postoperative perfusion deficits. *Critical Care Nursing Clinics of North America, 2*(4), 567-578.

Client Satisfaction—3014

Domain-Perceived Health (V)

Class-Satisfaction with Care (e)

Scale(s)-Not at all satisfied to Completely satisfied (s)

Care Recipient:

Data Source:

C

Definition: Extent of positive perception of care provided by nursing staff

OUTCOME TARGET RATING: Maintain at_____   Increase to_____

Client Satisfaction Overall Rating	Not at all satisfied 1	Somewhat satisfied 2	Moderately satisfied 3	Very satisfied 4	Completely satisfied 5	
INDICATORS:						
301401 Access to nursing staff	1	2	3	4	5	NA
301402 Access to supplies and equipment needed for care	1	2	3	4	5	NA
301403 Knowledge and expertise of nursing staff	1	2	3	4	5	NA
301404 Competence of nursing staff to perform procedures	1	2	3	4	5	NA
301405 Protection of legal rights by nursing staff	1	2	3	4	5	NA
301406 Protection of human rights by nursing staff	1	2	3	4	5	NA
301407 Concern for the client by nursing staff	1	2	3	4	5	NA
301408 Concern for the family by nursing staff	1	2	3	4	5	NA
301409 Questions answered completely	1	2	3	4	5	NA
301410 Instruction to improve understanding of illness	1	2	3	4	5	NA
301411 Instruction to improve participation in care	1	2	3	4	5	NA
301412 Integration of cultural beliefs into nursing care	1	2	3	4	5	NA
301413 Integration of values into nursing care	1	2	3	4	5	NA
301414 Assistance to achieve mobility	1	2	3	4	5	NA
301415 Assistance to achieve self-care	1	2	3	4	5	NA
301416 Assistance to cope with emotional concerns	1	2	3	4	5	NA
301417 Assistance to address spiritual needs	1	2	3	4	5	NA
301418 Relief of symptoms of illness	1	2	3	4	5	NA
301419 Care to control pain	1	2	3	4	5	NA
301420 Care to prevent harm or injury	1	2	3	4	5	NA
301421 Care to maintain body functions	1	2	3	4	5	NA

Continued

C

		Not at all satisfied	Somewhat satisfied	Moderately satisfied	Very satisfied	Completely satisfied	
301422	Care to maintain cleanliness	1	2	3	4	5	NA
301423	Cleanliness of care environment	1	2	3	4	5	NA
301424	Coordination of care as the client moves from one care setting to another	1	2	3	4	5	NA
301425	Client/family included in discharge planning	1	2	3	4	5	NA

Outcome Content References:

Abdellah, F. G., & Levine, E. (1957). Developing a measure of patient and personnel satisfaction with nursing care. *Nursing Research, 5*, 100-108.

Abramowitz, S., Cote, A. A., & Berry, E. (1987). Analyzing patient satisfaction: A multianalytic approach. *Quality Review Bulletin, 13*(4), 122-130.

Davis, B. A., & Bush, H. A. (1995). Developing effective measurement tools: A case study of the consumer emergency care satisfaction scale. *Journal of Nursing Care Quality, 9*(2), 26-35.

Davis, J., Davis, M., & Riggs, H. (1999). Taking the measure of patient satisfaction. *Nursing Times, 95*(24), 52-53.

Eriksen, L. (1988). Measuring patient satisfaction with nursing care: A magnitude estimation approach. In C. F. Waltz & O. W. Stickland (Eds.), *Measurement of nursing outcomes* (Vol. 1, pp. 523-527). New York: Springer.

Gesell, S. B., & Gregory, N. (2003). Identifying priority actions for improving patient satisfaction with outpatient cancer care. *Journal of Nursing Care Quality, 19*(3), 226-233.

Hegedus, K. S. (1999). Providers' and consumers' perspective of nurses' caring behaviours. *Journal of Advanced Nursing, 30*(5), 1090-1096.

Hinshaw, A. S., & Atwood, J. R. (1982). A patient satisfaction instrument: Precision by replication. *Nursing Research, 31*(3), 170-175.

LaMonica, E. L., Oberst, M. T., Madea, A. R., & Wolf, R. M. (1986). Development of a patient satisfaction scale. *Research in Nursing and Health, 9*(1), 43-50.

Larrabee, J. H., Ostrow, C. L., Withrow, M. L., Janney, M. A., Hobbs, G. R., Jr. & Burant, C. (2004). Predictors of patient satisfaction with inpatient hospital nursing care. *Research in Nursing & Health, 27*, 254-268.

Laschinger, H. S., Hall, L. M., Pedersen, C., & Almost, J. (2004). A psychometric analysis of the patient satisfaction with nursing care quality questionnaire: An actionable approach to measuring patient satisfaction. *Journal of Nursing Care Quality, 20*(3), 220-230.

Mark, B. A., & Wan, T. T. H. (2005). Testing measurement equivalence in a patient satisfaction instrument. *Western Journal of Nursing Research, 27*(6), 772-787.

Marsh, G. W. (1999). Measuring patient satisfaction outcomes across provider disciplines. *Journal of Nursing Measurement, 7*(1), 47-62.

Nussbaum, G. B. (2003). Spirituality in critical care: Patient comfort and satisfaction. *Critical Care Nursing Quarterly, 26*(3), 214-220.

Risser, N. L. (1975). Development of an instrument to measure patient satisfaction with nurses and nursing care in primary care settings. *Nursing Research, 24*(1), 45-52.

Ryden, M. B., Gross, C. R., Savik, K., Snyder, M., Oh, H. L., Jang, Y., Wang, J., & Krichbaum, K. E. (2000). Development of a measure of resident satisfaction with the nursing home. *Research in Nursing & Health, 23*(3), 237-245.

Walsh, M., & Walsh, A. (1999). Measuring patient satisfaction with nursing care: Experience of using the Newcastle Satisfaction with Nursing Scale. *Journal of Advanced Nursing, 29*(2), 307-315.

Ware, J. E., Davies-Avery, A., & Stewart, A. I. (1978). The measurement and meaning of patient satisfaction. *Health & Medical Care Services Review, 1*(1), 1, 3-14.

Wolf, L. R., Giardino, E. R., Osborne, P. A., & Ambrose, M. S. (1994). Dimensions of nurse caring. *Image—The Journal of Nursing Scholarship, 26*(2), 107-111.

Client Satisfaction: Access to Care Resources—3000

Domain-Perceived Health (V)

Class-Satisfaction with Care (e)

Scale(s)-Not at all satisfied to Completely satisfied (s)

Care Recipient:

Data Source:

C

Definition: Extent of positive perception of access to nursing staff, supplies, and equipment needed for care

OUTCOME TARGET RATING: Maintain at_____   Increase to_____

Client Satisfaction: Access to Care Resources Overall Rating	Not at all satisfied 1	Somewhat satisfied 2	Moderately satisfied 3	Very satisfied 4	Completely satisfied 5	
INDICATORS:						
300001 Availability of registered nurses	1	2	3	4	5	NA
300002 Availability of assistive staff	1	2	3	4	5	NA
300003 Availability of supplies needed for care	1	2	3	4	5	NA
300004 Availability of equipment needed for care	1	2	3	4	5	NA
300005 Informed of registered nurse and assistive staff responsible for care	1	2	3	4	5	NA
300006 Access to registered nurse responsible for care	1	2	3	4	5	NA
300007 Assistance with access to health providers	1	2	3	4	5	NA
300008 Assistance with contacting physician	1	2	3	4	5	NA
300009 Coordination of health care resources	1	2	3	4	5	NA
300010 Coordination of health providers	1	2	3	4	5	NA
300011 Wait times for getting an appointment	1	2	3	4	5	NA
300012 Wait times to be seen at appointment	1	2	3	4	5	NA
300013 Access to support group	1	2	3	4	5	NA

3rd edition 2004

Outcome Content References:

Larrabee, J. H., Ostrow, C. L., Withrow, M. L., Janney, M. A., Hobbs, G. R., Jr. & Burant, C. (2004). Predictors of patient satisfaction with inpatient hospital nursing care. *Research in Nursing & Health, 27,* 254-268.

Laschinger, H. S., Hall, L. M., Pedersen, C., & Almost, J. (2004). A psychometric analysis of the patient satisfaction with nursing care quality questionnaire: An actionable approach to measuring patient satisfaction. *Journal of Nursing Care Quality, 20*(3), 220-230.

Linder-Pelz, S. (1982). Toward a theory of patient satisfaction. *Social Science & Medicine, 16*(5), 577-582.

Mark, B. A., & Wan, T. T. H. (2005). Testing measurement equivalence in a patient satisfaction instrument. *Western Journal of Nursing Research, 27*(6), 772-787.

Marsh, G. W. (1999). Measuring patient satisfaction outcomes across provider disciplines. *Journal of Nursing Measurement, 7*(1), 47-62.

Ware, J. E., Davies-Avery, A., & Stewart, A. I. (1978). The measurement and meaning of patient satisfaction. *Health & Medical Care Services Review, 1*(1), 1, 3-14.

Client Satisfaction: Caring—3001

Domain-Perceived Health (V)

Class-Satisfaction with Care (e)

Scale(s)-Not at all satisfied to Completely satisfied (s)

Care Recipient:

Data Source:

C

Definition: Extent of positive perception of nursing staff's concern for the client

OUTCOME TARGET RATING: Maintain at_____   Increase to_____

Client Satisfaction: Caring Overall Rating	Not at all satisfied 1	Somewhat satisfied 2	Moderately satisfied 3	Very satisfied 4	Completely satisfied 5	

INDICATORS:

300101	Courtesy shown by staff	1	2	3	4	5	NA
300102	Compassion shown by staff	1	2	3	4	5	NA
300103	Kindness shown by staff	1	2	3	4	5	NA
300104	Respect shown by staff	1	2	3	4	5	NA
300105	Consideration for feelings	1	2	3	4	5	NA
300106	Consideration for opinions	1	2	3	4	5	NA
300107	Concern shown for individual needs	1	2	3	4	5	NA
300108	Relationship with nursing staff	1	2	3	4	5	NA
300109	Frequency with which checked on by staff	1	2	3	4	5	NA
300110	Promptness answering call light	1	2	3	4	5	NA
300111	Promptness responding to inquires	1	2	3	4	5	NA
300123	Follow through with client request	1	2	3	4	5	NA
300112	Emotional support provided	1	2	3	4	5	NA
300124	Assistance to address spiritual needs	1	2	3	4	5	NA
300113	Appropriate use of touch	1	2	3	4	5	NA
300114	Orientation to room, equipment, and routines	1	2	3	4	5	NA
300115	Visiting arrangements	1	2	3	4	5	NA
300116	Family and friends made welcome	1	2	3	4	5	NA
300117	Assistance with letter writing	1	2	3	4	5	NA
300118	Leisure activities provided	1	2	3	4	5	NA
300119	Information provided about options of care	1	2	3	4	5	NA
300120	Consideration for cost of care	1	2	3	4	5	NA
300121	Supplies and equipment not wasted	1	2	3	4	5	NA

C

3rd edition 2004; Revised 4th edition

Outcome Content References:

Abdellah, F. G., & Levine, E. (1957). Developing a measure of patient and personnel satisfaction with nursing care. *Nursing Research, 5,* 100-108.

Davis, B. A., & Bush, H. A. (1995). Developing effective measurement tools: A case study of the consumer emergency care satisfaction scale. *Journal of Nursing Care Quality, 9*(2), 26-35.

Davis, J., Davis, M., & Riggs, H. (1999). Taking the measure of patient satisfaction. *Nursing Times, 95*(24), 52-53.

Deitrick, L., Bokovoy, J., Stern, G., & Panik, A. (2006). Dance of the call bells: Using ethnography to evaluate patient satisfaction with quality of care. *Journal of Nursing Care Quality 21*(4), 316-324.

Eriksen, L. (1988). Measuring patient satisfaction with nursing care: A magnitude estimation approach. In C. F. Waltz & O. W. Stickland (Eds.), *Measurement of nursing outcomes* (Vol. 1, pp. 523-527). New York: Springer.

Hegedus, K. S. (1999). Providers' and consumers' perspective of nurses' caring behaviours. *Journal of Advanced Nursing, 30*(5), 1090-1096.

Hinshaw, A. S., & Atwood, J. R. (1982). A patient satisfaction instrument: Precision by replication. *Nursing Research, 31*(3), 170-175.

LaMonica, E. L., Oberst, M. T., Madea, A. R., & Wolf, R. M. (1986). Development of a patient satisfaction scale. *Research in Nursing & Health, 9*(1), 43-50.

Larrabee, J. H., Ostrow, C. L., Withrow, M. L., Janney, M. A., Hobbs, G. R., Jr. & Burant, C. (2004). Predictors of patient satisfaction with inpatient hospital nursing care. *Research in Nursing & Health, 27,* 254-268.

Laschinger, H. S., Hall, L. M., Pedersen, C., & Almost, J. (2004). A psychometric analysis of the patient satisfaction with nursing care quality questionnaire: An actionable approach to measuring patient satisfaction. *Journal of Nursing Care Quality, 20*(3), 220-230.

Mark, B. A., & Wan, T. T. H. (2005). Testing measurement equivalence in a patient satisfaction instrument. *Western Journal of Nursing Research, 27*(6), 772-787.

Marsh, G. W. (1999). Measuring patient satisfaction outcomes across provider disciplines. *Journal of Nursing Measurement, 7*(1), 47-62.

Nussbaum, G. B. (2003). Spirituality in critical care: Patient comfort and satisfaction. *Critical Care Nursing Quarterly, 26*(3), 214-220.

Risser, N. L. (1975). Development of an instrument to measure patient satisfaction with nurses and nursing care in primary care settings. *Nursing Research, 24*(1), 45-52.

Ryden, M. B., Gross, C. R., Savik, K., Snyder, M., Oh, H. L., Jang, Y., Wang, J., & Krichbaum, K. E. (2000). Development of a measure of resident satisfaction with the nursing home. *Research in Nursing & Health, 23*(3), 237-245.

Walsh, M., & Walsh, A. (1999). Measuring patient satisfaction with nursing care: Experience of using the Newcastle Satisfaction with Nursing Scale. *Journal of Advanced Nursing, 29*(2), 307-315.

Ware, J. E., Davies-Avery, A., & Stewart, A. I. (1978). The measurement and meaning of patient satisfaction. *Health & Medical Care Services Review, 1*(1), 1, 3-14.

Wolf, L. R., Giardino, E. R., Osborne, P. A., & Ambrose, M. S. (1994). Dimensions of nurse caring. *Image—The Journal of Nursing Scholarship, 26*(2), 107-111.

C

Client Satisfaction: Case Management—3015

Domain-Perceived Health (V)

Class-Satisfaction with Care (e)

Scale(s)-Not at all satisfied to Completely satisfied (s)

Care Recipient:

Data Source:

Definition: Extent of positive perception of case management services

OUTCOME TARGET RATING: Maintain at_____   Increase to_____

Client Satisfaction: Case Management Overall Rating	Not at all satisfied 1	Somewhat satisfied 2	Moderately satisfied 3	Very satisfied 4	Completely satisfied 5	
INDICATORS:						
301501 Availability of case manager	1	2	3	4	5	NA
301502 Availability of supplies needed for care	1	2	3	4	5	NA
301503 Availability of equipment needed for care	1	2	3	4	5	NA
301504 Assistance with contacting physician	1	2	3	4	5	NA
301505 Assistance with gaining access to health providers	1	2	3	4	5	NA
301506 Referrals made to appropriate health providers	1	2	3	4	5	NA
301507 Coordination of health care resources	1	2	3	4	5	NA
301508 Coordination of health providers	1	2	3	4	5	NA
301509 Coordination of care	1	2	3	4	5	NA
301510 Wait times for getting an appointment	1	2	3	4	5	NA
301511 Information provided about support groups	1	2	3	4	5	NA
301512 Consideration for feelings	1	2	3	4	5	NA
301513 Consideration of opinions	1	2	3	4	5	NA
301514 Concern shown for individual needs	1	2	3	4	5	NA
301515 Information provided about options for care	1	2	3	4	5	NA
301516 Information provided about cost of care	1	2	3	4	5	NA
301517 Consideration of cost of care	1	2	3	4	5	NA
301518 Avoidance of unnecessary treatments and procedures	1	2	3	4	5	NA
301519 Referral regarding costs and finances	1	2	3	4	5	NA
301520 Consistent information provided	1	2	3	4	5	NA
301521 Personal values considered	1	2	3	4	5	NA
301522 Personal preferences considered in care plan	1	2	3	4	5	NA

		Not at all satisfied	Somewhat satisfied	Moderately satisfied	Very satisfied	Completely satisfied	
301523	Respect for cultural values	1	2	3	4	5	NA
301524	Respect for religious beliefs	1	2	3	4	5	NA
301525	Health providers work as a team	1	2	3	4	5	NA
301526	Safety issues are addressed	1	2	3	4	5	NA
301527	Family included in providing care	1	2	3	4	5	NA
301528	Confidentiality of client information maintained	1	2	3	4	5	NA
301529	Explanation provided in understandable terms	1	2	3	4	5	NA
301530	Quality of instructional material provided	1	2	3	4	5	NA
301531	Included in decisions about care	1	2	3	4	5	NA
301532	Support for finding own solutions to problems	1	2	3	4	5	NA
301533	Information provided about legal rights	1	2	3	4	5	NA
301534	Information provided about course of illness	1	2	3	4	5	NA

Outcome Content References:

Buck, P. W., & Alexander, L. B. (2005). Neglected voices: Consumers with serious mental illness speak about intensive case management. *Administration and Policy in Mental Health Services Research, 33*(4), 470-481.

Coffey, D. S. (2003). Connection and autonomy in the case management relationship. *Psychiatric Rehabilitation Journal, 26*(4), 404-412.

Finch, G. L., & Linderberg, J. (1999). Improving patient satisfaction through unit-based team case management. *Continuum (Chicago), 19*(2), 12-16.

Hadjistavropoulos, H. D., Sagan, M., Bierlein, C., & Lawson, K. (2003). Development of a case management quality questionnaire. *Case Management Journal, 4*(1), 8-17.

Huber, D. L. (Ed.). (2005). *Disease management: A guide for case managers.* St. Louis: Saunders.

Kopelman, T., Huber, D. L., Kopelman, B. C., Sarrazin, M. V., & Hall, J. A. (2006). Client satisfaction with rural substance abuse case management services. *Care Management Journal, 7*(4), 179-190.

Mark, B. A., & Wan, T. T. H. (2005). Testing measurement equivalence in a patient satisfaction instrument. *Western Journal of Nursing Research, 27*(6), 772-787.

Rossi, P. (1999). *Case management in health care: A practical guide.* Philadelphia: Saunders.

C

Client Satisfaction: Communication—3002

Domain-Perceived Health (V)

Class-Satisfaction with Care (e)

Scale(s)-Not at all satisfied to Completely satisfied (s)

Care Recipient:

Data Source:

Definition: Extent of positive perception of information exchanged between client and nursing staff

OUTCOME TARGET RATING: Maintain at_____   Increase to_____

Client Satisfaction: Communication Overall Rating	Not at all satisfied 1	Somewhat satisfied 2	Moderately satisfied 3	Very satisfied 4	Completely satisfied 5	
INDICATORS:						
300201 Staff introduce self	1	2	3	4	5	NA
300202 Use of client's preferred name	1	2	3	4	5	NA
300203 Staff speak clearly	1	2	3	4	5	NA
300204 Staff listen to client	1	2	3	4	5	NA
300205 Staff encourage questions	1	2	3	4	5	NA
300206 Staff repeat information as often as needed	1	2	3	4	5	NA
300207 Staff take time when communicating	1	2	3	4	5	NA
300208 Staff present information in understandable way	1	2	3	4	5	NA
300209 Staff make sure information understood	1	2	3	4	5	NA
300210 Staff use non-judgmental communication	1	2	3	4	5	NA
300211 Questions answered clearly	1	2	3	4	5	NA
300212 Questions answered completely	1	2	3	4	5	NA
300213 Questions answered in a reasonable length of time	1	2	3	4	5	NA
300214 Consistent information given by nursing staff	1	2	3	4	5	NA
300215 Personal values considered in communication	1	2	3	4	5	NA
300216 Personal preferences considered	1	2	3	4	5	NA
300217 Discrepancies in information are resolved in a timely manner	1	2	3	4	5	NA
300218 Alternative communication methods used as needed	1	2	3	4	5	NA

3rd edition 2004

Outcome Content References:

Davis, J., Davis, M., & Riggs, H. (1999). Taking the measure of patient satisfaction. *Nursing Times, 95*(24), 52-53.

Deitrick, L., Bokovoy, J., Stern, G., & Panik, A. (2006). Dance of the call bells: Using ethnography to evaluate patient satisfaction with quality of care. *Journal of Nursing Care Quality 21*(4), 316-324.

Hegedus, K. S. (1999). Providers' and consumers' perspective of nurses' caring behaviours. *Journal of Advanced Nursing, 30*(5), 1090-1096.

Hinshaw, A. S., & Atwood, J. R. (1982). A patient satisfaction instrument: Precision by replication. *Nursing Research, 31*(3), 170-175.

LaMonica, E. L., Oberst, M. T., Madea, A. R., & Wolf, R. M. (1986). Development of a patient satisfaction scale. *Research in Nursing & Health, 9*(1), 43-50.

Larrabee, J. H., Ostrow, C. L., Withrow, M. L., Janney, M. A., Hobbs, G. R., Jr., & Burant, C. (2004). Predictors of patient satisfaction with inpatient hospital nursing care. *Research in Nursing & Health, 27*, 254-268.

Laschinger, H. S., Hall, L. M., Pedersen, C., & Almost, J. (2004). A psychometric analysis of the patient satisfaction with nursing care quality questionnaire: An actionable approach to measuring patient satisfaction. *Journal of Nursing Care Quality, 20*(3), 220-230.

Lynn, M. R., & McMillen, B. J. (1999). Do nurses know what patients think is important in nursing care? *Journal of Nursing Care Quality, 13*(5), 65-74.

Mark, B. A., & Wan, T. T. H. (2005). Testing measurement equivalence in a patient satisfaction instrument. *Western Journal of Nursing Research, 27*(6), 772-787.

McCabe, C. (2004). Nurse-patient communication: An exploration of patients' experiences. *Issues in Clinical Nursing, 13*, 41-49.

McGilton, K., Boscart, V., Irwin-Robinson, H., & Spanjevic, L. (2006). Communication enhancement: Nurse and patient satisfaction outcomes in a complex continuing care facility. *Journal of Advanced Nursing, 54*(1), 35-44

Risser, N. L. (1975). Development of an instrument to measure patient satisfaction with nurses and nursing care in primary care settings. *Nursing Research, 24*(1), 45-52.

Walsh, M., & Walsh, A. (1999). Measuring patient satisfaction with nursing care: Experience of using the Newcastle Satisfaction with Nursing Scale. *Journal of Advanced Nursing, 29*(2), 307-315.

Ware, J. E., Davies-Avery, A., & Stewart, A. I. (1978). The measurement and meaning of patient satisfaction. *Health & Medical Care Services Review, 1*(1), 1, 3-14.

Wolf, L. R., Giardino, E. R., Osborne, P. A., & Ambrose, M. S. (1994). Dimensions of nurse caring. *Image—The Journal of Nursing Scholarship, 26*(2), 107-111.

Yellen, E. (2003). The influence of nurse-sensitive variables on patient satisfaction. *AORN Journal, 78*, 783-793.

Yellen, E., Davis, G. C., & Ricard, R. (2002). The measurement of patient satisfaction. *Journal of Nursing Care Quality, 16*(4), 23-29.

C

Client Satisfaction: Continuity of Care—3003

Domain-Perceived Health (V)

Class-Satisfaction with Care (e)

Scale(s)-Not at all satisfied to Completely satisfied (s)

Care Recipient:

Data Source:

Definition: Extent of positive perception of coordination of care as the client moves from one care setting to another

OUTCOME TARGET RATING: Maintain at_____   Increase to_____

Client Satisfaction: Continuity of Care Overall Rating	Not at all satisfied 1	Somewhat satisfied 2	Moderately satisfied 3	Very satisfied 4	Completely satisfied 5	
INDICATORS:						
300301 Coordination of care	1	2	3	4	5	NA
300302 Personal preferences included in care plan	1	2	3	4	5	NA
300303 Client/family included in planning care	1	2	3	4	5	NA
300321 Client/family included in discharge planning	1	2	3	4	5	NA
300304 Client resources identified in discharge planning	1	2	3	4	5	NA
300305 Safety issues are addressed in care plan	1	2	3	4	5	NA
300306 Time to prepare for transfer	1	2	3	4	5	NA
300307 Information provided about what to expect when transferred	1	2	3	4	5	NA
300308 Opportunity provided to express concerns about managing self-care	1	2	3	4	5	NA
300309 Information provided to manage self-care	1	2	3	4	5	NA
300310 Opportunity to demonstrate care activities	1	2	3	4	5	NA
300311 Staff offer suggestions for solutions to concerns and questions	1	2	3	4	5	NA
300312 Discussion of strategies to meet care needs	1	2	3	4	5	NA
300313 Discussion of strategies to meet household needs	1	2	3	4	5	NA
300314 Personal preparation to deal with potential health problems	1	2	3	4	5	NA
300315 Discussion of guidelines for returning to sexual activities	1	2	3	4	5	NA
300316 Discussion of strategies for returning to work	1	2	3	4	5	NA
300317 Discussion of strategies for returning to homemaking activities	1	2	3	4	5	NA

		Not at all satisfied	Somewhat satisfied	Moderately satisfied	Very satisfied	Completely satisfied	
300318	Discussion of strategies for returning to community activities	1	2	3	4	5	NA
300319	Assistance with managing relocation costs and finances	1	2	3	4	5	NA
300320	Health providers work as a team	1	2	3	4	5	NA

3rd edition 2004; Revised 4th edition

Outcome Content References:

Eriksen, L. (1988). Measuring patient satisfaction with nursing care: A magnitude estimation approach. In C. F. Waltz & O. W. Stickland (Eds.), *Measurement of nursing outcomes* (Vol. 1, pp. 523-527). New York: Springer.

Gesell, S. B., & Gregory, N. (2003). Identifying priority actions for improving patient satisfaction with outpatient cancer care. *Journal of Nursing Care Quality, 19*(3), 226-233.

Larrabee, J. H., Ostrow, C. L., Withrow, M. L., Janney, M. A., Hobbs, G. R., Jr. & Burant, C. (2004). Predictors of patient satisfaction with inpatient hospital nursing care. *Research in Nursing & Health, 27*, 254-268.

Laschinger, H. S., Hall, L. M., Pedersen, C., & Almost, J. (2004). A psychometric analysis of the patient satisfaction with nursing care quality questionnaire: An actionable approach to measuring patient satisfaction. *Journal of Nursing Care Quality, 20*(3), 220-230.

Mark, B. A., & Wan, T. T. H. (2005). Testing measurement equivalence in a patient satisfaction instrument. *Western Journal of Nursing Research, 27*(6), 772-787.

Ware, J. E., Davies-Avery, A., & Stewart, A. I. (1978). The measurement and meaning of patient satisfaction. *Health & Medical Care Services Review, 1*(1), 1, 3-14.

Client Satisfaction: Cultural Needs Fulfillment—3004

Domain-Perceived Health (V)

Class-Satisfaction with Care (e)

Scale(s)-Not at all satisfied to Completely satisfied (s)

Care Recipient:

Data Source:

Definition: Extent of positive perception of integration of cultural beliefs, values and social structures into nursing care

OUTCOME TARGET RATING: Maintain at_____   Increase to_____

Client Satisfaction: Cultural Needs Fulfillment Overall Rating	Not at all satisfied 1	Somewhat satisfied 2	Moderately satisfied 3	Very satisfied 4	Completely satisfied 5	
INDICATORS:						
300401 Respect for cultural beliefs	1	2	3	4	5	NA
300402 Respect for cultural health behaviors	1	2	3	4	5	NA
300403 Respect for personal values	1	2	3	4	5	NA
300404 Respect for personal perspectives	1	2	3	4	5	NA
300405 Respect for traditions	1	2	3	4	5	NA
300406 Respect for religious beliefs	1	2	3	4	5	NA
300407 Respect for spiritual beliefs	1	2	3	4	5	NA
300408 Incorporation of cultural beliefs in health teaching	1	2	3	4	5	NA
300409 Care consistent with cultural beliefs	1	2	3	4	5	NA
300410 Use of creative methods to establish communication due to language differences	1	2	3	4	5	NA
300411 Consideration for cultural expectations	1	2	3	4	5	NA
300412 Respect for family members' participation in care	1	2	3	4	5	NA
300413 Respect for family members' participation in decisions	1	2	3	4	5	NA

3rd edition 2004

Outcome Content References:

Ali, N. S., & Khalil, H. Z. (1993). A comparison of American and Egyptian cancer patients' attitudes and unmet needs. *Cancer Nursing, 16*(3), 193-203.

Arruda, E. N., Larson, P. J., & Meleis, A. I. (1992). Comfort: Immigrant Hispanic cancer patient's views. *Cancer Nursing, 15*(6), 387-394.

Austin, W., Gallop, R., McCay, E., Peternelj-Taylor, C., & Bayer, M. (1999). Culturally competent care for psychiatric clients who have a history of sexual abuse. *Clinical Nursing Research, 8*(1), 5-25.

Capers, C. F. (1994). Mental health issues and African-Americans. *Mental Health Nursing, 29*(1), 57-72.

Chmielarczyk, V. (1991). Transcultural nursing: Providing culturally congruent care to the Hausa of Northwest Africa. *Journal of Transcultural Nursing, 3*(1), 15-19.

Cravener, P. (1992). Establishing therapeutic alliance across cultural barriers. *Journal of Psychosocial Nursing, 30*(12), 10-14.

Denman-Vitale, S., & Murillo, E. K. (1999). Effective promotion of breastfeeding among Latin American women newly immigrated to the United States. *Holistic Nursing Practice, 13*(4), 51-60.

Granda-Cameron, C. (1999). The experience of having cancer in Latin America. *Cancer Nursing, 22*(1), 51-57.

Larrabee, J. H., Ostrow, C. L., Withrow, M. L., Janney, M. A., Hobbs, G. R., Jr. & Burant, C. (2004). Predictors of patient satisfaction with inpatient hospital nursing care. *Research in Nursing & Health, 27*, 254-268.

Laschinger, H. S., Hall, L. M., Pedersen, C., & Almost, J. (2004). A psychometric analysis of the patient satisfaction with nursing care quality questionnaire: An actionable approach to measuring patient satisfaction. *Journal of Nursing Care Quality, 20*(3), 220-230.

Mark, B. A., & Wan, T. T. H. (2005). Testing measurement equivalence in a patient satisfaction instrument. *Western Journal of Nursing Research, 27*(6), 772-787.

Sommer, B. (1995). How we do it: Special considerations for Orthodox Jewish patients in the emergency department. *Journal of Emergency Nursing, 21*(6), 569-570.

Tripp-Reimer, T., Choi, E., Skemp Kelly, L., & Enslein, J. C. (2001). Cultural barriers to care: Inverting the problem. *Diabetes Spectrum, 14*(1), 13-22.

Weaver, H. N. (1999). Transcultural nursing with Native Americans: Critical knowledge, skills, and attitudes. *Journal of Transcultural Nursing, 10*(3), 197-202.

Willis, W. O. (1999). Culturally competent nursing care during the perinatal period. *Journal of Perinatal and Neonatal Nursing, 13*(3), 45-59.

Wilson, A. H., Pittman, K., & Wold, J. L. (2000). Listening to the quiet voices of Hispanic migrant children about health. *Journal of Pediatric Nursing, 15*(3), 137-147.

Yellen, E. (2003). The influence of nurse-sensitive variables on patient satisfaction. *AORN Journal, 78*, 783-793.

Yellen, E., Davis, G. C., & Ricard, R. (2002). The measurement of patient satisfaction. *Journal of Nursing Care Quality, 16*(4), 23-29.

C

C

Client Satisfaction: Functional Assistance—3005

Domain-Perceived Health (V)   *Care Recipient:*

Class-Satisfaction with Care (e)   *Data Source:*

Scale(s)-Not at all satisfied to Completely satisfied (s)

Definition: Extent of positive perception of nursing assistance to achieve mobility and self-care

OUTCOME TARGET RATING: Maintain at_____   Increase to_____

Client Satisfaction: Functional Assistance Overall Rating	Not at all satisfied 1	Somewhat satisfied 2	Moderately satisfied 3	Very satisfied 4	Completely satisfied 5	

INDICATORS:

300501	Included in planning for optimal mobility and self-care	1	2	3	4	5	NA
300502	Included in planning time schedule for self-care	1	2	3	4	5	NA
300503	Encouraged to be as active as possible	1	2	3	4	5	NA
300504	Assistance with physical activity	1	2	3	4	5	NA
300505	Exercise routine provided to gain or maintain mobility	1	2	3	4	5	NA
300506	Exercise routine provided to gain or maintain flexibility	1	2	3	4	5	NA
300507	Equipment provided to enhance mobility	1	2	3	4	5	NA
300516	Information provided for correct use of other devices	1	2	3	4	5	NA
300509	Room space provided for equipment needed to support functional independence	1	2	3	4	5	NA
300510	Safety taught in all activities	1	2	3	4	5	NA
300511	Opportunity to do self care unless assistance requested	1	2	3	4	5	NA
300512	Assistance with care	1	2	3	4	5	NA
300513	Allowed to choose own clothing	1	2	3	4	5	NA
300514	Allowed to choose food for meals	1	2	3	4	5	NA
300515	Information provided to manage medication	1	2	3	4	5	NA

3rd edition 2004; Revised 4th edition

Outcome Content References:

Hinshaw, A. S., & Atwood, J. R. (1982). A patient satisfaction instrument: Precision by replication. *Nursing Research, 31*(3), 170-175.

LaMonica, E. L., Oberst, M. T., Madea, A. R., & Wolf, R. M. (1986). Development of a patient satisfaction scale. *Research in Nursing & Health, 9*(1), 43-50.

Larrabee, J. H., Ostrow, C. L., Withrow, M. L., Janney, M. A., Hobbs, G. R., Jr. & Burant, C. (2004). Predictors of patient satisfaction with inpatient hospital nursing care. *Research in Nursing & Health, 27*, 254-268.

Laschinger, H. S., Hall, L. M., Pedersen, C., & Almost, J. (2004). A psychometric analysis of the patient satisfaction with nursing care quality questionnaire: An actionable approach to measuring patient satisfaction. *Journal of Nursing Care Quality, 20*(3), 220-230.

Mark, B. A., & Wan, T. T. H. (2005). Testing measurement equivalence in a patient satisfaction instrument. *Western Journal of Nursing Research, 27*(6), 772-787.

Risser, N. L. (1975). Development of an instrument to measure patient satisfaction with nurses and nursing care in primary care settings. *Nursing Research, 24*(1), 45-52.

Ware, J. E., Davies-Avery, A., & Stewart, A. I. (1978). The measurement and meaning of patient satisfaction. *Health & Medical Care Services Review, 1*(1), 1, 3-14.

C

Client Satisfaction: Pain Management—3016

Domain-Perceived Health (V)

Class-Satisfaction with Care (e)

Scale(s)-Not at all satisfied to Completely satisfied (s)

Care Recipient:

Data Source:

Definition: Extent of positive perception of nursing care to relieve pain

OUTCOME TARGET RATING: Maintain at_____   Increase to_____

Client Satisfaction: Pain Management Overall Rating	Not at all satisfied 1	Somewhat satisfied 2	Moderately satisfied 3	Very satisfied 4	Completely satisfied 5	
INDICATORS:						
301601 Pain controlled	1	2	3	4	5	NA
301602 Pain level regularly monitored	1	2	3	4	5	NA
301603 Side effects of medication monitored	1	2	3	4	5	NA
301604 Actions taken to relieve pain	1	2	3	4	5	NA
301605 Actions taken to provide comfort	1	2	3	4	5	NA
301606 Information provided to manage medication use	1	2	3	4	5	NA
301607 Personal preferences considered	1	2	3	4	5	NA
301608 Information provided about options for pain management	1	2	3	4	5	NA
301609 Pain management consistent with cultural beliefs	1	2	3	4	5	NA
301610 Preventive approaches used for pain management	1	2	3	4	5	NA
301611 Information provided about activity restrictions	1	2	3	4	5	NA
301612 Information provided about pain relief	1	2	3	4	5	NA
301613 Information provided about options for pain management after discharge	1	2	3	4	5	NA
301614 Referrals made to support groups	1	2	3	4	5	NA
301615 Health providers work as a team to manage pain	1	2	3	4	5	NA
301616 Referral to pain management health professionals as needed	1	2	3	4	5	NA
301617 Safety issues addressed with pain medication use	1	2	3	4	5	NA

Outcome Content References:

Herr, K., & Kwekkeboom, K. (Eds.). (2003). Chronic pain management. *Nursing Clinics of North America, 38*, 403-560.

Hinshaw, A. S., & Atwood, J. R. (1982). A patient satisfaction instrument: Precision by replication. *Nursing Research, 31*(3), 170-175.

Hogan, S. L. (2005). Patient satisfaction with pain management in the emergency department. *Topics in Emergency Medicine, 27*(4), 284-294.

Continued

C

Innis, J., Bikaunieks, N., Petryshen, P., Zellermeyer, V., & Ciccarelli, L. (2004). Patient satisfaction and pain management: An educational approach. *Journal of Nursing Care Quality, 19*(4), 322-327.

LaMonica, E. L., Oberst, M. T., Madea, A. R., & Wolf, R. M. (1986). Development of a patient satisfaction scale. *Research in Nursing and Health, 9*(1), 43-50.

Larrabee, J. H., Ostrow, C. L., Withrow, M. L., Janney, M. A., Hobbs, G. R., Jr. & Burant, C. (2004). Predictors of patient satisfaction with inpatient hospital nursing care. *Research in Nursing & Health, 27*, 254-268.

Laschinger, H. S., Hall, L. M., Pedersen, C., & Almost, J. (2004). A psychometric analysis of the patient satisfaction with nursing care quality questionnaire: An actionable approach to measuring patient satisfaction. *Journal of Nursing Care Quality, 20*(3), 220-230.

Mark, B. A., & Wan, T. T. H. (2005). Testing measurement equivalence in a patient satisfaction instrument. *Western Journal of Nursing Research, 27*(6), 772-787.

Risser, N. L. (1975). Development of an instrument to measure patient satisfaction with nurses and nursing care in primary care settings. *Nursing Research, 24*(1), 45-52.

Sjoling, M., Nordahl, G., Olofsson, N., & Asplund, K. (2003). The impact of preoperative information on state anxiety, postoperative pain and satisfaction with pain management. *Patient Education and Counseling, 51*, 169-176.

Sterman, E., Gauker, S., & Krieger, J. (2003). A comprehensive approach to improving cancer pain management and patient satisfaction. *Oncology Nursing Forum, 30*(5), 857-864.

Ware, J. E., Davies-Avery, A., & Stewart, A. I. (1978). The measurement and meaning of patient satisfaction. *Health & Medical Care Services Review, 1*(1), 1, 3-14.

Client Satisfaction: Physical Care—3006

Domain-Perceived Health (V)

Class-Satisfaction with Care (e)

Scale(s)-Not at all satisfied to Completely satisfied (s)

Care Recipient:

Data Source:

C

Definition: Extent of positive perception of nursing care to maintain body functions and cleanliness

OUTCOME TARGET RATING: Maintain at_____   Increase to_____

Client Satisfaction: Physical Care Overall Rating	Not at all satisfied 1	Somewhat satisfied 2	Moderately satisfied 3	Very satisfied 4	Completely satisfied 5

INDICATORS:

300601	Assistance with selecting food and fluid	1	2	3	4	5	NA
300602	Assistance with eating	1	2	3	4	5	NA
300603	Time for meals	1	2	3	4	5	NA
300604	Fluids available within restriction	1	2	3	4	5	NA
300605	Assistance with mouth care	1	2	3	4	5	NA
300606	Assistance with toileting	1	2	3	4	5	NA
300607	Normal bowel habits maintained	1	2	3	4	5	NA
300608	Normal bladder habits maintained	1	2	3	4	5	NA
300609	Assistance with bathing	1	2	3	4	5	NA
300610	Assistance with hair care	1	2	3	4	5	NA
300611	Assistance with nail care	1	2	3	4	5	NA
300612	Skin care routine maintained	1	2	3	4	5	NA
300613	Special skin care followed	1	2	3	4	5	NA
300614	Assistance with maintaining comfort	1	2	3	4	5	NA
300615	Time for rest	1	2	3	4	5	NA
300616	Sleep routine maintained	1	2	3	4	5	NA
300617	Assistance with ambulation	1	2	3	4	5	NA
300618	Opportunity for exercise	1	2	3	4	5	NA
300619	Special exercises provided	1	2	3	4	5	NA
300620	Assistance with repositioning	1	2	3	4	5	NA
300621	Assistance with transfer	1	2	3	4	5	NA

3rd edition 2004

Outcome Content References:

Davis, B. A., & Bush, H. A. (1995). Developing effective measurement tools: A case study of the consumer emergency care satisfaction scale. *Journal of Nursing Care Quality, 9*(2), 26-35.

Hinshaw, A. S., & Atwood, J. R. (1982). A patient satisfaction instrument: Precision by replication. *Nursing Research, 31*(3), 170-175.

LaMonica, E. L., Oberst, M. T., Madea, A. R., & Wolf, R. M. (1986). Development of a patient satisfaction scale. *Research in Nursing & Health, 9*(1), 43-50.

Continued

Larrabee, J. H., Ostrow, C. L., Withrow, M. L., Janney, M. A., Hobbs, G. R., Jr. & Burant, C. (2004). Predictors of patient satisfaction with inpatient hospital nursing care. *Research in Nursing & Health, 27*, 254-268.

Laschinger, H. S., Hall, L. M., Pedersen, C., & Almost, J. (2004). A psychometric analysis of the patient satisfaction with nursing care quality questionnaire: An actionable approach to measuring patient satisfaction. *Journal of Nursing Care Quality, 20*(3), 220-230.

Lynn, M. R., & McMillen, B. J. (1999). Do nurses know what patients think is important in nursing care? *Journal of Nursing Care Quality, 13*(5), 65-74.

Mark, B. A., & Wan, T. T. H. (2005). Testing measurement equivalence in a patient satisfaction instrument. *Western Journal of Nursing Research, 27*(6), 772-787.

Ryden, M. B., Gross, C. R., Savik, K., Snyder, M., Oh, H. L., Jang, Y., Wang, J., & Krichbaum, K. E. (2000). Development of a measure of resident satisfaction with the nursing home. *Research in Nursing & Health, 23*(3), 237-245.

Ware, J. E., Davies-Avery, A., & Stewart, A. I. (1978). The measurement and meaning of patient satisfaction. *Health & Medical Care Services Review, 1*(1), 1, 3-14.

Wolf, L. R., Giardino, E. R., Osborne, P. A., & Ambrose, M. S. (1994). Dimensions of nurse caring. *Image—The Journal of Nursing Scholarship, 26*(2), 107-111.

Client Satisfaction: Physical Environment—3007

Domain-Perceived Health (V)

Class-Satisfaction with Care (e)

Scale(s)-Not at all satisfied to Completely satisfied (s)

Care Recipient:

Data Source:

C

Definition: Extent of positive perception of living environment, treatment environment, equipment and supplies in acute or long term care settings

OUTCOME TARGET RATING: Maintain at_____   Increase to_____

Client Satisfaction: Physical Environment Overall Rating	Not at all satisfied 1	Somewhat satisfied 2	Moderately satisfied 3	Very satisfied 4	Completely satisfied 5	
INDICATORS:						
300701 Cleanliness of room	1	2	3	4	5	NA
300702 Cleanliness of bathroom	1	2	3	4	5	NA
300703 Cleanliness of equipment	1	2	3	4	5	NA
300704 Control of room lighting	1	2	3	4	5	NA
300705 Comfort of room temperature	1	2	3	4	5	NA
300723 Control of odors	1	2	3	4	5	NA
300706 Comfort of bathroom temperature	1	2	3	4	5	NA
300707 Comfort of treatment room temperature	1	2	3	4	5	NA
300708 Comfort of room humidity	1	2	3	4	5	NA
300711 Control of noise	1	2	3	4	5	NA
300712 Control of number of people in room	1	2	3	4	5	NA
300713 Supplies and equipment within reach	1	2	3	4	5	NA
300714 Call light within reach	1	2	3	4	5	NA
300716 Access to telephone	1	2	3	4	5	NA
300717 Access to television	1	2	3	4	5	NA
300718 Access to radio	1	2	3	4	5	NA
300715 Attractiveness of room	1	2	3	4	5	NA
300719 Availability of chairs for family and visitors	1	2	3	4	5	NA
300720 Availability of space nearby for family and visitors	1	2	3	4	5	NA
300721 Orientation of family and visitors to facilities	1	2	3	4	5	NA
300722 Space in room for personal items	1	2	3	4	5	NA

3rd edition 2004; Revised 4th edition

Outcome Content References:

Abdellah, F. G., & Levine, E. (1957). Developing a measure of patient and personnel satisfaction with nursing care. *Nursing Research, 5*, 100-108.

Continued

Eriksen, L. (1988). Measuring patient satisfaction with nursing care: A magnitude estimation approach. In C. F. Waltz & O. W. Stickland (Eds.), *Measurement of nursing outcomes* (Vol. 1, pp. 523-527). New York: Springer.

Gesell, S. B., & Gregory, N. (2003). Identifying priority actions for improving patient satisfaction with outpatient cancer care. *Journal of Nursing Care Quality, 19*(3), 226-233.

Larrabee, J. H., Ostrow, C. L., Withrow, M. L., Janney, M. A., Hobbs, G. R., Jr., & Burant, C. (2004). Predictors of patient satisfaction with inpatient hospital nursing care. *Research in Nursing & Health, 27,* 254-268.

Laschinger, H. S., Hall, L. M., Pedersen, C., & Almost, J. (2004). A psychometric analysis of the patient satisfaction with nursing care quality questionnaire: An actionable approach to measuring patient satisfaction. *Journal of Nursing Care Quality, 20*(3), 220-230.

Lynn, M. R., & McMillen, B. J. (1999). Do nurses know what patients think is important in nursing care? *Journal of Nursing Care Quality, 13*(5), 65-74.

Mark, B. A., & Wan, T. T. H. (2005). Testing measurement equivalence in a patient satisfaction instrument. *Western Journal of Nursing Research, 27*(6), 772-787.

Ryden, M. B., Gross, C. R., Savik, K., Snyder, M., Oh, H. L., Jang, Y., Wang, J., & Krichbaum, K. E. (2000). Development of a measure of resident satisfaction with the nursing home. *Research in Nursing & Health, 23*(3), 237-245.

Ware, J. E., Davies-Avery, A., & Stewart, A. I. (1978). The measurement and meaning of patient satisfaction. *Health & Medical Care Services Review, 1*(1), 1, 3-14.

Client Satisfaction: Protection of Rights—3008

Domain-Perceived Health (V)

Class-Satisfaction with Care (e)

Scale(s)-Not at all satisfied to Completely satisfied (s)

Care Recipient:

Data Source:

C

Definition: Extent of positive perception of protection of a client's legal and moral rights provided by nursing staff

OUTCOME TARGET RATING: Maintain at_____   Increase to_____

Client Satisfaction: Protection of Rights Overall Rating	Not at all satisfied 1	Somewhat satisfied 2	Moderately satisfied 3	Very satisfied 4	Completely satisfied 5	
INDICATORS:						
300801 Maintenance of privacy	1	2	3	4	5	NA
300802 Care consistent with religious and spiritual needs	1	2	3	4	5	NA
300803 Confidentiality of client information maintained	1	2	3	4	5	NA
300804 Requests respected	1	2	3	4	5	NA
300805 Personal preferences for care considered	1	2	3	4	5	NA
300806 Use of client's preferred name	1	2	3	4	5	NA
300807 Introduced to staff	1	2	3	4	5	NA
300808 Introduced to roommate(s)	1	2	3	4	5	NA
300809 Information provided about available services of other disciplines	1	2	3	4	5	NA
300810 Information provided about support groups	1	2	3	4	5	NA
300811 Allowed to choose between care options	1	2	3	4	5	NA
300812 Included in decisions about care	1	2	3	4	5	NA
300813 Information provided about legal rights	1	2	3	4	5	NA
300814 Information provided about advance directives	1	2	3	4	5	NA
300815 Avoidance of repetitive questions by more than one provider	1	2	3	4	5	NA

3rd edition 2004

Outcome Content References:

Eriksen, L. (1988). Measuring patient satisfaction with nursing care: A magnitude estimation approach. In C. F. Waltz & O. W. Stickland (Eds.), *Measurement of nursing outcomes* (Vol. 1, pp. 523-527). New York: Springer.

Hegedus, K. S. (1999). Providers' and consumers' perspective of nurses' caring behaviours. *Journal of Advanced Nursing, 30*(5), 1090-1096.

LaMonica, E. L., Oberst, M. T., Madea, A. R., & Wolf, R. M. (1986). Development of a patient satisfaction scale. *Research in Nursing & Health, 9*(1), 43-50.

Continued

Larrabee, J. H., Ostrow, C. L., Withrow, M. L., Janney, M. A., Hobbs, G. R., Jr., & Burant, C. (2004). Predictors of patient satisfaction with inpatient hospital nursing care. *Research in Nursing & Health, 27,* 254-268.

Laschinger, H. S., Hall, L. M., Pedersen, C., & Almost, J. (2004). A psychometric analysis of the patient satisfaction with nursing care quality questionnaire: An actionable approach to measuring patient satisfaction. *Journal of Nursing Care Quality, 20*(3), 220-230.

Mark, B. A., & Wan, T. T. H. (2005). Testing measurement equivalence in a patient satisfaction instrument. *Western Journal of Nursing Research, 27*(6), 772-787.

Ryden, M. B., Gross, C. R., Savik, K., Snyder, M., Oh, H. L., Jang, Y., Wang, J., & Krichbaum, K. E. (2000). Development of a measure of resident satisfaction with the nursing home. *Research in Nursing & Health, 23*(3), 237-245.

Ware, J. E., Davies-Avery, A., & Stewart, A. I. (1978). The measurement and meaning of patient satisfaction. *Health & Medical Care Services Review, 1*(1), 1, 3-14.

Wolf, L. R., Giardino, E. R., Osborne, P. A., & Ambrose, M. S. (1994). Dimensions of nurse caring. *Image—The Journal of Nursing Scholarship, 26*(2), 107-111.

Client Satisfaction: Psychological Care—3009

Domain-Perceived Health (V)

Class-Satisfaction with Care (e)

Scale(s)-Not at all satisfied to Completely satisfied (s)

Care Recipient:

Data Source:

C

Definition: Extent of positive perception of nursing assistance to cope with emotional issues and perform mental activities

OUTCOME TARGET RATING: Maintain at_____ Increase to_____

Client Satisfaction: Psychological Care Overall Rating	Not at all satisfied 1	Somewhat satisfied 2	Moderately satisfied 3	Very satisfied 4	Completely satisfied 5	
INDICATORS:						
300901 Information provided about course of illness	1	2	3	4	5	NA
300902 Information provided about expected improvement	1	2	3	4	5	NA
300917 Information provided about usual emotional responses to disease	1	2	3	4	5	NA
300918 Information provided about usual emotional responses to treatment regimen	1	2	3	4	5	NA
300904 Assistance with identifying community support groups for client	1	2	3	4	5	NA
300905 Assistance with identifying community support groups for family	1	2	3	4	5	NA
300906 Discussion of strategies to cope with mental impairments	1	2	3	4	5	NA
300907 Emotional support provided	1	2	3	4	5	NA
300908 Counseling provided to improve mental functioning	1	2	3	4	5	NA
300909 Counseling provided to improve emotional stability	1	2	3	4	5	NA
300910 Counseling provided to improve social interactions	1	2	3	4	5	NA
300919 Assistance with finding counseling services	1	2	3	4	5	NA
300912 Support for finding own solutions to problems	1	2	3	4	5	NA
300913 Support for expressing feelings	1	2	3	4	5	NA
300914 Support for working through feelings of loss	1	2	3	4	5	NA
300915 Support for identifying ways to cope with stress	1	2	3	4	5	NA
300916 Support for adjusting to functional changes	1	2	3	4	5	NA
300920 Assistance to address spiritual needs	1	2	3	4	5	NA

Continued

C

3rd edition 2004; Revised 4th edition

Outcome Content References:

Davis, B. A., & Bush, H. A. (1995). Developing effective measurement tools: A case study of the consumer emergency care satisfaction scale. *Journal of Nursing Care Quality, 9*(2), 26-35.

Gesell, S. B., & Gregory, N. (2003). Identifying priority actions for improving patient satisfaction with outpatient cancer care. *Journal of Nursing Care Quality, 19*(3), 226-233.

Larrabee, J. H., Ostrow, C. L., Withrow, M. L., Janney, M. A., Hobbs, G. R., Jr., & Burant, C. (2004). Predictors of patient satisfaction with inpatient hospital nursing care. *Research in Nursing & Health, 27,* 254-268.

Laschinger, H. S., Hall, L. M., Pedersen, C., & Almost, J. (2004). A psychometric analysis of the patient satisfaction with nursing care quality questionnaire: An actionable approach to measuring patient satisfaction. *Journal of Nursing Care Quality, 20*(3), 220-230.

Lynn, M. R., & McMillen, B. J. (1999). Do nurses know what patients think is important in nursing care? *Journal of Nursing Care Quality, 13*(5), 65-74.

Mark, B. A., & Wan, T. T. H. (2005). Testing measurement equivalence in a patient satisfaction instrument. *Western Journal of Nursing Research, 27*(6), 772-787.

Nussbaum, G. B. (2003). Spirituality in critical care: Patient comfort and satisfaction. *Critical Care Nursing Quarterly, 26*(3), 214-220.

Ryden, M. B., Gross, C. R., Savik, K., Snyder, M., Oh, H. L., Jang, Y., Wang, J., & Krichbaum, K. E. (2000). Development of a measure of resident satisfaction with the nursing home. *Research in Nursing & Health, 23*(3), 237-245.

Ware, J. E., Davies-Avery, A., & Stewart, A. I. (1978). The measurement and meaning of patient satisfaction. *Health & Medical Care Services Review, 1*(1), 1, 3-14.

Client Satisfaction: Safety—3010

Domain-Perceived Health (V)

Class-Satisfaction with Care (e)

Scale(s)-Not at all satisfied to Completely satisfied (s)

Care Recipient:

Data Source:

C

Definition: Extent of positive perception of procedures, information and nursing care to prevent harm or injury

OUTCOME TARGET RATING: Maintain at_____   Increase to_____

Client Satisfaction: Safety Overall Rating	Not at all satisfied 1	Somewhat satisfied 2	Moderately satisfied 3	Very satisfied 4	Completely satisfied 5	
INDICATORS:						
301001 Explanation of safety rules and procedures	1	2	3	4	5	NA
301002 Prompt response to injury by staff	1	2	3	4	5	NA
301003 Client identified before receiving medication	1	2	3	4	5	NA
301014 Protective devices used to prevent harm	1	2	3	4	5	NA
301005 Assistance with transfer	1	2	3	4	5	NA
301006 Assistance with ambulation	1	2	3	4	5	NA
301007 Assistance with toileting	1	2	3	4	5	NA
301008 Assistance with bathing	1	2	3	4	5	NA
301009 Warning signs of high risk environment clearly displayed	1	2	3	4	5	NA
301015 Fall prevention strategies	1	2	3	4	5	NA
301011 Information provided about treatment risks and complications	1	2	3	4	5	NA
301012 Maintenance of safe environment when cognitive function is impaired	1	2	3	4	5	NA
301013 Maintenance of protective environment when at risk for self-injury	1	2	3	4	5	NA

3rd edition 2004; Revised 4th edition

Outcome Content References:

Abdellah, F. G., & Levine, E. (1957). Developing a measure of patient and personnel satisfaction with nursing care. *Nursing Research, 5,* 100-108.

Eriksen, L. (1988). Measuring patient satisfaction with nursing care: A magnitude estimation approach. In C. F. Waltz & O. W. Stickland (Eds.), *Measurement of nursing outcomes* (Vol. 1, pp. 523-527). New York: Springer.

Larrabee, J. H., Ostrow, C. L., Withrow, M. L., Janney, M. A., Hobbs, G. R., Jr., & Burant, C. (2004). Predictors of patient satisfaction with inpatient hospital nursing care. *Research in Nursing & Health, 27,* 254-268.

Laschinger, H. S., Hall, L. M., Pedersen, C., & Almost, J. (2004). A psychometric analysis of the patient satisfaction with nursing care quality questionnaire: An actionable approach to measuring patient satisfaction. *Journal of Nursing Care Quality, 20*(3), 220-230.

Lynn, M. R., & McMillen, B. J. (1999). Do nurses know what patients think is important in nursing care? *Journal of Nursing Care Quality, 13*(5), 65-74.

Mark, B. A., & Wan, T. T. H. (2005). Testing measurement equivalence in a patient satisfaction instrument. *Western Journal of Nursing Research, 27*(6), 772-787.

Ryden, M. B., Gross, C. R., Savik, K., Snyder, M., Oh, H. L., Jang, Y., Wang, J., & Krichbaum, K. E. (2000). Development of a measure of resident satisfaction with the nursing home. *Research in Nursing & Health, 23*(3), 237-245.

Ware, J. E., Davies-Avery, A., & Stewart, A. I. (1978). The measurement and meaning of patient satisfaction. *Health & Medical Care Services Review, 1*(1), 1, 3-14.

C

Client Satisfaction: Symptom Control—3011

Domain-Perceived Health (V)

Class-Satisfaction with Care (e)

Scale(s)-Not at all satisfied to Completely satisfied (s)

Care Recipient:

Data Source:

Definition: Extent of positive perception of nursing care to relieve symptoms of illness

OUTCOME TARGET RATING: Maintain at_____   Increase to_____

Client Satisfaction: Symptom Control Overall Rating	Not at all satisfied 1	Somewhat satisfied 2	Moderately satisfied 3	Very satisfied 4	Completely satisfied 5	
INDICATORS:						
301101 Patterns of symptoms identified	1	2	3	4	5	NA
301102 Severity of symptoms identified	1	2	3	4	5	NA
301103 Duration of symptoms identified	1	2	3	4	5	NA
301104 Investigation of cause of symptoms	1	2	3	4	5	NA
301105 Actions taken to prevent symptoms	1	2	3	4	5	NA
301106 Symptoms responded to promptly	1	2	3	4	5	NA
301115 Care to control symptoms	1	2	3	4	5	NA
301116 Care to control pain	1	2	3	4	5	NA
301109 Actions taken to provide comfort	1	2	3	4	5	NA
301110 Symptoms regularly monitored	1	2	3	4	5	NA
301111 Monitored for unusual symptoms	1	2	3	4	5	NA
301112 Monitored for control of symptoms	1	2	3	4	5	NA
301113 Monitored for comfort	1	2	3	4	5	NA
301114 Referrals made to other health providers	1	2	3	4	5	NA

3rd edition 2004; Revised 4th edition

Outcome Content References:

Hogan, S. L. (2005). Patient satisfaction with pain management in the emergency department. *Topics in Emergency Medicine, 27*(4), 284-294.

Innis, J., Bikaunieks, N., Petryshen, P., Zellermeyer, V., & Ciccarelli, L. (2004). Patient satisfaction and pain management: An educational approach. *Journal of Nursing Care Quality, 19*(4), 322-327.

Larrabee, J. H., Ostrow, C. L., Withrow, M. L., Janney, M. A., Hobbs, G. R., Jr., & Burant, C. (2004). Predictors of patient satisfaction with inpatient hospital nursing care. *Research in Nursing & Health, 27*, 254-268.

Laschinger, H. S., Hall, L. M., Pedersen, C., & Almost, J. (2004). A psychometric analysis of the patient satisfaction with nursing care quality questionnaire: An actionable approach to measuring patient satisfaction. *Journal of Nursing Care Quality, 20*(3), 220-230.

Mark, B. A., & Wan, T. T. H. (2005). Testing measurement equivalence in a patient satisfaction instrument. *Western Journal of Nursing Research, 27*(6), 772-787.

Marsh, G. W. (1999). Measuring patient satisfaction outcomes across provider disciplines. *Journal of Nursing Measurement, 7*(1), 47-62.

Ryden, M. B., Gross, C. R., Savik, K., Snyder, M., Oh, H. L., Jang, Y., Wang, J., & Krichbaum, K. E. (2000). Development of a measure of resident satisfaction with the nursing home. *Research in Nursing & Health, 23*(3), 237-245.

Sterman, E., Gauker, S., & Krieger, J. (2003). A comprehensive approach to improving cancer pain management and patient satisfaction. *Oncology Nursing Forum, 30*(5), 857-864.

Ware, J. E., Davies-Avery, A., & Stewart, A. I. (1978). The measurement and meaning of patient satisfaction. *Health & Medical Care Services Review, 1*(1), 1, 3-14.

Client Satisfaction: Teaching—3012

Domain-Perceived Health (V)

Class-Satisfaction with Care (e)

Scale(s)-Not at all satisfied to Completely satisfied (s)

Care Recipient:

Data Source:

C

Definition: Extent of positive perception of instruction provided by nursing staff to improve knowledge, understanding, and participation in care

OUTCOME TARGET RATING: Maintain at_____   Increase to_____

Client Satisfaction: Teaching Overall Rating	Not at all satisfied 1	Somewhat satisfied 2	Moderately satisfied 3	Very satisfied 4	Completely satisfied 5	

INDICATORS:

301210	Personal knowledge considered before teaching	1	2	3	4	5	NA
301219	Explanations provided in understandable terms	1	2	3	4	5	NA
301222	Explanation of medical diagnosis	1	2	3	4	5	NA
301223	Explanation of nursing care	1	2	3	4	5	NA
301203	Explanation of diagnostic tests and preparation	1	2	3	4	5	NA
301204	Explanation of results of diagnostic tests	1	2	3	4	5	NA
301205	Explanation of medication therapeutic effects	1	2	3	4	5	NA
301206	Explanation of medication side effects	1	2	3	4	5	NA
301207	Explanation of reasons for treatment	1	2	3	4	5	NA
301208	Explanation of self-care responsibilities for treatment	1	2	3	4	5	NA
301209	Explanation of self-care responsibilities for medication management	1	2	3	4	5	NA
301212	Explanation of activity restrictions	1	2	3	4	5	NA
301213	Discussion of strategies to improve physical strength	1	2	3	4	5	NA
301214	Discussion of strategies to improve physical endurance	1	2	3	4	5	NA
301215	Discussion of strategies to improve health	1	2	3	4	5	NA
301211	Information provided about signs of complications	1	2	3	4	5	NA
301216	Explanation of available health resources	1	2	3	4	5	NA
301217	Explanation of costs of care	1	2	3	4	5	NA
301218	Time for client learning	1	2	3	4	5	NA
301220	Quality of instruction material	1	2	3	4	5	NA
301221	Staff supportive of learning process	1	2	3	4	5	NA

Continued

3rd edition 2004; Revised 4th edition

Outcome Content References:

Abramowitz, S., Cote, A. A., & Berry, E. (1987). *Quality Review Bulletin, 13*(4), 122-130.

Davis, B. A., & Bush, H. A. (1995). Developing effective measurement tools: A case study of the consumer emergency care satisfaction scale. *Journal of Nursing Care Quality, 9*(2), 26-35.

Gesell, S. B., & Gregory, N. (2003). Identifying priority actions for improving patient satisfaction with outpatient cancer care. *Journal of Nursing Care Quality, 19*(3), 226-233.

Hinshaw, A. S., & Atwood, J. R. (1982). A patient satisfaction instrument: Precision by replication. *Nursing Research, 31*(3), 170-175.

Larrabee, J. H., Ostrow, C. L., Withrow, M. L., Janney, M. A., Hobbs, G. R., Jr., & Burant, C. (2004). Predictors of patient satisfaction with inpatient hospital nursing care. *Research in Nursing & Health, 27*, 254-268.

Laschinger, H. S., Hall, L. M., Pedersen, C., & Almost, J. (2004). A psychometric analysis of the patient satisfaction with nursing care quality questionnaire: An actionable approach to measuring patient satisfaction. *Journal of Nursing Care Quality, 20*(3), 220-230.

Mark, B. A., & Wan, T. T. H. (2005). Testing measurement equivalence in a patient satisfaction instrument. *Western Journal of Nursing Research, 27*(6), 772-787.

Marsh, G. W. (1999). Measuring patient satisfaction outcomes across provider disciplines. *Journal of Nursing Measurement, 7*(1), 47-62.

Risser, N. L. (1975). Development of an instrument to measure patient satisfaction with nurses and nursing care in primary care settings. *Nursing Research, 24*(1), 45-52.

Ryden, M. B., Gross, C. R., Savik, K., Snyder, M., Oh, H. L., Jang, Y., Wang, J., & Krichbaum, K. E. (2000). Development of a measure of resident satisfaction with the nursing home. *Research in Nursing & Health, 23*(3), 237-245.

Ware, J. E., Davies-Avery, A., & Stewart, A. I. (1978). The measurement and meaning of patient satisfaction. *Health & Medical Care Services Review, 1*(1), 1, 3-14.

Client Satisfaction: Technical Aspects of Care—3013

Domain-Perceived Health (V)

Class-Satisfaction with Care (e)

Scale(s)-Not at all satisfied to Completely satisfied (s)

Care Recipient:

Data Source:

C

Definition: Extent of positive perception of nursing staff's knowledge and expertise used in providing care

OUTCOME TARGET RATING: Maintain at_____   Increase to_____

Client Satisfaction: Technical Aspects of Care Overall Rating	Not at all satisfied 1	Somewhat satisfied 2	Moderately satisfied 3	Very satisfied 4	Completely satisfied 5	
INDICATORS:						
301301 Correct care provided	1	2	3	4	5	NA
301302 Organization of care	1	2	3	4	5	NA
301303 Thoroughness of care	1	2	3	4	5	NA
301304 Capability of staff	1	2	3	4	5	NA
301305 Registered nurse knowledge of disease process	1	2	3	4	5	NA
301316 Registered nurse knowledge of procedures	1	2	3	4	5	NA
301307 Registered nurse knowledge of medication	1	2	3	4	5	NA
301308 Registered nurse knowledge of health history	1	2	3	4	5	NA
301309 Consistency in performance of care	1	2	3	4	5	NA
301310 Consistency of staff providing care	1	2	3	4	5	NA
301311 Comfort attended to during treatments	1	2	3	4	5	NA
301312 Gentleness of staff	1	2	3	4	5	NA
301317 Competence of staff	1	2	3	4	5	NA
301314 Responsiveness of staff to emergencies	1	2	3	4	5	NA
301315 Supplies and equipment not wasted	1	2	3	4	5	NA

3rd edition 2004; Revised 4th edition

Outcome Content References:

Abdellah, F. G., & Levine, E. (1957). Developing a measure of patient and personnel satisfaction with nursing care. *Nursing Research, 5,* 100-108.

Eriksen, L. (1988). Measuring patient satisfaction with nursing care: A magnitude estimation approach. In C. F. Waltz & O. W. Stickland (Eds.), *Measurement of nursing outcomes* (Vol. 1, pp. 523-527). New York: Springer.

Hinshaw, A. S., & Atwood, J. R. (1982). A patient satisfaction instrument: Precision by replication. *Nursing Research, 31*(3), 170-175.

LaMonica, E. L., Oberst, M. T., Madea, A. R., & Wolf, R. M. (1986). Development of a patient satisfaction scale. *Research in Nursing and Health, 9*(1), 43-50.

Larrabee, J. H., Ostrow, C. L., Withrow, M. L., Janney, M. A., Hobbs, G. R., Jr., & Burant, C. (2004). Predictors of patient satisfaction with inpatient hospital nursing care. *Research in Nursing & Health, 27,* 254-268.

Continued

Mark, B. A., & Wan, T. T. H. (2005). Testing measurement equivalence in a patient satisfaction instrument. *Western Journal of Nursing Research, 27*(6), 772-787.

Marsh, G. W. (1999). Measuring patient satisfaction outcomes across provider disciplines. *Journal of Nursing Measurement, 7*(1), 47-62.

Risser, N. L. (1975). Development of an instrument to measure patient satisfaction with nurses and nursing care in primary care settings. *Nursing Research, 24*(1), 45-52.

Laschinger, H. S., Hall, L. M., Pedersen, C., & Almost, J. (2004). A psychometric analysis of the patient satisfaction with nursing care quality questionnaire: An actionable approach to measuring patient satisfaction. *Journal of Nursing Care Quality, 20*(3), 220-230.

Ware, J. E., Davies-Avery, A., & Stewart, A. I. (1978). The measurement and meaning of patient satisfaction. *Health & Medical Care Services Review, 1*(1), 1, 3-14.

Wolf, L. R., Giardino, E. R., Osborne, P. A., & Ambrose, M. S. (1994). Dimensions of nurse caring. *Image—The Journal of Nursing Scholarship, 26*(2), 107-111.

C

Cognition—0900

Domain-Physiologic Health (II)

Class-Neurocognitive (J)

Scale(s)-Severely compromised to Not compromised (a)

Care Recipient:

Data Source:

Definition: Ability to execute complex mental processes

OUTCOME TARGET RATING: Maintain at_____   Increase to_____

Cognition Overall Rating	Severely compromised 1	Substantially compromised 2	Moderately compromised 3	Mildly compromised 4	Not compromised 5	
INDICATORS:						
090014 Communication clear for age	1	2	3	4	5	NA
090015 Communication appropriate for age	1	2	3	4	5	NA
090013 Comprehension of the meaning of situations	1	2	3	4	5	NA
090003 Attentiveness	1	2	3	4	5	NA
090004 Concentration	1	2	3	4	5	NA
090005 Cognitive orientation	1	2	3	4	5	NA
090006 Immediate memory	1	2	3	4	5	NA
090007 Recent memory	1	2	3	4	5	NA
090008 Remote memory	1	2	3	4	5	NA
090009 Information processing	1	2	3	4	5	NA
090010 Alternatives weighed when making decisions	1	2	3	4	5	NA
090011 Appropriate decision-making	1	2	3	4	5	NA
090016 Complex calculations skills	1	2	3	4	5	NA

1st edition 1997; Revised 3rd edition 2004; Revised 4th edition

Outcome Content References:

Abraham, I., & Reel, S. (1993). Cognitive nursing interventions with long-term care residents: Effects on neurocognitive dimensions. *Archives of Psychiatric Nursing, 6*(6), 356-365.

Dellasega, C. (1992). Home health nurses' assessments of cognition. *Applied Nursing Research, 5*(3), 127-133.

Erlanger, D. M., Kaushik, T., Broshek, D., Freeman, J., Feldman, D., & Festa, J. (2002). Development and validation of a web-based screening tool for monitoring cognitive status. *Journal of Head Trauma Rehabilitation 17*(5), 458-476.

+Folstein, M. F., Folstein, S. E., & McHugh, P. R. (1975). "Mini-Mental State": A practical method for grading the cognitive state of patients for the clinician. *Journal of Psychiatric Research, 12*(3), 189-198.

Foreman, M., Gilles, D., & Wagner, D. (1989). Impaired cognition in the critically ill elderly patient: Clinical implications. *Critical Care Nursing Quarterly, 12*(1), 61-73.

Gerdner, L. A., & Hall, G. R. (2001). Chronic confusion. In M. Maas, K. Buckwalter, M. Hardy, T. Tripp-Reimer, M. Titler, & J. Specht (Eds.), *Nursing care of older adults: Diagnoses, outcomes & interventions* (pp. 421-441). St. Louis: Mosby.

Inaba-Roland, K., & Maricle, R. (1992). Assessing delirium in the acute care setting. *Heart & Lung, 21*(1), 48-55.

Kupferer, S., Uebele, J., & Levin, D. (1988). Geriatric ambulatory surgery patients: Assessing cognitive functions. *AORN Journal, 47*(3), 752-766.

Mason, P. (1989). Cognitive assessment parameters and tools for the critically injured adult. *Critical Care Nursing Clinics of North America, 1*(1), 45-53.

Shih, R. A., Glass, T. A., Bandeen-Roche, K., Carlson, M. C., Bolla, K. I., Todd, A. C., & Schwartz, B. S. (2006). Environmental lead exposure and cognitive function in community-dwelling older adults. *Neurology, 67*(9), 1556-1562.

Souder, E., & O'Sullivan, P. S. (2000). Nursing documentation versus standardized assessment of cognitive status in hospitalized medical patients. *Applied Nursing Research, 13*(1), 29-36.

Continued

Strub, R. L., & Black, F. W. (2000). *The mental status examination in neurology* (4th ed.). Philadelphia: F.A. Davis.

Vellinga, A., Smit, J. H., van Leeuwen, E., van Tilburg W., & Jonker, C. (2004). Instruments to assess decision-making capacity: An overview. *International Psychogeriatrics 16*(4), 397-419.

Wakefield, B., Mentes, J., Mobily, P., Tripp-Reimer, T., Culp, K. R., Rapp, C. G., Gaspar, P., Kundrat, M., Wadle, K. R., & Akins, J. (2001). Acute confusion. In M. Maas, K. Buckwalter, M. Hardy, T. Tripp-Reimer, M. Titler, & J. Specht (Eds.), *Nursing care of older adults: Diagnoses, outcomes & interventions* (pp. 442-454). St. Louis: Mosby.

C

Cognitive Orientation—0901

Domain-Physiologic Health (II)

Class-Neurocognitive (J)

Scale(s)-Severely compromised to Not compromised (a)

Care Recipient:

Data Source:

Definition: Ability to identify person, place, and time accurately

OUTCOME TARGET RATING: Maintain at_____   Increase to_____

Cognitive Orientation Overall Rating	Severely compromised 1	Substantially compromised 2	Moderately compromised 3	Mildly compromised 4	Not compromised 5	
INDICATORS:						
090101 Identifies self	1	2	3	4	5	NA
090102 Identifies significant other	1	2	3	4	5	NA
090103 Identifies current place	1	2	3	4	5	NA
090104 Identifies correct day	1	2	3	4	5	NA
090105 Identifies correct month	1	2	3	4	5	NA
090106 Identifies correct year	1	2	3	4	5	NA
090107 Identifies correct season	1	2	3	4	5	NA
090109 Identifies significant current events	1	2	3	4	5	NA

1st edition 1997; Revised 3rd edition 2004

Outcome Content References:

Abraham, I. L., & Reel, S. J. (1993). Cognitive nursing interventions and long-term care residents: Effects on neurocognitive dimensions. *Archives of Psychiatric Nursing, 6*(6), 356-365.

Agostinelli, B., Demers, K., Garrigan, D., & Waszynski, C. (1994). Targeted interventions: Use of the mini-mental state exam. *Journal of Gerontological Nursing, 20*(8), 15-23.

Aird, T., & McIntosh, M. (2004). Nursing assessment. Nursing tools and strategies to assess cognition and confusion. *British Journal of Nusing 13*(10), 621-625.

Crimlisk, J. T. & Grande, M. M. (2004). Neurologic assessment skills for the acute medical surgical nurse. *ORTHOP NURS 23*(1), 3-11.

Critical Care Network. (2003). Check mental status or risk missing problems: quick assessment checks for neurological deficit. *Hospital Case Management 11*(5), 72-4.

Dellasega, C. (1992). Home health nurses' assessments of cognition. *Applied Nursing Research, 5*(3), 127-133.

Foreman, M., Theis, S., & Anderson, M. A. (1993). Adverse events in the hospitalized elderly. *Clinical Nursing Research, 2*(3) 360-370.

Foreman, M., Gilles, D., & Wagner, D. (1989). Impaired cognition in the critically ill elderly patient: Clinical implications. *Critical Care Nursing Quarterly, 12*(1), 61-73.

Gerdner, L. A., & Hall, G. R. (2001). Chronic confusion. In M. Maas, K. Buckwalter, M. Hardy, T. Tripp-Reimer, M. Titler, & J. Specht (Eds.), *Nursing care of older adults: Diagnoses, outcomes & interventions* (pp. 421-441). St. Louis: Mosby.

Hickey, J. V. (2003). *The clinical practice of neurological and neurosurgical nursing* (5th ed.). Philadelphia: Lippincott Williams & Wilkins.

Inaba-Roland, K., & Maricle, R. (1992). Assessing delirium in the acute care setting. *Heart & Lung, 21*(1), 48-55.

Mason, P. (1989). Cognitive assessment parameters and tools for the critically injured adult. *Critical Care Nursing Clinics of North America, 1*(1), 45-53.

Meyer, J., Xu, G., Thornby, J., Chowdhury, M., & Quach, M. (2002). Longitudinal analysis of abnormal domains comprising mild cognitive impairment (MCI) during aging. *Journal of Neurological Sciences, 201*(1-2), 19-25.

+Pfeiffer, E. (1975). A short portable mental status questionnaire for the assessment of organic brain deficit in elderly patients. *American Geriatrics Society, 23*(10), 433-441.

Souder, E., & O'Sullivan, P. S. (2000). Nursing documentation versus standardized assessment of cognitive status in hospitalized medical patients. *Applied Nursing Research, 13*(1), 29-36.

Strub, R. L., & Black, F. W. (2000). *The mental status examination in neurology* (4th ed.). Philadelphia: F.A. Davis.

Thibault, J. M., & Steiner, R. W. P. (2004). Efficient identification of adults with depression and dementia. *American Family Physician, 70*(6), 1101-10, 1023-5.

Comfort Status—2008

Domain-Perceived Health (V)

Class-Health & Life Quality (U)

Scale(s)-Severely compromised to Not compromised (a)

Care Recipient:

Data Source:

Definition: Overall physical, psychospiritual, sociocultural, and environmental ease and safety of an individual

OUTCOME TARGET RATING: Maintain at_____ Increase to_____

Comfort Status Overall Rating	Severely compromised 1	Substantially compromised 2	Moderately compromised 3	Mildly compromised 4	Not compromised 5	
INDICATORS:						
200801 Physical well-being	1	2	3	4	5	NA
200802 Symptom control	1	2	3	4	5	NA
200803 Psychological well-being	1	2	3	4	5	NA
200804 Physical surroundings	1	2	3	4	5	NA
200805 Room temperature	1	2	3	4	5	NA
200806 Social support from family	1	2	3	4	5	NA
200807 Social support from friends	1	2	3	4	5	NA
200808 Social relationships	1	2	3	4	5	NA
200809 Spiritual life	1	2	3	4	5	NA
200810 Care consistent with cultural beliefs	1	2	3	4	5	NA
200811 Care consistent with needs	1	2	3	4	5	NA
200812 Ability to communicate needs	1	2	3	4	5	NA

Outcome Content References:

Gropper, E. (1992). Promoting health by promoting comfort. *Nursing Forum, 27*(2), 5-8.

Hamilton, J. (1989). Comfort and the hospitalized chronically ill. *Journal of Gerontological Nursing, 15*(4), 28-33.

Kennedy, G. (1991). *A nursing investigation of comfort and comforting care of the acutely ill patient.* Unpublished doctoral dissertation, The University of Texas, Austin.

Kolcaba, K. (2003). *Comfort theory and practice: A vision for holistic health care and research.* New York: Springer.

Kolcaba, K., & DiMarco, M. (2005). Comfort theory and its application to pediatric nursing. *Pediatric Nursing, 31*(3), 187-194.

Kolcaba, K., Panno, J., & Holder, C. (2000). Acute care for elders (ACE): A holistic model for geriatric orthopaedic nursing care. *Journal of Orthopaedic Nursing, 19*(6), 53-60.

Tipton, L. (2001). A qualitative study of hope and the environment of persons living with cancer. *Dissertation Abstracts International, 62*(03), 1326B. (UMI No. 3008460).

Comfort Status: Environment—2009

Domain-Perceived Health (V)

Class-Health & Life Quality (U)

Scale(s)-Severely compromised to Not compromised (a)

Care Recipient:

Data Source:

C

Definition: Environmental ease, comfort, and safety of surroundings

OUTCOME TARGET RATING: Maintain at_____   Increase to_____

Comfort Status: Environment Overall Rating	Severely compromised 1	Substantially compromised 2	Moderately compromised 3	Mildly compromised 4	Not compromised 5	
INDICATORS:						
200901 Needed supplies and equipment within reach	1	2	3	4	5	NA
200902 Room temperature	1	2	3	4	5	NA
200903 Environment conducive to sleep	1	2	3	4	5	NA
200904 Contentment with physical surroundings	1	2	3	4	5	NA
200905 Orderliness of environment	1	2	3	4	5	NA
200906 Cleanliness of environment	1	2	3	4	5	NA
200907 Floor free of clutter	1	2	3	4	5	NA
200908 Safety devices used appropriately	1	2	3	4	5	NA
200909 Room lighting	1	2	3	4	5	NA
200910 Privacy	1	2	3	4	5	NA
200911 Availability of space for visitors	1	2	3	4	5	NA
200912 Comfortable bed	1	2	3	4	5	NA
200913 Comfortable furniture	1	2	3	4	5	NA
200914 Needed environmental adaptations	1	2	3	4	5	NA
200915 Peaceful environment	1	2	3	4	5	NA
200916 Control of noise	1	2	3	4	5	NA
200917 Control of odors	1	2	3	4	5	NA

Outcome Content References:

Gropper, E. (1992). Promoting health by promoting comfort. *Nursing Forum, 27*(2), 5-8.

Hamilton, J. (1989). Comfort and the hospitalized chronically ill. *Journal of Gerontological Nursing, 15*(4), 28-33.

Kennedy, G. (1991). *A nursing investigation of comfort and comforting care of the acutely ill patient.* Unpublished doctoral dissertation, The University of Texas, Austin.

Kolcaba, K. (2003). *Comfort theory and practice: A vision for holistic health care and research.* New York: Springer.

Kolcaba, K., Panno, J., & Holder, C. (2000). Acute care for elders (ACE): A holistic model for geriatric orthopaedic nursing care. *Journal of Orthopaedic Nursing, 19*(6), 53-60.

Oliver, D., Daly, F., Martin, F. C., & McMurdo, M. E. T. (2004). Risk factors and risk assessment tools for falls in hospital in-patients: A systematic review. *Age and Ageing, 33*(2), 122-130.

Sherwood, G., Thomas, E., Bennett, D., & Lewis, P. (2002). A teamwork model to promote patient safety in critical care. *Critical Care Nursing Clinics of North America, 14*(4), 333-340.

Tipton, L. (2001). *A qualitative study of hope and the environment of persons living with cancer. Dissertation Abstracts International, 62*(03), 1326B. (UMI No. 3008460).

C

Comfort Status: Physical—2010

Domain-Perceived Health (V)

Class-Health & Life Quality (U)

Scale(s)-Severely compromised to Not compromised (a) and Severe to None (n)

Care Recipient:

Data Source:

Definition: Physical ease related to bodily sensations and homeostatic mechanisms

OUTCOME TARGET RATING: Maintain at_____   Increase to_____

Comfort Status: Physical Overall Rating	Severely compromised 1	Substantially compromised 2	Moderately compromised 3	Mildly compromised 4	Not compromised 5	
INDICATORS:						
201001 Symptom control	1	2	3	4	5	NA
201002 Physical well-being	1	2	3	4	5	NA
201003 Muscular relaxation	1	2	3	4	5	NA
201004 Comfortable position	1	2	3	4	5	NA
201005 Comfortable clothing	1	2	3	4	5	NA
201006 Personal grooming and hygiene	1	2	3	4	5	NA
201007 Food intake	1	2	3	4	5	NA
201008 Fluid intake	1	2	3	4	5	NA
201009 Energy level	1	2	3	4	5	NA
201010 Body temperature	1	2	3	4	5	NA
201011 Airway patency	1	2	3	4	5	NA
201012 Oxygen saturation	1	2	3	4	5	NA

	Severe	Substantial	Moderate	Mild	None	
201013 Itching	1	2	3	4	5	NA
201014 Labored breathing	1	2	3	4	5	NA
201015 Air hunger	1	2	3	4	5	NA
201016 Restless legs syndrome	1	2	3	4	5	NA
201017 Muscle aches	1	2	3	4	5	NA
201018 Headache	1	2	3	4	5	NA
201019 Nausea	1	2	3	4	5	NA
201020 Vomiting	1	2	3	4	5	NA
201021 Urinary incontinence	1	2	3	4	5	NA
201022 Bowel incontinence	1	2	3	4	5	NA
201023 Diarrhea	1	2	3	4	5	NA
201024 Constipation	1	2	3	4	5	NA

Outcome Content References:

Dowd, T., Kolcaba, K., & Steiner, R. (2000). Cognitive strategies to enhance comfort and decrease episodes of urinary incontinence. *Holistic Nursing Practice, 14*(2), 91-102.

Gropper, E. (1992). Promoting health by promoting comfort. *Nursing Forum, 27*(2), 5-8.

Hamilton, J. (1989). Comfort and the hospitalized chronically ill. *Journal of Gerontological Nursing, 15*(4), 28-33.

Kennedy, G. (1991). *A nursing investigation of comfort and comforting care of the acutely ill patient.* Unpublished doctoral dissertation, The University of Texas, Austin.

Kolcaba, K. (2003). *Comfort theory and practice: A vision for holistic health care and research.* New York: Springer.

Tipton, L. (2001). A qualitative study of hope and the environment of persons living with cancer. *Dissertation Abstracts International, 62*(03), 1326B. (UMI No. 3008460).

Comfort Status: Psychospiritual—2011

Domain-Perceived Health (V)

Class-Health & Life Quality (U)

Scale(s)-Severely compromised to Not compromised (a) and Severe to None (n)

Care Recipient:

Data Source:

C

Definition: Psychospiritual ease related to self-concept, emotional well-being, source of inspiration, and meaning and purpose in one's life

OUTCOME TARGET RATING: Maintain at_____   Increase to_____

Comfort Status: Psychospiritual Overall Rating	Severely compromised 1	Substantially compromised 2	Moderately compromised 3	Mildly compromised 4	Not compromised 5	
INDICATORS:						
201101 Psychological well-being	1	2	3	4	5	NA
201102 Faith	1	2	3	4	5	NA
201103 Hope	1	2	3	4	5	NA
201104 Self-concept	1	2	3	4	5	NA
201105 Internal picture of self	1	2	3	4	5	NA
201106 Calm and tranquil affect	1	2	3	4	5	NA
201107 Expressions of optimism	1	2	3	4	5	NA
201108 Goal setting	1	2	3	4	5	NA
201109 Meaning and purpose in life	1	2	3	4	5	NA
201110 Spiritual contentment	1	2	3	4	5	NA
201111 Connectedness with inner-self	1	2	3	4	5	NA
	Severe	Substantial	Moderate	Mild	None	
201112 Depression	1	2	3	4	5	NA
201113 Anxiety	1	2	3	4	5	NA
201114 Stress	1	2	3	4	5	NA
201115 Fear	1	2	3	4	5	NA
201116 Loss of faith	1	2	3	4	5	NA
201117 Sense of spiritual abandonment	1	2	3	4	5	NA
201118 Suicidal thoughts	1	2	3	4	5	NA

Outcome Content References:

Gropper, E. (1992). Promoting health by promoting comfort. *Nursing Forum, 27*(2), 5-8.

Hamilton, J. (1989). Comfort and the hospitalized chronically ill. *Journal of Gerontological Nursing, 15*(4), 28-33.

Kennedy, G. (1991). *A nursing investigation of comfort and comforting care of the acutely ill patient.* Unpublished doctoral dissertation, The University of Texas, Austin.

Kolcaba, K., & Fisher, E. (1996). A holistic perspective on comfort care as an advance directive. *Critical Care Nursing Quarterly, 18*(4), 66-76.

Kolcaba, K. (2003). *Comfort theory and practice: A vision for holistic health care and research.* New York: Springer.

Puchalski, C., Kilpatrick, S., McCullough, M., & Larson, D. (2003). A systematic review of spiritual and religious variables in Palliative Medicine, American Journal of Hospice and Palliative Care, Hospice Journal, Journal of Palliative Care, and Journal of Pain and Symptom Management. *Palliative and Supportive Care, 1*, 7-13.

Tipton, L. (2001). A qualitative study of hope and the environment of persons living with cancer. *Dissertation Abstracts International, 62*(03), 1326B. (UMI No. 3008460).

Comfort Status: Sociocultural—2012

Domain-Perceived Health (V)

Class-Health & Life Quality (U)

Scale(s)-Severely compromised to Not compromised (a)

Care Recipient:

Data Source:

Definition: Social ease related to interpersonal, family, and societal relationships within a cultural context

OUTCOME TARGET RATING: Maintain at_____ Increase to_____

Comfort Status: Sociocultural Overall Rating	Severely compromised 1	Substantially compromised 2	Moderately compromised 3	Mildly compromised 4	Not compromised 5	
INDICATORS:						
201201 Social support from family	1	2	3	4	5	NA
201202 Social support from friends	1	2	3	4	5	NA
201203 Relationships with family	1	2	3	4	5	NA
201204 Relationships with friends	1	2	3	4	5	NA
201205 Trust in relationships with family	1	2	3	4	5	NA
201206 Trust in relationships with friends	1	2	3	4	5	NA
201207 Social interactions with others	1	2	3	4	5	NA
201208 Care consistent with cultural beliefs	1	2	3	4	5	NA
201209 Availability of culture-specific foods	1	2	3	4	5	NA
201210 Incorporation of cultural beliefs into daily activities	1	2	3	4	5	NA
201211 Use of spoken language	1	2	3	4	5	NA
201212 Ability to communicate needs	1	2	3	4	5	NA
201213 Use of strategies to enhance communication	1	2	3	4	5	NA
201214 Willingness to call on others for help	1	2	3	4	5	NA
201215 Use of disclosure	1	2	3	4	5	NA

Outcome Content References:

Gropper, E. (1992). Promoting health by promoting comfort. *Nursing Forum, 27*(2), 5-8.

Hamilton, J. (1989). Comfort and the hospitalized chronically ill. *Journal of Gerontological Nursing, 15*(4), 28-33.

Kennedy, G. (1991). *A nursing investigation of comfort and comforting care of the acutely ill patient.* Unpublished doctoral dissertation, The University of Texas, Austin.

Kolcaba, K. (2003). *Comfort theory and practice: A vision for holistic health care and research.* New York: Springer.

Leininger, M., & McFarland, M. (2002). *Transcultural nursing concepts, theories, research, & practices* (3rd ed.). New York: McGraw-Hill.

Tipton, L. (2001). A qualitative study of hope and the environment of persons living with cancer. *Dissertation Abstracts International, 62*(03), 1326B. (UMI No. 3008460).

Comfortable Death—2007

Domain-Perceived Health (V)   *Care Recipient:*

Class-Health & Life Quality (U)   *Data Source:*

Scale(s)-Severely compromised to Not compromised (a) and Severe to None (n)

C

Definition: Physical, psychospiritual, sociocultural and environmental ease with the impending end of life

OUTCOME TARGET RATING: Maintain at_____   Increase to_____

Comfortable Death Overall Rating	Severely compromised 1	Substantially compromised 2	Moderately compromised 3	Mildly compromised 4	Not compromised 5	
INDICATORS:						
200701 Calm affect	1	2	3	4	5	NA
200720 Physical environment	1	2	3	4	5	NA
200721 Room temperature	1	2	3	4	5	NA
200722 Psychological well-being	1	2	3	4	5	NA
200703 Airway patency	1	2	3	4	5	NA
200704 Body temperature	1	2	3	4	5	NA
200705 Comfortable position	1	2	3	4	5	NA
200723 Muscular relaxation	1	2	3	4	5	NA
200724 Support from family	1	2	3	4	5	NA
200725 Support from friends	1	2	3	4	5	NA
200726 Spiritual life	1	2	3	4	5	NA
200708 Personal hygiene	1	2	3	4	5	NA
200709 Oral hygiene	1	2	3	4	5	NA
200710 Food and fluid intake as desired	1	2	3	4	5	NA
200727 Expression of readiness for impending death	1	2	3	4	5	NA

	Severe	Substantial	Moderate	Mild	None	
200711 Moaning	1	2	3	4	5	NA
200712 Suffering	1	2	3	4	5	NA
200713 Thrashing	1	2	3	4	5	NA
200714 Pain	1	2	3	4	5	NA
200715 Itching	1	2	3	4	5	NA
200716 Retching or vomiting	1	2	3	4	5	NA
200717 Diarrhea	1	2	3	4	5	NA
200718 Labored breathing	1	2	3	4	5	NA
200719 Air hunger	1	2	3	4	5	NA
200728 Hyperactivity	1	2	3	4	5	NA
200729 Grimacing	1	2	3	4	5	NA
200730 Rebound tenderness	1	2	3	4	5	NA
200731 Jerking	1	2	3	4	5	NA
200732 Restlessness	1	2	3	4	5	NA

3rd edition 2004; Revised 4th edition

Continued

C

Outcome Content References:

Byock, I. (1997). *Dying well: The prospect for growth at the end of life.* New York: Riverhead Books.

Ferrell, B. R. (1999). Caring at the end of life. *Reflections, 25*(4), 31-37.

Gropper, E. (1992). Promoting health by promoting comfort. *Nursing Forum, 27*(2), 5-8.

Hamilton, J. (1989). Comfort and the hospitalized chronically ill. *Journal of Gerontological Nursing, 15*(4), 28-33.

Kennedy, G. (1991). A nursing investigation of comfort and comforting care of the acutely ill patient. Unpublished doctoral dissertation, The University of Texas, Austin.

Kolcaba, K. (2003). *Comfort theory and practice: A vision for holistic health care and research.* New York: Springer.

Kolcaba, K., & DiMarco, M. (2005). Comfort theory and its application to pediatric nursing. *Pediatric Nursing, 31*(3), 187-194.

Kolcaba, K., & Fisher, E. (1996). A holistic perspective on comfort care as an advance directive. *Critical Care Nursing Quarterly, 18*(4), 66-76.

Communication—0902

Domain-Physiologic Health (II)

Class-Neurocognitive (J)

Scale(s)-Severely compromised to Not compromised (a)

Care Recipient:

Data Source:

Definition: Reception, interpretation, and expression of spoken, written and non-verbal messages

OUTCOME TARGET RATING: Maintain at_____ Increase to_____

Communication Overall Rating	Severely compromised 1	Substantially compromised 2	Moderately compromised 3	Mildly compromised 4	Not compromised 5	
INDICATORS:						
090201 Use of written language	1	2	3	4	5	NA
090202 Use of spoken language	1	2	3	4	5	NA
090203 Use of pictures and drawings	1	2	3	4	5	NA
090204 Use of sign language	1	2	3	4	5	NA
090205 Use of non-verbal language	1	2	3	4	5	NA
090206 Acknowledgment of messages received	1	2	3	4	5	NA
090210 Accurate interpretation of messages received	1	2	3	4	5	NA
090207 Directs messages to correct recipient	1	2	3	4	5	NA
090208 Exchanges messages accurately with others	1	2	3	4	5	NA

1st edition 1997; Revised 3rd edition 2004

Outcome Content References:

Arnold, E., & Boggs, K. (1999). *Interpersonal relationships: Professional communications skills for nurses* (3rd ed.). Philadelphia: W.B. Saunders.

Emick-Herring, B. (2001). Impaired communication. In M. Maas, K. Buckwalter, M. Hardy, T. Tripp-Reimer, M. Titler, & J. Specht (Eds.), *Nursing care of older adults: Diagnoses, outcomes & interventions* (pp. 664-678). St. Louis: Mosby.

+Harvey, R., & Jellinek, H. (1981). Functional performance assessment: A program approach. *Archives Physical Medicine & Rehabilitation*, 62(9), 456-460.

Potter, P. A., & Perry, A. G. (2001). *Fundamentals of nursing* (5th ed.). St. Louis: Mosby.

Strub, R. L., & Black, F. W. (2000). *The mental status examination in neurology* (4th ed.). Philadelphia: F.A. Davis.

Communication: Expressive—0903

Domain-Physiologic Health (II)

Class-Neurocognitive (J)

Scale(s)-Severely compromised to Not compromised (a)

Care Recipient:

Data Source:

C

Definition: Expression of meaningful verbal and/or non-verbal messages

OUTCOME TARGET RATING: Maintain at_____   Increase to_____

Communication: Expressive Overall Rating	Severely compromised 1	Substantially compromised 2	Moderately compromised 3	Mildly compromised 4	Not compromised 5	
INDICATORS:						
090301 Use of written language	1	2	3	4	5	NA
090302 Use of spoken language: vocal	1	2	3	4	5	NA
090303 Use of spoken language: esophageal	1	2	3	4	5	NA
090304 Clarity of speech	1	2	3	4	5	NA
090305 Use of pictures and drawings	1	2	3	4	5	NA
090306 Use of sign language	1	2	3	4	5	NA
090307 Use of non-verbal language	1	2	3	4	5	NA
090308 Directs messages to correct recipient	1	2	3	4	5	NA

1st edition 1997; Revised 3rd edition 2004

Outcome Content References:

Arnold, E., & Boggs, K. (1999). *Interpersonal relationships: Professional communications skills for nurses* (3rd ed.). Philadelphia: W.B. Saunders.

Emick-Herring, B. (2001). Impaired communication. In M. Maas, K. Buckwalter, M. Hardy, T. Tripp-Reimer, M. Titler, & J. Specht (Eds.), *Nursing care of older adults: Diagnoses, outcomes & interventions* (pp. 664-678). St. Louis: Mosby.

+Harvey, R., & Jellinek, H. (1981). Functional performance assessment: A program approach. *Archives Physical Medicine & Rehabilitation, 62*(9), 456-460.

Potter, P. A., & Perry, A. G. (2001). *Fundamentals of nursing* (5th ed.). St. Louis: Mosby.

Strub, R. L., & Black, F. W. (2000). *The mental status examination in neurology* (4th ed.). Philadelphia: F.A. Davis.

Communication: Receptive—0904

Domain-Physiologic Health (II)

Class-Neurocognitive (J)

Scale(s)-Severely compromised to Not compromised (a)

Care Recipient:

Data Source:

C

Definition: Reception and interpretation of verbal and/or non-verbal messages

OUTCOME TARGET RATING: Maintain at_____   Increase to_____

Communication: Receptive Overall Rating	Severely compromised 1	Substantially compromised 2	Moderately compromised 3	Mildly compromised 4	Not compromised 5	
INDICATORS:						
090401 Interpretation of written language	1	2	3	4	5	NA
090402 Interpretation of spoken language	1	2	3	4	5	NA
090403 Interpretation of pictures and drawings	1	2	3	4	5	NA
090404 Interpretation of sign language	1	2	3	4	5	NA
090405 Interpretation of non-verbal language	1	2	3	4	5	NA
090406 Acknowledgment of messages received	1	2	3	4	5	NA

1st edition 1997; Revised 2nd edition 2000; Revised 3rd edition 2004

Outcome Content References:

Arnold, E., & Boggs, K. (1999). *Interpersonal relationships: Professional communications skills for nurses* (3rd ed.). Philadelphia: W.B. Saunders.

Emick-Herring, B. (2001). Impaired communication. In M. Maas, K. Buckwalter, M. Hardy, T. Tripp-Reimer, M. Titler, & J. Specht (Eds.), *Nursing care of older adults: Diagnoses, outcomes & interventions* (pp. 664-678). St. Louis: Mosby.

+Harvey, R., & Jellinek, H. (1981). Functional performance assessment: A program approach. *Archives Physical Medicine & Rehabilitation, 62*(9), 456-460.

Potter, P. A., & Perry, A. G. (2001). *Fundamentals of nursing* (5th ed.). St. Louis: Mosby.

Strub, R. L., & Black, F. W. (2000). *The mental status examination in neurology* (4th ed.). Philadelphia: F.A. Davis.

Community Competence—2700

Domain-Community Health (VII)

Class-Community Well-Being (b)

Scale(s)-Poor to Excellent (r)

Care Recipient:

Data Source:

C

Definition: Capacity of a community to collectively problem solve to achieve community goals

OUTCOME TARGET RATING: Maintain at_____   Increase to_____

Community Competence Overall Rating	**Poor 1**	**Fair 2**	**Good 3**	**Very good 4**	**Excellent 5**	

INDICATORS:

270001	Participation rates in community activities	1	2	3	4	5	NA
270003	Consideration of common and competing interests among groups when solving problems	1	2	3	4	5	NA
270004	Representation of all segments of the community in problem solving	1	2	3	4	5	NA
270005	Community issues articulated in media	1	2	3	4	5	NA
270006	Community issues articulated in community forums	1	2	3	4	5	NA
270007	Focus on community versus individual agendas	1	2	3	4	5	NA
270021	Collaboration among community groups to resolve problems	1	2	3	4	5	NA
270009	Consensus on goals and priorities	1	2	3	4	5	NA
270010	Consensus on actions to implement the goals	1	2	3	4	5	NA
270011	Communication among members and groups	1	2	3	4	5	NA
270012	Effective use of conflict management strategies	1	2	3	4	5	NA
270013	Procurement of resources	1	2	3	4	5	NA
270014	Use of external resources to meet goals	1	2	3	4	5	NA
270015	Flexibility of structures and processes that guide community decision-making	1	2	3	4	5	NA
270016	Participation rate in local government elections	1	2	3	4	5	NA
270017	Participation rate in school elections	1	2	3	4	5	NA
270018	Members attendance at community forums	1	2	3	4	5	NA
270019	Attainment of community goals	1	2	3	4	5	NA

2nd edition 2000; Revised 3rd edition 2004; Revised 4th edition

Outcome Content References:

Denham, A., Quinn, S., & Gamble, D. (1998). Community organizing for health promotion in the rural south: An exploration of community competence. *Family and Community Health, 21*(1), 1-21.

Eng, E., & Parker, E. (1994). Measuring community competence in the Mississippi Delta: The interface between program evaluation and empowerment. *Health Education Quarterly, 21*(2), 119-120.

Goeppinger, L., Lassiter, P., & Wilcox, B. (1982). Community health is community competence. *Nursing Outlook, 30*(8), 464-467.

Stanhope, M., & Lancaster, J. (2000). *Community health nursing* (5th ed.). St. Louis: Mosby.

Community Disaster Readiness—2804

Domain-Community Health (VII)

Class-Community Health Protection (c)

Scale-Not adequate to Totally adequate (f)

Care Recipient:

Data Source:

C

Definition: Community preparedness to respond to a natural or man-made calamitous event

OUTCOME TARGET RATING: Maintain at_____   Increase to_____

Community Disaster Readiness Overall Rating	Not adequate 1	Slightly adequate 2	Moderately adequate 3	Substantially adequate 4	Totally adequate 5	
INDICATORS:						
280401 Identification of potential types of disasters	1	2	3	4	5	NA
280432 Plan to protect water	1	2	3	4	5	NA
280433 Plan to protect food supplies	1	2	3	4	5	NA
280404 Policy designating temporary administrative authority	1	2	3	4	5	NA
280405 Public health laboratory facilities	1	2	3	4	5	NA
280406 Public health disease surveillance system	1	2	3	4	5	NA
280434 Plan to access electronic health records	1	2	3	4	5	NA
280408 Mass immunization plan	1	2	3	4	5	NA
280409 Surge capacity of hospital resources	1	2	3	4	5	NA
280435 Written plan for mobilization of personnel	1	2	3	4	5	NA
280436 Written plan for evacuation	1	2	3	4	5	NA
280437 Written plan for triage	1	2	3	4	5	NA
280438 Current written plan for communication	1	2	3	4	5	NA
280439 Current written plan for resource appropriation	1	2	3	4	5	NA
280411 Essential agency involvement in planning	1	2	3	4	5	NA
280412 Assignment of agency responsibilities in the event of disaster	1	2	3	4	5	NA
280413 Ongoing training for disaster response personnel	1	2	3	4	5	NA
280414 Plan to protect health and safety of response personnel	1	2	3	4	5	NA
280415 Notification network to alert response personnel	1	2	3	4	5	NA
280416 Notification network to alert government and support agencies	1	2	3	4	5	NA

Continued

C

	Not adequate	Slightly adequate	Moderately adequate	Substantially adequate	Totally adequate	
280417 Operational communication equipment	1	2	3	4	5	NA
280440 Plan for alternative communication among disaster personnel	1	2	3	4	5	NA
280441 Plan for alternative communication among agency networks	1	2	3	4	5	NA
280419 Functional warning mechanisms	1	2	3	4	5	NA
280420 Operational alternative utility resources	1	2	3	4	5	NA
280421 Emergency power backup	1	2	3	4	5	NA
280422 Equipment and supply availability	1	2	3	4	5	NA
280423 Equipment and supply maintenance	1	2	3	4	5	NA
280424 Designated, equipped shelters	1	2	3	4	5	NA
280425 Emergency shelter capacity	1	2	3	4	5	NA
280442 Plan to protect animals	1	2	3	4	5	NA
280426 Regular mass casualty drills with evaluation	1	2	3	4	5	NA
280427 Public education on disaster warning and response	1	2	3	4	5	NA
280428 Media plan for public information updates	1	2	3	4	5	NA
280443 Plan for coordination of victim health care	1	2	3	4	5	NA
280444 Plan for documentation of victim health care	1	2	3	4	5	NA
280430 Plan for availability of mental health care services	1	2	3	4	5	NA
280431 Written post disaster plan	1	2	3	4	5	NA

3rd edition 2004; Revised 4th edition

Outcome Content References:

American Public Health Association. (2002). *One year after the terrorist attacks: Is public health prepared?* Washington, DC: Author.

American Red Cross. (2006). *Disaster services.* Available from http://www.redcross.org/services/disaster

Chaffee, M. W. (2005). Hospital response to acute-onset disasters: The state of the science in 2005. *Nursing Clinics of North America, 40,* 565-577.

Hassmiller, S. (2000). Disaster management. In M. Stanhope & J. Lancaster (Eds.), *Community and public health nursing* (5th ed.). St. Louis: Mosby.

Landesman, L. Y. (2001). *Public health management of disasters: The practice guide.* Washington, DC: American Public Health Association.

Millin, M. G., Jenkins, J. L., & Kirsch, T. (2006), A comparative analysis of two external health care disaster responses following hurricane Katrina. *Prehospital Emergency Care, 10,* 451-456.

Rowney, R. (2005). The role of public health nursing in emergency preparedness and response. *Nursing Clinics of North America, 40,* 499-509.

Santamaria, B. (1995). Nursing in a disaster. In C. M. Smith & F. A. Maurer (Eds.), *Community health nursing: Theory and practice.* Philadelphia: W.B. Saunders.

Stratton, S. J., & Tyler, R. D. (2006). Characteristics of medical surge capacity demand for sudden-impact disasters. *Society for Academic Emergency Medicine, 13,* 1193-1197.

Community Disaster Response—2806

Domain-Community Health (VII)

Class-Community Health Protection (c)

Scale-Not adequate to Totally adequate (f)

Care Recipient:

Data Source:

Definition: Community response following a natural or man-made calamitous event

OUTCOME TARGET RATING: Maintain at_____   Increase to_____

Community Disaster Response Overall Rating	Not adequate 1	Slightly adequate 2	Moderately adequate 3	Substantially adequate 4	Totally adequate 5	
INDICATORS:						
280601 Availability of safe water	1	2	3	4	5	NA
280602 Availability of safe food	1	2	3	4	5	NA
280603 Availability of medication	1	2	3	4	5	NA
280604 Availability of supplies	1	2	3	4	5	NA
280605 Availability of shelters	1	2	3	4	5	NA
280606 Availability of hospital resources	1	2	3	4	5	NA
280607 Availability of personnel	1	2	3	4	5	NA
280608 Mobilization of personnel	1	2	3	4	5	NA
280609 Command authority identified	1	2	3	4	5	NA
280610 Evacuation of population	1	2	3	4	5	NA
280611 Triage of injured individuals	1	2	3	4	5	NA
280612 Evacuation of injured individuals	1	2	3	4	5	NA
280613 Operation of communication system	1	2	3	4	5	NA
280614 Government agencies notified of needs	1	2	3	4	5	NA
280615 Support agencies notified of needs	1	2	3	4	5	NA
280616 Timely notification of response personnel	1	2	3	4	5	NA
280617 Information provided to public in a timely manner	1	2	3	4	5	NA
280618 Response of government agencies in carrying out responsibilities	1	2	3	4	5	NA
280619 Response of support agencies in carrying out responsibilities	1	2	3	4	5	NA
280620 Coordination efforts of local, state, federal, international and non-governmental agencies	1	2	3	4	5	NA
280621 Performance of response personnel	1	2	3	4	5	NA
280622 Operation of emergency power	1	2	3	4	5	NA

Continued

		Not adequate	Slightly adequate	Moderately adequate	Substantially adequate	Totally adequate	
280623	Availability of functional equipment	1	2	3	4	5	NA
280624	Availability of decontamination equipment	1	2	3	4	5	NA
280625	Access to electronic health records	1	2	3	4	5	NA
280626	Mental health care available for population	1	2	3	4	5	NA
280627	Mental health care available for response personnel	1	2	3	4	5	NA
280628	Response of public health laboratory facilities	1	2	3	4	5	NA
280629	Accurate disposition logs of patient and evacuees	1	2	3	4	5	NA
280630	Data collected on injury patterns	1	2	3	4	5	NA
280631	Data collected on disease incidence	1	2	3	4	5	NA
280632	Mass immunization plan	1	2	3	4	5	NA
280633	Availability of morgue facilities	1	2	3	4	5	NA
280634	Provision of care for animals	1	2	3	4	5	NA
280635	Replacement of prescribed medication for individuals with chronic illness	1	2	3	4	5	NA
280636	Post disaster follow-up	1	2	3	4	5	NA

Outcome Content References:

Bass, M. L., Freidhoff, T., & Murphy, E. (2006). Providing consistent medical coverage at community events: North Carolina Rex Hospital's emergency response team. *Journal of Emergency Nursing, 32*, 75-77.

Chaffee, M. W. (2005). Hospital response to acute-onset disasters: The state of the science in 2005. *Nursing Clinics of North America, 40*, 565-577.

Millin, M. G., Jenkins, J. L., & Kirsch, T. (2006), A comparative analysis of two external health care disaster responses following hurricane Katrina. *Prehospital Emergency Care, 10*, 451-456.

Milsten, A. (2000). Hospital responses to acute-onset disasters: A review. *Prehospital Disaster Medicine, 15*(1), 32-45.

Mitchell, A. M., Sakraida, T. J., & Zalice, K. K. (2005). Disaster care: Psychological considerations. *Nursing Clinics of North America, 40*, 535-550.

Tarantino, D. (2006). Asian tsunami relief: Department of defense public health response: Policy and strategic coordination considerations. *Military Medicine, 171*(10), 15-18.

Community Health Status—2701

Domain-Community Health (VII)

Class-Community Well-Being (b)

Scale(s)-Poor to Excellent (r)

Care Recipient:

Data Source:

C

Definition: General state of well-being of a community or population

OUTCOME TARGET RATING: Maintain at_____   Increase to_____

Community Health Status Overall Rating	Poor 1	Fair 2	Good 3	Very good 4	Excellent 5	
INDICATORS:						
270111 Health status of infants	1	2	3	4	5	NA
270112 Health status of children	1	2	3	4	5	NA
270113 Health status of adolescents	1	2	3	4	5	NA
270114 Health status of adults	1	2	3	4	5	NA
270115 Health status of elders	1	2	3	4	5	NA
270132 Health status of minority populations	1	2	3	4	5	NA
270101 Participation rates in preventive health care services	1	2	3	4	5	NA
270102 Prevalence of health promotion programs	1	2	3	4	5	NA
270103 Prevalence of health protection programs	1	2	3	4	5	NA
270104 School enrollment rate	1	2	3	4	5	NA
270105 School attendance rate	1	2	3	4	5	NA
270106 Participation rates in worksite health programs	1	2	3	4	5	NA
270107 Participation rates in community health programs	1	2	3	4	5	NA
270108 Participation rates in school health programs	1	2	3	4	5	NA
270109 Evidence of health protection measures	1	2	3	4	5	NA
270110 Members with adequate health insurance coverage	1	2	3	4	5	NA
270116 Attendance at programs for healthy pregnancy	1	2	3	4	5	NA
270117 Compliance with environmental health standards	1	2	3	4	5	NA
270124 Mortality rates	1	2	3	4	5	NA
270133 Maternal mortality rates	1	2	3	4	5	NA
270119 Morbidity rates	1	2	3	4	5	NA
270120 Mental health illness rates	1	2	3	4	5	NA

Continued

		Poor	Fair	Good	Very good	Excellent	
270125	Chronic disease rates	1	2	3	4	5	NA
270134	Substance abuse rates adults	1	2	3	4	5	NA
270135	Substance abuse rates adolescents	1	2	3	4	5	NA
270136	Smoking rates	1	2	3	4	5	NA
270126	Sexually transmitted disease rates	1	2	3	4	5	NA
270137	Preterm birth rates	1	2	3	4	5	NA
270138	Low birth weight rates	1	2	3	4	5	NA
270121	Injury rates	1	2	3	4	5	NA
270122	Crime statistics	1	2	3	4	5	NA
270139	Homicide rates	1	2	3	4	5	NA
270127	Health surveillance data systems in place	1	2	3	4	5	NA
270128	Community health standards for health measurement and evaluation are defined	1	2	3	4	5	NA
270129	Monitoring of community health standards for health measurement and evaluation	1	2	3	4	5	NA
270130	Community demographics represented in health care planning and evaluation	1	2	3	4	5	NA

2nd edition 2000; Revised 3rd edition 2004; Revised 4th edition

Outcome Content References:

Deal, L. (1994). The effectiveness of community health nursing interventions: A literature review. *Public Health Nursing, 2*(5), 315-322.

Stanhope, M., & Lancaster, J. (2000). *Community health nursing* (5th ed.). St. Louis: Mosby.

Stoto, M. (1997). Sharing responsibility for the public's health: A new perspective from the Institute of Medicine. *Journal of Public Health Management and Practice, 3*(5), 22-34.

U.S. Department of Health and Human Services. (2000). *Healthy People 2010*. Washington, DC: Government Printing Office.

U.S. Department of Health and Human Services. (1998). *Clinician's handbook of preventive services: Put prevention into practice* (2nd ed.). Washington, DC: Government Printing Office.

U.S. Department of Health and Human Services. (1991). *Healthy People 2000: National health promotion and disease prevention objectives*. (DHHS Pub No (PHS) 91-50012). Washington, DC: Government Printing Office.

U.S. Preventive Services Task Force. (1996). *Guide to clinical preventive services* (2nd ed.). Baltimore: Williams & Wilkins.

Community Health Status: Immunity—2800

Domain-Community Health (VII)

Class-Community Well-Being (b)

Scale(s)-Poor to Excellent (r)

Care Recipient:

Data Source:

C

Definition: Resistance of community members to the invasion and spread of an infectious agent that could threaten public health

OUTCOME TARGET RATING: Maintain at_____   Increase to_____

Community Health Status: Immunity Overall Rating	Poor 1	Fair 2	Good 3	Very good 4	Excellent 5	

INDICATORS:

		Poor 1	Fair 2	Good 3	Very good 4	Excellent 5	
280001	Immunization rates equal to or greater than current national standards	1	2	3	4	5	NA
280002	Incidence of vaccine preventable disease at or below recommended national rate	1	2	3	4	5	NA
280003	Prevalence of vaccine preventable disease at or below recommended national rate	1	2	3	4	5	NA
280004	Surveillance of immunization status in schools	1	2	3	4	5	NA
280005	Surveillance of immunization status in group living facilities (e.g., jails, group homes)	1	2	3	4	5	NA
280006	Surveillance of communicable disease	1	2	3	4	5	NA
280007	Screening of at-risk populations for infections	1	2	3	4	5	NA
280008	Compliance with immunization recommendations	1	2	3	4	5	NA
280009	Culturally appropriate public education on the risks and benefits of immunization	1	2	3	4	5	NA
280010	Availability of low cost immunizations	1	2	3	4	5	NA
280011	Enforcement of preschool immunizations	1	2	3	4	5	NA

2nd edition 2000; Revised 3rd edition 2004

Outcome Content References:

Stanhope, M., & Lancaster, J. (2000). *Community health nursing* (5th ed.). St. Louis: Mosby.

U.S. Department of Health and Human Services. (2000). *Healthy People 2010*. Washington, DC: Government Printing Office.

U.S. Department of Health and Human Services. (1998). *Clinician's handbook of preventive services: Put prevention into practice* (2nd ed.). Washington, DC: Government Printing Office.

U.S. Department of Health and Human Services. (1991). *Healthy People 2000: National health promotion and disease prevention objectives* (DHHS Pub No (PHS) 91-50012). Washington, DC: Government Printing Office.

U.S. Preventive Services Task Force. (1996). *Guide to clinical preventive services* (2nd ed.). Baltimore: Williams & Wilkins.

Community Risk Control: Chronic Disease—2801

Domain-Community Health (VII)

Class-Community Health Protection (c)

Scale(s)-Poor to Excellent (r)

Care Recipient:

Data Source:

Definition: Community actions to reduce the risk of chronic diseases and related complications

OUTCOME TARGET RATING: Maintain at_____   Increase to_____

Community Risk Control: Chronic Disease Overall Rating	Poor 1	Fair 2	Good 3	Very good 4	Excellent 5	

INDICATORS:

280101	Provision of public education programs on chronic disease	1	2	3	4	5	NA
280102	Target population participation rates in risk reduction programs	1	2	3	4	5	NA
280103	Availability of preventive screening programs	1	2	3	4	5	NA
280104	Target population participation rates in preventive screening programs	1	2	3	4	5	NA
280105	Availability of chronic disease self-management education programs	1	2	3	4	5	NA
280106	Proportion of target population participation rates in chronic disease self-management education programs	1	2	3	4	5	NA
280107	Availability of health care services to treat chronic disease	1	2	3	4	5	NA
280118	Provision of health care services to fit target population	1	2	3	4	5	NA
280119	Monitoring of incidence of chronic disease	1	2	3	4	5	NA
280120	Monitoring of prevalence of chronic disease	1	2	3	4	5	NA
280121	Monitoring of chronic disease morbidity	1	2	3	4	5	NA
280122	Monitoring of chronic disease mortality	1	2	3	4	5	NA
280123	Monitoring of chronic disease complications	1	2	3	4	5	NA
280111	Compliance with national standards for chronic disease prevention and management	1	2	3	4	5	NA
280112	Incidence of chronic disease at or below state or national rates	1	2	3	4	5	NA
280114	Prevalence of chronic disease at or below state or national rates	1	2	3	4	5	NA

		Poor	Fair	Good	Very good	Excellent	
280124	Public policies that promote health	1	2	3	4	5	NA
280125	Public policies that prevent disease	1	2	3	4	5	NA
280116	Procurement and allocation of funding for chronic disease prevention programs	1	2	3	4	5	NA
280126	Evidence of advocacy efforts for prevention of chronic illness	1	2	3	4	5	NA
280127	Evidence of advocacy efforts for management of chronic illness	1	2	3	4	5	NA

2nd edition 2000; Revised 3rd edition 2004; Revised 4th edition

Outcome Content References:

Clemen-Stone, S., McGuire, S. L., & Eigsti, D. G. (2002). *Comprehensive community health nursing: Family, aggregate, and community practice* (6th ed.). St. Louis: Mosby.

Robinson, K. L., Driedger, M. S., Elliot, S. J., & Eyles, J. (2006). Understanding facilitators of and barriers to health promotion practice. *Health Promotion Practice, 7*(4), 467-476.

Stanhope, M., & Lancaster, J. (2000). *Community health nursing* (5th ed.). St. Louis: Mosby.

U.S. Department of Health and Human Services. (2000). *Healthy People 2010*. Washington, DC: Government Printing Office.

U.S. Preventive Services Task Force. (1996). *Guide to clinical preventive services* (2nd ed.). Baltimore: Williams & Wilkins.

C

Community Risk Control: Communicable Disease—2802

Domain-Community Health (VII)

Class-Community Health Protection (c)

Scale(s)-Poor to Excellent (r)

Care Recipient:

Data Source:

C

Definition: Community actions to eliminate or reduce the spread of infectious agents that threaten public health

OUTCOME TARGET RATING: Maintain at_____   Increase to_____

Community Risk Control: Communicable Disease Overall Rating	Poor 1	Fair 2	Good 3	Very good 4	Excellent 5	

INDICATORS:

280201	Screening of all targeted high risk groups	1	2	3	4	5	NA
280202	Surveillance for infectious disease outbreaks including a system of data collection, reporting and follow-up	1	2	3	4	5	NA
280203	Investigation and notification of contacts concerning risk for infectious disease	1	2	3	4	5	NA
280204	Disease occurrences reported as mandated	1	2	3	4	5	NA
280205	Availability of treatment services for infected individuals	1	2	3	4	5	NA
280206	Provision of products to decrease disease spread	1	2	3	4	5	NA
280207	Established polices and surveillance for assuring safe food storage, handling, and preparation	1	2	3	4	5	NA
280208	Water testing consistent with local, state and federal regulations	1	2	3	4	5	NA
280209	Promotion of community wide immunization	1	2	3	4	5	NA
280220	Plan for mass immunization	1	2	3	4	5	NA
280210	Enforcement of infection surveillance programs	1	2	3	4	5	NA
280221	Enforcement of infection control programs	1	2	3	4	5	NA
280211	Availability of chemoprophylaxis for travelers	1	2	3	4	5	NA
280212	Evidence of environmental controls	1	2	3	4	5	NA
280213	Enforcement of environmental monitoring policies	1	2	3	4	5	NA
280214	Enforcement of domestic animal vaccination	1	2	3	4	5	NA
280215	Availability of health care services to treat communicable diseases	1	2	3	4	5	NA

	Poor	Fair	Good	Very good	Excellent	
280216 Access to health care services	1	2	3	4	5	NA
280217 Culturally appropriate public education about transmission of infectious disease	1	2	3	4	5	NA
280218 Policies supporting control of infectious disease	1	2	3	4	5	NA
280222 Monitoring of communicable disease morbidity	1	2	3	4	5	NA
280223 Monitoring of communicable disease mortality	1	2	3	4	5	NA
280224 Monitoring of communicable disease complications	1	2	3	4	5	NA

2nd edition 2000; Revised 3rd edition 2004; Revised 4th edition

Outcome Content References:

Stanhope, M., & Lancaster, J. (2000). *Community health nursing* (5th ed.). St. Louis: Mosby.

U.S. Department of Health and Human Services. (2000). *Healthy people 2010*. Washington, DC: Government Printing Office.

U.S. Department of Health and Human Services. (1998). *Clinician's handbook of preventive services: Put prevention into practice* (2nd ed.). Washington, DC: Government Printing Office.

U.S. Department of Health and Human Services. (1991). *Healthy People 2000: National health promotion and disease prevention objectives* (DHHS Pub No (PHS) 91-50012). Washington, DC: Government Printing Office.

U.S. Preventive Services Task Force. (1996). *Guide to clinical preventive services* (2nd ed.). Baltimore: Williams & Wilkins.

Veenema, T. G., & Toke, J. (2006). Early detection and surveillance for biopreparedness and emerging infectious diseases. *Online Journal of Issues in Nursing, 11*(1), Manuscript 2.

C

Community Risk Control: Lead Exposure—2803

Domain-Community Health (VII)

Class-Community Health Protection (c)

Scale(s)-Poor to Excellent (r)

Care Recipient:

Data Source:

C

Definition: Community actions to reduce lead exposure and poisoning

OUTCOME TARGET RATING: Maintain at_____   Increase to_____

Community Risk Control: Lead Exposure Overall Rating	Poor 1	Fair 2	Good 3	Very good 4	Excellent 5	
INDICATORS:						
280314 Problem assessment by community stakeholders and policy makers	1	2	3	4	5	NA
280315 Organization of lead screening programs that includes focus on preschools	1	2	3	4	5	NA
280316 Culturally appropriate marketing of screening programs to high-risk groups	1	2	3	4	5	NA
280301 Use of lead screening programs by targeted high risk group	1	2	3	4	5	NA
280317 Organization of referral and treatment services for exposed individuals	1	2	3	4	5	NA
280302 Referral of exposed individuals to treatment	1	2	3	4	5	NA
280318 Treatment of individuals with exposure to lead	1	2	3	4	5	NA
280303 Surveillance for sources of lead	1	2	3	4	5	NA
280304 Abatement of known lead sources in the community	1	2	3	4	5	NA
280305 Identification of programs to identify nutritional deficiencies in all targeted high-risk groups	1	2	3	4	5	NA
280306 Adequacy of programs to correct nutritional deficiencies in all targeted high-risk groups	1	2	3	4	5	NA
280307 Provision of culturally-appropriate public education about lead poisoning prevention	1	2	3	4	5	NA
280319 Participation rates of high-risk groups in education programs	1	2	3	4	5	NA
280308 Policies that require the removal of lead-based paint from all buildings	1	2	3	4	5	NA
280321 Funds dedicated to screening of lead hazards	1	2	3	4	5	NA
280322 Funds dedicated to elimination of lead hazards	1	2	3	4	5	NA

		Poor	Fair	Good	Very good	Excellent	
280310	Incidence of elevated lead levels at or below recommended national standards	1	2	3	4	5	NA
280311	Enforcement of home-buyer notification	1	2	3	4	5	NA
280320	Advocacy on behalf of renters of pre-1950 homes	1	2	3	4	5	NA
280312	Enforcement of emission standards	1	2	3	4	5	NA

2nd edition 2000; Revised 3rd edition 2004; Revised 4th edition

Outcome Content References:

Kincl, L. D., Dietrich, K. N., & Bhattacharya, A. (2006). Injury trends for adolescents with early childhood lead exposure. *Journal of Adolescent Health, 39*, 604-606.

Morgan, L. (1996). Children and lead: A model of care for community health providers. *Family and Community Health, 19*(1), 42-48.

Needleman, H. (1998). Childhood lead poisoning: The promise and abandonment of primary prevention. *American Journal of Public Health, 88*(12), 1871-1876.

Needleman, H., Schell. A., Bellinger, D., Leviton, A., & Allred, E. (1990). The long-term effects of exposure to low doses of lead in childhood. *The New England Journal of Medicine, 22*(2), 83-90.

Rischitelli, G., Nygren, P., Biougatsos, C., Feeman, M., & Helfand, M. (2006). Screening for elevated lead levels in childhood and pregnancy: An update summary of evidence for the US Preventive Services Task Force. *Pediatrics, 118*(6), 1867-1895.

Schwartz, J. (1994). Societal benefits of reducing lead exposure. *Environmental Research, 66*(1), 105-124.

Shih, R. A., Glass, T. A., Bandeen-Roche, K., Carlson, M. C., Bolla, K. I., Todd, A. C., & Schwartz, B. S. (2006). Environmental lead exposure and cognitive function in community-dwelling older adults. *Neurology, 67*(9), 1556-1562.

Community Risk Control: Violence—2805

Domain-Community Health (VII)

Class-Community Health Protection (c)

Scale(s)-Poor to Excellent (r)

Care Recipient:

Data Source:

Definition: Community actions to eliminate or reduce intentional violent acts resulting in serious physical or psychological harm

OUTCOME TARGET RATING:　　Maintain at_____　　　　Increase to_____

Community Risk Control: Violence Overall Rating	Poor 1	Fair 2	Good 3	Very good 4	Excellent 5	

INDICATORS:

280501	Systematic assessment of at-risk groups	1	2	3	4	5	NA
280502	Support programs for high-risk groups	1	2	3	4	5	NA
280503	Intervention programs for high-risk groups	1	2	3	4	5	NA
280504	Existence of weapon control policies	1	2	3	4	5	NA
280505	Enforcement of weapon control policies	1	2	3	4	5	NA
280506	Strategies to reduce violent content in the media	1	2	3	4	5	NA
280507	Control of violent content in the media	1	2	3	4	5	NA
280508	Educational programs on violence prevention	1	2	3	4	5	NA
280509	Competence in recognizing violence by community leaders	1	2	3	4	5	NA
280510	Competence in managing violence by community leaders	1	2	3	4	5	NA
280511	Acceptance of population diversity	1	2	3	4	5	NA
280512	Enforcement of laws against hate crimes by community leaders	1	2	3	4	5	NA
280513	Systematic monitoring of community violence levels	1	2	3	4	5	NA

3rd edition 2004

Outcome Content References:

Bell, C. C. (1997). Community violence: Causes, prevention, and intervention. *Journal of the National Medical Association, 89*(10), 657-662.

Campbell, J., & Landenburger, K. (2000). Violence and human abuse. In M. Stanhope & J. Lancaster (Eds.), *Community and public health nursing* (5th ed., pp. 747-778). St. Louis: Mosby.

Jones, F. C. (1997). Community violence, children and youth: Considerations for programs, policy and nursing roles. *Pediatric Nursing, 23*(2), 131-137.

Kroposki, M., & Alexander, J. (1998). Measuring community health nursing outcomes. *South Carolina Nurse, 5*(4), 17-18.

Community Violence Level—2702

Domain-Community Health (VII)

Class-Community Well-Being (b)

Scale(s)-Poor to Excellent (r)

Care Recipient:

Data Source:

C

Definition: Incidence of violent acts compared with local, state or national values

OUTCOME TARGET RATING: Maintain at_____   Increase to_____

Community Violence Level Overall Rating	Poor 1	Fair 2	Good 3	Very good 4	Excellent 5	
INDICATORS:						
270201 Homicide rate	1	2	3	4	5	NA
270202 Suicide rate	1	2	3	4	5	NA
270203 Sexual assault rate	1	2	3	4	5	NA
270204 Physical assault rate	1	2	3	4	5	NA
270205 Child abuse rate	1	2	3	4	5	NA
270206 Elder abuse rate	1	2	3	4	5	NA
270207 Partner abuse rate	1	2	3	4	5	NA
270208 Hate crime rate	1	2	3	4	5	NA

3rd edition 2004

Outcome Content References:

Bell, C. C. (1997). Community violence: Causes, prevention, and intervention. *Journal of the National Medical Association, 89*(10), 657-662.

Campbell, J., & Landenburger, K. (2000). Violence and human abuse. In M. Stanhope & J. Lancaster (Eds.), *Community and public health nursing* (5th ed., pp. 747-778). St. Louis: Mosby.

Jones, F. C. (1997). Community violence, children and youth: Considerations for programs, policy and nursing roles. *Pediatric Nursing, 23*(2), 131-137.

Lutenbacher, M., Cooper, W. O., & Faccia, K. (2002). Planning youth violence prevention efforts: Decision-making across community sectors. *Journal of Adolescent Health, 30*(5), 346-354.

U.S. Department of Health and Human Services. (2000). *Healthy People 2010.* Washington, DC: Government Printing Office.

Compliance Behavior—1601

Domain-Health Knowledge & Behavior (IV)

Class-Health Behavior (Q)

Scale(s)-Never demonstrated to Consistently demonstrated (m)

Care Recipient:

Data Source:

> **Definition:** Personal actions to promote wellness, recovery, and rehabilitation recommended by a health professional

OUTCOME TARGET RATING   Maintain at_____   Increase to_____

Compliance Behavior Overall Rating	Never demonstrated 1	Rarely demonstrated 2	Sometimes demonstrated 3	Often demonstrated 4	Consistently demonstrated 5	
INDICATORS:						
160104 Accepts diagnosis	1	2	3	4	5	NA
160114 Seeks reputable information about diagnosis	1	2	3	4	5	NA
160115 Seeks reputable information about treatment	1	2	3	4	5	NA
160102 Discusses prescribed treatment regimen with health professional	1	2	3	4	5	NA
160103 Performs treatment regimen as prescribed	1	2	3	4	5	NA
160105 Keeps appointments with health professional	1	2	3	4	5	NA
160111 Reports changes in symptoms to health professional	1	2	3	4	5	NA
160106 Modifies treatment regimen as directed by health professional	1	2	3	4	5	NA
160112 Monitors treatment response	1	2	3	4	5	NA
160113 Monitors medication therapeutic effects	1	2	3	4	5	NA
160107 Performs self-screening when directed	1	2	3	4	5	NA
160108 Performs activities of daily living as prescribed	1	2	3	4	5	NA
160109 Seeks external reinforcement for performance of health behaviors	1	2	3	4	5	NA

1st edition 1997; Revised 3rd edition 2004; Revised 4th edition

Outcome Content References:

Barotsky, I., Sergenbaker, P., & Mills, M. (1979). Compliance and quality of life assessment. In J. Cohen (Ed.), *New directions in patient compliance* (pp. 59-74). Lexington, MA: D.C. Health.

Burkhart, P. V., Dunbar-Jacob, J. M., & Rohay, J. M. (2001). Accuracy of children's self-reported adherence to treatment. *Journal of Nursing Scholarship, 33*(1), 27-32.

+DiMatteo, M. R., Hays, R. D., & Sherbourne, C. D. (1992). Adherence to cancer regimens: Implications for treating the older patient. *Oncology, 6*(2 Suppl.), 50-57.

Epstein, L., & Cluss, P. A. (1982). A behavioral perspective on adherence to long-term medical regimens. *Journal of Consulting and Clinical Psychology, 50*, 950-971.

Folden, S. L. (1993). Definitions of health and health goals of participants in a community-based pulmonary rehabilitation program. *Public Health Nursing, 10*(1), 31-35.

Heiby, E., & Carlson, J. (1986). The health compliance model. *The Journal of Compliance in Health Care, 1*(2), 135-152.

Jensen, L., & Allen, M. (1993). Wellness: The dialect of illness. *Image—The Journal of Nursing Scholarship, 25*(3), 220-224.

King, I. M. (1988). Measuring health goal attainment in patients. In C. F. Waltz & O. L. Strickland (Eds.), *Measurement of nursing outcomes* (Vol. I, pp. 108-127). New York: Springer.

Kravits, R., Hays, R. D., Sherbourne, C. D., DiMatteo, M. R., Rogers, W. H., Ordway, L., & Greenfield, S. (1993). Recall of recommendations and adherence to advice among patients with chronic medical conditions. *Archives of Internal Medicine, 153*(16), 1869-1878.

Oldridge, N. (1982). Compliance and exercise in primary and secondary prevention of coronary heart disease: A review. *Preventive Medicine, 11*(1), 56-70.

C

Compliance Behavior: Prescribed Diet—1622

Domain-Health Knowledge & Behavior (IV)

Class-Health Behavior (Q)

Scale(s)-Never demonstrated to Consistently demonstrated (m)

Care Recipient:

Data Source:

Definition: Personal actions to follow food and fluid intake recommended by a health professional for a specific health condition

OUTCOME TARGET RATING: Maintain at_____   Increase to_____

Compliance Behavior: Prescribed Diet Overall Rating	Never demonstrated 1	Rarely demonstrated 2	Sometimes demonstrated 3	Often demonstrated 4	Consistently demonstrated 5	
INDICATORS:						
162201 Participates in setting achievable dietary goals with health professional	1	2	3	4	5	NA
162202 Selects food and fluid consistent with prescribed diet	1	2	3	4	5	NA
162203 Uses nutritional information on labels to guide selections	1	2	3	4	5	NA
162204 Selects portions consistent with prescribed diet	1	2	3	4	5	NA
162205 Eats food consistent with prescribed diet	1	2	3	4	5	NA
162206 Drinks fluid consistent with prescribed diet	1	2	3	4	5	NA
162207 Avoids food and fluid not allowed on diet	1	2	3	4	5	NA
162208 Follows recommendations for between meal food and fluid	1	2	3	4	5	NA
162209 Prepares food and fluid following dietary restrictions	1	2	3	4	5	NA
162210 Follows recommendations for number of meals per day	1	2	3	4	5	NA
162211 Plans meals consistent with prescribed diet	1	2	3	4	5	NA
162212 Plans strategies for situations that affect food and fluid intake	1	2	3	4	5	NA
162213 Alters diet within restrictions when activity level changes	1	2	3	4	5	NA
162214 Follows recommendations for diet staging	1	2	3	4	5	NA
162215 Uses a diary to monitor food and fluid intake over time	1	2	3	4	5	NA
162216 Aligns diet with cultural beliefs	1	2	3	4	5	NA
162217 Chooses foods consistent with cultural beliefs	1	2	3	4	5	NA

C

		Never demonstrated	Rarely demonstrated	Sometimes demonstrated	Often demonstrated	Consistently demonstrated	
162218	Avoids food and fluid that interact with medications	1	2	3	4	5	NA
162219	Avoids food and fluid that interact with herbal remedies	1	2	3	4	5	NA
162220	Avoids food and fluid that trigger allergic reactions	1	2	3	4	5	NA

Outcome Content References:

American Diabetes Association. (2004). Nutrition principles and recommendations in diabetes. *Diabetes Care, 27*(Suppl. 1), S36-S46.

Brownell, K., & Fairburn, C. (Eds.). (2002). *Eating disorders and obesity: A comprehensive handbook* (2nd ed.). New York: Guilford Press.

Dudek, S. G. (2007). *Nutrition essentials for nursing practice* (5th rev. ed.). Philadelphia: Lippincott Williams & Wilkins.

Frandsen, K. B., & Kristensen, J. S. (2002). Diet and lifestyle in the type 2 diabetes: The patient's perspective. *Practical Diabetes International, 19*(3), 77-80.

Lee, A., & Newman, J. (2003). Celiac diet: Its impact on quality of life. *Journal of the American Dietetic Association, 103*, 1533-1535.

Rosenberg, I. (Ed.). (2002). The 5 lifestyle steps for lowering blood pressure. *Tufts University Health & Nutrition Letter, 21*(6), 7.

C

Compliance Behavior: Prescribed Medication—1623

Domain-Health Knowledge & Behavior (IV)

Class-Health Behavior (Q)

Scale(s)-Never demonstrated to Consistently demonstrated (m)

Care Recipient:

Data Source:

C

| **Definition:** Personal actions to administer medication safely to meet therapeutic goals as recommended by a health professional |

OUTCOME TARGET RATING: Maintain at_____   Increase to_____

Compliance Behavior: Prescribed Medication Overall Rating	Never demonstrated 1	Rarely demonstrated 2	Sometimes demonstrated 3	Often demonstrated 4	Consistently demonstrated 5	

INDICATORS:

162301	Keeps a list of all medication with dose and frequency	1	2	3	4	5	NA
162302	Obtains required medication	1	2	3	4	5	NA
162303	Informs health professional of all medication being taken	1	2	3	4	5	NA
162304	Takes all medication at intervals prescribed	1	2	3	4	5	NA
162305	Takes correct dose	1	2	3	4	5	NA
162306	Modifies dose as instructed	1	2	3	4	5	NA
162307	Takes medication with or without food as prescribed	1	2	3	4	5	NA
162308	Avoids alcohol if contraindicated	1	2	3	4	5	NA
162309	Avoids food and fluids that are contraindicated	1	2	3	4	5	NA
162310	Administers topical medication correctly	1	2	3	4	5	NA
162311	Follows medication precautions	1	2	3	4	5	NA
162312	Monitors medication therapeutic effects	1	2	3	4	5	NA
162313	Monitors medication side effects	1	2	3	4	5	NA
162314	Monitors medication adverse effects	1	2	3	4	5	NA
162315	Uses strategies to minimize side effects	1	2	3	4	5	NA
162316	Reports therapeutic response to health professional	1	2	3	4	5	NA
162317	Reports adverse effects to health professional	1	2	3	4	5	NA
162318	Stores medication properly	1	2	3	4	5	NA
162319	Arranges for refills to ensure adequate supply	1	2	3	4	5	NA
162320	Monitors medication expiration date	1	2	3	4	5	NA

		Never demonstrated	Rarely demonstrated	Sometimes demonstrated	Often demonstrated	Consistently demonstrated	
162321	Disposes of medication properly	1	2	3	4	5	NA
162322	Disposes of syringes and needles properly	1	2	3	4	5	NA
162323	Administers subcutaneous medication correctly	1	2	3	4	5	NA
162324	Administers intramuscular medication correctly	1	2	3	4	5	NA
162325	Administers intravenous medication correctly	1	2	3	4	5	NA
162326	Maintains asepsis with non-parenteral medication	1	2	3	4	5	NA
162327	Monitors injection insertion sites	1	2	3	4	5	NA
162328	Rotates injection sites	1	2	3	4	5	NA
162329	Maintains needed supplies	1	2	3	4	5	NA
162330	Stores supplies correctly	1	2	3	4	5	NA
162331	Disposes of sharps correctly	1	2	3	4	5	NA
162332	Obtains required laboratory tests	1	2	3	4	5	NA

Outcome Content References:

Janssen, B., Gaebel, W., Haerter, M., Komaharadi, F., Lindel, B., & Weinmann, S. (2006). Evaluation of factors influencing medication compliance in inpatient treatment of psychotic disorders. *Psychoparmacology, 187,* 229-236.

Johnson, M. J. (2006). Development of the purposeful action medication-taking questionnaire. *Western Journal of Nursing Research, 28,* 335-351.

Roose, S. P. (2003). Compliance: The impact of adverse events and tolerability on the physician's treatment decisions. *European Neruopsychoparmacology, 13,* S85-S92.

Schmitz, J. M., Sayre, S. L., Stotts, A. L., Rothfleisch, J., & Mooney, M. E. (2005). Medication compliance during a smoking cessation clinical trial: A brief intervention using MEMS feedback. *Journal of Behavioral Medicine, 28*(2), 139-147.

C

C

Concentration—0905

Domain-Physiologic Health (II)

Class-Neurocognitive (J)

Scale(s)-Severely compromised to Not compromised (a)

Care Recipient:

Data Source:

Definition: Ability to focus on a specific stimulus

OUTCOME TARGET RATING: Maintain at_____   Increase to_____

Concentration Overall Rating	Severely compromised 1	Substantially compromised 2	Moderately compromised 3	Mildly compromised 4	Not compromised 5	
INDICATORS:						
090501 Maintains attention	1	2	3	4	5	NA
090502 Maintains focus	1	2	3	4	5	NA
090503 Responds to visual cues	1	2	3	4	5	NA
090504 Responds to auditory cues	1	2	3	4	5	NA
090505 Responds to tactile cues	1	2	3	4	5	NA
090506 Responds to olfactory cues	1	2	3	4	5	NA
090507 Responds to language cues	1	2	3	4	5	NA
090508 Spells 'world' backwards	1	2	3	4	5	NA
090515 Counts backward from 20 by 3s	1	2	3	4	5	NA
090516 Counts backward from 100 by 7s	1	2	3	4	5	NA
090510 Names the months of the year backward, starting with January	1	2	3	4	5	NA
090511 Draws a circle	1	2	3	4	5	NA
090514 Draws a triangle	1	2	3	4	5	NA
090512 Draws a pentagon	1	2	3	4	5	NA

1st edition 1997; Revised 3rd edition 2004; Revised 4th edition

Outcome Content References:

Abraham, I., & Reel, S. (1993). Cognitive nursing interventions with long-term care residents: Effects on neurocognitive dimensions. *Archives of Psychiatric Nursing, 6*(6), 356-365.

Agostinelli, B., Demers, K., Garrigan, D., & Waszynski, C. (1994). Targeted interventions: Use of the Mini-Mental State Exam. *Journal of Gerontological Nursing, 20*(8), 15-23.

Dellasega, C. (1992). Home health nurses' assessments of cognition. *Applied Nursing Research, 5*(3), 127-133.

+Folstein, M. F., Folstein, S. E., & McHugh, P. R. (1975). "Mini-Mental State"—A practical method for grading the cognitive state of patients for the clinician. *Journal of Psychiatric Research, 12*(3), 189-198.

Foreman, M., Gilles, D., & Wagner, D. (1989). Impaired cognition in the critically ill elderly patient: Clinical implications. *Critical Care Nursing Quarterly, 12*(1), 61-73.

Kupferer, S., Uebele, J., & Levin, D. (1988). Geriatric ambulatory surgery patients: Assessing cognitive functions. *AORN Journal, 47*(3), 752-766.

Mason, P. (1989). Cognitive assessment parameters and tools for the critically injured adult. *Critical Care Nursing Clinics of North America, 1*(1), 45-53.

Norris, J. A., & Hoffman, P. R. (1996). Attaining, sustaining, and focusing attention: Intervention for children with ADHD. *Seminars in Speech & Language, 17*(1), 59-71.

O'Keeffe, S. T., & Gosney, M. A. (1997). Assessing attentiveness in older hospital patients: Global assessment versus tests of attention. *Journal of the American Geriatrics Society, 45*(4), 470-473.

Strub, R. L., & Black, F. W. (2000). *The mental status examination in neurology* (4th ed.). Philadelphia: F.A. Davis.

Coordinated Movement—0212

Domain-Functional Health (I)

Class-Mobility (C)

Scale(s)-Severely compromised to Not compromised (a)

Care Recipient:

Data Source:

Definition: Ability of muscles to work together voluntarily for purposeful movement

OUTCOME TARGET RATING: Maintain at_____   Increase to_____

Coordinated Movement Overall Rating	Severely compromised 1	Substantially compromised 2	Moderately compromised 3	Mildly compromised 4	Not compromised 5	
INDICATORS:						
021201 Strength of muscle contraction	1	2	3	4	5	NA
021202 Muscle tone	1	2	3	4	5	NA
021203 Speed of movement	1	2	3	4	5	NA
021204 Smooth movement	1	2	3	4	5	NA
021205 Control of movement	1	2	3	4	5	NA
021206 Steadiness of movement	1	2	3	4	5	NA
021207 Balanced movement	1	2	3	4	5	NA
021208 Muscle tension	1	2	3	4	5	NA
021209 Movement in desired direction	1	2	3	4	5	NA
021210 Movement with desired timing	1	2	3	4	5	NA
021211 Movement at desired speed	1	2	3	4	5	NA
021212 Movement with desired precision	1	2	3	4	5	NA

3rd edition 2004

Outcome Content References:

Buchner, D. M. (1995). Clinical assessments of physical activity in older adults. In L. Z. Rubenstein, D. Wieland, & R. Bernabei (Eds.), *Geriatric assessment technology: The state of the art* (pp. 147-159). New York: Springer.

Crawford, S. G., Wilson, B. N., & Dewey, D. (2001). Identifying developmental coordination disorder: Consistency between tests. *Physical & Occupational Therapy in Pediatrics, 20*(2/3), 29-50.

DiFabio, R. P., Paul, S., Emasithi, A., & Greany, J. F. (2001). Evaluating eye-body coordination during unrestrained functional activity in older persons. *The Journals of Gerontology. Series A, Biological Sciences & Medical Sciences, 56*(9), M571-M574.

Guyton, A. C. (1992). *Human physiology and mechanisms of disease* (5th ed.). Philadelphia: W.B. Saunders.

Harris, T. (1997). Muscle mass and strength: Relation to function in population studies. *Journal of Nutrition, 127*(Suppl. 5), 1004S-1006S.

Junaid, K., Harris, S. R., Fulmer, K. A., & Carswell, A. (2000). Teachers' use of the MABC checklist to identify children with motor coordination difficulties. *Pediatric Physical Therapy, 12*(4), 158-163.

Matteson, M. A., McConnell, E. S., & Linton, A. D. (1997). *Gerontological nursing: Concepts and practice* (2nd ed.). Philadelphia: W.B. Saunders.

Novy, D. M., Simmonds, M. J., & Lee, C. E. (2002). Physical performance tasks: What are the underlying constructs? *Archives of Physical Medicine & Rehabilitation, 83*(1), 44-47.

Riggio, S., & Jagoda, A. (1999). The rapid neurologic examination, Part 2: Movement, reflexes, sensation, balance: Know the signs that lead to the site of the pathologic response. *Journal of Critical Illness, 14*(7), 368-372.

Schmitz, T. J. (2001). Coordination assessment. In S. B. O'Sullivan & T. J. Schmitz (Eds.), *Physical rehabilitation: Assessment and treatment* (4th ed., pp. 157-175). Philadelphia: F.A. Davis.

Coping—1302

Domain-Psychosocial Health (III)

Class-Psychosocial Adaptation (N)

Scale(s)-Never demonstrated to Consistently demonstrated (m)

Care Recipient:

Data Source:

Definition: Personal actions to manage stressors that tax an individual's resources

OUTCOME TARGET RATING: Maintain at_____   Increase to_____

Coping Overall Rating	Never demonstrated 1	Rarely demonstrated 2	Sometimes demonstrated 3	Often demonstrated 4	Consistently demonstrated 5	
INDICATORS:						
130201 Identifies effective coping patterns	1	2	3	4	5	NA
130202 Identifies ineffective coping patterns	1	2	3	4	5	NA
130203 Verbalizes sense of control	1	2	3	4	5	NA
130204 Reports decrease in stress	1	2	3	4	5	NA
130205 Verbalizes acceptance of situation	1	2	3	4	5	NA
130220 Seeks reputable information about diagnosis	1	2	3	4	5	NA
130221 Seeks reputable information about treatment	1	2	3	4	5	NA
130207 Modifies lifestyle to reduce stress	1	2	3	4	5	NA
130208 Adapts to life changes	1	2	3	4	5	NA
130222 Uses personal support system	1	2	3	4	5	NA
130210 Uses behaviors to reduce stress	1	2	3	4	5	NA
130211 Identifies multiple coping strategies	1	2	3	4	5	NA
130212 Uses effective coping strategies	1	2	3	4	5	NA
130213 Avoids unduly stressful situations	1	2	3	4	5	NA
130214 Verbalizes need for assistance	1	2	3	4	5	NA
130223 Obtains assistance from health professional	1	2	3	4	5	NA
130216 Reports decrease in physical symptoms of stress	1	2	3	4	5	NA
130217 Reports decrease in negative feelings	1	2	3	4	5	NA
130218 Reports increase in psychological comfort	1	2	3	4	5	NA

1st edition 1997; Revised 3rd edition 2004; Revised 4th edition

Outcome Content References:

Baldree, K., Murphy, S., & Powers, M. (1982). Stress identification and coping patterns in patients on hemodialysis. *Nursing Research, 31*(2), 107-112.

+Carver, C. S. (1997). You want to measure coping but your protocol's too long: Consider the Brief COPE. *International Journal of Behavioral Medicine, 4*, 92-100.

+Carver, C. S., Scheier, M. F., & Weintraub, J. K. (1989). Assessing coping strategies: A theoretically based approach. *Journal of Personality and Social Psychology, 56*(2), 267-283.

Folkman, S., Lazarus, R., Gruen, R., & Delongis, A. (1986). Appraisal, coping, health status, and psychological symptoms. *Journal of Personality and Social Psychology, 50*(3), 571-579.

McHaffie, H. (1992). The assessment of coping. *Clinical Nursing Research, 1*(1), 67-79.

Panzarine, S. (1985). Coping: Conceptual and methodological issues. *Advances in Nursing Science, 7*(4), 49-57.

Stolley, J. M. (2001). Ineffective individual coping. In M. Maas, K. Buckwalter, M. Hardy, T. Tripp-Reimer, M. Titler, & J. Specht (Eds.), *Nursing care of older adults: Diagnoses, outcomes & interventions* (pp. 766-777). St. Louis: Mosby.

Whiting, G., & Buckwalter, K. C. (2001). Grieving. In M. Maas, K. Buckwalter, M. Hardy, T. Tripp-Reimer, M. Titler, & J. Specht (Eds.), *Nursing care of older adults: Diagnoses, outcomes & interventions* (pp. 631-650). St. Louis: Mosby.

C

Decision-Making—0906

Domain-Physiologic Health (II)

Class-Neurocognitive (J)

Scale(s)-Severely compromised to Not compromised (a)

Care Recipient:

Data Source:

D

| **Definition:** Ability to make judgments and choose between two or more alternatives |

OUTCOME TARGET RATING: Maintain at_____   Increase to_____

Decision-Making Overall Rating	Severely compromised 1	Substantially compromised 2	Moderately compromised 3	Mildly compromised 4	Not compromised 5	
INDICATORS:						
090601 Identifies relevant information	1	2	3	4	5	NA
090602 Identifies alternatives	1	2	3	4	5	NA
090603 Identifies potential consequences of each alternative	1	2	3	4	5	NA
090604 Identifies needed resources to support each alternative	1	2	3	4	5	NA
090611 Identifies time frame necessary to support each alternative	1	2	3	4	5	NA
090612 Identifies sequence necessary to support each alternative	1	2	3	4	5	NA
090605 Recognizes contradiction with others' desires	1	2	3	4	5	NA
090606 Acknowledges social context of the situation	1	2	3	4	5	NA
090607 Acknowledges relevant legal implications	1	2	3	4	5	NA
090608 Weighs alternatives	1	2	3	4	5	NA
090609 Selects among alternatives	1	2	3	4	5	NA

1st edition 1997; Revised 3rd edition 2004; Revised 4th edition

Outcome Content References:

Abraham, I., & Reel, S. (1993). Cognitive nursing interventions with long-term care residents: Effects on neurocognitive dimensions. *Archives of Psychiatric Nursing, 6*(6), 356-365.

Agostinelli, B., Demers, K., Garrigan, D., & Waszynski, C. (1994). Targeted interventions: Use of the Mini-Mental State Exam. *Journal of Gerontological Nursing, 20*(8), 15-23.

Dellasega, C. (1992). Home health nurses' assessments of cognition. *Applied Nursing Research, 5*(3), 127-133.

Foreman, M., Gilles, D., & Wagner, D. (1989). Impaired cognition in the critically ill elderly patient: Clinical implications. *Critical Care Nursing Quarterly, 12*(1), 61-73.

+Uniform Data System for Medical Rehabilitation. (1997). *Guide for the Uniform Data Set for Medical Rehabilitation* (including the FIM™ instrument) (version 5.1). Buffalo, NY: UDSMR.

Jubeck, M. (1992). Are you sensitive to the cognitive needs of the elderly? *Home Healthcare Nurse, 10*(5), 20-25.

Kendall, E., Shum, D., Halson, D., Bunning, S., & Teb, M. (1997). The assessment of social problem-solving ability following traumatic brain injury. *Journal of Head Trauma Rehabilitation, 12*(3), 68-78.

Kupferer, S., Uebele, J., & Levin, D. (1988). Geriatric ambulatory surgery patients: Assessing cognitive functions. *AORN Journal, 47*(3), 752-766.

Mason, P. (1989). Cognitive assessment parameters and tools for the critically injured adult. *Critical Care Nursing Clinics of North America, 1*(1), 45-53.

Strub, R. L., & Black, F. W. (2000). *The mental status examination in neurology* (4th ed.). Philadelphia: F.A. Davis.

Vellinga, A., Smit, J. H., van Leeuwen, E., van Tilburg, W., & Jonker, C. (2004). Instruments to assess decision-making capacity: An overview. *International Psychogeriatrics, 16*(4), 397-419.

Depression Level—1208

Domain-Psychosocial Health (III)

Class-Psychological Well-Being (M)

Scale(s)-Severe to None (n)

Care Recipient:

Data Source:

D

Definition: Severity of melancholic mood and loss of interest in life events						

OUTCOME TARGET RATING: Maintain at_____   Increase to_____

Depression Level Overall Rating	Severe 1	Substantial 2	Moderate 3	Mild 4	None 5	

INDICATORS:

		Severe 1	Substantial 2	Moderate 3	Mild 4	None 5	
120801	Depressed mood	1	2	3	4	5	NA
120802	Loss of interest in activities	1	2	3	4	5	NA
120827	Negative life events	1	2	3	4	5	NA
120803	Lack of pleasure in activities	1	2	3	4	5	NA
120804	Impaired concentration	1	2	3	4	5	NA
120805	Inappropriate guilt	1	2	3	4	5	NA
120828	Excessive guilt	1	2	3	4	5	NA
120806	Fatigue	1	2	3	4	5	NA
120807	Feelings of worthlessness	1	2	3	4	5	NA
120808	Psychomotor retardation	1	2	3	4	5	NA
120829	Psychomotor agitation	1	2	3	4	5	NA
120809	Insomnia	1	2	3	4	5	NA
120830	Hypersomnia	1	2	3	4	5	NA
120810	Weight gain	1	2	3	4	5	NA
120831	Weight loss	1	2	3	4	5	NA
120811	Increased appetite	1	2	3	4	5	NA
120832	Decreased appetite	1	2	3	4	5	NA
120835	Recurrent thoughts of death	1	2	3	4	5	NA
120836	Recurrent thoughts of suicide	1	2	3	4	5	NA
120813	Indecisiveness	1	2	3	4	5	NA
120814	Sadness	1	2	3	4	5	NA
120815	Crying spells	1	2	3	4	5	NA
120816	Anger	1	2	3	4	5	NA
120817	Hopelessness	1	2	3	4	5	NA
120818	Loneliness	1	2	3	4	5	NA
120819	Low self-esteem	1	2	3	4	5	NA
120820	Decreased libido	1	2	3	4	5	NA
120821	Decreased activity level	1	2	3	4	5	NA
120822	Lack of spontaneity	1	2	3	4	5	NA
120823	Irritability	1	2	3	4	5	NA
120833	Recreational drug use	1	2	3	4	5	NA
120834	Increased alcohol use	1	2	3	4	5	NA
120825	Poor personal hygiene/grooming	1	2	3	4	5	NA

2nd edition 2000; Revised 3rd edition 2004; Revised 4th edition

Continued

D

Outcome Content References:

American Psychiatric Association. (2000). *Diagnostic and statistical manual of mental disorders* (4th ed. text revision). Washington, DC: Author.

Brink, T. L., Yesavage, J. A., Lum, O., Heersema, P. H., Adey, M., & Rose, T. L. (1982). Screening tests for geriatric depression. *Clinical Gerontologist, 1*(1), 37-43.

Kendler, K. S., Karkowski, L. M., & Prescott, C. A. (1999). Causal relationship between stressful life events and the onset of major depression. *American Journal of Psychiatry, 156*(6), 837-841.

Kraaij, V., Arensman, E., & Spinhoven, P. (2002). Negative life events and depression in elderly persons: A meta-analysis. *Journal of Gerontology Series B—Psychological Sciences, 57*(1), P87-P94.

Lloyd-Williams, M., Friedman, T., & Rudd, N. (2001). An analysis of the validity of the Hospital Anxiety and Depression Scale as a screening tool in patients with advanced metastatic cancer. *Journal of Pain & Symptom Management, 22*(6), 990-996.

Oakley, L. D., & Kane, J. (1999). Personal and social illness demands related to depression. *Archives of Psychiatric Nursing, 13*(6), 294-302.

Raue, P. J., Brown, E. L., & Bruce, M. L. (2002). Assessing behavior health using OASIS: Part 1: Depression and suicidality. *Home Healthcare Nurse, 20*(3), 154-162.

U.S. Department of Health and Human Services. (1993). *Depression and primary care: Detection and diagnosis* (Vol. 1) (AHCPR publication No. 93-0550). Rockville, MD: Government Printing Office.

U.S. Department of Health and Human Services. (1993). *Depression and primary care: Treatment of major depression* (Vol. 2) (AHCPR publication No. 93-0551). Rockville, MD: Government Printing Office.

Depression Self-Control—1409

Domain-Psychosocial Health (III)

Class-Self-Control (O)

Scale(s)-Never demonstrated to Consistently demonstrated (m)

Care Recipient:

Data Source:

D

Definition: Personal actions to minimize melancholy and maintain interest in life events

OUTCOME TARGET RATING: Maintain at_____   Increase to_____

Depression Self-Control Overall Rating	Never demonstrated 1	Rarely demonstrated 2	Sometimes demonstrated 3	Often demonstrated 4	Consistently demonstrated 5	
INDICATORS:						
140901 Monitors ability to concentrate	1	2	3	4	5	NA
140902 Monitors intensity of depression	1	2	3	4	5	NA
140903 Identifies precursors of depression	1	2	3	4	5	NA
140904 Plans strategies to reduce effects of precursors	1	2	3	4	5	NA
140905 Monitors behavioral manifestations of depression	1	2	3	4	5	NA
140906 Reports adequate sleep	1	2	3	4	5	NA
140907 Reports improved libido	1	2	3	4	5	NA
140908 Monitors physical manifestations of depression	1	2	3	4	5	NA
140909 Reports improved mood	1	2	3	4	5	NA
140910 Maintains stable weight	1	2	3	4	5	NA
140911 Follows treatment regimen	1	2	3	4	5	NA
140923 Uses medication as prescribed	1	2	3	4	5	NA
140924 Sets realistic goals	1	2	3	4	5	NA
140925 Delays big decision until feeling better	1	2	3	4	5	NA
140926 Participates in enjoyable activities	1	2	3	4	5	NA
140913 Follows exercise plan	1	2	3	4	5	NA
140914 Adheres to therapy schedule	1	2	3	4	5	NA
140915 Reports changes in symptoms to a health provider	1	2	3	4	5	NA
140920 Avoids alcohol misuse	1	2	3	4	5	NA
140921 Avoids non-prescription drug misuse	1	2	3	4	5	NA
140922 Avoids recreational drug use	1	2	3	4	5	NA
140918 Maintains personal hygiene and grooming	1	2	3	4	5	NA

2nd edition 2000; Revised 3rd edition 2004; Revised 4th edition

Continued

Outcome Content References:

Adams, P. (2000). Insight: A mental health prevention intervention. *Nursing Clinics of North America, 35*(2), 329-338.

American Psychiatric Association. (2000). *Diagnostic and statistical manual of mental disorders* (4th ed. text revision). Washington, DC: Author.

Cronin, J., Nash, V., Ray-Mihm, R., & Tucker, S. (2001). Relationship between psychiatric clinical assessment scores and patients' daily activities. *Journal of the American Psychiatric Nurses Association, 7*(5), 145-154.

Jaret, P. (1999). Fitness. Move the body, heal the mind. *Health, 13*(1), 50-51.

Johnson, C. D. (1999). Therapeutic recreation treats depression in the elderly. *Home Health Care Services Quarterly, 18*(2), 79-90.

Laliberte, R. (1999). How to manage your moods. *New Choices: Living Even Better After 50, 39*(6), 44-47.

Lantz, M. S. (2001). The psychiatric consultant. Suicide in late life: Identifying and managing at-risk older patients. *Geriatrics, 56*(7), 47-48.

Peden, A. R., Hall, L. A., Rayens, M. K., & Beebe, L. L. (2000). Reducing negative thinking and depressive symptoms in college women. *Journal of Nursing Scholarship, 32*(2), 145-151.

Tucker, S., & Darley, J. (2001). How to detect and manage depression in older people. *Nursing Times, 97*(45), 36-37.

U.S. Department of Health and Human Services. (1993). *Depression and primary care: Detection and diagnosis* (Vol. 1) (AHCPR publication No. 93-0550). Rockville, MD: Government Printing Office.

U.S. Department of Health and Human Services. (1993). *Depression and primary care: Treatment of major depression* (Vol. 2) (AHCPR publication No. 93-0551). Rockville, MD: Government Printing Office.

D

Development: Late Adulthood—0121

Domain-Functional Health (I)   Care Recipient:

Class-Growth & Development (B)   Data Source:

Scale(s)-Never demonstrated to Consistently demonstrated (m) and Consistently demonstrated to Never demonstrated (t)

Definition: Cognitive, psychosocial, and moral progression from 65 years of age and older

OUTCOME TARGET RATING: Maintain at_____   Increase to_____

Development: Late Adulthood Overall Rating	Never demonstrated 1	Rarely demonstrated 2	Sometimes demonstrated 3	Often demonstrated 4	Consistently demonstrated 5	

INDICATORS:

012101	Maintains cognitive function	1	2	3	4	5	NA
012102	Maintains language skills	1	2	3	4	5	NA
012103	Maintains problem solving skills	1	2	3	4	5	NA
012104	Maintains lifelong learning	1	2	3	4	5	NA
012105	Exhibits realistic outlook about abilities	1	2	3	4	5	NA
012106	Compensates if deterioration in memory occurs	1	2	3	4	5	NA
012107	Copes with personal loss	1	2	3	4	5	NA
012108	Copes with own mortality	1	2	3	4	5	NA
012109	Maintains life interests	1	2	3	4	5	NA
012110	Exhibits sense of pride	1	2	3	4	5	NA
012111	Exhibits sense of accomplishment	1	2	3	4	5	NA
012112	Maintains relationships with immediate family	1	2	3	4	5	NA
012113	Maintains relationships with extended family	1	2	3	4	5	NA
012114	Maintains close relationships with friends	1	2	3	4	5	NA
012115	Copes with adult children in the home	1	2	3	4	5	NA
012116	Performs positive role in lives of grandchildren	1	2	3	4	5	NA
012117	Adjusts to parenting role of grandchildren	1	2	3	4	5	NA
012118	Adjusts to retirement	1	2	3	4	5	NA
012119	Develops new interests	1	2	3	4	5	NA
012120	Adapts to changing needs for assistance	1	2	3	4	5	NA
012121	Accepts assistance from others	1	2	3	4	5	NA
012122	Adjusts to change in financial income	1	2	3	4	5	NA

D

Continued

D

		Never demonstrated	Rarely demonstrated	Sometimes demonstrated	Often demonstrated	Consistently demonstrated	
012123	Adjusts to change in living arrangements	1	2	3	4	5	NA
012124	Adjusts to change in marital status	1	2	3	4	5	NA
012125	Adjusts to change in marital relationship	1	2	3	4	5	NA
012126	Adjusts to sexual function changes	1	2	3	4	5	NA
012127	Practices safe sex	1	2	3	4	5	NA
012128	Adapts to functional impairment	1	2	3	4	5	NA
012129	Avoids substance misuse	1	2	3	4	5	NA
012130	Challenges ageism stereotypes	1	2	3	4	5	NA
012131	Derives support from religious or spiritual beliefs	1	2	3	4	5	NA
012132	Seeks understanding to meaning of own life	1	2	3	4	5	NA
012133	Adheres to laws that protect welfare of others	1	2	3	4	5	NA
012134	Acknowledges personal values	1	2	3	4	5	NA
012135	Acknowledges values of others	1	2	3	4	5	NA
012136	Acknowledges personal opinions	1	2	3	4	5	NA
012137	Acknowledges opinions of others	1	2	3	4	5	NA
012138	Refrains from violating the rights of others	1	2	3	4	5	NA
012139	Respects others	1	2	3	4	5	NA
012140	Respects the environment	1	2	3	4	5	NA
012141	Supports equality in treatment of others	1	2	3	4	5	NA
012142	Recognizes that mutual trust is necessary in healthy relationships	1	2	3	4	5	NA

		Consistently demonstrated	Often demonstrated	Sometimes demonstrated	Rarely demonstrated	Never demonstrated	
012143	Exhibits anger	1	2	3	4	5	NA
012144	Exhibits inappropriate trust in others	1	2	3	4	5	NA
012145	Exhibits loneliness	1	2	3	4	5	NA
012146	Exhibits depression	1	2	3	4	5	NA
012147	Exhibits anxiety	1	2	3	4	5	NA
012148	Dwells on past	1	2	3	4	5	NA

4th edition

Outcome Content References:

Andreoletti, C., Weratti, B. W., & Lachan, M. E. (2006). Age differences in the relationship between anxiety and recall. *Aging & Mental Health, 10*(3), 265-271.

Eva, K. W. (2003). Stemming the tide: Cognitive aging theories and their implications for continuing education in the health professions. *Journal of Continuing Education in the Health, 23*(3), 133-140.

Isaacowitz, D. M., Vaillant, G. E., & Seligman, M. E. P. (2003). Strengths and satisfaction across the adult lifespan. *International Journal of Aging & Human Development, 57*(2), 181-201.

Newman, R. S., & German, D. J. (2005). Life span effects of lexical factors on oral naming. *Language & Speech, 48*(Part 2), 123-156.

Papalia, D. E., Olds, S. W., & Feldman, R. D. (2007). *Human development* (10th ed.). New York: McGraw Hill.

Skultety, K. M., & Whitbourne, S. K. (2004). Gender differences in identity processes and self-esteem in middle and later adulthood. *Journal of Women & Aging, 16*(1/2), 175-188.

Spira, M. (2006). Mapping your future—A proactive approach to aging. *Journal of Gerontological Social Work, 47*(1/2), 71-87.

Troyer, A. K., Hafliger, A., Cadieux, M. J., & Craik, F. I. M. (2006). Name and face learning in older adults effects of level of processing, self-generation, and intention to learn. *Journals of Gerontology Series B: Psychological Sciences & Social Sciences, 61B*(2), 67-74.

Valentjin, S. A., van Boxtel, M. P., van Hooren, S. A., Bosma, H., Beckers, H. J., Ponds, R. W., Jolles, J. (2005). Change in sensory functioning predicts change in cognitive functioning: Results from a 6-year follow-up in the Maastricht aging study. *Journal of the American Geriatrics Society, 53*(3), 374-380.

D

Development: Middle Adulthood—0122

Domain-Functional Health (I)

Class-Growth & Development (B)

Scale(s)-Never demonstrated to Consistently demonstrated (m) and Consistently demonstrated to Never demonstrated (t)

Care Recipient:

Data Source:

D

Definition: Cognitive, psychosocial, and moral progression from 40 through 64 years of age

OUTCOME TARGET RATING: Maintain at_____   Increase to_____

Development: Middle Adulthood Overall Rating	Never demonstrated 1	Rarely demonstrated 2	Sometimes demonstrated 3	Often demonstrated 4	Consistently demonstrated 5	
INDICATORS:						
012201 Exhibits high level cognitive function	1	2	3	4	5	NA
012202 Uses expanded language skills	1	2	3	4	5	NA
012203 Uses accumulated knowledge in decision-making	1	2	3	4	5	NA
012204 Exhibits high level problem solving skills	1	2	3	4	5	NA
012205 Exhibits creativity	1	2	3	4	5	NA
012206 Maintains lifelong learning	1	2	3	4	5	NA
012207 Exhibits success in chosen occupation	1	2	3	4	5	NA
012208 Exhibits occupational flexibility	1	2	3	4	5	NA
012209 Copes with personal loss	1	2	3	4	5	NA
012210 Copes with career burnout	1	2	3	4	5	NA
012211 Expresses optimism about the present	1	2	3	4	5	NA
012212 Expresses optimism about the future	1	2	3	4	5	N
012213 Adjusts to children leaving home	1	2	3	4	5	NA
012214 Copes with adult children in the home	1	2	3	4	5	NA
012215 Performs positive role in lives of grandchildren	1	2	3	4	5	NA
012216 Adjusts to parenting role of grandchildren	1	2	3	4	5	NA
012217 Exhibits strong sense of self	1	2	3	4	5	NA
012218 Maintains a healthy intimate relationship with partner	1	2	3	4	5	NA
012219 Maintains relationships with immediate family	1	2	3	4	5	NA
012220 Maintains relationships with extended family	1	2	3	4	5	NA
012221 Develops close relationships with friends	1	2	3	4	5	NA

	Never demonstrated	Rarely demonstrated	Sometimes demonstrated	Often demonstrated	Consistently demonstrated	
012222 Adjusts to sexual function changes	1	2	3	4	5	NA
012223 Practices safe sex	1	2	3	4	5	NA
012224 Adjusts to midlife changes	1	2	3	4	5	NA
012225 Avoids substance misuse	1	2	3	4	5	NA
012226 Adheres to laws that protect welfare of others	1	2	3	4	5	NA
012227 Acknowledges personal values	1	2	3	4	5	NA
012228 Acknowledges values of others	1	2	3	4	5	NA
012229 Acknowledges personal opinions	1	2	3	4	5	NA
012230 Acknowledges opinions of others	1	2	3	4	5	NA
012231 Refrains from violating rights of others	1	2	3	4	5	NA
012232 Respects others	1	2	3	4	5	NA
012233 Respects the environment	1	2	3	4	5	NA
012234 Supports equality in treatment of others	1	2	3	4	5	NA
012235 Recognizes that mutual trust is necessary in healthy relationships	1	2	3	4	5	NA

	Consistently demonstrated	Often demonstrated	Sometimes demonstrated	Rarely demonstrated	Never demonstrated	
012236 Dwells on past	1	2	3	4	5	NA
012237 Exhibits unresolved anger	1	2	3	4	5	NA
012238 Exhibits unresolved emotional issues	1	2	3	4	5	NA
012239 Exhibits incapacitating fear	1	2	3	4	5	NA
012240 Exhibits unsafe risk taking behaviors	1	2	3	4	5	NA
012241 Exhibits impulsivity	1	2	3	4	5	NA

4th edition

Outcome Content References:

Hartman-Stein, P. E., & Potkanowicz, E. S. (2003). Behavioral determinants of healthy aging: Good news for the baby boomer generation. *Online Journal of Issues in Nursing, 8*(2), 6.

Isaacowitz, D. M., Vaillant, G. E., & Seligman, M. E. P. (2003). Strengths and satisfaction across the adult lifespan. *International Journal of Aging & Human Development, 57*(2), 181-201.

Newman, R. S., & German, D. J. (2005). Life span effects of lexical factors on oral naming. *Language & Speech, 48*(Part 2), 123-156.

Papalia, D. E., Olds, S. W., & Feldman, R. D. (2007). *Human development* (10th ed.). New York: McGraw Hill.

Skultety, K. M., & Whitbourne, S. K. (2004). Gender differences in identity processes and self-esteem in middle and later adulthood. *Journal of Women & Aging, 16*(1/2), 175-188.

Development: Young Adulthood—0123

Domain-Functional Health (I)
Class-Growth & Development (B)
Scale(s)-Never demonstrated to Consistently demonstrated (m) and Consistently Demonstrated to Never Demonstrated (t)

Care Recipient:
Data Source:

D

Definition: Cognitive, psychosocial, and moral progression from 18 through 39 years of age

OUTCOME TARGET RATING: Maintain at_____   Increase to_____

Development: Young Adulthood Overall Rating	Never demonstrated 1	Rarely demonstrated 2	Sometimes demonstrated 3	Often demonstrated 4	Consistently demonstrated 5	
INDICATORS:						
012301 Expresses complex thoughts	1	2	3	4	5	NA
012302 Expands language skills	1	2	3	4	5	NA
012303 Makes educational choices	1	2	3	4	5	NA
012304 Makes occupational choices	1	2	3	4	5	NA
012305 Establishes gainful employment	1	2	3	4	5	NA
012306 Establishes pattern of lifelong learning	1	2	3	4	5	NA
012307 Exhibits stable personality traits	1	2	3	4	5	NA
012308 Adjusts lifestyle according to life events	1	2	3	4	5	NA
012309 Embraces sexual identity	1	2	3	4	5	NA
012310 Practices safe sex	1	2	3	4	5	NA
012311 Maintains a healthy intimate relationship with partner	1	2	3	4	5	NA
012312 Maintains relationships with immediate family	1	2	3	4	5	NA
012313 Maintains relationships with extended family	1	2	3	4	5	NA
012314 Develops new friendships	1	2	3	4	5	NA
012315 Copes with personal loss	1	2	3	4	5	NA
012316 Adapts to parental role	1	2	3	4	5	NA
012317 Exhibits autonomy	1	2	3	4	5	NA
012318 Exhibits self-control	1	2	3	4	5	NA
012319 Exhibits personal responsibility	1	2	3	4	5	NA
012320 Avoids substance misuse	1	2	3	4	5	NA
012321 Adheres to laws that protect the welfare of others	1	2	3	4	5	NA
012322 Acknowledges personal values	1	2	3	4	5	NA
012323 Acknowledges values of others	1	2	3	4	5	NA
012324 Acknowledges personal opinions	1	2	3	4	5	NA
012325 Acknowledges opinions of others	1	2	3	4	5	NA
012326 Refrains from violating the rights of others	1	2	3	4	5	NA
012327 Respects others	1	2	3	4	5	NA
012328 Respects the environment	1	2	3	4	5	NA

		Consistently demonstrated	Often demonstrated	Sometimes demonstrated	Rarely demonstrated	Never demonstrated	
012329	Dwells on past	1	2	3	4	5	NA
012330	Exhibits unresolved anger	1	2	3	4	5	NA
012331	Exhibits unresolved emotional issues	1	2	3	4	5	NA
012332	Exhibits incapacitating fear	1	2	3	4	5	NA
012333	Exhibits inappropriate mistrust in others	1	2	3	4	5	NA
012334	Exhibits unsafe risk taking behaviors	1	2	3	4	5	NA
012335	Exhibits impulsivity	1	2	3	4	5	NA

4th edition

D

Outcome Content References:

Andreoletti, C., Weratti, B. W., & Lachan, M. E. (2006). Age differences in the relationship between anxiety and recall. *Aging & Mental Health, 10*(3), 265-271.

Isaacowitz, D. M., Vaillant, G. E., & Seligman, M. E. P. (2003). Strengths and satisfaction across the adult lifespan. *International Journal of Aging & Human Development, 57*(2), 181-201.

McLaren, L., Kuh, D., Hardy, R., & Gauvin, L. (2004). Positive and negative body-related comments and their relationship with body dissatisfaction in middle-aged women. *Psychology & Health, 19*(2), 261-272.

Newman, R. S., & German, D. J. (2005). Life span effects of lexical factors on oral naming. *Language & Speech, 48*(Part 2), 123-156.

Papalia, D. E., Olds, S. W., & Feldman, R. D. (2007). *Human development* (10th ed.). New York: McGraw Hill.

Diabetes Self-Management—1619

Domain-Health Knowledge & Behavior (IV)

Class-Health Behavior (Q)

Scale(s)-Never demonstrated to Consistently demonstrated (m)

Care Recipient:

Data Source:

D

Definition: Personal actions to manage diabetes mellitus, its treatment, and prevent disease progression

OUTCOME TARGET RATING: Maintain at_____   Increase to_____

Diabetes Self-Management Overall Rating	Never demonstrated 1	Rarely demonstrated 2	Sometimes demonstrated 3	Often demonstrated 4	Consistently demonstrated 5	
INDICATORS:						
161901 Accepts health provider's diagnosis	1	2	3	4	5	NA
161902 Seeks information about methods to prevent complications	1	2	3	4	5	NA
161903 Follows preventive foot care practices	1	2	3	4	5	NA
161904 Obtains dilated vision examination as recommended	1	2	3	4	5	NA
161905 Adjusts medication when acutely ill	1	2	3	4	5	NA
161906 Reports non-healing breaks in skin to primary care provider	1	2	3	4	5	NA
161907 Participates in health care decision making process	1	2	3	4	5	NA
161908 Participates in prescribed educational program	1	2	3	4	5	NA
161909 Performs treatment regimen as prescribed	1	2	3	4	5	NA
161910 Performs correct procedure for blood glucose testing	1	2	3	4	5	NA
161911 Monitors blood glucose	1	2	3	4	5	NA
161912 Treats symptoms of hyperglycemia	1	2	3	4	5	NA
161913 Treats symptoms of hypoglycemia	1	2	3	4	5	NA
161914 Monitors frequency of hypoglycemia episodes	1	2	3	4	5	NA
161915 Reports symptoms of complications	1	2	3	4	5	NA
161916 Uses diary to monitor blood glucose level over time	1	2	3	4	5	NA
161917 Uses preventive measures to reduce risk of complications	1	2	3	4	5	NA

		Never demonstrated	Rarely demonstrated	Sometimes demonstrated	Often demonstrated	Consistently demonstrated	
161941	Obtains health care if blood glucose levels fluctuate outside of recommended parameters	1	2	3	4	5	NA
161919	Monitors urinary glucose and ketones	1	2	3	4	5	NA
161920	Follows recommended diet	1	2	3	4	5	NA
161921	Follows recommended activity level	1	2	3	4	5	NA
161922	Monitors body weight	1	2	3	4	5	NA
161923	Uses effective weight control strategies	1	2	3	4	5	NA
161924	Maintains optimum weight	1	2	3	4	5	NA
161925	Follows restrictions for alcohol use	1	2	3	4	5	NA
161926	Participates in smoking cessation regimen	1	2	3	4	5	NA
161927	Participates in recommended exercise program	1	2	3	4	5	NA
161928	Performs usual life routine	1	2	3	4	5	NA
161929	Uses correct procedure for insulin administration	1	2	3	4	5	NA
161930	Stores insulin correctly	1	2	3	4	5	NA
161931	Obtains required medication	1	2	3	4	5	NA
161932	Uses medication as prescribed	1	2	3	4	5	NA
161933	Monitors medication therapeutic effects	1	2	3	4	5	NA
161934	Rotates injection sites	1	2	3	4	5	NA
161935	Uses only over-the-counter medication approved by health professional	1	2	3	4	5	NA
161936	Obtains flu and pneumonia immunizations	1	2	3	4	5	NA
161937	Uses health care services congruent with needs	1	2	3	4	5	NA
161938	Reports need for financial assistance	1	2	3	4	5	NA
161939	Keeps appointments with health professional	1	2	3	4	5	NA
161940	Maintains plan for medical emergencies	1	2	3	4	5	NA
161943	Obtains preconception counseling	1	2	3	4	5	NA
161944	Monitors for depression	1	2	3	4	5	NA
161942	Adjusts life routine for optimum health	1	2	3	4	5	NA

D

Continued

3rd edition 2004; Revised 4th edition

Outcome Content References:

American Diabetes Association. (1998). Standards of medical care for patients with diabetes mellitus. *Diabetes Care, 21* (Suppl. 1), S23-S31.

American Diabetes Association. (1998). Testing of glycemia in diabetes. *Diabetes Care, 21*(Suppl. 1), S69-S71.

Cryer, P. E. (2001). Hypoglycemia risk reduction in Type I Diabetes. *Experimental & Clinical Endocrinology & Diabetes, 109*(Suppl. 2), S412-S423.

Dalewitz, J., Khan, N., & Hershey, C. O. (2000). Barriers to control blood glucose in diabetes mellitus. *American Journal of Medical Quality, 15*(1), 16-25.

Funnell, M. M., Hunt, C., Kulkarni, K., Rubin, R. R., & Yarborough, P. C. (Eds.). (1998). *A core curriculum for Association of Diabetes educators.* Chicago: American Association of Diabetes Educators.

Kelley, D. B. (Ed.). (1998). *Intensive diabetes management.* (2nd ed.). Alexandria, VA: American Diabetes Association.

Lebovitz, H. E. (Ed.). (1998). *Therapy for diabetes mellitus and related disorders* (3rd ed.). Alexandria, VA: American Diabetes Association.

Lewis, S. M., Collier, I. C., Heitkemper, M. M., & Dirksen, S. R. (2000). *Medical-surgical nursing: Assessment & management of clinical problems* (5th ed.). St. Louis: Mosby.

McCance, K. L., & Huether, S. E. (2002). *Pathophysiology: The biologic basis for disease in adults and children* (4th ed.). St. Louis: Mosby.

Miller, D. K., & Fain, J. A. (2006). Diabetes self-management education. *Nursing Clinics of North America, 41,* 655-666.

D

Dignified Life Closure—1307

Domain-Psychosocial Health (III)

Class-Psychosocial Adaptation (N)

Scale(s)-Never demonstrated to Consistently demonstrated (m)

Care Recipient:

Data Source:

D

Definition: Personal actions to maintain control during approaching end of life					

OUTCOME TARGET RATING: Maintain at_____   Increase to_____

Dignified Life Closure Overall Rating	Never demonstrated 1	Rarely demonstrated 2	Sometimes demonstrated 3	Often demonstrated 4	Consistently demonstrated 5

INDICATORS:

130701	Puts affairs in order	1	2	3	4	5	NA
130702	Expresses hopefulness	1	2	3	4	5	NA
130703	Participates in decisions related to care	1	2	3	4	5	NA
130704	Participates in decisions about hospitalization	1	2	3	4	5	NA
130705	Participates in decisions about resuscitation status	1	2	3	4	5	NA
130706	Controls decisions about organ donation	1	2	3	4	5	NA
130707	Participates in planning funeral	1	2	3	4	5	NA
130708	Maintains current will	1	2	3	4	5	NA
130709	Maintains advance directives	1	2	3	4	5	NA
130710	Resolves important issues	1	2	3	4	5	NA
130711	Shares feelings about dying	1	2	3	4	5	NA
130712	Reconciles relationships	1	2	3	4	5	NA
130713	Completes meaningful goals	1	2	3	4	5	NA
130714	Maintains sense of control of remaining time	1	2	3	4	5	NA
130715	Exchanges affection with others	1	2	3	4	5	NA
130716	Disengages gradually from significant others	1	2	3	4	5	NA
130717	Recalls lifetime memories	1	2	3	4	5	NA
130718	Reviews life's accomplishments	1	2	3	4	5	NA
130719	Discusses spiritual experiences	1	2	3	4	5	NA
130720	Discusses spiritual concerns	1	2	3	4	5	NA
130721	Maintains physical independence	1	2	3	4	5	NA
130722	Controls treatment choices	1	2	3	4	5	NA
130723	Controls food/drink intake	1	2	3	4	5	NA
130724	Controls personal possessions	1	2	3	4	5	NA
130725	Expresses readiness for death	1	2	3	4	5	NA

Continued

3rd edition 2004

Outcome Content References:

Callanan, M., & Kelley, P. (1992). *Final gifts*. New York: Poseidon Press.

Cicirelli, V. G. (1997). Elders' end-of-life decisions: Implications for hospice care. *Hospice Journal Physical, Psychosocial, & Pastoral Care of the Dying, 12*(1), 57-72.

Ferrell, B. R. (1993). To know suffering. *Oncology Nursing Forum, 20*(10), 1471-1477.

McCanse, R. P. (1995). The McCanse Readiness for Death Instrument (MRDI): A reliable and valid measure for hospice care. *Hospice Journal, 10*(1), 15-26.

Potter, P. A., & Perry, A. G. (2001). *Fundamentals of nursing* (5th ed.). St. Louis: Mosby.

Quill, T. E. (1993). *Death and dignity: Making choices and taking charge*. New York: W. W. Norton & Co.

Schmele, J. A. (1995). Perceptions of a dying patient of the quality of care and caring: An interview with Ivan Hanson. *Journal of Nursing Care Quality, 9*(4), 31-42.

D

Discharge Readiness: Independent Living—0311

Domain-Functional Health (I)   Care Recipient:

Class-Self-Care (D)   Data Source:

Scale-Never demonstrated to Consistently demonstrated (m) and Consistently demonstrated to Never demonstrated (t)

D

Definition: Readiness of a patient to relocate from a health care institution to living independently

OUTCOME TARGET RATING: Maintain at_____   Increase to_____

Discharge Readiness: Independent Living Overall Rating	Never demonstrated 1	Rarely demonstrated 2	Sometimes demonstrated 3	Often demonstrated 4	Consistently demonstrated 5	
INDICATORS:						
031113 Obtains needed assistance	1	2	3	4	5	NA
031114 Uses personal support system	1	2	3	4	5	NA
031106 Describes signs & symptoms to health professional	1	2	3	4	5	NA
031107 Describes prescribed treatments	1	2	3	4	5	NA
031108 Describes risks for complications	1	2	3	4	5	NA
031115 Manages own non-parenteral medication	1	2	3	4	5	NA
031116 Manages own parenteral medication	1	2	3	4	5	NA
031110 Performs activities of daily living (ADLs) independently	1	2	3	4	5	NA
031111 Performs instrumental activities of daily living (IADLs) independently	1	2	3	4	5	NA
031112 Makes appropriate judgments	1	2	3	4	5	NA
031117 Participates in discharge planning	1	2	3	4	5	NA

	Consistently demonstrated	Often demonstrated	Sometimes demonstrated	Rarely demonstrated	Never demonstrated	
031101 Fever	1	2	3	4	5	NA
031102 Infection	1	2	3	4	5	NA
031103 Confusion	1	2	3	4	5	NA

3rd edition 2004; Revised 4th edition

Outcome Content References:

Barnes, S. (2000). Ambulatory surgery. Are you watching the clock? Let criteria define discharge readiness. *Journal of Perianesthesia Nursing, 15*(3), 174-176.

Bull, M. J., Hansen, H. E., & Gross, C. R. (2000). Differences in family caregiver outcomes by their level of involvement in discharge planning. *Applied Nursing Research, 13*(2), 76-82.

Costa, M. J. (2001). The lived perioperative experience of ambulatory surgery patients. *AORN Journal, 74*(6), 874-876, 878-881.

Harris, M. D. (1999). Medicare & the nurse. 10 DRGs that can affect home care referrals. *Home Healthcare Nurse, 17*(2), 127-129.

Higson, J., & Bolland, R. (2001). Paediatric discharge criteria lead to improved outcomes. *Times, 97*(35), 30-31.

Kuc, J. A., & Pietro, J. (1999). Safe discharge from the PACU and ambulatory care setting. *Journal of Nursing Law, 6*(2), 7-14.

Walker, C. R., Watters, N., Nadon, C., Graham, K., & Niday, P. (1999). Discharge of mothers and babies from hospital after birth of a healthy full-term infant: Developing criteria through a community-wide consensus process. *Canadian Journal of Public Health, 90*(5), 313-315.

Discharge Readiness: Supported Living—0312

Domain-Functional Health (I)

Class-Self-Care (D)

Scale-Never demonstrated to Consistently demonstrated (m)

Care Recipient:

Data Source:

D

| **Definition:** Readiness of a patient to relocate from a health care institution to a lower level of supported living |

OUTCOME TARGET RATING: Maintain at_____   Increase to_____

Discharge Readiness: Supported Living Overall Rating	Never demonstrated 1	Rarely demonstrated 2	Sometimes demonstrated 3	Often demonstrated 4	Consistently demonstrated 5	

INDICATORS:

		Never 1	Rarely 2	Sometimes 3	Often 4	Consistently 5	
031201	Patient needs consistent with staff support	1	2	3	4	5	NA
031202	Patient needs consistent with family support	1	2	3	4	5	NA
031203	Oriented to care at new residence	1	2	3	4	5	NA
031204	Accepts transfer to new residence	1	2	3	4	5	NA
031205	Describes special needs	1	2	3	4	5	NA
031206	Describes short term plan	1	2	3	4	5	NA
031207	Describes long term plan	1	2	3	4	5	NA
031208	Describes plan for continuity of care	1	2	3	4	5	NA
031209	Participates in discharge planning	1	2	3	4	5	NA

3rd edition 2004; Revised 4th edition

Outcome Content References:

Bosek, M. S. D., Burton, L. A., & Savage, T. A. (1999). The patient who could not be discharged: How far should patient autonomy extend? *JONA's Healthcare Law, Ethics, & Regulation, 1*(4), 23-30.

Bull, M. J., Hansen, H. E., & Gross, C. R. (2000). Differences in family caregiver outcomes by their level of involvement in discharge planning. *Applied Nursing Research, 13*(2), 76-82.

Chan, L., & Ciol, M. (2000). Medicare's payment system: Its effect on discharges to skilled nursing facilities from rehabilitation hospitals. *Archives of Physical Medicine & Rehabilitation, 81*(6), 715-719.

Discomfort Level—2109

Domain-Perceived Health (V)
Class-Symptom Status (V)
Scale(s)-Severe to None (n)

Care Recipient:
Data Source:

Definition: Severity of observed or reported mental or physical discomfort

OUTCOME TARGET RATING: Maintain at_____   Increase to_____

Discomfort Level Overall Rating		Severe 1	Substantial 2	Moderate 3	Mild 4	None 5	
INDICATORS:							
210901	Pain	1	2	3	4	5	NA
210902	Anxiety	1	2	3	4	5	NA
210903	Moaning	1	2	3	4	5	NA
210904	Suffering	1	2	3	4	5	NA
210905	Thrashing	1	2	3	4	5	NA
210906	Stress	1	2	3	4	5	NA
210907	Fear	1	2	3	4	5	NA
210908	Depression	1	2	3	4	5	NA
210909	Hallucinations	1	2	3	4	5	NA
210910	Delusions	1	2	3	4	5	NA
210911	Paranoid thoughts	1	2	3	4	5	NA
210912	Obsessive compulsive behaviors	1	2	3	4	5	NA
210913	Hyperactivity	1	2	3	4	5	NA
210914	Restlessness	1	2	3	4	5	NA
210915	Restless legs syndrome	1	2	3	4	5	NA
210916	Itching	1	2	3	4	5	NA
210917	Muscle aches	1	2	3	4	5	NA
210918	Grimacing	1	2	3	4	5	NA
210919	Facial tension	1	2	3	4	5	NA
210920	Rebound tenderness	1	2	3	4	5	NA
210921	Jerking	1	2	3	4	5	NA
210922	Poor body positioning	1	2	3	4	5	NA
210923	Labored breathing	1	2	3	4	5	NA
210924	Air hunger	1	2	3	4	5	NA
210925	Loss of appetite	1	2	3	4	5	NA
210926	Chilling	1	2	3	4	5	NA
210927	Hypothermia	1	2	3	4	5	NA
210928	Nausea	1	2	3	4	5	NA
210929	Vomiting	1	2	3	4	5	NA
210930	Diarrhea	1	2	3	4	5	NA

Continued

		Severe	Substantial	Moderate	Mild	None	
210931	Bowel incontinence	1	2	3	4	5	NA
210932	Constipation	1	2	3	4	5	NA
210933	Urinary incontinence	1	2	3	4	5	NA
210934	Inability to communicate	1	2	3	4	5	NA
210935	Suicidal thoughts	1	2	3	4	5	NA
210936	Loss of faith	1	2	3	4	5	NA
210937	Sense of spiritual abandonment	1	2	3	4	5	NA

4th edition

Outcome Content References:

Gropper, E. I. (1992). Promoting health by promoting comfort. *Nursing Forum, 27*(2), 5-8.

Hamilton, J. (1989). Comfort and the hospitalized chronically ill. *Journal of Gerontological Nursing, 15*(4), 28-33.

Kennedy, G. T. (1991). *A nursing investigation of comfort and comforting care of the acutely ill patient.* Unpublished doctoral dissertation, The University of Texas, Austin.

Kolcaba, K. (2003). *Comfort theory and practice: A vision for holistic health care and research.* New York: Springer.

Kolcaba, K., & DiMarco, M. (2005). Comfort theory and its application to pediatric nursing. *Pediatric Nursing, 31*(3), 187-194.

Tipton, L. (2001). *A qualitative study of hope and the environment of persons living with cancer. Dissertation Abstracts International, 62*(03), 1326B. (UMI No. 3008460).

Distorted Thought Self-Control—1403

Domain-Psychosocial Health (III)

Class-Self-Control (O)

Scale(s)-Never demonstrated to Consistently demonstrated (m)

Care Recipient:

Data Source:

D

Definition: Self-restraint of disruptions in perception, thought processes, and thought content

OUTCOME TARGET RATING: Maintain at_____   Increase to_____

Distorted Thought Self-Control Overall Rating	Never demonstrated 1	Rarely demonstrated 2	Sometimes demonstrated 3	Often demonstrated 4	Consistently demonstrated 5	
INDICATORS:						
140301 Recognizes hallucinations or delusions are occurring	1	2	3	4	5	NA
140302 Refrains from attending to hallucinations or delusions	1	2	3	4	5	NA
140303 Refrains from responding to hallucinations or delusions	1	2	3	4	5	NA
140304 Monitors frequency of hallucinations or delusions	1	2	3	4	5	NA
140305 Describes content of hallucinations or delusions	1	2	3	4	5	NA
140306 Reports decrease in hallucinations or delusions	1	2	3	4	5	NA
140307 Asks for validation of reality	1	2	3	4	5	NA
140308 Maintains affect consistent with mood	1	2	3	4	5	NA
140309 Interacts with others appropriately	1	2	3	4	5	NA
140310 Perceives environment accurately	1	2	3	4	5	NA
140311 Exhibits logical thought flow patterns	1	2	3	4	5	NA
140312 Exhibits reality-based thinking	1	2	3	4	5	NA
140313 Exhibits appropriate thought content	1	2	3	4	5	NA
140314 Exhibits ability to grasp ideas of others	1	2	3	4	5	NA

1st edition 1997; Revised 2nd edition 2000; Revised 3rd edition 2004

Outcome Content References:

Andreasen, N. C., & Black, D. (2001). *Introductory textbook of psychiatry* (3rd ed.). Washington, DC: American Psychiatric Publishing.

Buccheri, R., Trygstad, L., Kanas, N., & Dowling, G. (1997). Symptom management of auditory hallucinations in schizophrenia: Results of 1-year follow up. *Journal of Psychosocial Nursing & Mental Health Services, 35*(12), 20-28, 37-38.

Buccheri, R., Trygstad, L., Kanas, N., Waldron, B., & Dowling, G. (1996). Auditory hallucinations in schizophrenia: Group experience in examining symptom management and behavioral strategies. *Journal of Psychosocial Nursing & Mental Health Services, 34*(2), 12-26, 44-45.

+Cummings, J. L.(1997). The Neuropsychiatric Inventory: Assessing psychopathology in dementia patients. *Neurology, 48*(Suppl. 6), S10-S16.

Frederick, J., & Cotanch, P. (1995). Self-help techniques for auditory hallucinations in schizophrenia. *Issues in Mental Health Nursing, 16*(3), 213-224.

Grimaldi, D., & Cousins, A. (1985). Paranoia. *Journal of Emergency Nursing, 11*(4), 201-204.

MacRae, A. (1997). The model of functional deficits associated with hallucinations. *American Journal of Occupational Therapy, 51*(1), 57-63.

Rosenthal, T. T., & McGuinness, T. M. (1986). Dealing with delusional patients: Discovering the distorted truth. *Issues in Mental Health Nursing, 8*(2), 143-154.

Stuart, G. W., & Laraia, M. T. (2001). *Principles and practice of psychiatric nursing* (7th ed.). St. Louis: Mosby.

Drug Abuse Cessation Behavior—1630

Domain-Health Knowledge & Behavior (IV)

Class-Health Behavior (Q)

Scale(s)-Never demonstrated to Consistently demonstrated (m)

Care Recipient:

Data Source:

D

Definition: Personal actions to eliminate drug use that poses a threat to health

OUTCOME TARGET RATING: Maintain at_____   Increase to_____

Drug Abuse Cessation Behavior Overall Rating	Never demonstrated 1	Rarely demonstrated 2	Sometimes demonstrated 3	Often demonstrated 4	Consistently demonstrated 5	
INDICATORS:						
163001 Expresses willingness to stop drug use	1	2	3	4	5	NA
163002 Expresses belief in the ability to stop drug use	1	2	3	4	5	NA
163003 Identifies benefits of eliminating harmful drug use	1	2	3	4	5	NA
163004 Identifies negative consequences of drug use	1	2	3	4	5	NA
163005 Develops effective strategies to eliminate drug use	1	2	3	4	5	NA
163006 Identifies barriers to harmful drug use elimination	1	2	3	4	5	NA
163007 Adjusts drug use elimination strategies as needed	1	2	3	4	5	NA
163008 Commits to drug elimination strategies	1	2	3	4	5	NA
163009 Follows selected drug elimination strategies	1	2	3	4	5	NA
163010 Participates in screening for associated health problems	1	2	3	4	5	NA
163011 Uses strategies to cope with withdrawal symptoms	1	2	3	4	5	NA
163012 Uses behavior modification strategies	1	2	3	4	5	NA
163013 Uses effective coping strategies	1	2	3	4	5	NA
163014 Obtains assistance from health professional	1	2	3	4	5	NA
163015 Uses personal support system	1	2	3	4	5	NA
163016 Uses reputable sources of information	1	2	3	4	5	NA
163017 Uses drug replacement therapy	1	2	3	4	5	NA
163018 Uses alternative therapy	1	2	3	4	5	NA
163019 Identifies emotional states that affect drug use	1	2	3	4	5	NA
163020 Adjusts lifestyle to promote drug elimination	1	2	3	4	5	NA

		Never demonstrated	Rarely demonstrated	Sometimes demonstrated	Often demonstrated	Consistently demonstrated	
163021	Participates in drug withdrawal program	1	2	3	4	5	NA
163022	Participates in counseling	1	2	3	4	5	NA
163023	Monitors for signs of depression	1	2	3	4	5	NA
163024	Uses prescribed medication as recommended	1	2	3	4	5	NA
163025	Uses non-prescription medication as recommended	1	2	3	4	5	NA
163026	Uses available support groups	1	2	3	4	5	NA
163027	Uses available community resources	1	2	3	4	5	NA
163028	Eliminates harmful drug use	1	2	3	4	5	NA

4th edition

Outcome Content References:

Giesbrecht, N., & Haydon, E. (2006). Community-based interventions and alcohol, tobacco and other drugs: Foci, outcomes and implications, *Drug and Alcohol Review, 25*, 633-646.

Gossop, M., Marsden, J., Stewart, D., Treacy, S. (2002). Change and stability of change after treatment of drug misuse 2-year outcomes from the national treatment outcomes research study (UK). *Addicitive Behaviors, 27*, 155-166.

Kaminer, Y., Burleson, J. A., & Goldberger, R. (2002). Cognitive-behavioral coping skills and psychoeducation therapies for adolescent substance abuse. *Journal of Nervous and Mental Disease, 190*, 737-745.

Kenna, G. A., Nielsen, D. M., Mello, P., Schiesl, A., & Swift, R. M. (2007). Pharmacotherapy of dual substance abuse and dependence. *CNS Drugs, 21*(3), 213-237.

Litten, R. Z., & Allen, J. P. (1999). Medications for alcohol, illicit drug, and tobacco dependence: An update of research findings. *Journal of Substance Abuse Treatement, 16*(2), 105-112.

Simpson, D. D. (1997). Effectivencess of drug abuse treatment: A review of research from field settings. In J. A. Egertson, D.M. Fox, & A.I. Leshner (Eds.), *Treating drug abusers effectively.* Oxford: Blackwell.

Williams, R. J., Chang, S. Y., & Addiction Center Adolescent Research Group (2000). A comprehensive and compartive review of adolescent substance abuse treatment outcome, *Clinical Psychology: Science and Practice, 7*, 138-166.

Winters, K. C., Stinchfield, R., Latimer, W. W., & Lee, S. (2007). Long-term outcome of substance-dependent youth following 12-step treatment. *Journal of Substance Abuse Treatment, 33*, 61-69.

Electrolyte & Acid/Base Balance—0600

Domain-Physiologic Health (II)   Care Recipient:

Class-Fluid & Electrolytes (G)   Data Source:

Scale(s)-Severe deviation from normal range to No deviation from normal range (b) and Severe to None (n)

E

Definition: Balance of electrolytes and non-electrolytes in the intracellular and extracellular compartments of the body

OUTCOME TARGET RATING: Maintain at_____   Increase to_____

Electrolyte & Acid/Base Balance Overall Rating	Severe deviation from normal range 1	Substantial deviation from normal range 2	Moderate deviation from normal range 3	Mild deviation from normal range 4	No deviation from normal range 5	
INDICATORS:						
060001 Apical heart rate	1	2	3	4	5	NA
060002 Apical heart rhythm	1	2	3	4	5	NA
060003 Respiratory rate	1	2	3	4	5	NA
060004 Respiratory rhythm	1	2	3	4	5	NA
060005 Serum sodium	1	2	3	4	5	NA
060006 Serum potassium	1	2	3	4	5	NA
060007 Serum chloride	1	2	3	4	5	NA
060008 Serum calcium	1	2	3	4	5	NA
060009 Serum magnesium	1	2	3	4	5	NA
060010 Serum pH	1	2	3	4	5	NA
060011 Serum albumin	1	2	3	4	5	NA
060012 Serum creatinine	1	2	3	4	5	NA
060013 Serum bicarbonate	1	2	3	4	5	NA
060024 Serum carbon dioxide	1	2	3	4	5	NA
060025 Serum osmolarity	1	2	3	4	5	NA
060026 Serum glucose	1	2	3	4	5	NA
060027 Serum hematocrit	1	2	3	4	5	NA
060014 Blood urea nitrogen	1	2	3	4	5	NA
060028 Blood urea nitrogen to creatinine ratio	1	2	3	4	5	NA
060015 Urine pH	1	2	3	4	5	NA
060029 Urine sodium	1	2	3	4	5	NA
060030 Urine chloride	1	2	3	4	5	NA
060031 Urine creatinine	1	2	3	4	5	NA
060032 Urine osmolarity	1	2	3	4	5	NA
060022 Urine specific gravity	1	2	3	4	5	NA
060019 Neuromuscular non-irritability	1	2	3	4	5	NA
060023 Sensation in extremities	1	2	3	4	5	NA

E

		Severe	Substantial	Moderate	Mild	None	
060033	Impaired cognition	1	2	3	4	5	NA
060034	Fatigue	1	2	3	4	5	NA
060035	Muscle weakness	1	2	3	4	5	NA
060036	Muscle cramps	1	2	3	4	5	NA
060037	Abdominal cramps	1	2	3	4	5	NA
060038	Nausea	1	2	3	4	5	NA
060039	Dysrhythmia	1	2	3	4	5	NA
060040	Restlessness	1	2	3	4	5	NA
060041	Paresthesia	1	2	3	4	5	NA

1st edition 1997; Revised 3rd edition 2004; Revised 4th edition

Outcome Content References:

Cherry, R. (1992). Furosemide facts. *Emergency Medical Services, 21*(9), 79.

Cullen, L. (1992). Interventions related to fluid and electrolytes. *Nursing Clinics of North America, 27*(2), 60, 62, 79.

Innerarity, S. A. (1997). *Fluids and electrolytes* (3rd ed.). Springhouse, PA: Springhouse.

McCance, K. L., & Huether, S. E. (2002). *Pathophysiology: The biologic basis for disease in adults and children* (4th ed.). St. Louis: Mosby.

Methany, N. (2000). *Fluid and electrolyte balance: Nursing considerations* (4th ed.). Philadelphia: Lippincott Williams & Wilkins.

Norris, C. (1982). *Concept clarification in nursing*. Rockville, MD: Aspen.

Schuller, D., Mitchell, J., Calendrino, F., & Schuster, D. (1991). Fluid balance during pulmonary edema: Is fluid gain a marker or a cause of post-operative outcome? *Chest, 100*(4), 1068-1075.

Vullo-Navich, K., Smith, S., Andrews, M., Levine, A. M., Tischer, J. F., & Veglia, J. M. (1998). Comfort and incidence of abnormal serum sodium, BUN, creatinine and osmolality in dehydration of terminal illness. *The American Journal of Hospice & Palliative Care, 15*(2), 77-84.

Elopement Occurrence—1919

Domain-Health Knowledge & Behavior (IV)

Class-Risk Control & Safety (T)

Scale(s)-10 and over to None (g)

Care Recipient:

Data Source:

E

Definition: Number of times in the past 24 hours / 1 week / 1 month (select one) that an individual with a cognitive impairment escapes a secure area

OUTCOME TARGET RATING: Maintain at_____   Increase to_____

Elopement Occurrence Overall Rating	10 and over 1	7-9 2	4-6 3	1-3 4	None 5	

INDICATORS:

191901	Left place of residence unattended	1	2	3	4	5	NA
191902	Left secure area unattended	1	2	3	4	5	NA
191903	Opened exterior door	1	2	3	4	5	NA
191904	Slipped away from group activities	1	2	3	4	5	NA
191905	Climbed out window	1	2	3	4	5	NA

4th edition

Outcome Content References:

Algase, D. L., Son, G., Beattie, E., Song, J., Leitsch, S., & Yao, L. (2004). The interrelatedness of wandering and wayfinding in a community sample of persons with dementia. *Dementia and Geriatric Cognitive Disorders, 17*(3), 231-239.

Aud, M. A. (2004). Dangerous wandering: Elopements of older adults with dementia from long-term care facilities. *American Journal of Alzheimer's Disorders and Other Dementias, 19*(6), 361-368.

Dewing, J. (2006). Wandering into the future: Reconceptualizing wandering 'a natural and good thing'. *International Journal of Older People Nursing, 1*(4), 239–249.

Lai, C. K. Y., & Arthur, D. G. (2003). Wandering behavior in persons with dementia. *Journal of Advanced Nursing, 44*(2), 173–182.

Elopement Propensity Risk—1920

Domain-Health Knowledge & Behavior (IV)

Class-Risk Control & Safety (T)

Scale(s)-Consistently demonstrated to Never demonstrated (m)

Care Recipient:

Data Source:

E

Definition: The propensity of an individual with cognitive impairment to escape a secure area

OUTCOME TARGET RATING: Maintain at_____   Increase to_____

Elopement Propensity Risk Overall Rating	Consistently demonstrated 1	Often demonstrated 2	Sometimes demonstrated 3	Rarely demonstrated 4	Never demonstrated 5	
INDICATORS:						
192001 Wanders	1	2	3	4	5	NA
192002 Appears agitated	1	2	3	4	5	NA
192003 Refuses to remove coat	1	2	3	4	5	NA
192004 Packs bag to leave	1	2	3	4	5	NA
192005 Attempts to leave secure area	1	2	3	4	5	NA
192006 Leaves secure area unobserved	1	2	3	4	5	NA
192007 Leaves yard when outside	1	2	3	4	5	NA
192008 Appears sad	1	2	3	4	5	NA
192009 Weeps	1	2	3	4	5	NA
192010 Appears frightened	1	2	3	4	5	NA
192011 Asks others for assistance to leave	1	2	3	4	5	NA
192012 Attempts to leave with visitors	1	2	3	4	5	NA
192013 States wants to go home	1	2	3	4	5	NA
192014 Threatens to leave	1	2	3	4	5	NA
192015 Attempts to disengage alarm	1	2	3	4	5	NA

4th edition

Outcome Content References:

Algase, D. L., Son, G., Beattie, E., Song, J., Leitsch, S., & Yao, L. (2004). The interrelatedness of wandering and wayfinding in a community sample of persons with dementia. *Dementia and Geriatric Cognitive Disorders, 17*(3), 231-239.

Aud, M. A. (2004). Dangerous wandering: Elopements of older adults with dementia from long-term care facilities. *American Journal of Alzheimer's Disorders and Other Dementias, 19*(6), 361-368.

Dewing, J. (2006). Wandering into the future: Reconceptualizing wandering 'a natural and good thing'. *International Journal of Older People Nursing, 1*(4), 239–249.

Greenberg, H., Blank, H. R., & Argrett, S. (1968). The anatomy of elopement from an acute adolescent service: Escape from engagement. *Psychiatric Quarterly, 42*(1), 28-47.

Lai, C. K. Y., & Arthur, D. G. (2003). Wandering behavior in persons with dementia. *Journal of Advanced Nursing, 44*(2), 173–182.

Endurance—0001

Domain-Functional Health (I)

Class-Energy Maintenance (A)

Scale(s)-Severely compromised to Not compromised (a) and Severe to None (n)

Care Recipient:

Data Source:

E

Definition: Capacity to sustain activity

OUTCOME TARGET RATING: Maintain at_____   Increase to_____

Endurance Overall Rating	Severely compromised 1	Substantially compromised 2	Moderately compromised 3	Mildly compromised 4	Not compromised 5	

INDICATORS:

000101	Performance of usual routine	1	2	3	4	5	NA
000102	Activity	1	2	3	4	5	NA
000104	Concentration	1	2	3	4	5	NA
000106	Muscle endurance	1	2	3	4	5	NA
000107	Eating pattern	1	2	3	4	5	NA
000108	Libido	1	2	3	4	5	NA
000109	Energy restored after rest	1	2	3	4	5	NA
000112	Blood oxygen level	1	2	3	4	5	NA
000113	Hemoglobin	1	2	3	4	5	NA
000114	Hematocrit	1	2	3	4	5	NA
000115	Blood glucose	1	2	3	4	5	NA
000116	Serum electrolytes	1	2	3	4	5	NA

		Severe	Substantial	Moderate	Mild	None	
000110	Exhaustion	1	2	3	4	5	NA
000111	Lethargy	1	2	3	4	5	NA
000118	Fatigue	1	2	3	4	5	NA

1st edition 1997; Revised 3rd edition 2004; Revised 4th edition

Outcome Content References:

Ades, P. A., Ballor, D. L., Ashikaga, T., Utton, J. L., & Streekumaran Nair, K. (1996). Weight training improves walking endurance in healthy elderly persons, *Annals of Internal Medicine, 124*(6), 568-572.

+Dartmouth Primary Care Cooperative Information Project. (1987). *COOP Charts.* Hanover, NH: Department of Community and Family Medicine, Dartmouth Medical School.

Ellis, J. R., & Nowlis, E. A. (1994). *Providing nursing care within the nursing process* (5th ed.). Philadelphia: J.B. Lippincott.

Johns, M. E. (1991). Activity and exercise. In S. Wingate (Ed.), *Cardiac nursing: A clinical management and patient care resource* (pp. 141-145). Gaithersburg, MD: Aspen.

Lubkin, I. M. (2002). *Chronic illness: Impact and interventions* (5th ed.). Sudbury, MA: Jones and Bartlett.

Potter, P. A., & Perry, A. G. (2001). *Fundamentals of nursing* (5th ed.). St. Louis: Mosby.

Pugh, L. C., & Milligan, R. (1993). A framework for the study of childbearing fatigue. *Advances in Nursing Science, 15*(4), 60-70.

Tiesinga, L. J., Dassen, T. W. N., & Halfens, R. J. G. (1996). Fatigue: A summary of the definitions, dimensions, and indicators. *Nursing Diagnosis, 7*(2), 51-62.

Titler, M. G. (2001). Activity intolerance. In M. Maas, K. Buckwalter, M. Hardy, T. Tripp-Reimer, M. Titler, & J. Specht (Eds.), *Nursing care of older adults: Diagnoses, outcomes & interventions* (pp. 324-336). St. Louis: Mosby.

Topf, M. (1992). Effects of personal control over hospital noise on sleep. *Research in Nursing & Health, 15*(1), 19-28.

Energy Conservation—0002

Domain-Functional Health (I)

Class-Energy Maintenance (A)

Scale(s)-Never demonstrated to Consistently demonstrated (m)

Care Recipient:

Data Source:

E

Definition: Personal actions to manage energy for initiating and sustaining activity

OUTCOME TARGET RATING: Maintain at_____   Increase to_____

Energy Conservation Overall Rating	Never demonstrated 1	Rarely demonstrated 2	Sometimes demonstrated 3	Often demonstrated 4	Consistently demonstrated 5	
INDICATORS:						
000201 Balances activity and rest	1	2	3	4	5	NA
000202 Uses naps to restore energy	1	2	3	4	5	NA
000203 Recognizes energy limitations	1	2	3	4	5	NA
000204 Uses energy conservation techniques	1	2	3	4	5	NA
000209 Organizes activities to conserve energy	1	2	3	4	5	NA
000205 Adapts lifestyle to energy level	1	2	3	4	5	NA
000206 Maintains adequate nutrition	1	2	3	4	5	NA
000207 Reports adequate endurance for activity	1	2	3	4	5	NA

1st edition 1997; Revised 3rd edition 2004

Outcome Content References:

Dixon, J. K., Dixon, J. P., & Hickey, M. (1993). Energy as a central factor in the self assessment of health. *Advances in Nursing Science, 15*(4), 1-12.

+Lee, K. A., Hicks, G., & Nino-Murcia, G. (1991). Validity and reliability of a scale to assess fatigue. *Psychiatry Research, 36(3)*, 291-298.

Lubkin, I. M. (2002). *Chronic illness: Impact and interventions* (5th ed.). Sudbury, MA: Jones and Bartlett.

McCane, K. L., & Huether, S. E. (2002). *Pathophysiology: The biologic basis for disease in adults and children* (4th ed.). St. Louis: Mosby.

Potter, P. A., & Perry, A. G. (2001). *Fundamentals of nursing* (5th ed.). St. Louis: Mosby.

Fall Prevention Behavior—1909

Domain-Health Knowledge & Behavior (IV)

Class-Risk Control & Safety (T)

Scale(s)-Never demonstrated to Consistently demonstrated (m)

Care Recipient:

Data Source:

Definition: Personal or family caregiver actions to minimize risk factors that might precipitate falls in the personal environment

OUTCOME TARGET RATING: Maintain at_____   Increase to_____

Fall Prevention Behavior Overall rating	Never demonstrated 1	Rarely demonstrated 2	Sometimes demonstrated 3	Often demonstrated 4	Consistently demonstrated 5	

INDICATORS:

190903	Places barriers to prevent falls	1	2	3	4	5	NA
190905	Uses handrails as needed	1	2	3	4	5	NA
190915	Uses grab bars as needed	1	2	3	4	5	NA
190914	Uses rubber mats in tub/shower	1	2	3	4	5	NA
190910	Uses well-fitting tied shoes	1	2	3	4	5	NA
190901	Uses assistive devices correctly	1	2	3	4	5	NA
190918	Uses vision correcting devices	1	2	3	4	5	NA
190902	Provides assistance with mobility	1	2	3	4	5	NA
190919	Uses safe transfer procedure	1	2	3	4	5	NA
190922	Provides adequate lighting	1	2	3	4	5	NA
190909	Uses stools and ladders safely	1	2	3	4	5	NA
190906	Eliminates clutter, spills, glare from floors	1	2	3	4	5	NA
190907	Removes rugs	1	2	3	4	5	NA
190908	Arranges for removal of snow and ice from walking surfaces	1	2	3	4	5	NA
190911	Adjusts toilet height as needed	1	2	3	4	5	NA
190912	Adjusts chair height as needed	1	2	3	4	5	NA
190913	Adjusts bed height as needed	1	2	3	4	5	NA
190916	Controls restlessness	1	2	3	4	5	NA
190917	Uses precautions when taking medication that increase risk for falls	1	2	3	4	5	NA

1st edition 1997; Revised 3rd edition 2004

Outcome Content References:

Abreu, N., Hutchins, J., Matson, J., Polizzi, N., & Seymour, C. J. (1998). Effect of group versus home visit safety education and prevention strategies for falling in community-dwelling elderly persons. *Home Health Care Management & Practice, 10*(4), 57-65.

Johnson, M., Cusick, A., & Chang, S. (2001). Home-screen: A short scale to measure fall risk in the home. *Public Health Nursing, 18*(3), 169-177.

Kilpack, V., Boehm, J., Smith, N., & Mudge, B. (1991). Using research-based interventions to decrease patient falls. *Applied Nursing Research, 4*(2), 50-56.

Meller, J. L., & Shermeta, D. W. (1987). Falls in urban children. *American Journal of Diseases of Children, 14*(12), 1271-1275.

Moss, A. B. (1992). Are the elderly safe at home? *Journal of Community Health Nursing, 9*(1), 13-19.

O'Connor, M. S., Boyle, W. E., O'Connor, G. T., & Letellier, R. (1992). Self-reported safety practices in child care facilities. *American Journal of Preventative Medicine, 8*(1), 14-18.

Scott, V. J., Votova, K., & Gallagher, E. (2006). Falls prevention training for community health workers: Strategies and actions for independent living (SAIL). *Journal of Gerontological Nursing, 32*(10), 48-56.

Urton, M. M. (1991). A community home inspection approach to preventing falls among the elderly. *Public Health Reports, 106*(2), 192-196.

F

Falls Occurrence—1912

Domain-Health Knowledge & Behavior (IV)

Class-Risk Control & Safety (T)

Scale(s)-10 and over to None (g)

Care Recipient:

Data Source:

Definition: Number of times an individual falls

OUTCOME TARGET RATING: Maintain at_____   Increase to_____

Falls Occurrence Overall Rating	10 and over 1	7-9 2	4-6 3	1-3 4	None 5	
INDICATORS:						
191201 Falls while standing still	1	2	3	4	5	NA
191202 Falls while walking	1	2	3	4	5	NA
191203 Falls while sitting	1	2	3	4	5	NA
191204 Falls from bed	1	2	3	4	5	NA
191205 Falls while transferring	1	2	3	4	5	NA
191206 Falls climbing steps	1	2	3	4	5	NA
191207 Falls descending steps	1	2	3	4	5	NA
191209 Falls going to bathroom	1	2	3	4	5	NA
191210 Falls while bending over specify period of the time 24 hours/1 week/1 month	1	2	3	4	5	NA

1st edition 1997; Revised 3rd edition 2004; Revised 4th edition

F

Outcome Content References:

Baker, L. (1992). Developing a safety plan that works for patients and nurses. *Rehabilitation Nursing, 17*(5), 264-266.

Nelson, R. C., & Amin, M. A. (1990). Falls in the elderly. *Emergency Care of the Elderly, 8*(2), 309-323.

Schoenfelder, D. P., & Van Why, K. (1997). A fall prevention educational program for community dwelling seniors. *Public Health Nursing, 14*(6), 383-390.

Schroeder, P. (1995). Benchmarking patient falls. *Nursing Quality Connection, 4*(5), 5.

Sorock, G. S. (1988). Falls among the elderly: Epidemiology and prevention. *American Journal of Preventive Medicine, 4*(5), 282-288.

Family Coping—2600

Domain-Family Health (VI)

Class-Family Well-Being (X)

Scale(s)-Never demonstrated to Consistently demonstrated (m)

Care Recipient:

Data Source:

Definition: Family actions to manage stressors that tax family resources

OUTCOME TARGET RATING: Maintain at_____   Increase to_____

Family Coping Overall Rating	Never demonstrated 1	Rarely demonstrated 2	Sometimes demonstrated 3	Often demonstrated 4	Consistently demonstrated 5	

INDICATORS:

260020	Establishes role flexibility	1	2	3	4	5	NA
260002	Enables member role flexibility	1	2	3	4	5	NA
260003	Confronts family problems	1	2	3	4	5	NA
260005	Manages family problems	1	2	3	4	5	NA
260006	Involves family members in decision making	1	2	3	4	5	NA
260007	Expresses feelings and emotions openly among members	1	2	3	4	5	NA
260021	Uses strategies to manage family conflict	1	2	3	4	5	NA
260009	Uses family-centered stress reduction strategies	1	2	3	4	5	NA
260010	Cares for needs of all family members	1	2	3	4	5	NA
260011	Establishes family priorities	1	2	3	4	5	NA
260012	Establishes schedule for family routines and activities	1	2	3	4	5	NA
260019	Shares responsibility for family tasks	1	2	3	4	5	NA
260013	Arranges for respite care	1	2	3	4	5	NA
260014	Plans for emergencies	1	2	3	4	5	NA
260015	Maintains financial stability	1	2	3	4	5	NA
260022	Reports need for family assistance	1	2	3	4	5	NA
260023	Obtains family assistance	1	2	3	4	5	NA
260024	Uses available family support system	1	2	3	4	5	NA
260025	Uses available community resources	1	2	3	4	5	NA

2nd edition 2000; Revised 3rd edition 2004; Revised 4th edition

Outcome Content References:

Friedman, M. (1991). An instrument to evaluate effectiveness in family functioning. *Western Journal of Nursing Research, 13*(2), 220-241.

Hymovich, D. P. (1983). The Chronicity Impact and Coping Instrument: Parent Questionnaire. *Nursing Research, 32*(5), 275-281.

Lohan, J. A., & Murphy, S. A. (2002). Family functioning and family typology after an adolescent or young adult's sudden violent death. *Journal of Family Nursing, 8*(1), 32-49.

McCubbin, H. I. (1987). Family Coping Inventory. In H. I. McCubbin, & A. I. Thomas (Eds.), *Family assessment: Research and practice.* Madison, WI: University of Wisconsin-Madison.

Ryan-Wenger, N. M. (1990). Development and psychometric properties of the Schoolagers' Coping Strategies Inventory. *Nursing Research, 39*(6), 344-349.

F

Family Functioning—2602

Domain-Family Health (VI)

Class-Family Well-Being (X)

Scale(s)-Never demonstrated to Consistently demonstrated (m)

Care Recipient:

Data Source:

Definition: Capacity of the family system to meet the needs of its members during developmental transitions

OUTCOME TARGET RATING: Maintain at_____ Increase to_____

Family Functioning Overall Rating	Never demonstrated 1	Rarely demonstrated 2	Sometimes demonstrated 3	Often demonstrated 4	Consistently demonstrated 5	

INDICATORS:

260201	Socializes new family members	1	2	3	4	5	NA
260202	Cares for dependent members	1	2	3	4	5	NA
260203	Regulates behavior of members	1	2	3	4	5	NA
260204	Allocates responsibilities among members	1	2	3	4	5	NA
260206	Maintains stable core of traditions	1	2	3	4	5	NA
260208	Adapts to developmental transitions	1	2	3	4	5	NA
260209	Adapts to unexpected crises	1	2	3	4	5	NA
260210	Obtains adequate resources to meet needs of members	1	2	3	4	5	NA
260211	Creates environment where members can openly express feelings	1	2	3	4	5	NA
260212	Accepts diversity among members	1	2	3	4	5	NA
260213	Involves members in problem solving	1	2	3	4	5	NA
260214	Involves members in conflict resolution	1	2	3	4	5	NA
260221	Members receptive to new ideas	1	2	3	4	5	NA
260205	Members perform expected roles	1	2	3	4	5	NA
260222	Members support one another	1	2	3	4	5	NA
260223	Members assist one another	1	2	3	4	5	NA
260216	Members spend time with one another	1	2	3	4	5	NA
260217	Members express commitment to family	1	2	3	4	5	NA
260218	Members express loyalty to family	1	2	3	4	5	NA
260219	Members participate in community activities	1	2	3	4	5	NA

F

Continued

2nd edition 2000; Revised 3rd edition 2004; Revised 4th edition

Outcome Content References:

Friedman, M. M., Bowden, V., & Jones, E. (2003). *Family nursing: Research theory & practice* (5th ed.). New Jersey: Prentice Hall.

Friedman, M. (1991). An instrument to evaluate effectiveness in family functioning. *Western Journal of Nursing Research, 13*(2), 220-241.

Nishka, K. J. (2001). Mexican American family survival, continuity, and growth: The parental perspective. *Nursing Science Quarterly, 14*(4), 322-329.

Quayhagen, M. P., & Roth, P. A. (1989). From models to measures in assessment of mature families. *Journal of Professional Nursing, 5*(3), 144-151.

Roberts, C. S., & Feetham, S. A. (1982). Assessing family functioning across three areas of relationships. *Nursing Research, 31*(4), 231-235.

Swain, K. J., & Harrigan, M. P. (1995). *Measures of family functioning for research and practice*. New York: Springer.

Tamplin, A., & Goodyer, I. M. (2001). Family functioning in adolescents at high and low risk for major depressive disorder. *European Child & Adolescent Psychiatry, 10*(3), 170-190.

F

Family Health Status—2606

Domain-Family Health (VI)

Class-Family Well-Being (X)

Scale(s)-Severely compromised to Not compromised (a) and Severe to None (n)

Care Recipient:

Data Source:

Definition: Overall health and social competence of family unit

OUTCOME TARGET RATING: Maintain at_____   Increase to_____

F

Family Health Status Overall Rating	Severely compromised 1	Substantially compromised 2	Moderately compromised 3	Mildly compromised 4	Not compromised 5	
INDICATORS:						
260605 Physical health of members	1	2	3	4	5	NA
260606 Physical activity of members	1	2	3	4	5	NA
260618 Mental health of members	1	2	3	4	5	NA
260601 Immunization of members	1	2	3	4	5	NA
260628 Screening for infections of members	1	2	3	4	5	NA
260612 Physical development of members	1	2	3	4	5	NA
260613 Psychosocial development of members	1	2	3	4	5	NA
260617 Adjustment to disabilities	1	2	3	4	5	NA
260602 Appropriate child care provisions	1	2	3	4	5	NA
260603 Appropriate dependent adult care provisions	1	2	3	4	5	NA
260604 Access to health care	1	2	3	4	5	NA
260607 School attendance of members	1	2	3	4	5	NA
260608 School achievement of members	1	2	3	4	5	NA
260609 Parental employment	1	2	3	4	5	NA
260610 Appropriate housing	1	2	3	4	5	NA
260611 Nutritious food supply	1	2	3	4	5	NA
260630 Financial resources	1	2	3	4	5	NA
260615 Appropriate health care resources	1	2	3	4	5	NA
260616 Appropriate social services resources	1	2	3	4	5	NA
	Severe	**Substantial**	**Moderate**	**Mild**	**None**	
260620 Domestic violence	1	2	3	4	5	NA
260621 Physical abuse of members	1	2	3	4	5	NA
260624 Psychological abuse of members	1	2	3	4	5	NA
260625 Alcohol abuse	1	2	3	4	5	NA
260626 Tobacco use	1	2	3	4	5	NA
260627 Recreational drug use	1	2	3	4	5	NA

Continued

	Severe	Substantial	Moderate	Mild	None	
260631 Gambling addiction	1	2	3	4	5	NA

2nd edition 2000; Revised 3rd edition 2004; Revised 4th edition

Outcome Content References:

Children's Defense Fund. (1997). *The state of America's children: Leave no child behind—Yearbook 1997*. Washington, DC: Author.

Cody, W. K. (1999). The view of family within the human becoming theory. In R. R. Parse (Ed.), *Illuminations: The human becoming theory in practice and research*. Sudbury, MA: Jones and Bartlett.

DeVoe, E. R., & Kantor, G. K. (2002). Measurement issues in child maltreatment and family violence prevention programs. *Trauma Violence & Abuse, 3*(1), 15-39.

Donnelly, E. (1993). Family health assessment. *Home Healthcare Nurse, 11*(2), 30-37.

Ford-Gilboe, M. (2002). Developing knowledge about family health promotion by testing the development model of health and nursing. *Journal of Family Nursing, 8*(2), 140-156.

Friedman, M. (1991). An instrument to evaluate effectiveness in family functioning. *Western Journal of Nursing Research, 13*(2), 220-241.

Garwick, A. W., Patterson, J. M., Meschke, L. L., Bennett, F. C., & Blum, R. W. (2002). The uncertainty of preadolescents' chronic health conditions and family distress. *Journal of Family Nursing, 8*(1), 11-31.

Graham, K. Y. (1995). Childbearing family health: A wake up call. *Public Health Nursing, 12*(3), 141.

Nishka, K. J. (2001). Mexican American family survival, continuity, and growth: The parental perspective. *Nursing Science Quarterly, 14*(4), 322-329.

Quayhagen, M. P., & Roth, P. A. (1989). From models to measures in assessment of mature families. *Journal of Professional Nursing, 5*(3), 144-151.

Reutter, L. (1984). Family health assessment—An integrated approach. *Journal of Advanced Nursing, 9*(4), 391-399.

Family Integrity—2603

Domain-Family Health (VI)

Class-Family Well-Being (X)

Scale(s)-Never demonstrated to Consistently demonstrated (m)

Care Recipient:

Data Source:

Definition: Family members' behaviors that collectively demonstrate cohesion, strength, and emotional bonding

OUTCOME TARGET RATING: Maintain at_____   Increase to_____

Family Integrity Overall Rating	Never demonstrated 1	Rarely demonstrated 2	Sometimes demonstrated 3	Often demonstrated 4	Consistently demonstrated 5	
INDICATORS:						
260305 Interacts frequently with extended family	1	2	3	4	5	NA
260308 Involves members in conflict resolution	1	2	3	4	5	NA
260309 Involves members in problem solving	1	2	3	4	5	NA
260310 Encourages individual autonomy and independence	1	2	3	4	5	NA
260311 Prepares and eats meals together	1	2	3	4	5	NA
260312 Participates in leisure-time activities together	1	2	3	4	5	NA
260313 Participates in family rituals	1	2	3	4	5	NA
260314 Participates in family traditions	1	2	3	4	5	NA
260315 Members provide support during times of crisis	1	2	3	4	5	NA
260301 Members express loyalty	1	2	3	4	5	NA
260302 Members express strong ties to family	1	2	3	4	5	NA
260303 Members express affection to one another	1	2	3	4	5	NA
260304 Members assist one another in performing roles and daily tasks	1	2	3	4	5	NA
260306 Members share thoughts, feelings, interests, concerns	1	2	3	4	5	NA
260307 Members communicate openly and honestly with one another	1	2	3	4	5	NA

2nd edition 2000; Revised 3rd edition 2004

Outcome Content References:

Friedman, M. M., Bowden, V., & Jones, E. (2003). *Family nursing: Research theory & practice* (5th ed.). New Jersey: Prentice Hall.

Swain, K. J., & Harrigan, M. P. (1995). *Measures of family functioning for research and practice.* New York: Springer.

Thomasgard, M., & Metz, W. P. (1999). Parent-child relationship disorders: What do the Child Vulnerability Scale and the Parent Protection Scale measure? *Clinical Pediatrics, 38*(6), 347-356.

F

Family Normalization—2604

Domain-Family Health (VI)

Class-Family Well-Being (X)

Scale(s)-Never demonstrated to Consistently demonstrated (m)

Care Recipient:

Data Source:

> **Definition:** Capacity of the family system to develop strategies for optimal functioning when a member has a chronic illness or disability

OUTCOME TARGET RATING: Maintain at_____   Increase to_____

Family Normalization Overall Rating	Never demonstrated 1	Rarely demonstrated 2	Sometimes demonstrated 3	Often demonstrated 4	Consistently demonstrated 5	
INDICATORS:						
260417 Acknowledges potential of impairment to alter family routines	1	2	3	4	5	NA
260403 Maintains usual family routines	1	2	3	4	5	NA
260405 Adapts family routines to accommodate needs of affected member	1	2	3	4	5	NA
260406 Meets physical needs of family members	1	2	3	4	5	NA
260407 Meets psychosocial needs of family members	1	2	3	4	5	NA
260408 Meets developmental needs of family members	1	2	3	4	5	NA
260418 Reports family life returned to precrisis state	1	2	3	4	5	NA
260419 Maintains activities and routines as appropriate	1	2	3	4	5	NA
260420 Maintains usual expectations for member	1	2	3	4	5	NA
260412 Provides activities appropriate to age and ability for affected member	1	2	3	4	5	NA
260413 Structures activities to avoid embarrassment of affected member	1	2	3	4	5	NA
260414 Structures environment to avoid embarrassment of affected member	1	2	3	4	5	NA
260415 Uses community support groups	1	2	3	4	5	NA

2nd edition 2000; Revised 3rd edition 2004; Revised 4th edition

Outcome Content References:

Bossert, E., Holaday, B., Harkins, A., & Turner-Henson, A. (1990). Strategies of normalization used by parents of chronically ill school age children. *Journal of Child Psychiatric Nursing, 3*(2), 57-61.

Knafl, K., Brietmayer, B., Gallo, A., & Zoeller, L. (1996). Family response to childhood chronic illness: Description of management styles. *Journal of Pediatric Nursing, 11*(5), 315-316.

Knafl, K. A., & Deatrick, J. A. (1986). How families manage chronic conditions: An analysis of the concept of normalization. *Research in Nursing and Health, 9*(3), 215-222.

Knafl, K. A., & Gilliss, C. L. (2002). Families and chronic illness: A synthesis of current research. *Journal of Family Nursing, 8*(3), 178-198.

Wade, S. L., Taylor, H. G., Drotar, D., Stancin, T., Yeates, K. O., & Minich, N. M. (2002). A prospective study of long-term caregiver and family adaptation following brain injury in children. *Journal of Health Trauma Rehabilitation, 17*(2), 96-111.

F

Family Participation in Professional Care—2605

Domain-Family Health (VI)   Care Recipient:

Class-Family Well-Being (X)   Data Source:

Scale(s)-Never demonstrated to Consistently demonstrated (m)

F

Definition: Family involvement in decision-making, delivery, and evaluation of care provided by health care personnel

OUTCOME TARGET RATING: Maintain at_____   Increase to_____

Family Participation in Professional Care Overall Rating	Never demonstrated 1	Rarely demonstrated 2	Sometimes demonstrated 3	Often demonstrated 4	Consistently demonstrated 5	
INDICATORS:						
260501 Participates in planning care	1	2	3	4	5	NA
260502 Participates in providing care	1	2	3	4	5	NA
260503 Provides relevant information	1	2	3	4	5	NA
260504 Obtains required information	1	2	3	4	5	NA
260505 Identifies factors that affect care	1	2	3	4	5	NA
260506 Collaborates in determining treatment	1	2	3	4	5	NA
260507 Defines needs and problems relevant to care	1	2	3	4	5	NA
260508 Makes decisions when patient is unable to do so	1	2	3	4	5	NA
260509 Participates in decisions with patient	1	2	3	4	5	NA
260510 Participates in mutual goal setting for care	1	2	3	4	5	NA
260511 Evaluates effectiveness of care	1	2	3	4	5	NA
260513 Participates in discharge planning	1	2	3	4	5	NA

2nd edition 2000; Revised 4th edition

Outcome Content References:

Biley, F. C. (1992). Some determinants that effect patient participation in decision-making about nursing care. *Journal of Advanced Nursing, 17,* 414-421.

Brownlea, A. (1987). Participation: Myths, realities and prognosis. *Social Science and Medicine, 25*(6), 605-614.

Ende, J., Kazis, L., Ash, A., & Moskowitz, M. A. (1989). Measuring patients' desire for autonomy: Decision making and information-seeking preferences among medical patients. *Journal of General Internal Medicine, 4*(1), 23-30.

Janis, I. L., & Rodin, J. (1979). Attribution, control and decision making: Social psychology and health care. In G. D. Stone, F. Cohen & N. E. Adler (Eds.), *Health psychology.* San Francisco: Josey-Bass.

McEwen, J. (1985). Primary health care: The challenge of participation. In U. Laaser, R. Senault, & H. Viefhues (Eds.), *Primary health care in the making.* Hiedelberg: Springer-Verlag.

Richardson, A., & Bray, C. (1987). *Promoting health through participation.* London: Policy Studies Institute.

Stanhope, M., & Lancaster, J. (2000). *Community health nursing* (5th ed.). St Louis: Mosby.

Family Resiliency—2608

Domain-Family Health (VI)

Class-Family Well-Being (X)

Scale-Never demonstrated to Consistently demonstrated (m)

Care Recipient:

Data Source:

Definition: Positive adaptation and function of the family system following significant adversity or crisis

OUTCOME TARGET RATING: Maintain at_____   Increase to_____

Family Resiliency Overall Rating	Never demonstrated 1	Rarely demonstrated 2	Sometimes demonstrated 3	Often demonstrated 4	Consistently demonstrated 5	
INDICATORS:						
260801 Mobilizes quickly following adversity	1	2	3	4	5	NA
260802 Proposes practical, constructive solutions for disputes	1	2	3	4	5	NA
260803 Adapts to adversities as challenges	1	2	3	4	5	NA
260804 Tolerates separations when required	1	2	3	4	5	NA
260805 Discusses meaning of crisis	1	2	3	4	5	NA
260806 Expresses confidence in overcoming adversities	1	2	3	4	5	NA
260807 Maintains values, goals, and dreams	1	2	3	4	5	NA
260809 Supports members	1	2	3	4	5	NA
260810 Cooperates to meet challenges	1	2	3	4	5	NA
260811 Nurtures members	1	2	3	4	5	NA
260812 Protects members	1	2	3	4	5	NA
260813 Communicates clearly among members	1	2	3	4	5	NA
260814 Clarifies ambiguous communication	1	2	3	4	5	NA
260815 Uses conflict resolution strategies	1	2	3	4	5	NA
260816 Shares humor	1	2	3	4	5	NA
260817 Reports learning and growth	1	2	3	4	5	NA
260818 Maintains usual family routines	1	2	3	4	5	NA
260819 Prepares for future challenges	1	2	3	4	5	NA
260820 Supports individuality and independence among members	1	2	3	4	5	NA
260821 Accepts respite from extended family	1	2	3	4	5	NA
260822 Accepts respite from friends	1	2	3	4	5	NA
260823 Accepts assistance with direct care from extended family	1	2	3	4	5	NA
260824 Accepts assistance with direct care from friends	1	2	3	4	5	NA

		Never demonstrated	Rarely demonstrated	Sometimes demonstrated	Often demonstrated	Consistently demonstrated	
260825	Accepts assistance with instrumental activities of daily living from extended family	1	2	3	4	5	NA
260826	Accepts assistance with instrumental activities of daily living from friends	1	2	3	4	5	NA
260827	Seeks emotional support from extended family	1	2	3	4	5	NA
260828	Seeks emotional support from friends	1	2	3	4	5	NA
260829	Uses community resources for assistance	1	2	3	4	5	NA
260830	Uses community groups for emotional support	1	2	3	4	5	NA
260831	Adjusts schedules to support and assist members	1	2	3	4	5	NA
260832	Uses health care team for information and assistance	1	2	3	4	5	NA

3rd edition 2004; Revised 4th edition

Outcome Content References:

Armstrong, M., I. Birnie-Lefcovitch, S. & Ungar, M. (2005). Pathways between social support, family well being, quality of parenting, and child resilience: What we know. *Journal of Child & Family Studies, 14*(2), 269-281.

Black, C., & Ford-Gilboe, M. (2004). Adolescent mothers: Resilience, family health work and health-promoting practices. *Journal of Advanced Nursing, 48*(4), 351-360.

McCubbin, M., Balling, K., Possin, P., Frierdich, S., & Bryne, B. (2002). Family resiliency in childhood cancer. *Family Relations, 51*, 103-111.

Patterson, J. M. (2002). Integrating family resilience and family stress theory. *Journal of Marriage and Family, 64*, 349-360.

Walsh, F. (2002). A family resilience framework: Innovative practice applications. *Family Relations, 51*, 130-137.

F

Family Social Climate—2601

Domain-Family Health (VI)

Class-Family Well-Being (X)

Scale(s)-Never demonstrated to Consistently demonstrated (m)

Care Recipient:

Data Source:

F

Definition: Supportive milieu as characterized by family member relationships and goals

OUTCOME TARGET RATING: Maintain at_____   Increase to_____

Family Social Climate Overall Rating	Never demonstrated 1	Rarely demonstrated 2	Sometimes demonstrated 3	Often demonstrated 4	Consistently demonstrated 5	

INDICATORS:

260101	Participates in activities together	1	2	3	4	5	NA
260102	Participates in family traditions	1	2	3	4	5	NA
260103	Attends religious services together	1	2	3	4	5	NA
260121	Maintains relationships with extended family members	1	2	3	4	5	NA
260122	Maintains relationships with friends	1	2	3	4	5	NA
260105	Participates in leisure activities	1	2	3	4	5	NA
260119	Participates in community events	1	2	3	4	5	NA
260106	Establishes family rules	1	2	3	4	5	NA
260123	Establishes family routine	1	2	3	4	5	NA
260124	Maintains family routine	1	2	3	4	5	NA
260108	Maintains clean home	1	2	3	4	5	NA
260109	Supports one another	1	2	3	4	5	NA
260110	Provides privacy for members	1	2	3	4	5	NA
260111	Encourages individual autonomy and independence	1	2	3	4	5	NA
260125	Encourages maturity-enhancing activities	1	2	3	4	5	NA
260126	Encourages life-long learning	1	2	3	4	5	NA
260112	Shares the decision-making process	1	2	3	4	5	NA
260113	Works cooperatively to meet family goals	1	2	3	4	5	NA
260114	Shares feelings with one another	1	2	3	4	5	NA
260120	Shares problems with one another	1	2	3	4	5	NA
260115	Discusses issues relevant to family	1	2	3	4	5	NA
260116	Solves problems together	1	2	3	4	5	NA
260117	Promotes cohesion	1	2	3	4	5	NA

2nd edition 2000; Revised 3rd edition 2004; Revised 4th edition

Outcome Content References:

Burston, A., Puckering, C., & Kearney, E. (2005). At HOME in Scotland: Validation of the home observation for measurement of the environment inventory. *Child: Care, Health & Development, 31*(5), 533-538.

Folden, S. L. (2001). The politics of the family. In P. L. Munhall (Ed.), *The emergence of family into the 21st century*. Sudbury, MA: Jones and Bartlett.

Moos, R. H. (1974). *Family Environment Scale—Form R*. Palo Alto, CA: Consulting Psychologists Press.

Soubhi, H., Potvin, L., & Paradis, G. (2004). Family process and parent's leisure time physical activity. *American Journal of Health Behavior, 28*(3), 218-230.

Swain, K. J., & Harrigan, M. P. (1995). *Measures of family functioning for research and practice*. New York: Springer.

Family Support During Treatment—2609

Domain-Family Health (VI)

Class-Family Well-Being (X)

Scale(s)-Never demonstrated to Consistently demonstrated (m)

Care Recipient:

Data Source:

Definition: Family presence and emotional support for an individual undergoing treatment

OUTCOME TARGET RATING: Maintain at_____   Increase to_____

Family Support During Treatment Overall Rating	Never demonstrated 1	Rarely demonstrated 2	Sometimes demonstrated 3	Often demonstrated 4	Consistently demonstrated 5	
INDICATORS:						
260901 Members express desire to support ill member	1	2	3	4	5	NA
260902 Members express feelings and emotions of concern for ill member	1	2	3	4	5	NA
260903 Members ask how they may assist	1	2	3	4	5	NA
260904 Requests information about procedure	1	2	3	4	5	NA
260905 Requests information about patient condition	1	2	3	4	5	NA
260906 Members maintain communication with ill member	1	2	3	4	5	NA
260907 Members encourage ill member	1	2	3	4	5	NA
260908 Members provide comforting touch to ill member	1	2	3	4	5	NA
260915 Seeks social support for ill member	1	2	3	4	5	NA
260916 Seeks spiritual support for ill member	1	2	3	4	5	NA
260910 Collaborates with ill member in determining care	1	2	3	4	5	NA
260911 Collaborates with health providers in determining care	1	2	3	4	5	NA
260912 Members verbalize meaning of health crisis	1	2	3	4	5	NA
260913 Contacts other members as desired by ill member	1	2	3	4	5	NA
260914 Provides accurate information to other members	1	2	3	4	5	NA
260917 Participates in discharge planning	1	2	3	4	5	NA

3rd edition 2004; Revised 4th edition

F

Continued

Outcome Content References:

American Heart Association. (2000). Part 2: Ethical aspects of CPR and ECC. *Circulation, 102*(Suppl. 8), I12-I21.

Bull, M. J., Hansen, H. E., & Gross, C. R. (2000). Differences in family caregiver outcomes by their level of involvement in discharge planning. *Applied Nursing Research, 13*(2), 76-82.

Eichhorn, D. J., Meyers, T. A., Guzzetta, C. E., Clark, A. P., Klein, J. D., & Calvin, A. O. (2001). During invasive procedures and resuscitation: Hearing the voice of the patient. *American Journal of Nursing, 101*(5), 48-55.

Emergency Nurses Association. (1998). Emergency Nurses Association position statement: Family presence at the bedside during invasive procedures and/or resuscitation. *Journal of Emergency Nursing, 21*(2), 26A.

Emergency Nurses Association. (2000). *Presenting the option for family presence* (2nd ed.). Des Plaines, IL: Author.

Friedman, M. (1991). An instrument to evaluate effectiveness in family functioning. *Western Journal of Nursing Research, 13*(2), 220-241.

Hampe, S. O. (1975). Needs of a grieving spouse in a hospital setting. *Nursing Research, 24*(2), 113-120.

McPhee, A. T. (1983). Let the family in. *Nursing, 13*(1), 120.

Meyers, T. A., Eichhorn, D. J., & Guzzetta, C. E. (1998). Do families want to be present during CPR? A retrospective survey. *Journal of Emergency Nursing, 24*(5), 400-405.

Meyers, T. A., Eichhorn, D. J., Guzzetta, C. E., Clark, A. P., Klein, J. D., Taliaferro, E., & Calvin, A. (2000). Family presence during invasive procedures and resuscitation. *American Journal of Nursing, 100*(2), 32-42.

F

Fatigue Level—0007

Domain-Functional Health (I)

Class-Energy Maintenance (A)

Scale(s)-Severe to None (n) Severely compromised to Not compromised (a)

Care Recipient:

Data Source:

F

Definition: Severity of observed or reported prolonged generalized fatigue

OUTCOME TARGET RATING: Maintain at_____   Increase to_____

Fatigue Level Overall Rating	Severe 1	Substantial 2	Moderate 3	Mild 4	None 5	
INDICATORS:						
000701 Exhaustion	1	2	3	4	5	NA
000702 Lassitude	1	2	3	4	5	NA
000703 Depressed mood	1	2	3	4	5	NA
000704 Loss of appetite	1	2	3	4	5	NA
000705 Decreased libido	1	2	3	4	5	NA
000706 Impaired concentration	1	2	3	4	5	NA
000707 Decreased motivation	1	2	3	4	5	NA
000708 Headaches	1	2	3	4	5	NA
000709 Sore throat	1	2	3	4	5	NA
000710 Tender lymph nodes	1	2	3	4	5	NA
000711 Muscle pain	1	2	3	4	5	NA
000712 Joint pain	1	2	3	4	5	NA
000713 Post exertional malaise	1	2	3	4	5	NA
000714 Stress level	1	2	3	4	5	NA

	Severely compromised	Substantially compromised	Moderately compromised	Mildly compromised	Not compromised	
000715 Activities of daily living	1	2	3	4	5	NA
000716 Instrumental activities of daily living	1	2	3	4	5	NA
000717 Work performance	1	2	3	4	5	NA
000718 Lifestyle performance	1	2	3	4	5	NA
000719 Rest quality	1	2	3	4	5	NA
000720 Sleep quality	1	2	3	4	5	NA
000721 Balance of activity and rest	1	2	3	4	5	NA
000722 Alertness	1	2	3	4	5	NA
000723 Hematocrit	1	2	3	4	5	NA
000724 Oxygen saturation	1	2	3	4	5	NA
000725 Thyroid function	1	2	3	4	5	NA
000726 Immune function	1	2	3	4	5	NA
000727 Neurological function	1	2	3	4	5	NA
000728 Metabolism	1	2	3	4	5	NA

4th edition

Continued

Outcome Content References:

Aaronson, L. S., Teel, C., Cassmeyer, V., Neuberger, G. B., Pallikkathayil, L., Pierce, J., Press, A. N., Williams, P. D., & Wingate, A. (1999). Defining and measuring fatigue. *Image: Journal of Nursing Scholarship, 31*(1), 45-51.

Chalder, T., Berelowitz, K., Pawlikowska, T., Watts, L., Wessely, S., Wright, D., & Wallace, J. P. (1993). Development of a fatigue scale. *Journal of Psychosomatic Research, 37,* 147-153.

Hampton, T. (2006). Chronic fatigue syndrome answers sought. *JAMA: Journal of the American Medical Association, 296*(24), 2915.

Jason, L. A., Corradi, K., Gress, S., Williams, S., & Torres-Harding, S. (2006). Causes of death among patients with chronic fatigue syndrome. *Health Care for Women International, 27,* 615-626.

Krupp, L. B., LaRocca, N. G., Muir Nash, J., & Steinberg, A. D. (1989). The fatigue severity scale, Application to patients with multiple sclerosis and systemic lupus erythematosus. *Archives of Neurology, 46,* 1121-1123.

Piper, B. F., Dibble, S. L., Dodd, M. J., Weiss, M. C., Slaughter, R. E., & Paul, S. M. (1998). The revised Piper Fatigue Scale: Psychometric evaluation in women with breast cancer. *Oncology Nursing Forum, 25*(4), 67-84.

Smets, E. M. A., Garssen, B., Bonke, B., & De Haes, J. C. J. M. (1995). The Multidimensional Fatigue Inventory (MFI) psychometric qualities of an instrument to assess fatigue. *Journal of Psychosomatic Research, 39,* 315-325.

Tiesinga, L. J., Dassen, T. W. N., Halfens, R. J. G., & Van Den Heuvel, W. J. A. (2001). Sensitivity, specificity, and usefulness of the Dutch Fatigue Scale. *Nursing Diagnosis, 12*(3), July-September, 93-106.

Tiesinga, L. J., Dassen, T. W. N., Reid, J. H., & Van Dentleuvel, J. A. in Michielsen, H. J., DeVries, J., VanHeck, G., VandeViyven, Foms, J. A., Sijtsmak (2004). Examination of the dimensionality of fatigue: The construction of the Fatigue Assessment Scale (FAS). *European Journal of Psychological Assessment 20*(1), 39-48.

F

Fear Level—1210

Domain-Psychosocial Health (III)

Class-Psychological Well-Being (M)

Scale(s)-Severe to None (n)

Care Recipient:

Data Source:

Definition: Severity of manifested apprehension, tension, or uneasiness arising from an identifiable source

OUTCOME TARGET RATING: Maintain at_____   Increase to_____

Fear Level Overall Rating	Severe 1	Substantial 2	Moderate 3	Mild 4	None 5	

INDICATORS:

121001	Distress	1	2	3	4	5	NA
121002	Tendency to blame others	1	2	3	4	5	NA
121003	Self-absorption	1	2	3	4	5	NA
121004	Lack of self-confidence	1	2	3	4	5	NA
121005	Restlessness	1	2	3	4	5	NA
121006	Irritability	1	2	3	4	5	NA
121007	Outbursts of anger	1	2	3	4	5	NA
121008	Difficulty concentrating	1	2	3	4	5	NA
121009	Difficulty learning	1	2	3	4	5	NA
121010	Difficulty problem solving	1	2	3	4	5	NA
121011	Decreased perceptual field	1	2	3	4	5	NA
121012	Perceived inadequacy in interpersonal relationships	1	2	3	4	5	NA
121013	Exaggerated concern about life events	1	2	3	4	5	NA
121014	Preoccupation with life events	1	2	3	4	5	NA
121015	Preoccupation with source of fear	1	2	3	4	5	NA
121016	Increased blood pressure	1	2	3	4	5	NA
121017	Increased radial pulse rate	1	2	3	4	5	NA
121018	Increased respiratory rate	1	2	3	4	5	NA
121019	Dilated pupils	1	2	3	4	5	NA
121020	Sweating	1	2	3	4	5	NA
121021	Feeling faint	1	2	3	4	5	NA
121022	Muscle tension	1	2	3	4	5	NA
121023	Facial tension	1	2	3	4	5	NA
121024	Frequent urination	1	2	3	4	5	NA
121025	Diarrhea	1	2	3	4	5	NA
121026	Inability to sleep	1	2	3	4	5	NA
121027	Skin pallor	1	2	3	4	5	NA
121028	Fatigue	1	2	3	4	5	NA
121029	Withdrawal	1	2	3	4	5	NA
121030	Avoidance behavior	1	2	3	4	5	NA
121031	Verbalized fear	1	2	3	4	5	NA
121032	Crying	1	2	3	4	5	NA

Continued

	Severe	Substantial	Moderate	Mild	None	
121033 Dread	1	2	3	4	5	NA
121034 Panic	1	2	3	4	5	NA
121035 Terror	1	2	3	4	5	NA

3rd edition 2004; Revised 4th edition

Outcome Content References:

American Psychiatric Association. (2000). *Diagnostic and statistical manual of mental disorders* (4th ed. text revision). Washington, DC: Author.

Charron, H. S. (1998). Anxiety disorders. In E. M. Varcarolis (Ed.), *Foundations of psychiatric mental health nursing* (3rd ed., pp. 443-477). Philadelphia: W.B. Saunders.

Kim, M., Sertella, R., Gulanick, M., Moyer, K., Parsons, E., Scherbel, J., Stafford, M., Suhayada, R., & Yocum, C. (1984). Clinical validation of cardiovascular nursing diagnoses. In M. Kim, G. McFarland, & A. McLane (Eds.), *Classification of nursing diagnoses: Proceedings of the fifth national conference* (pp. 128-137). St. Louis: Mosby.

Taylor-Loughran, A. E., O'Brien, M. E., Lachapelle, R., & Rangel, S. (1989). Defining characteristics of the nursing diagnoses fear and anxiety: A validation study. *Applied Nursing Research, 2*(4), 178-186.

Whitley, G. G., & Tousman, S. A. (1996). A multivariate approach for validation of anxiety and fear. *Nursing Diagnoses, 7*(3), 116-124.

F

Fear Level: Child—1213

Domain-Psychological Health (III)

Class-Psychological Well-Being (M)

Scale(s)-Severe to None (n)

Care Recipient:

Data Source:

Definition: Severity of manifested apprehension, tension, or uneasiness arising from an identifiable source in a child from 1 year through 17 years of age

OUTCOME TARGET RATING: Maintain at_____   Increase to_____

Fear Level: Child Overall Rating	Severe 1	Substantial 2	Moderate 3	Mild 4	None 5	
INDICATORS:						
121302 Increased heart rate	1	2	3	4	5	NA
121303 Headaches	1	2	3	4	5	NA
121304 Stomachaches	1	2	3	4	5	NA
121305 Frequent urination	1	2	3	4	5	NA
121306 Frequent diarrhea	1	2	3	4	5	NA
121307 Fatigue	1	2	3	4	5	NA
121308 Weight loss	1	2	3	4	5	NA
121310 Sweating	1	2	3	4	5	NA
121311 Crying	1	2	3	4	5	NA
121312 Emotional lability	1	2	3	4	5	NA
121313 Stammering	1	2	3	4	5	NA
121314 Irritability	1	2	3	4	5	NA
121315 Excessive giggling	1	2	3	4	5	NA
121316 Avoidance behavior	1	2	3	4	5	NA
121317 Withdrawal	1	2	3	4	5	NA
121318 Increased school absence	1	2	3	4	5	NA
121319 Cheating	1	2	3	4	5	NA
121320 Difficulty staying on task	1	2	3	4	5	NA
121321 Difficulty concentrating	1	2	3	4	5	NA
121322 Tics	1	2	3	4	5	NA
121323 Nail biting	1	2	3	4	5	NA
121324 Finger sucking	1	2	3	4	5	NA
121325 Hair chewing	1	2	3	4	5	NA
121326 Chewing clothing	1	2	3	4	5	NA
121327 Fidgeting	1	2	3	4	5	NA
121328 Rocking motion	1	2	3	4	5	NA
121329 Shaking	1	2	3	4	5	NA
121330 Violent behavior	1	2	3	4	5	NA
121331 Violence displayed in drawings	1	2	3	4	5	NA

F

Continued

		Severe	Substantial	Moderate	Mild	None	
121332	Destructive behavior	1	2	3	4	5	NA
121333	Stealing	1	2	3	4	5	NA
121334	Regressive behavior	1	2	3	4	5	NA
121335	Excessive approval seeking behavior	1	2	3	4	5	NA
121336	Demanding behavior	1	2	3	4	5	NA
121337	Fabrication of stories	1	2	3	4	5	NA
121338	Continuous questioning	1	2	3	4	5	NA
121339	Clinging behavior	1	2	3	4	5	NA
121340	Injury faking behavior	1	2	3	4	5	NA
121341	Self-destructive behavior	1	2	3	4	5	NA
121342	Recreational drug use	1	2	3	4	5	NA
121343	Alcohol use	1	2	3	4	5	NA
121344	Excessive self-denigration	1	2	3	4	5	NA
121345	Dread	1	2	3	4	5	NA
121346	Panic	1	2	3	4	5	NA
121347	Terror	1	2	3	4	5	NA

3rd edition 2004; Revised 4th edition

Outcome Content References:

Berliner, L., & Saunders, B. E. (1996). Treating fear and anxiety in sexually abused children. *Child Maltreatment, 1*(4), 294-310.

Byrne, B. (2000). Relationships between anxiety, fear, self-esteem and coping strategies in adolescence. *Adolescence, 35*(137), 201-216.

Carlson, K. L., Broome, M., & Vessey, J. A. (2000). Using distraction to reduce reported pain, fear and behavioral distress in children and adolescents: A multisite study. *Journal of the Society of Pediatric Nursing, 5*(2), 75-85.

Carr, T. D., Lemanek, K. L., & Armstrong, F. D. (1998). Pain and fear ratings: Clinical implications of age and gender differences. *Journal of Pain and Symptom Management, 15*(5), 305-313.

Carroll, M. K., & Ryan-Wenger, N. A. (1999). School-age children's fears, anxiety and human figure drawings. *Journal of Pediatric Health Care, 13*(1), 24-31.

Nicastro, E. A., & Whetsell, M. V. (1999). Children's fears. *Journal of Pediatric Nursing, 14*(6), 392-402.

Potter, P. A., & Perry, A. G. (2001). *Fundamentals of nursing* (5th ed.). St. Louis: Mosby.

Wilson, A. H., & Yorker, B. (1996). Fears of medical events among school-age children with emotional disorders, parents, and health care providers. *Issues in Mental Health Nursing, 18*(1), 57-71.

Wong, D. L., Hockenberry-Eaton, M., Wilson, D., Winkelstein, M. L., Ahmann, E., & DiVito-Thomas, P. A. (1999). *Whaley & Wong's nursing care of infants and children* (6th ed.). St. Louis: Mosby.

Fear Self-Control—1404

Domain-Psychosocial Health (III)

Class-Self-Control (O)

Scale(s)-Never demonstrated to Consistently demonstrated (m)

Care Recipient:

Data Source:

> **Definition:** Personal actions to eliminate or reduce disabling feelings of apprehension, tension, or uneasiness from an identifiable source

OUTCOME TARGET RATING: Maintain at_____   Increase to_____

Fear Self-Control Overall Rating	Never demonstrated 1	Rarely demonstrated 2	Sometimes demonstrated 3	Often demonstrated 4	Consistently demonstrated 5	
INDICATORS:						
140401 Monitors intensity of fear	1	2	3	4	5	NA
140402 Eliminates precursors of fear	1	2	3	4	5	NA
140403 Seeks information to reduce fear	1	2	3	4	5	NA
140404 Avoids source of fear when possible	1	2	3	4	5	NA
140405 Plans coping strategies for fearful situations	1	2	3	4	5	NA
140406 Uses effective coping strategies	1	2	3	4	5	NA
140407 Uses relaxation techniques to reduce fear	1	2	3	4	5	NA
140408 Monitors duration of episodes	1	2	3	4	5	NA
140409 Monitors length of time between episodes	1	2	3	4	5	NA
140410 Maintains role performance	1	2	3	4	5	NA
140411 Maintains social relationships	1	2	3	4	5	NA
140412 Maintains concentration	1	2	3	4	5	NA
140413 Maintains control over life	1	2	3	4	5	NA
140414 Maintains physical functioning	1	2	3	4	5	NA
140415 Maintains a sense of purpose despite fear	1	2	3	4	5	NA
140416 Remains productive	1	2	3	4	5	NA
140417 Controls fear response	1	2	3	4	5	NA

1st edition 1997; Revised 2nd edition 2000; Revised 3rd edition 2004

Outcome Content References:

+Marks, I. M., & Mathews, A. M. (1979). Brief standard self-rating for phobic patients. *Behavior Research and Therapy,* 17(3), 263-267.

McAuley, E., Mihalko, S. L., & Rosengren K. (1997). Self-efficacy and balance correlates of fear of falling in the elderly. *Journal of Aging and Physical Activity,* 5(4), 329-340.

McFarland, G. K., & McFarlane, E. A. (1997). *Nursing diagnosis & intervention: Planning for patient care* (3rd ed.). St. Louis: Mosby.

Moorhead, S. A., & Brighton, V. A. (2001). Anxiety and fear. In M. Maas, K. Buckwalter, M. Hardy, T. Tripp-Reimer, M. Titler, & J. Specht (Eds.), *Nursing care of older adults: Diagnoses, outcomes & interventions* (pp. 571-592). St. Louis: Mosby.

Stuart, G. W., & Laraia, M. T. (2001). *Principles and practice of psychiatric nursing* (7th ed.). St. Louis: Mosby.

Whitley, G. G., & Tousman, S. A. (1996). A multivariate approach for validation of anxiety and fear. *Nursing Diagnosis,* 7(3), 116-124.

Wilson, A. H., & Yorker, B. (1997). Fears of medical events among school-age children with emotional disorders, parents, and health care providers. *Issues in Mental Health Nursing,* 18(1), 57-71.

F

Fetal Status: Antepartum—0111

Domain-Functional Health (I)

Class-Growth & Development (B)

Scale(s)-Severe deviation from normal range to No deviation from normal range (b)

Care Recipient:

Data Source:

> **Definition:** Extent to which fetal signs are within normal limits from conception to the onset of labor

OUTCOME TARGET RATING: Maintain at_____   Increase to_____

Fetal Status: Antepartum Overall Rating	Severe deviation from normal range 1	Substantial deviation from normal range 2	Moderate deviation from normal range 3	Mild deviation from normal range 4	No deviation from normal range 5

INDICATORS:

011101	Fetal heart rate (120-160 bpm)	1	2	3	4	5	NA
011102	Deceleration patterns in electronic fetal monitor findings	1	2	3	4	5	NA
011103	Variability in electronic fetal monitor findings	1	2	3	4	5	NA
011104	Fetal ultrasound growth measurements	1	2	3	4	5	NA
011105	Fetal movement frequency	1	2	3	4	5	NA
011106	Fetal movement pattern	1	2	3	4	5	NA
011107	Nonstress test	1	2	3	4	5	NA
011108	Contraction stress test	1	2	3	4	5	NA
011109	Auscultated acceleration test	1	2	3	4	5	NA
011110	Biophysical profile score	1	2	3	4	5	NA
011111	Amniotic fluid sample findings	1	2	3	4	5	NA
011112	Umbilical artery blood flow velocity	1	2	3	4	5	NA

2nd edition 2000; Revised 3rd edition 2004

Outcome Content References:

Armour, K. (2004). Using surveillance to improve maternal and fetal outcomes: Antepartum maternal-fetal assessment. *AWHONN Lifelines, 8*(3), 232-240.

Association of Women's Health, Obstetric and Neonatal Nurses. (1998). *Clinical competencies and education guide: Limited ultrasound examinations in obstetric and gynecologic/infertility settings.* Washington, DC: Author.

Calhoun, S. (1990). "Ask the Experts": Daily fetal movement counts. *NAACOG Newsletter, 17*(8), p. 6.

Chez, B. F., Skurnick, J. H., Chez, R. A., Verklan, M. T., Biggs, S., & Hage, M. L. (1990). Interpretations of nonstress tests by obstetric nurses. *Journal of Obstetric, Gynecologic, and Neonatal Nursing, 19*(3), 227-232.

Gaffney, S., Solinger, L., & Vinzileos, A. (1990). The biophysical profile for fetal surveillance. *MCN: American Journal of Maternal Child Nursing, 15*(6), 356-360.

Gebauer, C., & Lowe, N. (1993). The biophysical profile: Antepartal assessment of fetal well-being. *Journal of Obstetric, Gynecologic, and Neonatal Nursing, 22*(2), 115-123.

Gegor, C. L., & Paine, L. L. (1992). Antepartum fetal assessment techniques: An update for today's perinatal nurse. *Journal of Perinatal and Neonatal Nursing, 5*(4), 1-15.

Givens, S. R., & Moore, M. L. (1995). Status report on maternal and child health indicators. *Journal of Perinatal and Neonatal Nursing, 9*(1), 8-18.

Lowdermilk, D. L., & Perry, S. E. (2004). *Maternity & women's health care* (8th ed.). St. Louis: Mosby.

Paine, L. L., Benedict, M. I., Strobino, D. M., Gegor, C. L., & Larson, E. L. (1992). A comparison of the auscultated acceleration test and the nonstress test as predicators of perinatal outcomes. *Nursing Research, 41*(2), 87-91.

Petrikovsky, B. M. (1991). Antepartum fetal evaluation. A search for the ideal test. *Neonatal Intensive Care, 4*(5), 38-39.

Tucker, S. M. (2004). *Pocket guide to fetal monitoring and assessment* (5th ed.). St. Louis: Mosby.

F

Fetal Status: Intrapartum—0112

Domain-Functional Health (I)

Class-Growth & Development (B)

Scale(s)-Severe deviation from normal range to No deviation from normal range (b)

Care Recipient:

Data Source:

F

Definition: Extent to which fetal signs are within normal limits from onset of labor to delivery

OUTCOME TARGET RATING: Maintain at_____   Increase to_____

Fetal Status: Intrapartum Overall Rating	Severe deviation from normal range 1	Substantial deviation from normal range 2	Moderate deviation from normal range 3	Mild deviation from normal range 4	No deviation from normal range 5	
INDICATORS:						
011201 Fetal heart rate (120-160 bpm)	1	2	3	4	5	NA
011202 Deceleration patterns in electronic fetal monitor findings	1	2	3	4	5	NA
011203 Variability in electronic fetal monitor findings	1	2	3	4	5	NA
011204 Amniotic fluid color	1	2	3	4	5	NA
011205 Amniotic fluid amount	1	2	3	4	5	NA
011206 Fetal position	1	2	3	4	5	NA
011207 Fetal presenting part	1	2	3	4	5	NA
011209 Fetal scalp blood pH	1	2	3	4	5	NA
011210 Fetal scalp stimulation response	1	2	3	4	5	NA
011212 Fetal pulse oximetry	1	2	3	4	5	NA

2nd edition 2000; Revised 3rd edition 2004; Revised 4th edition

Outcome Content References:

Dickason, E. J., Schultz, M. O., & Silverman, B. L. (1998). *Maternal-infant nursing care* (3rd ed.). St. Louis: Mosby.

East, C. E., Chan, F. Y., & Colditz, P. B. (2004). Fetal pulse oximetry for fetal assessment in labour. *Cochrane Database of Systematic Review 2004*, Issue 4, Art. No.: CD004075. DOI: 10.102/14651858. CD004075. pub 2.

Hodnett, E. (1996). Nursing support of the laboring woman. *Journal of Obstetric, and Neonatal Nursing, 25*(3), 257-263.

Lowdermilk, D. L., & Perry, S. E. (2004). *Maternity & women's health care* (8th ed.). St. Louis: Mosby.

Lowe, N. K. (1996). The pain and discomfort of labor and birth. *Journal of Obstetric, and Neonatal Nursing, 25*(1), 82-92.

Mattson, S. (Ed.). (2000). *Core curriculum for maternal-newborn nursing* (2nd ed.). Philadelphia: W.B. Saunders.

Tucker, S. M. (2004). *Pocket guide to fetal monitoring and assessment* (5th ed.). St. Louis: Mosby.

Fluid Balance—0601

Domain-Physiologic Health (II)

Class-Fluid & Electrolytes (G)

Scale(s)-Severely compromised to Not compromised (a) and Severe to None (n)

Care Recipient:

Data Source:

Definition: Water balance in the intracellular and extracellular compartments of the body

OUTCOME TARGET RATING: Maintain at_____   Increase to_____

Fluid Balance Overall Rating	Severely compromised 1	Substantially compromised 2	Moderately compromised 3	Mildly compromised 4	Not compromised 5	

INDICATORS:

060101	Blood pressure	1	2	3	4	5	NA
060122	Radial pulse rate	1	2	3	4	5	NA
060102	Mean arterial pressure	1	2	3	4	5	NA
060103	Central venous pressure	1	2	3	4	5	NA
060104	Pulmonary wedge pressure	1	2	3	4	5	NA
060105	Peripheral pulses	1	2	3	4	5	NA
060107	24-hour intake and output balance	1	2	3	4	5	NA
060109	Stable body weight	1	2	3	4	5	NA
060116	Skin turgor	1	2	3	4	5	NA
060117	Moist mucous membranes	1	2	3	4	5	NA
060118	Serum electrolytes	1	2	3	4	5	NA
060119	Hematocrit	1	2	3	4	5	NA
060120	Urine specific gravity	1	2	3	4	5	NA

		Severe	Substantial	Moderate	Mild	None	
060106	Orthostatic hypotension	1	2	3	4	5	NA
060108	Adventitious breath sounds	1	2	3	4	5	NA
060110	Ascites	1	2	3	4	5	NA
060111	Neck vein distention	1	2	3	4	5	NA
060112	Peripheral edema	1	2	3	4	5	NA
060113	Soft, sunken eyeballs	1	2	3	4	5	NA
060114	Confusion	1	2	3	4	5	NA
060115	Thirst	1	2	3	4	5	NA
060123	Muscle cramps	1	2	3	4	5	NA
060124	Dizziness	1	2	3	4	5	NA

1st edition 1997; Revised 3rd edition 2004

Outcome Content References:

Bosquet, G. L. (1990). Congestive heart failure: A review of nonpharmacologic therapies. *Journal of Cardiovascular Nursing,* *4*(3), 35-46.

Coats, A. J. S., Adamopoulos, S., Meyer, T. E., Conway, J., & Sleight, P. (1990). Effects of physical training in chronic heart failure. *The Lancet, 335*(8681), 63-66.

Coyle, E. F. (2004). Fluid and fuel intake during exercise. *Journal of Sports Sciences, 22*, 39-55.

Fukada, N. (1990). Outcome standards for the client with congestive heart failure. *Journal of Cardiovascular Nursing, 4*(3), 59-70.

Johanson, B. C. (1988). *Standards for critical care* (3rd ed.). St. Louis: Mosby.

Kraft, P. A. (2000). The osmotic shift. *Journal of Intravenous Nursing, 23*(4), 220-224.

Medina, J. (2000). *Standards for acute and critical care nursing practice* (3rd ed.). Irvine, CA: American Association of Critical-Care Nurses.

Reese, J. L. (2001). Fluid volume deficit—dehydration: Isotonic, hypotonic, and hypertonic. In M. Maas, K. Buckwalter, M. Hardy, T. Tripp-Reimer, M. Titler, & J. Specht (Eds.), *Nursing care of older adults: Diagnoses, outcomes & interventions* (pp. 183-200). St. Louis: Mosby.

Toto, K. H. (1998). Fluid balance assessment: The total perspective. *Critical Care Clinics of North America, 10*(4), 383-400.

Vullo-Navich, K., Smith, S., Andrews, M., Levine, A. M., Tischer, J. F., & Veglia, J. M. (1998). Comfort and incidence of abnormal serum sodium, BUN, creatinine and osmolality in dehydration of terminal illness. *The American Journal of Hospice & Palliative Care, 15*(2), 77-84.

F

Fluid Overload Severity—0603

Domain-Physiologic Health (II)

Class-Fluid & Electrolytes (G)

Scale(s)-Severe to None (n)

Care Recipient:

Data Source:

F

Definition: Severity of excess fluids in the intracellular and extracellular compartments of the body

OUTCOME TARGET RATING: Maintain at_____   Increase to_____

Fluid Overload Severity Overall Rating	Severe 1	Substantially 2	Moderately 3	Mild 4	None 5	
INDICATORS:						
060301 Periorbital edema	1	2	3	4	5	NA
060302 Hand edema	1	2	3	4	5	NA
060303 Sacral edema	1	2	3	4	5	NA
060304 Ankle edema	1	2	3	4	5	NA
060305 Leg edema	1	2	3	4	5	NA
060306 Ascites	1	2	3	4	5	NA
060307 Increased abdominal girth	1	2	3	4	5	NA
060308 Generalized edema	1	2	3	4	5	NA
060309 Venous congestion	1	2	3	4	5	NA
060310 Rales	1	2	3	4	5	NA
060311 Malaise	1	2	3	4	5	NA
060312 Lethargy	1	2	3	4	5	NA
060313 Headache	1	2	3	4	5	NA
060314 Confusion	1	2	3	4	5	NA
060315 Seizures	1	2	3	4	5	NA
060316 Coma	1	2	3	4	5	NA
060317 Increased blood pressure	1	2	3	4	5	NA
060318 Weight gain	1	2	3	4	5	NA
060319 Decreased urine output	1	2	3	4	5	NA
060320 Decreased specific urine gravity	1	2	3	4	5	NA
060321 Decreased urine color	1	2	3	4	5	NA
060322 Decreased serum sodium	1	2	3	4	5	NA
060323 Increased serum sodium	1	2	3	4	5	NA

3rd edition 2004

Outcome Content References:

Edwards, S. L. (2000). Fluid overload and monitoring indices. *Professional Nurse, 15*(9), 568-572.

Kelly, A. L. (1999). Left ventricular systolic heart failure resulting in acute pulmonary edema: Pathophysiology and nursing management in the emergency department. *Australian Emergency Nursing Journal, 2*(1), 5-9.

Smeltzer, S. C., & Bare, B. G. (Eds.). (2003). *Brunner and Suddarth's textbook of medical-surgical nursing* (10th ed.). Philadelphia: Lippincott Williams & Wilkins.

Gastrointestinal Function—1015

Domain-Physiologic Health (II)   Care Recipient:

Class-Digestion & Nutrition (K)   Data Source:

Scale(s)-Severely compromised to Not compromised (a) and Severe to None (n)

Definition: Extent to which foods (ingested or tube-fed) are moved from ingestion to excretion

OUTCOME TARGET RATING: Maintain at_____   Increase to_____

Gastrointestinal Function Overall Rating	Severely compromised 1	Substantially compromised 2	Moderately compromised 3	Mildly compromised 4	Not compromised 5	
INDICATORS:						
101501 Food / feeding tolerance	1	2	3	4	5	NA
101502 Abdominal girth	1	2	3	4	5	NA
101503 Frequency of stools	1	2	3	4	5	NA
101504 Color of stool	1	2	3	4	5	NA
101505 Consistency of stool	1	2	3	4	5	NA
101506 Amount of stool	1	2	3	4	5	NA
101507 Axillary temperature	1	2	3	4	5	NA
101508 Bowel sounds	1	2	3	4	5	NA
101509 Gastric aspirates: color	1	2	3	4	5	NA
101510 Gastric aspirates: amount of residuals	1	2	3	4	5	NA
101511 Skin color over abdomen	1	2	3	4	5	NA
101512 Activity level	1	2	3	4	5	NA

	Severe	Substantial	Moderate	Mild	None	
101513 Pain	1	2	3	4	5	NA
101514 Abdominal distention	1	2	3	4	5	NA
101515 Abdominal tenderness	1	2	3	4	5	NA
101516 Regurgitation	1	2	3	4	5	NA
101517 Increase in visible peristalsis	1	2	3	4	5	NA
101518 Thrashing	1	2	3	4	5	NA
101519 Fist clenching	1	2	3	4	5	NA
101520 Blood in stool	1	2	3	4	5	NA
101521 White blood count elevation	1	2	3	4	5	NA
101522 White blood count depression	1	2	3	4	5	NA
101523 White blood count differential	1	2	3	4	5	NA

4th edition

Outcome Content References:

Black, J., & Hawks, J. (2005). *Medical surgical nursing: Clinical management for positive outcomes* (7th ed.). St. Louis: Saunders.

Carlson, S., Montalto, M. B., Ponder, D. L., Werkman, S. H., & Korones, S. B. (1998). Lower incidence of necrotizing entero-colitis in infants fed a preterm formula with egg phospholipids. *Pediatric Research, 44*(4), 491-498.

Continued

Carlos, M., Babyn, P., Marcon, M., Moore, A. (1997). Changes in gastric emptying in early postnatal life. *Journal of Pediatrics, 130*(6), 931-937.

Pilliteri, A. (2003). *Maternal and child health nursing: Care of the childbearing and childrearing family* (4th ed.). Philadelphia: Williams & Wilkins.

Stevens, B. Johnston, C., Franck, L., Petryshen, P., Jack, A., & Foster, G. (1999). The efficacy of developmentally sensitive interventions and sucrose for relieving procedural pain in very low birth weight neonates. *Journal of Nursing Research, 48*(1), 35-43.

Wong, D., and Hockenberry, M. (2003). *Nursing care of infants and children* (7th ed.). St. Louis: Mosby.

Kenner, C., Lott, J., & Flandermeyer, A. (2003). *Comprehensive neonatal nursing: A physiologic perspective* (3rd ed.). Philadelphia: W.B. Saunders.

G

Grief Resolution—1304

Domain-Psychosocial Health (III)

Class-Psychosocial Adaptation (N)

Scale(s)-Never demonstrated to Consistently demonstrated (m)

Care Recipient:

Data Source:

Definition: Adjustment to actual or impending loss

OUTCOME TARGET RATING: Maintain at_____   Increase to_____

Grief Resolution Overall Rating	Never demonstrated 1	Rarely demonstrated 2	Sometimes demonstrated 3	Often demonstrated 4	Consistently demonstrated 5	

INDICATORS:

130401	Resolves feelings about loss	1	2	3	4	5	NA
130402	Expresses spiritual beliefs about death	1	2	3	4	5	NA
130403	Verbalizes reality of loss	1	2	3	4	5	NA
130404	Verbalizes acceptance of loss	1	2	3	4	5	NA
130405	Describes meaning of the loss	1	2	3	4	5	NA
130406	Participates in planning funeral	1	2	3	4	5	NA
130409	Discusses unresolved conflict(s)	1	2	3	4	5	NA
130410	Reports absence of somatic distress	1	2	3	4	5	NA
130411	Reports decreased preoccupation with loss	1	2	3	4	5	NA
130412	Maintains living environment	1	2	3	4	5	NA
130413	Maintains personal grooming and hygiene	1	2	3	4	5	NA
130414	Reports adequate sleep	1	2	3	4	5	NA
130415	Reports adequate nutrition intake	1	2	3	4	5	NA
130416	Reports normal sexual desire	1	2	3	4	5	NA
130417	Seeks social support	1	2	3	4	5	NA
130418	Shares loss with significant others	1	2	3	4	5	NA
130419	Reports involvement in social activities	1	2	3	4	5	NA
130420	Progresses through stages of grief	1	2	3	4	5	NA
130421	Expresses positive expectations about the future	1	2	3	4	5	NA

1st edition 1997; Revised 3rd edition 2004

Outcome Content References:

Batemen, A., Broderick, D., Gleason, L., Kardon, R., Flaherty, C., & Anderson, S. (1992). Dysfunctional grieving. *Journal of Psychosocial Nursing*, 30(12), 5-9.

Cooley, M. E. (1992). Bereavement care: A role for nurses. *Cancer Nursing*, 15(2), 125-129.

Continued

Freitag-Koontz, M. J. (1988). Parents' grief reaction to the diagnosis of their infants' severe neurologic impairment and static encephalopathy. *Journal of Perinatal and Neonatal Nursing, 2*(2), 45-57.

Gibbons, M. B. (1992). A child dies, a child survives: The impact of sibling loss. *Journal of Pediatric Health Care, 6*(2), 45-57.

Harrigan, R., Naber, M., Jensen, K., Tse, A., & Perez, D. (1993). Perinatal grief: Response to the loss of an infant. *Neonatal Network, 12*(5), 25-31.

Kallenberg, K., & Soderfeldt, B. (1992). Three years later: Grief, view of life, and personal crisis after the death of a family member. *Journal of Palliative Care, 8*(4), 13-19.

Kirschling, J. M., & McBride, A. B. (1989). Effects of age and sex on the experience of widowhood. *Western Journal of Nursing Research, 11*(2), 207-218.

Kuntz, B. (1991). Exploring the grief of adolescents after the death of a parent. *Journal of Child and Adolescent Psychiatric and Mental Health Nursing, 4*(3), 105-109.

+Prigerson, H. G., Maciejewski, P. K., Reynolds, C. F., Bierhals, A., Newsom, J. T., Fasiczka, A., Frank, E., Doman, J., & Miller, M. (1995). Inventory of complicated grief: A scale to measure maladaptive symptoms of loss. *Psychiatry Research, 59*(1-2), 65-79.

Whiting, G., & Buckwalter, K. C. (2001). Grieving. In M. Maas, K. Buckwalter, M. Hardy, T. Tripp-Reimer, M. Titler, & J. Specht (Eds.), *Nursing care of older adults: Diagnoses, outcomes & interventions* (pp. 631-650). St. Louis: Mosby.

G

Growth—0110

Domain-Functional Health (I)
Class-Growth & Development (B)
Scale(s)-Severe deviation from normal range to No deviation from normal range (b)

Care Recipient:
Data Source:

Definition: Normal increase in bone size and body weight during growth years

OUTCOME TARGET RATING: Maintain at_____   Increase to_____

Growth Overall Rating	Severe deviation from normal range 1	Substantial deviation from normal range 2	Moderate deviation from normal range 3	Mild deviation from normal range 4	No deviation from normal range 5	
INDICATORS:						
011001 Weight percentile for sex	1	2	3	4	5	NA
011002 Weight percentile for age	1	2	3	4	5	NA
011003 Weight percentile for height	1	2	3	4	5	NA
011004 Rate of weight gain	1	2	3	4	5	NA
011005 Rate of height gain	1	2	3	4	5	NA
011006 Length/height percentile for age	1	2	3	4	5	NA
011007 Length/height percentile for sex	1	2	3	4	5	NA
011008 Head circumference percentile for age	1	2	3	4	5	NA
011009 Bone mass index	1	2	3	4	5	NA
011010 Mean body mass	1	2	3	4	5	NA

1st edition 1997; Revised 3rd edition 2004

Outcome Content References:

Allen, K. D., Warzak, W. J., Greger, N. G., Bernotas, T. D., & Huseman, C. A. (1993). Psychosocial adjustment of children with isolated growth hormone deficiency. *Children's Health Care, 22*(1), 61-72.

Blinkin, N. J., Yip, R., Fleshood, L., & Trowbridge, F. L. (1988). Birth weight and childhood growth. *Pediatrics, 82*(6), 828-834.

Georgieff, M. K., Hoffman, J. S., Pereira, G. R., Bernbaum, J., & Hoffman-Williamson, M. (1985). Effect of neonatal caloric deprivation on head growth and 1-year developmental status in preterm infants. *Journal of Pediatrics, 107*, 581-587.

Hockenberry, M. J., Wilson, D., Winkelstein, M. L., & Kline, N. E. (2003). *Wong's nursing care of infants and children* (7th ed.). St. Louis: Mosby.

Jung, E., & Czajka-Narins, D. M. (1985). Birth weight doubling and tripling times: An updated look at the effects of birth weight, sex, race and type of feeding. *The American Journal of Clinical Nutrition, 42*(8), 182-189.

Sapala, S. (1994). Pediatric management problems. *Pediatric Nursing, 20*(1), 54-55.

Tanner, J. M., & Davies, P. S. W. (1985). Clinical longitudinal standards for height and height velocity for North American children. *The Journal of Pediatrics, 107*(3), 317-329.

G

Health Beliefs—1700

Domain-Health Knowledge & Behavior (IV)

Class-Health Beliefs (R)

Scale(s)-Very weak to Very strong (l)

Care Recipient:

Data Source:

Definition: Personal convictions that influence health behaviors

OUTCOME TARGET RATING: Maintain at_____   Increase to_____

Health Beliefs Overall Rating	Very weak 1	Weak 2	Moderate 3	Strong 4	Very strong 5	
INDICATORS:						
170001 Perceived importance of taking action	1	2	3	4	5	NA
170002 Perceived threat from inaction	1	2	3	4	5	NA
170003 Perceived benefits of action	1	2	3	4	5	NA
170004 Perceived internal control of action	1	2	3	4	5	NA
170005 Perceived control of health outcome	1	2	3	4	5	NA
170006 Perceived reduction of threat from action	1	2	3	4	5	NA
170007 Perceived improvement in lifestyle from action	1	2	3	4	5	NA
170008 Perceived ability to perform action	1	2	3	4	5	NA
170009 Perceived resources to perform action	1	2	3	4	5	NA
170010 Perceived absence of barriers to action	1	2	3	4	5	NA

1st edition 1997

Outcome Content References:

+Champion, V. L. (1993). Instrument refinement for breast cancer screening behaviors. *Nursing Research, 42*(3), 139-143.

Clarke, V. A., Lovegrove, H., Williams, A., & Machperson, M. (2000). *Journal of Behavioral Medicine, 23*(4), 367-376.

Gillis, A. J. (1993). Determinants of health promoting lifestyle: An integrative review. *Journal of Advanced Nursing, 18*(3), 345-353.

Glick, O. J., & Ressler, C. (2001). Altered health maintenance. In M. Maas, K. Buckwalter, M. Hardy, T. Tripp-Reimer, M. Titler, & J. Specht (Eds.), *Nursing care of older adults: Diagnoses, outcomes & interventions* (pp. 6-22). St. Louis: Mosby.

Hayes, D., & Ross, C. (1987). Concern with appearance, health beliefs, and eating habits. *Journal of Health and Social Behavior, 28*(6), 120-130.

+Kim, K. K., Horan, M. L., Gendler, P., & Patel, M. K. (1991). Development and evaluation of the osteoporosis health belief scale. *Research in Nursing & Health, 14*(2), 155-163.

Robertson, D., & Keller, C. (1992). Relationships among health beliefs, self-efficacy, and exercise adherence in patients with coronary artery disease. *Heart & Lung, 21*(1), 56-63.

Thompson, J., McFarland, G. K., & Hirsch, J. E. (2002). *Mosby's clinical nursing* (5th ed.). St. Louis: Mosby.

Health Beliefs: Perceived Ability to Perform—1701

Domain-Health Knowledge & Behavior (IV)

Class-Health Beliefs (R)

Scale(s)-Very weak to Very strong (l)

Care Recipient:

Data Source:

Definition: Personal conviction that one can carry out a given health behavior

OUTCOME TARGET RATING: Maintain at_____   Increase to_____

Health Beliefs: Perceived Ability to Perform Overall Rating	Very weak 1	Weak 2	Moderate 3	Strong 4	Very strong 5	
INDICATORS:						
170101 Perception that health behavior is not too complex	1	2	3	4	5	NA
170102 Perception that health behavior requires reasonable effort	1	2	3	4	5	NA
170103 Perception that the frequency of health behavior is not excessive	1	2	3	4	5	NA
170104 Perception of likelihood of performing health behavior over time	1	2	3	4	5	NA
170105 Confidence related to past experience with health behavior	1	2	3	4	5	NA
170106 Confidence related to past experience with similar health behaviors	1	2	3	4	5	NA
170107 Confidence related to observation of successful experiences of others	1	2	3	4	5	NA
170108 Confidence in ability to perform health behavior	1	2	3	4	5	NA

1st edition 1997; Revised 3rd edition 2004

Outcome Content References:

Bauer, M. S., Williford, W. O., McBride, L., McBride, K., & Shea, N. M. (2005). Perceived barriers to health care access in a treated population. *International Journal of Psychiatry in Medicine, 35*(1), 13-26.

Calfee, C. S., Katz, P. P., Yelin, E. H., Iribarren, C., & Eisner, M. D. (2007). The influence of perceived control of asthma on health outcomes. *Chest, 130*, 1312-1318.

+Champion, V. L. (1993). Instrument refinement for breast cancer screening behaviors. *Nursing Research, 42*(3), 139-143.

Clarke, V. A., Lovegrove, H., Williams, A., & Machperson, M. (2000). *Journal of Behavioral Medicine, 23*(4), 367-376.

De Weerdt, I., Visser, A., & Van der Veen, E. (1989). Attitude behavior theories and diabetes education programs. *Patient Education and Counseling, 14*, 3-19.

Hayes, D., & Ross, C. (1987). Concern with appearance, health beliefs, and eating habits. *Journal of Health and Social Behavior, 28*(6), 120-130.

Jemmot, L., & Jemmot, J. (1992). Increasing condom-use intentions among sexually active black adolescent women. *Nursing Research, 41*(5), 273-278.

Jensen, K., Banwart, L., Venhaus, R., Popkess-Vawter, S., & Perkins, S. B. (1993). Advanced rehabilitation nursing care of coronary angioplasty patients using self-efficacy theory. *Journal of Advanced Nursing, 18*(6), 926-931.

Kim, K. K., Horan, M. L., Gendler, P., & Patel, M. K. (1991). Development and evaluation of the Osteoporosis Health Belief Scale. *Research in Nursing & Health, 14*(2), 155-163.

Lowe, N. K. (1993). Maternal confidence for labor: Development of the Childbirth Self-Efficacy Inventory. *Research in Nursing & Health, 16*(2), 141-149.

Robertson, D., & Keller, C. (1992). Relationships among health beliefs, self-efficacy, and exercise adherence in patients with coronary artery disease. *Heart & Lung, 21*(1), 56-63.

+Smith, M. S., Wallston, K. A., & Smith, C. A. (1995). The development and validation of the Perceived Health Competence Scale. *Health Education Research, 10*(1), 51-64.

H

Health Beliefs: Perceived Control—1702

Domain-Health Knowledge & Behavior (IV)

Class-Health Beliefs (R)

Scale(s)-Very weak to Very strong (l)

Care Recipient:

Data Source:

Definition: Personal conviction that one can influence a health outcome

OUTCOME TARGET RATING: Maintain at_____   Increase to_____

Health Beliefs: Perceived Control Overall Rating	Very weak 1	Weak 2	Moderate 3	Strong 4	Very strong 5	
INDICATORS:						
170201 Perceived responsibility for health decisions	1	2	3	4	5	NA
170202 Requested involvement in health decisions	1	2	3	4	5	NA
170203 Efforts at gathering information	1	2	3	4	5	NA
170204 Belief that own decisions control health outcomes	1	2	3	4	5	NA
170205 Belief that own actions control health outcomes	1	2	3	4	5	NA
170206 Willingness to designate surrogate decision maker	1	2	3	4	5	NA
170207 Willingness to have current living will	1	2	3	4	5	NA

1st edition 1997

Outcome Content References:

Calnan, M., & Moss, S. (1984). The Health Belief Model and compliance with education given at a class in breast self-examination. *Journal of Health and Social Behavior, 25*(2), 198-210.

+Champion, V. L. (1993). Instrument refinement for breast cancer screening behaviors. *Nursing Research, 42*(3), 139-143.

Clarke, V. A., Lovegrove, H., Williams, A., & Machperson, M. (2000). *Journal of Behavioral Medicine, 23*(4), 367-376.

Gillis, A. J. (1993). Determinants of health promoting lifestyle: An integrative review. *Journal of Advanced Nursing, 18*(3), 345-353.

Hayes, D., & Ross, C. (1987). Concern with appearance, health beliefs, and eating habits. *Journal of Health and Social Behavior, 28*(6), 120-130.

+Wallston, K. A., & Wallston, B. S. (1981). Health Locus of Control Scales. In H. Lefcourt (Ed.), *Research with the locus of control construct* (Vol. 1, pp. 189-243). New York: Academic Press.

+Wallston, K. A., Wallston, B. S., & DeVellis, R. (1978). Development of the Multidimensional Health Locus of Control (MHLC) Scales. *Health Education Monographs, 6,* 160-170.

Health Beliefs: Perceived Resources—1703

Domain-Health Knowledge & Behavior (IV)   *Care Recipient:*

Class-Health Beliefs (R)   *Data Source:*

Scale(s)-Very weak to Very strong (l)

Definition: Personal conviction that one has adequate means to carry out a health behavior

OUTCOME TARGET RATING: Maintain at_____   Increase to_____

Health Beliefs: Perceived Resources Overall Rating		Very weak 1	Weak 2	Moderate 3	Strong 4	Very strong 5	
INDICATORS:							
170301	Perceived support of significant others	1	2	3	4	5	NA
170302	Perceived support of friends	1	2	3	4	5	NA
170303	Perceived support of neighbors	1	2	3	4	5	NA
170304	Perceived support of health provider	1	2	3	4	5	NA
170305	Perceived support of self-help groups	1	2	3	4	5	NA
170306	Perceived functional ability	1	2	3	4	5	NA
170307	Perceived energy to act	1	2	3	4	5	NA
170309	Perceived adequacy of time	1	2	3	4	5	NA
170310	Perceived adequacy of personal finances	1	2	3	4	5	NA
170311	Perceived adequacy of health insurance	1	2	3	4	5	NA
170318	Perceived access to medication	1	2	3	4	5	NA
170312	Perceived access to equipment	1	2	3	4	5	NA
170313	Perceived access to supplies	1	2	3	4	5	NA
170314	Perceived access to health care services	1	2	3	4	5	NA
170315	Perceived access to transportation	1	2	3	4	5	NA
170316	Perceived access to physical assistance	1	2	3	4	5	NA

1st edition 1997; Revised 3rd edition 2004

Outcome Content References:

+Becker, H., Stuifbergen, A. K., & Sands, D. (1991). Development of a scale to measure barriers to health promotion activities among persons with disabilities. *American Journal of Health Promotion, 5*(6), 449-454.

+Champion, V. L. (1993). Instrument refinement for breast cancer screening behaviors. *Nursing Research, 42*(3), 139-143.

Clarke, V. A., Lovegrove, H., Williams, A., & Machperson, M. (2000). *Journal of Behavioral Medicine, 23*(4), 367-376.

Gillis, A. J. (1993). Determinants of health promoting lifestyle: An integrative review. *Journal of Advanced Nursing, 18*(3), 345-353.

Kim, K. K., Horan, M. L., Gendler, P., & Patel, M. K. (1991). Development and evaluation of the osteoporosis health belief scale. *Research in Nursing & Health, 14*(2), 155-163.

Robertson, D., & Keller, C. (1992). Relationships among health beliefs, self-efficacy, and exercise adherence in patients with coronary artery disease. *Heart & Lung, 21*(1), 56-63.

H

Health Beliefs: Perceived Threat—1704

Domain-Health Knowledge & Behavior (IV)

Class-Health Beliefs (R)

Scale(s)-Very weak to Very strong (l)

Care Recipient:

Data Source:

Definition: Personal conviction that a threatening health problem is serious and has potential negative consequences for lifestyle

OUTCOME TARGET RATING:　　Maintain at_____　　　Increase to_____

Health Beliefs: Perceived Threat Overall Rating	Very weak 1	Weak 2	Moderate 3	Strong 4	Very strong 5	
INDICATORS:						
170401 Perceived threat to health	1	2	3	4	5	NA
170403 Perceived vulnerability to progressive health problems	1	2	3	4	5	NA
170404 Concern regarding illness or injury	1	2	3	4	5	NA
170405 Concern regarding potential complications	1	2	3	4	5	NA
170406 Perceived severity of illness or injury	1	2	3	4	5	NA
170407 Perceived severity of complications	1	2	3	4	5	NA
170408 Perceived threat of discomfort from illness or injury	1	2	3	4	5	NA
170409 Perception that condition may be of long duration	1	2	3	4	5	NA
170410 Perceived impact on current lifestyle	1	2	3	4	5	NA
170411 Perceived impact on future lifestyle	1	2	3	4	5	NA
170412 Perceived impact on functional status	1	2	3	4	5	NA
170414 Perceived threat of death	1	2	3	4	5	NA

1st edition 1997; Revised 3rd edition 2004

Outcome Content References:

+Champion, V. L. (1993). Instrument refinement for breast cancer screening behaviors. *Nursing Research, 42*(3), 139-143.

Calnan, M., & Moss, S. (1984). The health belief model and compliance with education given at a class in breast self-examination. *Journal of Health and Social Behavior, 25*(2), 198-210.

Clarke, V. A., Lovegrove, H., Williams, A., & Machperson, M. (2000). *Journal of Behavioral Medicine, 23*(4), 367-376.

De Weerdt, I., Visser, A., & Van Der Veen, E. (1989). Attitude behavior theories and diabetes education programs. *Patient Education and Counseling, 14*, 3-19.

Dunn, S., Beeney, L., Hoskins, P., & Turtle, J. (1990). Knowledge and attitude change as predictors of metabolic improvement in diabetes education. *Social Science and Medicine, 31*(10), 1135-1141.

+Kim, K. K., Horan, M. L., Gendler, P., & Patel, M. K. (1991). Development and evaluation of the osteoporosis health belief scale. *Research in Nursing & Health, 14*(2), 155-163.

Robertson, D., & Keller, C. (1992). Relationships among health beliefs, self-efficacy, and exercise adherence in patients with coronary artery disease. *Heart & Lung, 21*(1), 56-63.

Thompson, J., McFarland, G., & Hirsch, J. (2002). *Mosby's clinical nursing* (5th ed.). St. Louis: Mosby.

H

Health Orientation—1705

Domain-Health Knowledge & Behavior (IV)

Class-Health Beliefs (R)

Scale(s)-Very weak to Very strong (l)

Care Recipient:

Data Source:

Definition: Personal commitment to health behaviors as lifestyle priorities

OUTCOME TARGET RATING: Maintain at_____   Increase to_____

Health Orientation Overall Rating		Very weak 1	Weak 2	Moderate 3	Strong 4	Very strong 5	
INDICATORS:							
170501	Focus on wellness	1	2	3	4	5	NA
170514	Focus on maintaining health behaviors	1	2	3	4	5	NA
170502	Focus on disease prevention	1	2	3	4	5	NA
170503	Focus on maintaining role performance	1	2	3	4	5	NA
170504	Focus on maintaining functional abilities	1	2	3	4	5	NA
170505	Focus on adjustment to life situations	1	2	3	4	5	NA
170506	Focus on overall well-being	1	2	3	4	5	NA
170507	Expectation that individual is responsible for health-related choices	1	2	3	4	5	NA
170508	Perception that health behavior is relevant to one's health	1	2	3	4	5	NA
170515	Perceived importance of incorporating health behaviors with cultural beliefs	1	2	3	4	5	NA
170512	Perception that health is a high priority in making lifestyle choices	1	2	3	4	5	NA

1st edition 1997; Revised 3rd edition 2004

Outcome Content References:

Gillis, A. J. (1993). Determinants of health promoting lifestyle: An integrative review. *Journal of Advanced Nursing, 18*(3), 345-353.

Glick, O. J., & Ressler, C. (2001). Altered health maintenance. In M. Maas, K. Buckwalter, M. Hardy, T. Tripp-Reimer, M. Titler, & J. Specht (Eds.), *Nursing care of older adults: Diagnoses, outcomes & interventions* (pp. 6-22). St. Louis: Mosby.

Kulbok, P., & Baldwin, J. (1992). From preventive health behavior to health promotion: Advancing a positive construct of health. *Advances in Nursing Science, 14*(4), 50-64.

Palank, C. (1991). Determinants of health promoting behavior. *Nursing Clinics of North America, 26*(4), 815-832.

Pender, N. J. (1990). Expressing health through lifestyle patterns. *Nursing Science Quarterly, 3*(3), 115-122.

+Walker, S. N., Sechrist, K. R., & Pender, N. J. (1995). *The Health-Promoting Lifestyle Profile II*. Omaha, NE: University of Nebraska at Omaha.

+Walker, S. N., Sechrist, K. R., & Pender, N. J. (1987). The Health-Promoting Lifestyle Profile: Development and psychometric characteristics. *Nursing Research, 36*(2), 76-81.

Ziebland, S., Evans, J., McPherson, A. (2006). The choice is yours? How women with ovarian cancer make sense of treatment choices. *Patient Education and Counseling, 62*, 361-367.

H

Health Promoting Behavior—1602

Domain-Health Knowledge & Behavior (IV)   *Care Recipient:*

Class-Health Behavior (Q)   *Data Source:*

Scale(s)-Never demonstrated to Consistently demonstrated (m)

Definition: Personal actions to sustain or increase wellness

OUTCOME TARGET RATING: Maintain at_____   Increase to_____

Health Promoting Behavior Overall Rating	Never demonstrated 1	Rarely demonstrated 2	Sometimes demonstrated 3	Often demonstrated 4	Consistently demonstrated 5	
INDICATORS:						
160201 Uses risk avoidance behaviors	1	2	3	4	5	NA
160202 Monitors environment for risks	1	2	3	4	5	NA
160203 Monitors personal behavior for risks	1	2	3	4	5	NA
160221 Balances activity and rest	1	2	3	4	5	NA
160222 Maintains adequate sleep	1	2	3	4	5	NA
160205 Uses effective stress reduction techniques	1	2	3	4	5	NA
160206 Maintains social relationships	1	2	3	4	5	NA
160207 Performs healthy behaviors routinely	1	2	3	4	5	NA
160208 Supports healthful public policy	1	2	3	4	5	NA
160209 Uses financial resources to promote health	1	2	3	4	5	NA
160210 Uses social support to promote health	1	2	3	4	5	NA
160212 Obtains recommended immunizations	1	2	3	4	5	NA
160213 Obtains recommended health screenings	1	2	3	4	5	NA
160214 Follows healthy diet	1	2	3	4	5	NA
160223 Drinks eight glasses of water daily	1	2	3	4	5	NA
160224 Obtains regular check-ups	1	2	3	4	5	NA
160215 Uses effective weight control strategies	1	2	3	4	5	NA
160216 Uses effective exercise routine	1	2	3	4	5	NA
160217 Avoids exposure to infectious disease	1	2	3	4	5	NA
160225 Avoids exposure to second-hand smoke	1	2	3	4	5	NA
160218 Avoids alcohol misuse	1	2	3	4	5	NA
160219 Avoids tobacco use	1	2	3	4	5	NA
160220 Avoids recreational drug use	1	2	3	4	5	NA

H

1st edition 1997; Revised 3rd edition 2004; Revised 4th edition

Outcome Content References:

Green, L., & Raeburn, J. (1990). Contemporary development in health promotion. In N. Bracht (Ed.), *Health promotion at the community level* (pp. 29-44). Thousand Oaks, CA: Sage.

Johnson, P. H., & Kittleson, M. J. (2003). A qualitative exploration of health behaviors and the associated factor among university students from different cultures. *The International Journal of Health Education, 6,* 14-25.

Kulbok, P., & Baldwin, J. (1992). From preventive health behavior to health promotion: Advancing a positive construct of health. *Advances in Nursing Science, 14*(4), 50-64.

Leenerts, M. H., Teel, C. S., & Pendleton, M. K. (2002). Building a model of self-care for health promotion in aging. *Journal of Nursing Scholarship, 34*(4), 355-361.

Mechanic, D., & Cleary, P. (1980). Factors associated with maintenance of positive behavior. *Preventive Medicine, 9*(6), 805-814.

Resnick, B. (2000). Health promotion practices of the older adult. *Public Health Nursing, 17*(3), 160-168.

Seeman, T. E. (2000). Health promoting effects of friends and family on health outcomes in older adults. *American Journal of Health Promotion, 14*(6), 362-370.

Simons-Morton, D. G., Mullen, P. D., Mains, D. A., Tabak, E. R., & Green, L. W. (1992). Characteristics of controlled studies of patient education and counseling for preventive health behavior. *Patient Education and Counseling, 19*(2), 175-204.

Stevenson, J. S. (2001). Health seeking behaviors. In M. Maas, K. Buckwalter, M. Hardy, T. Tripp-Reimer, M. Titler, & J. Specht (Eds.), *Nursing care of older adults: Diagnoses, outcomes & interventions* (pp. 75-85). St. Louis: Mosby.

+Walker, S. N., Sechrist, K. R., & Pender, N. J. (1995). *The Health-Promoting Lifestyle Profile II*. Omaha, NE: University of Nebraska at Omaha.

+Walker, S. N., Sechrist, K. R., & Pender, N. J. (1987). The Health Promoting Lifestyle Profile: Development and psychometric characteristics. *Nursing Research, 36*(2), 76-81.

H

Health Seeking Behavior—1603

Domain-Health Knowledge & Behavior (IV)

Class-Health Behavior (Q)

Scale(s)-Never demonstrated to Consistently demonstrated (m)

Care Recipient:

Data Source:

Definition: Personal actions to promote optimal wellness, recovery, and rehabilitation

OUTCOME TARGET RATING: Maintain at_____   Increase to_____

Health Seeking Behavior Overall Rating	Never demonstrated 1	Rarely demonstrated 2	Sometimes demonstrated 3	Often demonstrated 4	Consistently demonstrated 5	
INDICATORS:						
160301 Asks health-related questions	1	2	3	4	5	NA
160302 Completes health-related tasks	1	2	3	4	5	NA
160303 Performs self-screening	1	2	3	4	5	NA
160313 Obtains assistance from health professional	1	2	3	4	5	NA
160305 Performs activities of daily living consistent with tolerance	1	2	3	4	5	NA
160306 Describes strategies to eliminate unhealthy behavior	1	2	3	4	5	NA
160314 Performs self-developed health behavior	1	2	3	4	5	NA
160308 Performs prescribed health behavior	1	2	3	4	5	NA
160315 Uses reputable health information	1	2	3	4	5	NA
160310 Describes strategies to optimize health	1	2	3	4	5	NA
160316 Seeks assistance from family members when needed	1	2	3	4	5	NA

1st edition 1997; Revised 3rd edition 2004; Revised 4th edition

Outcome Content References:

Folden, S. L. (1993). Definitions of health and health goals of participants in a community-based pulmonary rehabilitation program. *Public Health Nursing, 10*(1), 31-35.

Frich, J. C., Ose, L., Malterud, K., & Fugelli, P. (2006). Perceived vulnerability to heart disease in patients with familial hypercholesterolemia: A qualitative interview study. *Annals of Family Medicine, 4*(3), 198-204.

Jensen, L., & Allen, M. (1993). Wellness: The dialect of illness. *Image-The Journal of Nursing Scholarship, 25*(3), 220-224.

Kaplan, M., Kiernan, N. E., & James, L. (2006). Intergenerational family conversations and decision making about eating healthfully. *Journal of Nutrition Education & Behavior, 38*(5), 298-306.

Macnee, C. L., Edwards, J., Kaplan, A., Reed, S., Bradford, S., Walls, J., & Schaller-Ayers, J. M. (2006). Evaluation of NOC standardized outcome of "health seeking behavior" in nurse-managed clinics. *Journal of Nursing Care quality, 21*(3), 242-247.

Mansfield, A. K., Addis, M. E., Mahalik, J. R. (2003). "Why won't he go to the doctor?": The psychology of men's help seeking. *International Journal of Men's Health, 2*(2), 93-109.

Nicoteri, J. A., & Arnold, E. C. (2005). The development of health care-seeking behaviors in traditional-age undergraduate college students. *Journal of the American Academy of Nurse Practitioners, 17*(10), 411-415.

Pender, N. J. (1990). Expressing health through lifestyle patterns. *Nursing Science Quarterly, 3*(3), 115-122.

Pender, N. J., & Pender, A. R. (1986). Attitudes, subjective norms, and intentions of engage in health behaviors. *Nursing Research, 35*(1), 15-18.

Stevenson, J. S. (2001). Health seeking behaviors. In M. Maas, K. Buckwalter, M. Hardy, T. Tripp-Reimer, M. Titler, & J. Specht (Eds.), *Nursing care of older adults: Diagnoses, outcomes & interventions* (pp. 75-85). St. Louis: Mosby.

+Walker, S. N., Sechrist, K. R., & Pender, N. J. (1995). *The Health-Promoting Lifestyle Profile II.* Omaha, NE: University of Nebraska at Omaha.

+Walker, S. N., Sechrist, K. R., & Pender, N. J. (1987). The Health Promoting Lifestyle Profile: Development and psychometric characteristics. *Nursing Research, 36*(2), 76-81.

Woods, N. (1989). Conceptualizations of self-care: Toward health-oriented models. *Advances in Nursing Science, 12*(1), 1-13.

H

Hearing Compensation Behavior—1610

Domain-Health Knowledge & Behavior (IV)

Class-Health Behavior (Q)

Scale(s)-Never demonstrated to Consistently demonstrated (m)

Care Recipient:

Data Source:

Definition: Personal actions to identify, monitor, and compensate for hearing loss

OUTCOME TARGET RATING: Maintain at_____   Increase to_____

Hearing Compensation Behavior Overall Rating	Never demonstrated 1	Rarely demonstrated 2	Sometimes demonstrated 3	Often demonstrated 4	Consistently demonstrated 5	
INDICATORS:						
161001 Monitors symptoms of hearing deterioration	1	2	3	4	5	NA
161002 Positions self to advantage hearing	1	2	3	4	5	NA
161003 Reminds others to use techniques that advantage hearing	1	2	3	4	5	NA
161004 Eliminates background noise	1	2	3	4	5	NA
161005 Uses sign language	1	2	3	4	5	NA
161006 Uses lip reading	1	2	3	4	5	NA
161007 Uses closed captioning for television viewing	1	2	3	4	5	NA
161009 Uses hearing supportive devices	1	2	3	4	5	NA
161012 Uses hearing aids correctly	1	2	3	4	5	NA
161010 Cares for internal hearing assistive devices correctly	1	2	3	4	5	NA
161011 Cares for external hearing assistive devices correctly	1	2	3	4	5	NA
161013 Uses support services for hearing impaired	1	2	3	4	5	NA

2nd edition 2000; Revised 3rd edition 2004; Revised 4th edition

Outcome Content References:

Burrell, L. O. (Ed.). (1992). *Adult nursing in hospital and community settings*. Norwalk, CT: Appleton & Lange.

Phipps, W. J., Monahan, F. D., Sands J. K., Marek, J., & Neighbors, M. (Eds.). (2003). *Medical-surgical nursing: Concepts and clinical practice* (7th ed.). St. Louis: Mosby.

Smeltzer, S. C., & Bare, B. G. (Eds.). (2003). *Brunner and Suddarth's textbook of medical-surgical nursing* (10th ed.). Philadelphia: Lippincott Williams & Wilkins.

H

Heedfulness of Affected Side—0918

Domain-Physiologic Health (II)

Class-Neurocognitive (J)

Scale(s)-Never demonstrated to Consistently demonstrated (m)

Care Recipient:

Data Source:

Definition: Personal actions to acknowledge, protect, and cognitively integrate affected body part(s) into self

OUTCOME TARGET RATING: Maintain at_____   Increase to_____

Heedfulness of Affected Side Overall Rating	Never demonstrated 1	Rarely demonstrated 2	Sometimes demonstrated 3	Often demonstrated 4	Consistently demonstrated 5	
INDICATORS:						
091801 Acknowledges affected side as being integral to self	1	2	3	4	5	NA
091802 Protects affected side when ambulating	1	2	3	4	5	NA
091803 Protects affected side when positioning	1	2	3	4	5	NA
091804 Protects affected side when transferring	1	2	3	4	5	NA
091805 Protects affected side during rest or sleep	1	2	3	4	5	NA
091806 Performs activities of daily living to affected side	1	2	3	4	5	NA
091807 Arranges environment to compensate for physical or sensory deficits	1	2	3	4	5	NA
091808 Changes body orientation to enable unaffected side to compensate for physical or sensory deficits	1	2	3	4	5	NA
091809 Uses visual scanning as a compensatory strategy	1	2	3	4	5	NA
091810 Promotes strength and dexterity of affected limb	1	2	3	4	5	NA
091811 Prevents under use of affected limb	1	2	3	4	5	NA
091812 Maintains postural control	1	2	3	4	5	NA

4th edition

Outcome Content References:

Duncan, P. W., Zorowitz, R., Bates, B., Choi, J. Y., Glasberg, J. J., Graham, G. D., Katz, R. C., Lamberty, K., & Reker, D. (2005). Management of adult stroke rehabilitation care: A clinical practice guideline. *Stroke, 36*(9), e100-143.

Intercollegiate Stroke Working Party. (2004). *National clinical guidelines for stroke* (2nd ed.). London: Clinical Effectiveness and Evaluation Unit of the Royal College of Physicians.

Punt, T. D., & Riddoch, M. J. (2006). Motor neglect: Implications for movement and rehabilitation following stroke. *Disability and Rehabilitation, 28*(13-14), 857-864.

Slater, D. I., Curtin, S., Johns, J. S., Schmidt, C., Tipton, J. L., & Newbury, R. E. (2006). *Middle cerebral artery stroke*. Retrieved January 22, 2007, from http://www.emedicine.com/pmr/topic77.htm

Perennou, D. A., Leblond, C., Amblard, B., Micallef, J. P., Herisson, C., & Pelissier, Y. (2001). Transcutaneous electric nerve stimulation reduces neglect-related postural instability after stroke. *Archives of Physical Medicine and Rehabilitation, 82*, 440-448.

Ringman, J. M., Saver, J. L., Woolson, R. F., Clarke, W. R., & Adams, H. P. (2004). Frequency, risk factors, anatomy, and course of unilateral neglect in an acute stroke cohort. *Neurology, 63*, 468-474.

Weitzel, E. A. (2001). Unilateral neglect. In M. Maas, K. Buckwalter, M. Hardy, T. Tripp-Reimer, M. Titler, & J. Specht (Eds.), *Nursing care of older adults: Diagnosis, outcomes, and interventions* (pp. 492-502). St Louis: Mosby.

H

Hemodialysis Access—1105

Domain-Physiologic Health (II)

Class-Tissue Integrity (L)

Scale(s)-Severely compromised to Not compromised (a) and Severe to None (n)

Care Recipient:

Data Source:

Definition: Functionality of a dialysis access site

OUTCOME TARGET RATING: Maintain at_____   Increase to_____

Hemodialysis Access Overall Rating	Severely compromised 1	Substantially compromised 2	Moderately compromised 3	Mildly compromised 4	Not compromised 5	

INDICATORS:

110501	Blood volume flow through fistula/shunt	1	2	3	4	5	NA
110502	Site skin color	1	2	3	4	5	NA
110517	Access site skin temperature	1	2	3	4	5	NA
110505	Bruit	1	2	3	4	5	NA
110506	Thrill	1	2	3	4	5	NA
110509	Distal peripheral pulses	1	2	3	4	5	NA
110510	Distal peripheral skin temperature	1	2	3	4	5	NA
110511	Distal peripheral skin color	1	2	3	4	5	NA
110514	Clotting time	1	2	3	4	5	NA

		Severe	Substantial	Moderate	Mild	None	
110503	Drainage at site	1	2	3	4	5	NA
110507	Hematoma at site	1	2	3	4	5	NA
110508	Bleeding at site	1	2	3	4	5	NA
110512	Distal peripheral edema	1	2	3	4	5	NA
110515	Tenderness at site	1	2	3	4	5	NA
110513	Cannula displacement	1	2	3	4	5	NA

2nd edition 2000; Revised 3rd edition 2004

Outcome Content References:

Broscious, S. K., & Castagnola, J. (2006). Chronic kidney disease: Acute manifestations and role of critical care nurses. *Critical Care Nurse, 26*(4), 17-28.

Eisenbud, M. D. (1996). *The handbook of dialysis access.* Columbus, OH: Anadem Publishing.

Lancaster, L. E. (Ed.). (1995). *ANNA's core curriculum for nephrology nurses* (3rd ed.) (Section X). Pitman, NJ: Anthony J. Janetti.

Levine, D. Z. (1997). *Caring for the renal patient* (3rd ed.). Philadelphia: W.B. Saunders.

Gutch, C. F., Stoner, M. H., & Corea, A. L. (1999). *Review of hemodialysis for nurses and dialysis personnel* (6th ed.). St. Louis: Mosby.

Rabani, A., & Jafarian, A. (2005). Function and complications of arteriovenous fistula in chronic hemodialysis patients (a report from two referral centers). *Journal of Medical Council of Islamic Republic of Iran, 22*(4), 369.

Hope—1201

Domain-Psychosocial Health (III)

Class-Psychological Well-Being (M)

Scale(s)-Never demonstrated to Consistently demonstrated (m)

Care Recipient:

Data Source:

Definition: Optimism that is personally satisfying and life-supporting

OUTCOME TARGET RATING: Maintain at_____   Increase to_____

Hope Overall Rating	Never demonstrated 1	Rarely demonstrated 2	Sometimes demonstrated 3	Often demonstrated 4	Consistently demonstrated 5	

INDICATORS:

120101	Expresses expectation of a positive future	1	2	3	4	5	NA
120102	Expresses faith	1	2	3	4	5	NA
120103	Expresses will to live	1	2	3	4	5	NA
120104	Expresses reasons to live	1	2	3	4	5	NA
120105	Expresses meaning in life	1	2	3	4	5	NA
120106	Expresses optimism	1	2	3	4	5	NA
120107	Expresses belief in self	1	2	3	4	5	NA
120108	Expresses belief in others	1	2	3	4	5	NA
120109	Expresses inner peace	1	2	3	4	5	NA
120110	Expresses sense of self-control	1	2	3	4	5	NA
120111	Exhibits a zest for life	1	2	3	4	5	NA
120112	Sets goals	1	2	3	4	5	NA

1st edition 1997; Revised 3rd edition 2004

Outcome Content References:

+Beckman, E. E., Leber, W. R., Watkins, J. T., Boyer, J. L., & Cook, J. B. (1986). Development of an instrument to measure Beck's cognitive triad: The Cognitive Triad Inventory. *Journal of Consulting and Clinical Psychology, 54*(4), 566-567.

Farran, C. J. (2001). Hopelessness. In M. Maas, K. Buckwalter, M. Hardy, T. Tripp-Reimer, M. Titler, & J. Specht (Eds.), *Nursing care of older adults: Diagnoses, outcomes & interventions* (pp. 601-612). St. Louis: Mosby.

Hall, B. (1990). The struggle of the diagnosed terminally ill person to maintain hope. *Nursing Science Quarterly, 3*(4), 177-184.

Herth, K. (1993). Hope in the family caregiver of terminally ill people. *Journal of Advanced Nursing, 18*(4), 538-548.

Hunt-Raleigh, E. (1992). Sources of hope in chronic illness. *Oncology Nursing Forum, 3*(19), 443-448.

Owen, D. (1989). Nurses perspectives on the meaning of hope in patients with cancer: A qualitative study. *Oncology Nursing Forum, 1*(16), 75-79.

Sowers, W. (2005). Transforming systems of care: The American Association of Community Psychiatrists guideline recovery oriented services. *Community Mental Health Journal, 41*(6), 757-774.

Stephenson, C. (1991). The concept of hope revisited for nursing. *Journal of Advanced Nursing, 16*(12), 1456-1461.

H

Hydration—0602

Domain-Physiologic Health (II)

Class-Fluid & Electrolytes (G)

Scale(s)-Severely compromised to Not compromised (a) and Severe to None (n)

Care Recipient:

Data Source:

Definition: Adequate water in the intracellular and extracellular compartments of the body

OUTCOME TARGET RATING:　　Maintain at_____　　　Increase to_____

Hydration Overall Rating	Severely compromised 1	Substantially compromised 2	Moderately compromised 3	Mildly compromised 4	Not compromised 5	
INDICATORS:						
060201　Skin turgor	1	2	3	4	5	NA
060202　Moist mucous membranes	1	2	3	4	5	NA
060215　Fluid intake	1	2	3	4	5	NA
060211　Urine output	1	2	3	4	5	NA
060216　Serum sodium	1	2	3	4	5	NA
060217　Tissue perfusion	1	2	3	4	5	NA
060218　Cognitive function	1	2	3	4	5	NA
	Severe	**Substantial**	**Moderate**	**Mild**	**None**	
060205　Thirst	1	2	3	4	5	NA
060219　Dark urine	1	2	3	4	5	NA
060208　Soft, sunken eyeballs	1	2	3	4	5	NA
060220　Sunken fontanel	1	2	3	4	5	NA
060212　Decreased blood pressure	1	2	3	4	5	NA
060221　Rapid, thready pulse	1	2	3	4	5	NA
060213　Increased hematocrit	1	2	3	4	5	NA
060222　Increased blood urea nitrogen	1	2	3	4	5	NA
060223　Weight loss	1	2	3	4	5	NA
060224　Muscle cramps	1	2	3	4	5	NA
060225　Muscle twitching	1	2	3	4	5	NA
060226　Diarrhea	1	2	3	4	5	NA

1st edition 1997; Revised 3rd edition 2004

Outcome Content References:

Arieff, A. (1986). Hyponatremia, convulsions, respiratory arrest, and permanent brain damage after elective surgery in healthy women. *The New England Journal of Medicine, 314*(24), 1529-1534.

Carcillo, J. A., Davis, A. L., & Zaritsky, A. (1991). Role of early fluid resuscitation in pediatric septic shock. *Journal of the American Medical Association, 266*(9), 1242-1245.

Gilski, D. (1993). Controversies in patient management after cardiac surgery. *Journal of Cardiovascular Nursing, 7*(4), 1-13.

Hill, P., & Aldag, J. (1991). Potential indicators of insufficient milk supply syndrome. *Research in Nursing & Health, 14*(1), 11-19.

Innerarity, S. A. (1997). *Fluids and electrolytes* (3rd ed.). Springhouse, PA: Springhouse.

The Joanna Briggs Institute for Evidence Based Nursing and Midwifery. (2000). Identification and nursing management of dysphagia in adults with neurological impairment. *Best Practice, 4*(2), Blackwell Science-Asia, Australia.

Mentes, J., Culp, K., Wakefield, B., Gaspar, P., Rapp, C., Mobily, P., & Tripp-Reimer, T. (1998). Dehydration as a precipitating factor in the development of acute confusion in the frail elderly. In B. Vellas, J. Albarde, & P. Garry (Eds.), *Facts, research, and intervention in geriatrics: Hydration and aging* (pp. 83-100). Paris: Serdi Publisher.

Reese, J. L. (2001). Fluid volume deficit—dehydration: Isotonic, hypotonic, and hypertonic. In M. Maas, K. Buckwalter, M. Hardy, T. Tripp-Reimer, M. Titler, & J. Specht (Eds.), *Nursing care of older adults: Diagnoses, outcomes & interventions* (pp. 183-200). St. Louis: Mosby.

Wakefield, B., Mentes, J., Digglemann, L., & Culp, K. (2002). Monitoring hydration status in elderly veterans. *Western Journal of Nursing Research, 24*(2), 132-142.

Hyperactivity Level—0915

Domain-Physiologic Health (II)

Class-Neurocognitive (J)

Scale-Severe to None (n)

Care Recipient:

Data Source:

| **Definition:** Severity of patterns of inattention or impulsivity in a child from 1 year through 17 years of age |

OUTCOME TARGET RATING: Maintain at_____   Increase to_____

Hyperactivity Level Overall Rating		Severe 1	Substantial 2	Moderate 3	Mild 4	None 5	
INDICATORS:							
091501	Inattention	1	2	3	4	5	NA
091524	Difficulty listening	1	2	3	4	5	NA
091503	Difficulty organizing tasks	1	2	3	4	5	NA
091504	Inability to stay on task	1	2	3	4	5	NA
091525	Difficulty completing tasks	1	2	3	4	5	NA
091506	Difficulty with tasks that require sustained cognitive effort	1	2	3	4	5	NA
091507	Careless mistakes	1	2	3	4	5	NA
091508	Frequency of losing things	1	2	3	4	5	NA
091509	Excessive distractibility	1	2	3	4	5	NA
091510	Excessive forgetfulness	1	2	3	4	5	NA
091511	Impulsivity	1	2	3	4	5	NA
091512	Excessive fidgeting	1	2	3	4	5	NA
091513	Inability to remain seated	1	2	3	4	5	NA
091526	Excessive running	1	2	3	4	5	NA
091527	Excessive climbing	1	2	3	4	5	NA
091515	Excessive motor behavior	1	2	3	4	5	NA
091516	Difficulty playing quietly	1	2	3	4	5	NA
091517	Excessive talking	1	2	3	4	5	NA
091518	Blurts out answers before the question is completed	1	2	3	4	5	NA
091519	Difficulty waiting turn	1	2	3	4	5	NA
091520	Excessive interrupting of others	1	2	3	4	5	NA
091521	Intrusive, abrasive, loud, interpersonal interactions	1	2	3	4	5	NA
091522	Inappropriate aggressive behavior	1	2	3	4	5	NA
091523	Difficulty keeping hands to self	1	2	3	4	5	NA

3rd edition 2004; Revised 4th edition

Outcome Content References:

American Psychiatric Association. (2000). *Diagnostic and statistical manual of mental disorders* (4th ed. text revision). Washington, DC: Author.

Caldwell, C. L., Wasson, D., Anderson, M. A., Brighton, V., & Dixon, L., 3rd. (2005). Development of the nursing outcome (NOC) label: Hyperactivity level. *Journal of Child and Adolescent Psychiatric Nursing, 18*(3), 95-102.

Caldwell, C. L., Wasson, D., Brighton, V., Dixon, L., & Anderson, M. A. (2003). Personal autonomy: Development of a NOC label. *International Journal of Nursing Terminologies & Classifications, 14*(4), 12-13.

Hechtman, L. (2000). Assessment and diagnosis of attention deficit/hyperactive disorder. *Child and Adolescent Psychiatric Clinics of North America, 9*(3), 481-498.

Novak, L. L. (1999). Attention deficit hyperactivity disorder. In M. R. Dambro (Ed.), *Griffith's 5-minute clinical consult.* Philadelphia: Lippincott Williams & Wilkins.

Sharma, V., Newcorn, J. H., Matier-Sharma, K., & Halperin, J. M. (1997). Attention-deficient and disruptive behavior disorders. In A. Tasman (Ed.), *Psychiatry.* Philadelphia: W.B. Saunders.

H

Identity—1202

Domain-Psychosocial Health (III)

Class-Psychological Well-Being (M)

Scale(s)-Never demonstrated to Consistently demonstrated (m)

Care Recipient:

Data Source:

Definition: Distinguishes between self and non-self and characterizes one's essence

OUTCOME TARGET RATING: Maintain at_____   Increase to_____

Identity Overall Rating	Never demonstrated 1	Rarely demonstrated 2	Sometimes demonstrated 3	Often demonstrated 4	Consistently demonstrated 5	
INDICATORS:						
120201 Verbalizes affirmations of personal identity	1	2	3	4	5	NA
120202 Exhibits congruent verbal and nonverbal behavior about self	1	2	3	4	5	NA
120203 Verbalizes clear sense of personal identity	1	2	3	4	5	NA
120204 Differentiates self from environment	1	2	3	4	5	NA
120205 Differentiates self from other human beings	1	2	3	4	5	NA
120206 Perceives environment accurately	1	2	3	4	5	NA
120207 Performs social roles	1	2	3	4	5	NA
120208 Verbalizes own value system	1	2	3	4	5	NA
120209 Challenges faulty beliefs about self	1	2	3	4	5	NA
120210 Challenges negative images of self	1	2	3	4	5	NA
120211 Recognizes interpersonal versus intrapersonal conflict	1	2	3	4	5	NA
120212 Establishes personal boundaries	1	2	3	4	5	NA
120213 Verbalizes trust in self	1	2	3	4	5	NA

1st edition 1997; Revised 3rd edition 2004

Outcome Content References:

Barnard, D. (1990). Healing the damaged self: Identity, intimacy, and meaning in the lives of the chronically ill. *Perspectives in Biology & Medicine, 33*(4), 535-546.

Erickson, E. (1968). *Identity, youth and crisis.* New York: W. W. Norton & Co.

Gara, M. A., Rosenberg, S., & Cohen, B. (1987). Personal identity and the schizophrenic process: An integration. *Psychiatry, 50*(3), 267-278.

Grotevant, H. D., & Adams, G. R. (1984). Development of an objective measure to assess ego identity in adolescence: Validation and replication. *Journal of Youth and Adolescence, 13*(5), 419-437.

Hernandez, J. T., & Diclemente, R. J. (1992). Self-control and ego identity development as predictors of unprotected sex in late adolescent males. *Journal of Adolescence, 15*(4), 437-447.

Marcia, J. E. (1966). Development and validations of ego identity status. *Journal of Personality and Social Psychology, 3*, 551-558.

Marcia, J. E. (1967). Ego identity status: Relationships to change in self-esteem, general adjustment, and authoritarianism. *Journal of Personality, 35*, 118-133.

Oldaker, S. (1985). Identity confusion: Nursing diagnoses for adolescents. *Nursing Clinics of North America, 20*(4), 763-773.

Streitmatter, J. (1993). Gender differences in identity development: An examination of longitudinal data. *Adolescence, 28*(109), 55-66.

Streitmatter, J. (1993). Identity status and identity style: A replication study. *Journal of Adolescence, 16*(2), 211-215.

Stuart, G. W., & Laraia, M. T. (2001). *Principles and practice of psychiatric nursing* (7th ed.). St. Louis: Mosby.

+Tan, A. L., Kendis, R. J., Fine, J. T., & Porac, J. (1977). A short measure of Eriksonian ego identity. *Journal of Personality Assessment, 41*, 279-284.

Immobility Consequences: Physiological—0204

Domain-Functional Health (I)

Class-Mobility (C)

Scale(s)-Severe to None (n) and Severely compromised to Not compromised (a)

Care Recipient:

Data Source:

Definition: Severity of compromise in physiological functioning due to impaired physical mobility

OUTCOME TARGET RATING: Maintain at_____   Increase to_____

Immobility Consequences: Physiological Overall Rating	Severe 1	Substantial 2	Moderate 3	Mild 4	None 5	

INDICATORS:

		Severe 1	Substantial 2	Moderate 3	Mild 4	None 5	
020401	Pressure sore(s)	1	2	3	4	5	NA
020402	Constipation	1	2	3	4	5	NA
020403	Stool impaction	1	2	3	4	5	NA
020405	Hypoactive bowel	1	2	3	4	5	NA
020406	Paralytic ileus	1	2	3	4	5	NA
020407	Urinary calculi	1	2	3	4	5	NA
020408	Urinary retention	1	2	3	4	5	NA
020409	Fever	1	2	3	4	5	NA
020410	Urinary tract infection	1	2	3	4	5	NA
020413	Bone fracture	1	2	3	4	5	NA
020415	Contracted joints	1	2	3	4	5	NA
020416	Ankylosed joints	1	2	3	4	5	NA
020417	Orthostatic hypotension	1	2	3	4	5	NA
020418	Venous thrombosis	1	2	3	4	5	NA
020419	Lung congestion	1	2	3	4	5	NA
020422	Pneumonia	1	2	3	4	5	NA

		Severely compromised	Substantially compromised	Moderately compromised	Mildly compromised	Not compromised	
020404	Nutritional status	1	2	3	4	5	NA
020411	Muscle strength	1	2	3	4	5	NA
020412	Muscle tone	1	2	3	4	5	NA
020414	Joint movement	1	2	3	4	5	NA
020420	Cough effectiveness	1	2	3	4	5	NA
020421	Vital capacity	1	2	3	4	5	NA

1st edition 1997; Revised 2nd edition 2000; Revised 3rd edition 2004

Outcome Content References:

Bloomfield, S. A. (1997). Changes in musculoskeletal structure and function with prolonged bed rest. *Medicine & Science in Sports & Exercise, 29*(2), 197-206.

Greenleaf, J. E. (1997). Intensive exercise training during bed rest attenuates deconditioning. *Medicine & Science in Sports & Exercise, 29*(2), 207-215.

Continued

Irvin, D. J., & White, M. (2004). The importance of accurately assessing orthostatic hypotension. *Geriatric Nursing, 25*(2), 99-101.

Kottke, F. J., & Lehmann, J. F. (1990). *Krusen's handbook of physical medicine and rehabilitation* (4th ed.). Philadelphia: W.B. Saunders.

Maas, M., & Specht, J. P. (2001). Impaired physical mobility. In M. Maas, K. Buckwalter, M. Hardy, T. Tripp-Reimer, M. Titler, & J. Specht (Eds.), *Nursing care of older adults: Diagnoses, outcomes & interventions* (pp. 337-365). St. Louis: Mosby.

Milde, F. K. (1981). Physiological immobilization. In L. Hart, J. Reese & M. Fearing (Eds.), *Concepts common to acute illness: Identification and management* (pp. 67-109). St. Louis: Mosby.

Olson, E. V., Johnson, B. J., Thompson, L. F., McCarthy, J. S., Edmonds, R. E., Schroeder, L. M., & Wade, M. (1967). The hazards of immobility. *American Journal of Nursing, 67*(4), 780-797.

Potter, P. A., & Perry, A. G. (1997). Mobility and immobility. In P. A. Potter & A. G. Perry (Eds.), *Fundamentals of nursing: Concepts, process, and practice* (4th ed., pp. 1460-1520). St. Louis: Mosby.

Rubin, M. (1988). The physiology of bedrest. *American Journal of Nursing, 88*(1), 50-55.

I

Immobility Consequences: Psycho-Cognitive—0205

Domain-Functional Health (I)

Class-Mobility (C)

Scale(s)-Severe to None (n) and Severely compromised to Not compromised (a)

Care Recipient:

Data Source:

Definition: Severity of compromise in psycho-cognitive functioning due to impaired physical mobility

OUTCOME TARGET RATING: Maintain at_____   Increase to_____

Immobility Consequences: Psycho-Cognitive Overall Rating	Severe 1	Substantial 2	Moderate 3	Mild 4	None 5	
INDICATORS:						
020504 Perceptual distortions	1	2	3	4	5	NA
020507 Exaggerated emotions	1	2	3	4	5	NA
020508 Sleep disturbance	1	2	3	4	5	NA
020510 Negative body image	1	2	3	4	5	NA
020513 Depression	1	2	3	4	5	NA
020514 Apathy	1	2	3	4	5	NA

	Severely compromised	Substantially compromised	Moderately compromised	Mildly compromised	Not compromised	
020501 Alertness	1	2	3	4	5	NA
020502 Cognitive status	1	2	3	4	5	NA
020503 Attentiveness	1	2	3	4	5	NA
020505 Kinesthetic sense	1	2	3	4	5	NA
020509 Self-esteem	1	2	3	4	5	NA
020511 Ability to act	1	2	3	4	5	NA

1st edition 1997; Revised 3rd edition 2004

Outcome Content References:

Friedrich, R. M., & Lively, S. I. (1981). Psychological immobilization. In L. Hart, J. Reese, & M. Fearing (Eds.), *Concepts common to acute illness: Identification and management* (pp. 51-66). St. Louis: Mosby.

Greenleaf, J. E. (1997). Intensive exercise training during bed rest attenuates deconditioning. *Medicine & Science in Sports & Exercise, 29*(2), 207-215.

Maas, M., & Specht, J. P. (2001). Impaired physical mobility. In M. Maas, K. Buckwalter, M. Hardy, T. Tripp-Reimer, M. Titler, & J. Specht (Eds.), *Nursing care of older adults: Diagnoses, outcomes & interventions* (pp. 337-365). St. Louis: Mosby.

Rubin, M. (1988). How bedrest changes perception. *American Journal of Nursing, 88*(1), 55-56.

Immune Hypersensitivity Response—0707

Domain-Physiologic Health (II)

Class-Immune Response (H)

Scale(s)-Severe to None (n) and Severely compromised to Not compromised (a)

Care Recipient:

Data Source:

Definition: Severity of inappropriate immune responses

OUTCOME TARGET RATING: Maintain at_____   Increase to_____

Immune Hypersensitivity Response Overall Rating	Severe 1	Substantial 2	Moderate 3	Mild 4	None 5	

INDICATORS:

		Severe 1	Substantial 2	Moderate 3	Mild 4	None 5	
070701	Alterations in skin	1	2	3	4	5	NA
070702	Alterations in mucosa	1	2	3	4	5	NA
070703	Allergic reactions	1	2	3	4	5	NA
070704	Localized inflammatory responses	1	2	3	4	5	NA
070705	Autoimmune events	1	2	3	4	5	NA
070706	Vasculitis	1	2	3	4	5	NA
070707	Transplant rejection	1	2	3	4	5	NA
070708	Graft versus host response	1	2	3	4	5	NA
070709	Itching	1	2	3	4	5	NA
070710	Jaundice	1	2	3	4	5	NA
070711	Level of auto-antibodies or auto-antigens	1	2	3	4	5	NA
070712	Increased bilirubin	1	2	3	4	5	NA
070713	Alterations in complete blood count	1	2	3	4	5	NA
070714	Alterations in differential white blood count	1	2	3	4	5	NA
070715	Alterations in complement levels	1	2	3	4	5	NA
070716	Alterations in T4-cell level	1	2	3	4	5	NA
070717	Alterations in T8-cell level	1	2	3	4	5	NA

		Severely compromised	Substantially compromised	Moderately compromised	Mildly compromised	Not compromised	
070718	Respiratory function	1	2	3	4	5	NA
070719	Cardiac function	1	2	3	4	5	NA
070720	Gastrointestinal function	1	2	3	4	5	NA
070721	Renal function	1	2	3	4	5	NA
070722	Neurological function	1	2	3	4	5	NA
070723	Joint mobility	1	2	3	4	5	NA

3rd edition 2004

Outcome Content References:

Birney, M. H. (1991). Psychoneuroimmunology: A holistic framework for the study of stress and illness. *Holistic Nursing Practice, 5*(4), 32-38.

Brandt, B. (1990). Nursing protocol for the patient with neutropenia. *Oncology Nursing Forum, 17*(Suppl. 1), 9-15.

McCance, K. L., & Huether, S. E. (2002). *Pathophysiology: The biologic basis for disease in adults and children* (4th ed.). St. Louis: Mosby.

Phillips, M. C., & Olson, L. R. (1993). The immunologic role of the gastrointestinal tract. *Critical Care Nursing Clinics of North America, 5*(1), 107-118.

Van Wynsberghe, D., Noback, C. R., & Carola, R. (1995). *Human anatomy and physiology* (3rd ed.). New York: McGraw-Hill.

Workman, M. L. (1993). The immune system: Your defensive partner and offensive foe. *AACN, 4*(3), 453-470.

Immune Status—0702

Domain-Physiologic Health (II)

Class-Immune Response (H)

Scale-Severely compromised to Not compromised (a) and Severe to None (n)

Care Recipient:

Data Source:

Definition: Natural and acquired appropriately targeted resistance to internal and external antigens

OUTCOME TARGET RATING: Maintain at_____   Increase to_____

Immune Status Overall Rating	Severely compromised 1	Substantially compromised 2	Moderately compromised 3	Mildly compromised 4	Not compromised 5	
INDICATORS:						
070203 Gastrointestinal function	1	2	3	4	5	NA
070204 Respiratory function	1	2	3	4	5	NA
070205 Genitourinary function	1	2	3	4	5	NA
070207 Body temperature	1	2	3	4	5	NA
070208 Skin integrity	1	2	3	4	5	NA
070209 Mucosa integrity	1	2	3	4	5	NA
070211 Immunizations current	1	2	3	4	5	NA
070220 Screening for infections current	1	2	3	4	5	NA
070212 Antibody titers	1	2	3	4	5	NA
070213 Skin test reaction with exposure	1	2	3	4	5	NA
070214 Absolute white blood count	1	2	3	4	5	NA
070215 Differential white blood count	1	2	3	4	5	NA
070216 T4-cell level	1	2	3	4	5	NA
070217 T8-cell level	1	2	3	4	5	NA
070218 Complement levels	1	2	3	4	5	NA
070219 Thymus x-ray findings	1	2	3	4	5	NA
	Severe	Substantial	Moderate	Mild	None	
070201 Recurrent infections	1	2	3	4	5	NA
070202 Tumors	1	2	3	4	5	NA
070206 Weight loss	1	2	3	4	5	NA
070210 Chronic fatigue	1	2	3	4	5	NA

1st edition 1997; Revised 3rd edition 2004; Revised 4th edition

Outcome Content References:

Birney, M. H. (1991). Psychoneuroimmunology: A holistic framework for the study of stress and illness. *Holistic Nursing Practice, 5*(4), 32-38.

Brandt, B. (1990). Nursing protocol for the patient with neutropenia. *Oncology Nursing Forum, 17*(Suppl. 1), 9-15.

Hymes, D. J. (1985). Primary immunodeficiency disorders in the neonate. *Neonatal Network—The Journal of Neonatal Nursing, 3*(4), 40-48.

Lentz, A. K., & Feezor, R. J. (2003). Principles of immunology. *Nutritional Clinical Practice, 18*(6), 451-460.

Mayer, L. (2003). Mucosal immunity. *Pediatrics, 111*(6), 1595-1600.

McCance, K. L., & Huether, S. E. (2002). *Pathophysiology: The biologic basis for disease in adults and children* (4th ed.). St. Louis: Mosby.

Phillips, M. C., & Olson, L. R. (1993). The immunologic role of the gastrointestinal tract. *Critical Care Nursing Clinics of North America, 5*(1), 107-118.

Ungvarski, P. J., & Flaskerud, J. H. (1999). *HIV/AIDS: A guide to primary care management* (4th ed.). Philadelphia: W.B. Saunders.

Urakawa, K., & Yokoyama, K. (2004). Can relaxation programs with music enhance human immune function? *Journal of Alternative and Complementary Medicine, 10*(4), 605-606

Van Wynsberghe, D., Noback, C. R., & Carola, R. (1995). *Human anatomy and physiology* (3rd ed.). New York: McGraw-Hill.

Weber, R. (2003). Our innate immune system: barking at the doorbell. *Dermatological Nursing, 15*(5), 471.

Workman, M. L. (1993). The immune system: Your defensive partner and offensive foe. *AACN, 4*(3), 453-470.

I

Immunization Behavior—1900

Domain-Health Knowledge & Behavior (IV)

Class-Risk Control & Safety (T)

Scale(s)-Never demonstrated to Consistently demonstrated (m)

Care Recipient:

Data Source:

Definition: Personal actions to obtain immunization to prevent a communicable disease

OUTCOME TARGET RATING: Maintain at_____   Increase to_____

Immunization Behavior Overall Rating	Never demonstrated 1	Rarely demonstrated 2	Sometimes demonstrated 3	Often demonstrated 4	Consistently demonstrated 5	
INDICATORS:						
190001 Acknowledges disease risk without immunization	1	2	3	4	5	NA
190002 Describes risks associated with specific immunization	1	2	3	4	5	NA
190003 Describes contraindications to specific immunization	1	2	3	4	5	NA
190004 Brings updated vaccination card to each visit	1	2	3	4	5	NA
190005 Obtains immunizations recommended for age by the American Academy of Pediatrics or United States Public Health Service	1	2	3	4	5	NA
190006 Describes relief measures for vaccine side effects	1	2	3	4	5	NA
190007 Reports any adverse reactions	1	2	3	4	5	NA
190009 Confirms date of next immunization	1	2	3	4	5	NA
190010 Obtains immunizations recommended with chronic illness by the American Academy of Pediatrics or United States Public Health Service	1	2	3	4	5	NA
190011 Obtains immunizations recommended for occupational risk by the American Academy of Pediatrics or United States Public Health Service	1	2	3	4	5	NA
190012 Obtains immunizations recommended for travel by the American Academy of Pediatrics or United States Public Health Service	1	2	3	4	5	NA
190013 Identifies community resources for immunization	1	2	3	4	5	NA

1st edition 1997; Revised 2nd edition 2000; Revised 3rd edition 2004

I

Continued

Outcome Content References:

Forshner, L., & Garza, A. (1999). Childhood vaccines: An update. *RN, 62*(4), 32-37.

Notice to readers: Recommended childhood immunization schedule—United States, 2002. (2002). *Morbidity and Mortality Weekly Report, 51*(2), 31-33.

Paulson, P. R., & Hammer, A. L. (2002). Updates & kidbits. Pediatric immunization update 2002. *Pediatric Nursing, 28*(2), 173-181.

Preboth, M. (2000). Practice guidelines. ACIP recommendations for the prevention of hepatitis A through immunization. *American Family Physician, 61*(7), 2246-2248.

Selekman, J. (1994). The guidelines for immunizations have changed again! *Pediatric Nursing, 20*(4), 376-378.

Sharts-Hopko, N. C. (1994). Current immunization guidelines. *MCN: American Journal of Maternal Child Nursing, 19*(2), 82-84.

Smith, C., & Maurer, F. (1995). *Community health nursing: Theory and practice*. Philadelphia: W.B. Saunders.

U.S. Department of Health and Human Services. (1994). *Clinician's handbook of preventive service: Put prevention into practice*. Washington, DC: Government Printing Office.

Zimmerman, R. K., & Ball, J. A. (2001). Adult vaccinations. *Primary Care: Clinics in Office Practice, 28*(4), 763-790.

I

Impulse Self-Control—1405

Domain-Psychosocial Health (III)

Class-Self-Control (O)

Scale(s)-Never demonstrated to Consistently demonstrated (m)

Care Recipient:

Data Source:

Definition: Self-restraint of compulsive or impulsive behaviors

OUTCOME TARGET RATING: Maintain at_____   Increase to_____

Impulse Self-Control Overall Rating	Never demonstrated 1	Rarely demonstrated 2	Sometimes demonstrated 3	Often demonstrated 4	Consistently demonstrated 5	

INDICATORS:

140501	Identifies harmful impulsive behaviors	1	2	3	4	5	NA
140502	Identifies feelings that lead to impulsive actions	1	2	3	4	5	NA
140503	Identifies behaviors that lead to impulsive actions	1	2	3	4	5	NA
140504	Identifies consequences of impulsive actions	1	2	3	4	5	NA
140505	Recognizes risks in environment	1	2	3	4	5	NA
140514	Avoids high risk environments	1	2	3	4	5	NA
140515	Avoids high risk situations	1	2	3	4	5	NA
140507	Controls impulses	1	2	3	4	5	NA
140516	Obtains assistance when experiencing impulses	1	2	3	4	5	NA
140509	Uses available social support	1	2	3	4	5	NA
140517	Keeps referral appointments	1	2	3	4	5	NA
140511	Upholds contract to control behavior	1	2	3	4	5	NA
140512	Maintains self-control without supervision	1	2	3	4	5	NA

1st edition 1997; Revised 2nd edition 2000; Revised 3rd edition 2004; Revised 4th edition

Outcome Content References:

American Psychiatric Association Practice Guidelines. (1993). Practice guidelines for eating disorders. *American Journal of Psychiatry, 150*(2), 207-228.

Dyckoff, D., Goldstein, L., & Levine-Schacht, L. (1996). The investigation of behavioral contracting in patients with borderline personality disorder. *Journal of the American Psychiatric Nurses Association, 2*(3), 71-76.

Gallop, R. (1992). Self-destructive and impulsive behavior in the patient with borderline personality disorder: Rethinking hospital treatment and management. *Archives of Psychiatric Nursing, 6*(6), 366-373.

Gallop, R., McCay, E., & Esplen, M. T. (1992). The conceptualization of impulsivity for psychiatric nursing practice. *Archives of Psychiatric Nursing, 6*(6), 366-373.

Ingram, T. N. (2001). Risk for violence: Self-Directed or directed at others. In M. Maas, K. Buckwalter, M. Hardy, T. Tripp-Reimer, M. Titler, & J. Specht (Eds.), *Nursing care of older adults: Diagnoses, outcomes & interventions* (pp. 696-705). St. Louis: Mosby.

+Lazzaro, T. A., Beggs, D. L., & McNeil, K. A. (1969). The development and validation of the Self-Report Test of Impulse Control. *Journal of Clinical Psychology, 25*(4), 434-438.

Miller, L. J. (1990). The formal treatment contract in the inpatient management of borderline personality disorder. *Hospital and Community Psychiatry, 41*(9), 985-987.

Staples, N. R., & Schwartz, M. (1990). Anorexia nervosa support group: Providing transitional support. *Journal of Psychosocial Nursing and Mental Health Services, 28*(2), 6-10.

Stuart, G. W., & Laraia, M. T. (2001). *Principles and practice of psychiatric nursing* (7th ed.). St. Louis: Mosby.

I

Infection Severity—0703

Domain-Physiologic Health (II)

Class-Immune Response (H)

Scale(s)-Severe to None (n)

Care Recipient:

Data Source:

Definition: Severity of infection and associated symptoms

OUTCOME TARGET RATING: Maintain at_____   Increase to_____

Infection Severity Overall Rating	Severe 1	Substantial 2	Moderate 3	Mild 4	None 5	
INDICATORS:						
070301 Rash	1	2	3	4	5	NA
070302 Uncrusted vesicles	1	2	3	4	5	NA
070303 Foul-smelling discharge	1	2	3	4	5	NA
070304 Purulent sputum	1	2	3	4	5	NA
070305 Purulent drainage	1	2	3	4	5	NA
070306 Pyuria	1	2	3	4	5	NA
070307 Fever	1	2	3	4	5	NA
070329 Hypothermia	1	2	3	4	5	NA
070330 Temperature instability	1	2	3	4	5	NA
070333 Pain	1	2	3	4	5	NA
070334 Tenderness	1	2	3	4	5	NA
070309 Gastrointestinal symptoms	1	2	3	4	5	NA
070310 Lymphadenopathy	1	2	3	4	5	NA
070311 Malaise	1	2	3	4	5	NA
070312 Chilling	1	2	3	4	5	NA
070313 Unexplained cognitive impairment	1	2	3	4	5	NA
070331 Lethargy	1	2	3	4	5	NA
070332 Loss of appetite	1	2	3	4	5	NA
070319 Chest x-ray infiltration	1	2	3	4	5	NA
070320 Blood culture colonization	1	2	3	4	5	NA
070321 Sputum culture colonization	1	2	3	4	5	NA
070322 Cerebrospinal fluid culture colonization	1	2	3	4	5	NA
070323 Wound site culture colonization	1	2	3	4	5	NA
070324 Urine culture colonization	1	2	3	4	5	NA
070325 Stool culture colonization	1	2	3	4	5	NA
070326 White blood count elevation	1	2	3	4	5	NA
070327 White blood count depression	1	2	3	4	5	NA

Site of infection_____

1st edition 1997; Revised 3rd edition 2004; Revised 4th edition

Outcome Content References:

Albrutyn, E., & Talbot, G. H. (1987). Surveillance strategies: A primer. *Infection Control, 8*(11), 459-464.

Birnbaum, D. (1987). Nosocomial infection surveillance programs. *Infection Control, 8*(11), 474-479.

Burns, M. V. (1998). *Pathophysiology: A self-instructional program* (pp. 151-207). Stamford, CT: Appleton & Lange.

Carter, C., & Pottinger, J. M. (2001). Risk for infection. In M. Maas, K. Buckwalter, M. Hardy, T. Tripp-Reimer, M. Titler, & J. Specht (Eds.), *Nursing care of older adults: Diagnoses, outcomes & interventions* (pp. 47-62). St. Louis: Mosby.

Haley, R. W., Aber, R. C., & Bennett, J. V. (1986). Surveillance of nosocomial infections. In J. V. Bennett & D. S. Brachman (Eds.), *Hospital infections* (2nd ed., pp. 51-71). Boston: Little, Brown & Company.

Levy, C. R., Eilertsen, T., Kramer, A. M., & Hutt, E. (2006). Which clinical indicators and resident characteristics are associated with health care practitioner nursing home visits or hospital transfer for urinary tract infections? *Journal of the American Medical Directors Association, 7*(8), 493-498.

Yamashita, H., Tsukayama, H., Hori, N., Kimura, T., & Tanno, Y. (2000). Incidence of adverse reactions associated with acupuncture. *Journal of Alternative & Complementary Medicine, 6*(4), 345-350.

I

Infection Severity: Newborn—0708

Domain-Physiologic Health (II)

Class-Immune Response (H)

Scale(s)-Severe to None (n)

Care Recipient:

Data Source:

Definition: Severity of infection and associated symptoms during the first 28 days of life

OUTCOME TARGET RATING: Maintain at_____   Increase to_____

Infection Severity: Newborn Overall Rating	Severe 1	Substantial 2	Moderate 3	Mild 4	None 5	
INDICATORS:						
070801 Temperature instability	1	2	3	4	5	NA
070802 Hypothermia	1	2	3	4	5	NA
070803 Tachypnea	1	2	3	4	5	NA
070804 Tachycardia	1	2	3	4	5	NA
070805 Bradycardia	1	2	3	4	5	NA
070806 Arrhythmias	1	2	3	4	5	NA
070807 Hypotension	1	2	3	4	5	NA
070808 Hypertension	1	2	3	4	5	NA
070809 Pale	1	2	3	4	5	NA
070810 Mottled skin	1	2	3	4	5	NA
070811 Cyanosis	1	2	3	4	5	NA
070812 Cold, clammy skin	1	2	3	4	5	NA
070813 Vomiting	1	2	3	4	5	NA
070814 Diarrhea	1	2	3	4	5	NA
070815 Abdominal distension	1	2	3	4	5	NA
070816 Feeding intolerance	1	2	3	4	5	NA
070817 Lethargy	1	2	3	4	5	NA
070818 Irritability	1	2	3	4	5	NA
070819 Seizures	1	2	3	4	5	NA
070820 Jitteriness	1	2	3	4	5	NA
070821 High-pitched cry	1	2	3	4	5	NA
070822 Rash	1	2	3	4	5	NA
070823 Uncrusted vesicles	1	2	3	4	5	NA
070824 Foul-smelling discharge	1	2	3	4	5	NA
070825 Purulent drainage	1	2	3	4	5	NA
070826 Conjunctivitis	1	2	3	4	5	NA
070827 Infected umbilicus	1	2	3	4	5	NA
070828 Blood culture colonization	1	2	3	4	5	NA
070829 Wound site culture colonization	1	2	3	4	5	NA
070830 Urine culture colonization	1	2	3	4	5	NA

I

		Severe	Substantial	Moderate	Mild	None	
070831	Stool culture colonization	1	2	3	4	5	NA
070832	Chest x-ray infiltration	1	2	3	4	5	NA
070833	Cerebrospinal fluid culture colonization	1	2	3	4	5	NA
070834	White blood count elevation	1	2	3	4	5	NA
070835	White blood count depression	1	2	3	4	5	NA

Site of infection_____

3rd edition 2004

Outcome Content References:

Albrutyn, E., & Talbot, G. H. (1987). Surveillance strategies: A primer. *Infection Control, 8*(11), 459-464.

Antonow, J. A., Smout, R. J., Gassaway, J., Horn, S. D., & Wilson, D. F. (2001). Variation among 10 pediatric hospitals: Sepsis evaluations for infants with bronchiolitis. *Journal of Nursing Care Quality, 15*(3), 39-49.

Deacon, J., & O'Neill, P. (Eds.). (1999). *Core curriculum for neonatal intensive care nursing* (2nd ed.). Philadelphia: W.B. Saunders.

Griffin, M. P., & Moorman, J. R. (2001). Toward the early diagnosis of neonatal sepsis and sepsis-like illness using novel heart rate analysis. *Pediatrics, 107*(1), 97-104.

Mattson, S., & Smith, J. E. (Eds.). (2000). *Core curriculum for maternal-newborn nursing* (2nd ed.). Philadelphia: W.B. Saunders.

Mullany, L. C., Darmstadt, G. L., Katz, J., Khatry, S. K., LeClerq, S. C., Adhikari, R. K., & Tielsch, J. M. (2006). *Archives of Disease in Childhood—Fetal & Neonatal Edition, 91*(2), F99-F104.

I

Information Processing—0907

Domain-Physiologic Health (II)

Class-Neurocognitive (J)

Scale(s)-Severely compromised to Not compromised (a)

Care Recipient:

Data Source:

Definition: Ability to acquire, organize, and use information

OUTCOME TARGET RATING: Maintain at_____   Increase to_____

Information Processing Overall Rating	Severely compromised 1	Substantially compromised 2	Moderately compromised 3	Mildly compromised 4	Not compromised 5	
INDICATORS:						
090701 Identifies common objects	1	2	3	4	5	NA
090709 Comprehends a sentence	1	2	3	4	5	NA
090710 Comprehends a paragraph	1	2	3	4	5	NA
090711 Comprehends a story	1	2	3	4	5	NA
090716 Comprehends universal symbols	1	2	3	4	5	NA
090703 Verbalizes a coherent message	1	2	3	4	5	NA
090704 Exhibits organized thought processes	1	2	3	4	5	NA
090705 Exhibits logical thought processes	1	2	3	4	5	NA
090712 Explains similarity between two items	1	2	3	4	5	NA
090713 Explains dissimilarity between two items	1	2	3	4	5	NA
090714 Adds several numbers	1	2	3	4	5	NA
090715 Subtracts several numbers	1	2	3	4	5	NA

1st edition 1997; Revised 3rd edition 2004; Revised 4th edition

Outcome Content References:

Abraham, I., & Reel, S. (1993). Cognitive nursing interventions with long-term care residents: Effects on neurocognitive dimensions. *Archives of Psychiatric Nursing, 6*(6), 356-365.

Agostinelli, B., Demers, K., Garrigan, D., & Waszynski, C. (1994). Targeted interventions: Use of the mini-mental state exam. *Journal of Gerontological Nursing, 20*(8), 15-23.

Dellasega, C. (1992). Home health nurses' assessments of cognition. *Applied Nursing Research, 5*(3), 127-133.

+Folstein, M. F., Folstein, S. E., & McHugh, P. R. (1975). "Mini-Mental State": A practical method for grading the cognitive state of patients for the clinician. *Journal of Psychiatric Research, 12*(3), 189-198.

Foreman, M., Theis, S., & Anderson, M. A. (1993). Adverse events in the hospitalized elderly. *Clinical Nursing Research, 2*(3), 360-370.

Gerdner, L. A., & Hall, G. R. (2001). Chronic confusion. In M. Maas, K. Buckwalter, M. Hardy, T. Tripp-Reimer, M. Titler, & J. Specht (Eds.), *Nursing care of older adults: Diagnoses, outcomes & interventions* (pp. 421-441). St. Louis: Mosby.

Inaba-Roland, K., & Maricle, R. (1992). Assessing delirium in the acute care setting. *Heart & Lung, 21*(1), 48-55.

Mason, P. (1989). Cognitive assessment parameters and tools for the critically injured adult. *Critical Care Nursing Clinics of North America, 1*(1), 45-53.

Prins, N. D., van Dijk, E. J., den Heijer, T., Vermeer, S. E., Jolles, J., Koudstaal, P. J., Hofman, A., & Breteler, M. M. B. (2005). Cerebral small-vessel disease and decline in information processing speed, executive function and memory. *Brain: A Journal of Neurology, 128*(part 9), 2034-2041.

Strub, R. L., & Black, F. W. (2000). *The mental status examination in neurology* (4th ed.). Philadelphia: F.A. Davis.

Joint Movement—0206

Domain-Functional Health (I)

Class-Mobility (C)

Scale(s)-Severe deviation from normal range to No deviation from normal range (b)

Care Recipient:

Data Source:

Definition: Active range of motion of all joints with self-initiated movement

OUTCOME TARGET RATING: Maintain at_____ Increase to_____

Joint Movement Overall Rating	Severe deviation from normal range 1	Substantial deviation from normal range 2	Moderate deviation from normal range 3	Mild deviation from normal range 4	No deviation from normal range 5	
INDICATORS:						
020601 Jaw	1	2	3	4	5	NA
020602 Neck	1	2	3	4	5	NA
020620 Spine	1	2	3	4	5	NA
020603 Fingers (right)	1	2	3	4	5	NA
020604 Fingers (left)	1	2	3	4	5	NA
020605 Thumb (right)	1	2	3	4	5	NA
020606 Thumb (left)	1	2	3	4	5	NA
020607 Wrist (right)	1	2	3	4	5	NA
020608 Wrist (left)	1	2	3	4	5	NA
020609 Elbow (right)	1	2	3	4	5	NA
020610 Elbow (left)	1	2	3	4	5	NA
020611 Shoulder (right)	1	2	3	4	5	NA
020612 Shoulder (left)	1	2	3	4	5	NA
020613 Ankle (right)	1	2	3	4	5	NA
020614 Ankle (left)	1	2	3	4	5	NA
020615 Knee (right)	1	2	3	4	5	NA
020616 Knee (left	1	2	3	4	5	NA
020617 Hip (right)	1	2	3	4	5	NA
020618 Hip (left)	1	2	3	4	5	NA

1st edition 1996; Revised 4th edition

Outcome Content References:

Bickley, L. (2002). *Bates' guide to physical examination and history taking* (8th ed.). Philadelphia: Lippincott Williams & Wilkins.

Hoeman, S. (2002). *Rehabilitation nursing: Process, application, and outcomes* (3rd ed.). St. Louis: Mosby.

Seidel, H. M., Ball, J. W., Dains, J. E., & Benedict, G. W. (2003). *Mosby's guide to physical examination* (5th ed.). St. Louis: Mosby.

J

Joint Movement: Ankle—0213

Domain-Functional Health (I)
Class-Mobility (C)
Scale(s)-Severe deviation from normal range to No deviation from normal range (b)

Care Recipient:
Data Source:

Definition: Active range of motion of the ankle with self-initiated movement

OUTCOME TARGET RATING: Maintain at_____   Increase to_____

Joint Movement: Ankle Overall Rating	Severe deviation from normal range 1	Substantial deviation from normal range 2	Moderate deviation from normal range 3	Mild deviation from normal range 4	No deviation from normal range 5	
INDICATORS:						
021301 Dorsal flexion 20 degrees (R)	1	2	3	4	5	NA
021302 Plantar flexion 45 degrees (R)	1	2	3	4	5	NA
021303 Inversion 30 degrees (R)	1	2	3	4	5	NA
021304 Eversion 20 degrees (R)	1	2	3	4	5	NA
021305 Rotation (R)	1	2	3	4	5	NA
021306 Dorsal flexion 20 degrees (L)	1	2	3	4	5	NA
021307 Plantar flexion 45 degrees (L)	1	2	3	4	5	NA
021308 Inversion 30 degrees (L)	1	2	3	4	5	NA
021309 Eversion 20 degrees (L)	1	2	3	4	5	NA
021310 Rotation (L)	1	2	3	4	5	NA

Specify: Right (R)____ Left (L)____ Both____

3rd edition 2004

Outcome Content References:

Bickley, L. (2002). *Bates' guide to physical examination and history taking* (8th ed.). Philadelphia: Lippincott Williams & Wilkins.
Hoeman, S. (2002). *Rehabilitation nursing: Process, application, and outcomes* (3rd ed.). St. Louis: Mosby.
Seidel, H. M., Ball, J. W., Dains, J. E., & Benedict, G. W. (2003). *Mosby's guide to physical examination* (5th ed.). St. Louis: Mosby.

Joint Movement: Elbow—0214

Domain-Functional Health (I)   Care Recipient:

Class-Mobility (C)   Data Source:

Scale(s)-Severe deviation from normal range to No deviation from normal range (b)

Definition: Active range of motion of the elbow with self-initiated movement

OUTCOME TARGET RATING: Maintain at_____   Increase to_____

Joint Movement: Elbow Overall Rating	Severe deviation from normal range 1	Substantial deviation from normal range 2	Moderate deviation from normal range 3	Mild deviation from normal range 4	No deviation from normal range 5	
INDICATORS:						
021401 Extension 0 degrees (R)	1	2	3	4	5	NA
021402 Flexion 160 degrees (R)	1	2	3	4	5	NA
021403 Supination 90 degrees (R)	1	2	3	4	5	NA
021404 Pronation 90 degrees (R)	1	2	3	4	5	NA
021405 Extension 0 degrees (L)	1	2	3	4	5	NA
021406 Flexion 160 degrees (L)	1	2	3	4	5	NA
021407 Supination 90 degrees (L)	1	2	3	4	5	NA
021408 Pronation 90 degrees (L)	1	2	3	4	5	NA

Specify: Right (R)____ Left (L)____ Both____

3rd edition 2004

Outcome Content References:

Bickley, L. (2002). *Bates' guide to physical examination and history taking* (8th ed.). Philadelphia: Lippincott Williams & Wilkins.
Hoeman, S. (2002). *Rehabilitation nursing: Process, application, and outcomes* (3rd ed.). St. Louis: Mosby.
Seidel, H. M., Ball, J. W., Dains, J. E., & Benedict, G. W. (2003). *Mosby's guide to physical examination* (5th ed.). St. Louis: Mosby.

J

Joint Movement: Fingers—0215

Domain-Functional Health (I)   *Care Recipient:*

Class-Mobility (C)   *Data Source:*

Scale(s)-Severe deviation from normal range to No deviation from normal range (b)

Definition: Active range of motion of the fingers with self-initiated movement

OUTCOME TARGET RATING: Maintain at_____   Increase to_____

Joint Movement: Fingers Overall Rating	Severe deviation from normal range 1	Substantial deviation from normal range 2	Moderate deviation from normal range 3	Mild deviation from normal range 4	No deviation from normal range 5	
INDICATORS:						
021501 Metacarpophalangeal extension 0 degrees (R)	1	2	3	4	5	NA
021502 Metacarpophalangeal flexion 90 degrees (R)	1	2	3	4	5	NA
021503 Metacarpophalangeal hyperflexion 30 degrees (R)	1	2	3	4	5	NA
021504 Proximal interphalangeal extension 0 degrees (R)	1	2	3	4	5	NA
021505 Proximal interphalangeal flexion 100-120 degrees (R)	1	2	3	4	5	NA
021506 Distal interphalangeal extension 0 degrees (R)	1	2	3	4	5	NA
021507 Distal interphalangeal flexion 45-80 degrees (R)	1	2	3	4	5	NA
021508 Metacarpophalangeal extension 0 degrees (L)	1	2	3	4	5	NA
021509 Metacarpophalangeal flexion 90 degrees (L)	1	2	3	4	5	NA
021510 Metacarpophalangeal hyperflexion 30 degrees (L)	1	2	3	4	5	NA
021511 Proximal interphalangeal extension 0 degrees (L)	1	2	3	4	5	NA
021512 Proximal interphalangeal flexion 100-120 degrees (L)	1	2	3	4	5	NA
021513 Distal interphalangeal extension 0 degrees (L)	1	2	3	4	5	NA
021514 Distal interphalangeal flexion 45-80 degrees (L)	1	2	3	4	5	NA

Specify: Right (R)____ Left (L)____ Both____

3rd edition 2004

Outcome Content References:

Bickley, L. (2002). *Bates' guide to physical examination and history taking* (8th ed.). Philadelphia: Lippincott Williams & Wilkins.
Hoeman, S. (2002). *Rehabilitation nursing: Process, application, and outcomes* (3rd ed.). St. Louis: Mosby.
Seidel, H. M., Ball, J. W., Dains, J. E., & Benedict, G. W. (2003). *Mosby's guide to physical examination* (5th ed.). St. Louis: Mosby.

Joint Movement: Hip—0216

Domain-Functional Health (I)

Class-Mobility (C)

Scale(s)-Severe deviation from normal range to No deviation from normal range (b)

Care Recipient:

Data Source:

Definition: Active range of motion of the hip with self-initiated movement

OUTCOME TARGET RATING: Maintain at_____   Increase to_____

Joint Movement: Hip Overall Rating	Severe deviation from normal range 1	Substantial deviation from normal range 2	Moderate deviation from normal range 3	Mild deviation from normal range 4	No deviation from normal range 5	
INDICATORS:						
021601 Flexion knee straight 90 degrees (R)	1	2	3	4	5	NA
021602 Extension knee straight 0 degrees (R)	1	2	3	4	5	NA
021603 Hyperextension knee straight 15 degrees (R)	1	2	3	4	5	NA
021604 Flexion knee bent 120 degrees (R)	1	2	3	4	5	NA
021605 Abduction 45 degrees (R)	1	2	3	4	5	NA
021606 Adduction 30 degrees (R)	1	2	3	4	5	NA
021607 Internal rotation 40 degrees (R)	1	2	3	4	5	NA
021608 External rotation 45 degrees (R)	1	2	3	4	5	NA
021609 Flexion knee straight 90 degrees (L)	1	2	3	4	5	NA
021610 Extension knee straight 0 degrees (L)	1	2	3	4	5	NA
021611 Hyperextension knee straight 15 degrees (L)	1	2	3	4	5	NA
021612 Flexion knee bent 120 degrees (L)	1	2	3	4	5	NA
021613 Abduction 45 degrees (L)	1	2	3	4	5	NA
021614 Adduction 30 degrees (L)	1	2	3	4	5	NA
021615 Internal rotation 40 degrees (L)	1	2	3	4	5	NA
021616 External rotation 45 degrees (L)	1	2	3	4	5	NA

Specify: Right (R)____ Left (L)____ Both____

3rd edition 2004

Outcome Content References:

Bickley, L. (2002). *Bates' guide to physical examination and history taking* (8th ed.). Philadelphia: Lippincott Williams & Wilkins.
Hoeman, S. (2002). *Rehabilitation nursing: Process, application, and outcomes* (3rd ed.). St. Louis: Mosby.
Seidel, H. M., Ball, J. W., Dains, J. E., & Benedict, G. W. (2003). *Mosby's guide to physical examination* (5th ed.). St. Louis: Mosby.

Joint Movement: Knee—0217

Domain-Functional Health (I)

Class-Mobility (C)

Scale(s)-Severe deviation from normal range to No deviation from normal range (b)

Care Recipient:

Data Source:

Definition: Active range of motion of the knee with self-initiated movement

OUTCOME TARGET RATING: Maintain at_____   Increase to_____

Joint Movement: Knee Overall Rating	Severe deviation from normal range 1	Substantial deviation from normal range 2	Moderate deviation from normal range 3	Mild deviation from normal range 4	No deviation from normal range 5	
INDICATORS:						
021701 Extension 0 degrees (R)	1	2	3	4	5	NA
021702 Flexion 130 degrees (R)	1	2	3	4	5	NA
021703 Hyperextension 15 degrees (R)	1	2	3	4	5	NA
021704 Extension 0 degrees (L)	1	2	3	4	5	NA
021705 Flexion 130 degrees (L)	1	2	3	4	5	NA
021706 Hyperextension 15 degrees (L)	1	2	3	4	5	NA

Specify: Right (R)____ Left (L)____ Both____

3rd edition 2004

Outcome Content References:

Bickley, L. (2002). *Bates' guide to physical examination and history taking* (8th ed.). Philadelphia: Lippincott Williams & Wilkins. Hoeman, S. (2002). *Rehabilitation nursing: Process, application, and outcomes* (3rd ed.). St. Louis: Mosby.

Seidel, H. M., Ball, J. W., Dains, J. E., & Benedict, G. W. (2003). *Mosby's guide to physical examination* (5th ed.). St. Louis: Mosby.

Joint Movement: Neck—0218

Domain-Functional Health (I)   Care Recipient:

Class-Mobility (C)   Data Source:

Scale(s)-Severe deviation from normal range to No deviation from normal range (b)

Definition: Active range of motion of the neck with self-initiated movement

OUTCOME TARGET RATING: Maintain at_____   Increase to_____

Joint Movement: Neck Overall Rating	Severe deviation from normal range 1	Substantial deviation from normal range 2	Moderate deviation from normal range 3	Mild deviation from normal range 4	No deviation from normal range 5	
INDICATORS:						
021801 Flexion 45 degrees	1	2	3	4	5	NA
021802 Extension 55 degrees	1	2	3	4	5	NA
021803 Lateral bending 40 degrees (R)	1	2	3	4	5	NA
021804 Lateral bending 40 degrees (L)	1	2	3	4	5	NA
021805 Rotation	1	2	3	4	5	NA

3rd edition 2004

Outcome Content References:

Bickley, L. (2002). *Bates' guide to physical examination and history taking* (8th ed.). Philadelphia: Lippincott Williams & Wilkins.

Hoeman, S. (2002). *Rehabilitation nursing: Process, application, and outcomes* (3rd ed.). St. Louis: Mosby.

Seidel, H. M., Ball, J. W., Dains, J. E., & Benedict, G. W. (2003). *Mosby's guide to physical examination* (5th ed.). St. Louis: Mosby.

J

Joint Movement: Passive—0207

Domain-Functional Health (I)

Class-Mobility (C)

Scale-Severe deviation from normal range to No deviation from normal range (b)

Care Recipient:

Data Source:

Definition: Joint movement with assistance

OUTCOME TARGET RATING: Maintain at_____   Increase to_____

Joint Movement: Passive Overall Rating	Severe deviation from normal range 1	Substantial deviation from normal range 2	Moderate deviation from normal range 3	Mild deviation from normal range 4	No deviation from normal range 5	
INDICATORS:						
020702 Neck	1	2	3	4	5	NA
020703 Fingers (right)	1	2	3	4	5	NA
020705 Thumb (right)	1	2	3	4	5	NA
020707 Wrist (right)	1	2	3	4	5	NA
020709 Elbow (right)	1	2	3	4	5	NA
020711 Shoulder (right)	1	2	3	4	5	NA
020713 Ankle (right)	1	2	3	4	5	NA
020715 Knee (right)	1	2	3	4	5	NA
020717 Hip (right)	1	2	3	4	5	NA
020704 Fingers (left)	1	2	3	4	5	NA
020706 Thumb (left)	1	2	3	4	5	NA
020708 Wrist (left)	1	2	3	4	5	NA
020710 Elbow (left)	1	2	3	4	5	NA
020712 Shoulder (left)	1	2	3	4	5	NA
020714 Ankle (left)	1	2	3	4	5	NA
020716 Knee (left)	1	2	3	4	5	NA
020718 Hip (left)	1	2	3	4	5	NA

1st edition 1997; Revised 3rd edition 2004

Outcome Content References:

Bickley, L. (2002). *Bates' guide to physical examination and history taking* (8th ed.). Philadelphia: Lippincott Williams & Wilkins. Hoeman, S. (2002). *Rehabilitation nursing: Process, application, and outcomes* (3rd ed.). St. Louis: Mosby.

Seidel, H. M., Ball, J. W., Dains, J. E., & Benedict, G. W. (2003). *Mosby's guide to physical examination* (5th ed.). St. Louis: Mosby.

Joint Movement: Shoulder—0219

Domain-Functional Health (I)   Care Recipient:

Class-Mobility (C)   Data Source:

Scale(s)-Severe deviation from normal range to No deviation from normal range (b)

Definition: Active range of motion of the shoulder with self-initiated movement

OUTCOME TARGET RATING: Maintain at_____   Increase to_____

Joint Movement: Shoulder Overall Rating	Severe deviation from normal range 1	Substantial deviation from normal range 2	Moderate deviation from normal range 3	Mild deviation from normal range 4	No deviation from normal range 5	

INDICATORS:

021901	Forward flexion 180 degrees (R)	1	2	3	4	5	NA
021902	Extension 50 degrees (R)	1	2	3	4	5	NA
021903	External rotation 90 degrees (R)	1	2	3	4	5	NA
021904	Internal rotation 90 degrees (R)	1	2	3	4	5	NA
021905	Abduction 180 degrees (R)	1	2	3	4	5	NA
021906	Adduction 50 degrees (R)	1	2	3	4	5	NA
021907	Forward flexion 180 degrees (L)	1	2	3	4	5	NA
021908	Extension 50 degrees (L)	1	2	3	4	5	NA
021909	External rotation 90 degrees (L)	1	2	3	4	5	NA
021910	Internal rotation 90 degrees (L)	1	2	3	4	5	NA
021911	Abduction 180 degrees (L)	1	2	3	4	5	NA
021912	Adduction 50 degrees (L)	1	2	3	4	5	NA

Specify: Right (R)____ Left (L)____ Both____

3rd edition 2004

Outcome Content References:

Bickley, L. (2002). *Bates' guide to physical examination and history taking* (8th ed.). Philadelphia: Lippincott Williams & Wilkins.
Hoeman, S. (2002). *Rehabilitation nursing: Process, application, and outcomes* (3rd ed.). St. Louis: Mosby.
Seidel, H. M., Ball, J. W., Dains, J. E., & Benedict, G. W. (2003). *Mosby's guide to physical examination* (5th ed.). St. Louis: Mosby.

J

Joint Movement: Spine—0220

Domain-Functional Health (I)

Class-Mobility (C)

Scale(s)-Severe deviation from normal range to No deviation from normal range (b)

Care Recipient:

Data Source:

Definition: Active range of motion of the spine with self-initiated movement

OUTCOME TARGET RATING: Maintain at_____   Increase to_____

Joint Movement: Spine Overall Rating	Severe deviation from normal range 1	Substantial deviation from normal range 2	Moderate deviation from normal range 3	Mild deviation from normal range 4	No deviation from normal range 5	
INDICATORS:						
022001 Extension 30 degrees	1	2	3	4	5	NA
022002 Flexion 90 degrees	1	2	3	4	5	NA
022003 Lateral bending 35 degrees (R)	1	2	3	4	5	NA
022004 Rotation (R)	1	2	3	4	5	NA
022005 Lateral bending 35 degrees (L)	1	2	3	4	5	NA
022006 Rotation (L)	1	2	3	4	5	NA

3rd edition 2004

Outcome Content References:

Bickley, L. (2002). *Bates' guide to physical examination and history taking* (8th ed.). Philadelphia: Lippincott Williams & Wilkins.
Hoeman, S. (2002). *Rehabilitation nursing: Process, application, and outcomes* (3rd ed.). St. Louis: Mosby.
Seidel, H. M., Ball, J. W., Dains, J. E., & Benedict, G. W. (2003). *Mosby's guide to physical examination* (5th ed.). St. Louis: Mosby.

Joint Movement: Wrist—0221

Domain-Functional Health (I)

Class-Mobility (C)

Scale(s)-Severe deviation from normal range to No deviation from normal range (b)

Care Recipient:

Data Source:

Definition: Active range of motion of the wrist with self-initiated movement

OUTCOME TARGET RATING:　　Maintain at_____　　　Increase to_____

Joint Movement: Wrist Overall Rating	Severe deviation from normal range 1	Substantial deviation from normal range 2	Moderate deviation from normal range 3	Mild deviation from normal range 4	No deviation from normal range 5	
INDICATORS:						
022101 Radial deviation 20 degrees (R)	1	2	3	4	5	NA
022102 Ulnar deviation 55 degrees (R)	1	2	3	4	5	NA
022103 Flexion 90 degrees (R)	1	2	3	4	5	NA
022104 Extension 70 degrees (R)	1	2	3	4	5	NA
022105 Radial deviation 20 degrees (L)	1	2	3	4	5	NA
022106 Ulnar deviation 55 degrees (L)	1	2	3	4	5	NA
022107 Flexion 90 degrees (L)	1	2	3	4	5	NA
022108 Extension 70 degrees (L)	1	2	3	4	5	NA

Specify: Right (R)____ Left (L)____ Both____

3rd edition 2004

Outcome Content References:

Bickley, L. (2002). *Bates' guide to physical examination and history taking* (8th ed.). Philadelphia: Lippincott Williams & Wilkins.

Hoeman, S. (2002). *Rehabilitation nursing: Process, application, and outcomes* (3rd ed.). St. Louis: Mosby.

Seidel, H. M., Ball, J. W., Dains, J. E., & Benedict, G. W. (2003). *Mosby's guide to physical examination* (5th ed.). St. Louis: Mosby.

Kidney Function—0504

Domain-Physiologic Health (II)

Class-Elimination (F)

Scale(s)-Severely compromised to Not compromised (a) and Severe to None (n)

Care Recipient:

Data Source:

Definition: Filtration of blood and elimination of metabolic waste products through the formation of urine

OUTCOME TARGET RATING: Maintain at_____   Increase to_____

Kidney Function Overall Rating	Severely compromised 1	Substantially compromised 2	Moderately compromised 3	Mildly compromised 4	Not compromised 5	
INDICATORS:						
050401 Fluid intake	1	2	3	4	5	NA
050402 24-hour intake and output balance	1	2	3	4	5	NA
050403 Blood urea nitrogen	1	2	3	4	5	NA
050404 Serum creatinine	1	2	3	4	5	NA
050405 Urine specific gravity	1	2	3	4	5	NA
050406 Urine color	1	2	3	4	5	NA
050407 Urine proteins	1	2	3	4	5	NA
050408 Urine pH	1	2	3	4	5	NA
050409 Urine electrolytes	1	2	3	4	5	NA
050410 Arterial bicarbonate (HCO_3)	1	2	3	4	5	NA
050411 Arterial pH	1	2	3	4	5	NA
050412 Serum electrolytes	1	2	3	4	5	NA
	Severe	Substantial	Moderate	Mild	None	
050413 Urine glucose	1	2	3	4	5	NA
050414 Hematuria	1	2	3	4	5	NA
050415 Urine ketones	1	2	3	4	5	NA
050416 Urine abnormal microscopic findings	1	2	3	4	5	NA
050417 Kidney stone formation	1	2	3	4	5	NA
050418 Weight gain	1	2	3	4	5	NA
050419 Hypertension	1	2	3	4	5	NA
050420 Nausea	1	2	3	4	5	NA
050421 Fatigue	1	2	3	4	5	NA
050422 Malaise	1	2	3	4	5	NA
050423 Anemia	1	2	3	4	5	NA

3rd edition 2004

Outcome Content References:

Broscious, S. K., & Castagnola, J. (2006). Chronic kidney disease: Acute manifestations and role of critical care nurses. *Critical Care Nurse, 26*(4), 17-28.

K

Brundage, D. J., & Linton, A. D. (1997). Age related changes in the genitourinary system. In M. A. Matteson, E. S. McConnell, & A. D. Linton (Eds.), *Gerontological nursing: Concepts in practice* (2nd ed.). Philadelphia: W.B. Saunders.

Culp, K., Flanigan, M., Dudley, J., Taylor, L., Bissen, T., & Garrison, S. (1998). Using the Quetelet Body Mass Index as a prognostic indicator for patients starting renal replacement therapy. *American Nephrology Nurses Association Journal, 25*(3), 321-332.

Culp, K., Flanigan, M., & Hayajneh, Y. (1999). Body weight and hemodialysis adequacy: An analysis of urea reduction ratios. *American Nephrology Nurses Association Journal, 26*(4), 391-402.

Culp, K., Flanigan, M., Lowie, E., Lew, N., & Zimmerman, B. (1996). Modeling mortality risk in hemodialysis patients using laboratory values as time-dependent covariates. *American Journal of Kidney Diseases, 28*(5), 741-746.

Guyton, A. C., Hall, J. E., & Schmitt, W. (1997). *Human physiology and mechanisms of disease* (6th ed.). New York: Harcourt Brace & Company.

Potter, P. A., & Perry, A. G. (2001). *Fundamentals of nursing* (5th ed.). St. Louis: Mosby.

Roth, C., & Culp, K. (2001). Renal osteodystrophy in elderly patients with end-stage renal disease. *Journal of Gerontological Nursing, 27*(7), 46-51.

K

Knowledge: Arthritis Management—1831

Domain-Health Knowledge & Behavior (IV)

Class-Health Knowledge (S)

Scale(s)-No knowledge to Extensive knowledge (u)

Care Recipient:

Data Source:

Definition: Extent of understanding conveyed about arthritis, its treatment, and the prevention of complications

OUTCOME TARGET RATING: Maintain at_____   Increase to_____

Knowledge: Arthritis Management Overall Rating	No knowledge 1	Limited knowledge 2	Moderate knowledge 3	Substantial knowledge 4	Extensive knowledge 5	
INDICATORS:						
183101 Cause and contributing factors	1	2	3	4	5	NA
183102 Usual course of disease process	1	2	3	4	5	NA
183103 Signs and symptoms of early disease	1	2	3	4	5	NA
183104 Signs and symptoms of worsening disease	1	2	3	4	5	NA
183105 Potential body changes due to disease	1	2	3	4	5	NA
183106 Benefits of disease management	1	2	3	4	5	NA
183107 Strategies to balance activity and rest	1	2	3	4	5	NA
183108 Energy conservation techniques	1	2	3	4	5	NA
183109 Benefits of exercise	1	2	3	4	5	NA
183110 Modification of daily activities	1	2	3	4	5	NA
183111 Factors that decrease the ability to perform activity	1	2	3	4	5	NA
183112 Effective exercise routine	1	2	3	4	5	NA
183113 Strategies to protect joints	1	2	3	4	5	NA
183114 Strategies to manage pain	1	2	3	4	5	NA
183115 Surgical treatment options	1	2	3	4	5	NA
183116 Medical treatment options	1	2	3	4	5	NA
183117 Medication therapeutic effects	1	2	3	4	5	NA
183118 Medication side effects	1	2	3	4	5	NA
183119 Medication adverse effects	1	2	3	4	5	NA
183120 When to obtain assistance from a health professional	1	2	3	4	5	NA
183121 Health beliefs that affect adherence to treatment plan	1	2	3	4	5	NA
183122 Effects of being overweight	1	2	3	4	5	NA
183123 Diet modifications	1	2	3	4	5	NA
183124 Correct use of assistive device	1	2	3	4	5	NA

		No knowledge	Limited knowledge	Moderate knowledge	Substantial knowledge	Extensive knowledge	
183125	Home safety measures	1	2	3	4	5	NA
183126	Fall prevention measures	1	2	3	4	5	NA
183127	Available support groups	1	2	3	4	5	NA
183128	Reputable sources of arthritis information	1	2	3	4	5	NA

4th edition

Outcome Content References:

Bellamy, N., Buchanan, W. W., Goldsmith, C. H., Campbell, J., & Stitt, L. W. (1988). Validation study of WOMAC: A health status instrument for measuring clinically important patient relevant outcomes to antirheumatic drug therapy in patients with osteoarthritis of the hip or knee. *Journal of Rheumatology, 15*, 1796-1840.

Branch, V. K., Lipsky, K., Nieman, T., & Lipsky, P. E. (1999). Positive impact of an intervention by arthritis patient educators on knowledge and satisfaction of patients in a rheumatology practice. *Arthritis Care and Research, 12*(6), 370-375.

Davies, G. M., Watson, D. J., & Bellamy, N. (1999). Comparison of the responsiveness and relative effect size of the Western Ontario and McMaster Universities Osteoarthritis Index and the Short-Form Medical Outcomes Study Survey in a randomized, clinical trial of osteoarthritis patients. *Arthritis Care Research, 12*, 172-179.

Edworthy, S. M., Devins, G. M., Watson, M. M. (1995). The Arthritis Knowledge Questionnaire. *Arthritis and Rheumatism, 38*, 590-600.

Figaro, M. K, Williams-Russo, P., Allegrante, J. P. (2005) Expectation and outlook: The impact of patient preference on arthritis care among African Americans. *Journal of Ambulatory Care Management, 28*(1), 41-48.

Hammond, A., & Lincoln, N. (1999). The Joint Protection Knowledge Assessment (JPKA): Reliability and validity. *British Journal of Occupational Therapy, 62*(3), 117-122.

Hill, J., & Bird, H. (2007). Patient knowledge and misconceptions of osteoarthritis assessed by a validated self-completed knowledge questionnaire (PKQ-OA). *Rheumatology, 46*(5), 796-800.

Memel, D. S., & Kirwan, J. R. (1999). General practitioners knowledge of functional and social factors in patients with rheumatoid arthritis. *Health and Social Care in the Community, 7*(6), 387-393.

Neame, R., & Hammond, A. (2005). Beliefs about medications: a questionnaire survey of people with rheumatoid arthritis. *Rheumatology, 44*, 762-767.

Neame, R., Hammond, A., & Deighton, C. (2005). Need for information and for involvement in decision making among patients with rheumatoid arthritis: A questionnaire survey. *Arthritis Care & Research, 53*(2), 249-255.

K

Knowledge: Asthma Management—1832

Domain-Health Knowledge & Behavior (IV)

Class-Health Knowledge (S)

Scale(s)-No knowledge to Extensive knowledge (u)

Care Recipient:

Data Source:

> **Definition:** Extent of understanding conveyed about asthma, its treatment, and the prevention of complications

OUTCOME TARGET RATING: Maintain at_____ Increase to_____

Knowledge: Asthma Management Overall Rating	No knowledge 1	Limited knowledge 2	Moderate knowledge 3	Substantial knowledge 4	Extensive knowledge 5	
INDICATORS:						
183201 Signs and symptoms of asthma	1	2	3	4	5	NA
183202 Benefits of disease management	1	2	3	4	5	NA
183203 Cause and contributing factors	1	2	3	4	5	NA
183204 Usual course of disease process	1	2	3	4	5	NA
183205 Potential complications of asthma	1	2	3	4	5	NA
183206 Strategies to manage asthma	1	2	3	4	5	NA
183207 Asthma management goals	1	2	3	4	5	NA
183208 Importance of continual access to inhaler	1	2	3	4	5	NA
183209 Effects on lifestyle	1	2	3	4	5	NA
183210 Relationship of physical and emotional stress to condition	1	2	3	4	5	NA
183211 Importance of complying with treatment regimen	1	2	3	4	5	NA
183212 Importance of complying with medication regimen	1	2	3	4	5	NA
183213 Actions to be taken in an emergency	1	2	3	4	5	NA
183214 Options for assistance with medical emergencies	1	2	3	4	5	NA
183215 Proper technique to measure peak expiratory flow	1	2	3	4	5	NA
183216 When to use peak flow meter	1	2	3	4	5	NA
183217 Conditions that trigger asthma	1	2	3	4	5	NA
183218 Strategies to manage controllable environmental risk factors	1	2	3	4	5	NA
183219 Benefits of ongoing monitoring	1	2	3	4	5	NA
183220 Effective breathing techniques	1	2	3	4	5	NA
183221 Recommended activity level	1	2	3	4	5	NA
183222 Activity restrictions	1	2	3	4	5	NA
183223 Leisure activity recommendations	1	2	3	4	5	NA
183224 Identification of medication used for asthma	1	2	3	4	5	NA

K

		No knowledge	Limited knowledge	Moderate knowledge	Substantial knowledge	Extensive knowledge	
183225	Strategies to balance activity and rest	1	2	3	4	5	NA
183226	Medication therapeutic effects	1	2	3	4	5	NA
183227	Medication side effects	1	2	3	4	5	NA
183228	Medication adverse effects	1	2	3	4	5	NA
183229	When to obtain assistance from a health professional	1	2	3	4	5	NA
183230	When to obtain emergency treatment	1	2	3	4	5	NA
183231	Available support groups	1	2	3	4	5	NA
183232	Available community resources	1	2	3	4	5	NA
183233	Reputable sources of asthma information	1	2	3	4	5	NA

4th edition

Outcome Content References:

American Academy of Allergy, Asthma, and Immunology (AAAAI). (1999). Pediatric asthma: Promoting best practice guide for managing asthma. Retrieved September 20, 2005, from http://www.aaaai.org/members/resources/initiatives/pediatricasthma.stm

Baker, V., Friedman, J., & Schmitt, R. (2002a). Asthma management, part I: An overview of the problem and current trends. *Journal of School Nursing, 18*(3), 128-137.

Baker, V., Friedman, J., & Schmitt, R. (2002b). Asthma management, part II: Pharmacologic management. *Journal of School Nursing, 18*(5), 257-269.

Lung, C. L., & Lung, M. L. (2003). General principles of asthma management: Symptom monitoring. *Nursing Clinics of North America, 38*, 585-596.

National Asthma Education and Prevention Program (NAEPP). (1997). *Expert panel report II. Guidelines for the diagnosis and management of asthma* (Publication No. 97-4051). Bethesda, MD: U.S. Department of Health and Human Services.

Yawn, B. P. (2005). Asthma. In D. L. Huber (Ed.), *Disease management: A guide for case managers* (pp. 100-131). St. Louis: Saunders.

Yoos, H. L., Philipson, E., McMullen, A. (2003). Asthma management across the life span: The child with asthma. *Nursing Clinics of North America, 38*(4), 635-652.

K

Knowledge: Body Mechanics—1827

Domain-Health Knowledge & Behavior (IV)

Class-Health Knowledge (S)

Scale(s)-No knowledge to Extensive knowledge (u)

Care Recipient:

Data Source:

Definition: Extent of understanding conveyed about proper body alignment, balance and coordinated movement

OUTCOME TARGET RATING: Maintain at_____   Increase to_____

Knowledge: Body Mechanics Overall Rating	No knowledge 1	Limited knowledge 2	Moderate knowledge 3	Substantial knowledge 4	Extensive knowledge 5	
INDICATORS:						
182701 Natural spinal curves	1	2	3	4	5	NA
182702 Proper standing posture	1	2	3	4	5	NA
182703 Proper sitting posture	1	2	3	4	5	NA
182704 Proper lying posture	1	2	3	4	5	NA
182705 Proper lifting techniques	1	2	3	4	5	NA
182706 Exercises to improve posture	1	2	3	4	5	NA
182707 Exercises to improve muscle flexibility	1	2	3	4	5	NA
182708 Exercises to improve joint mobility	1	2	3	4	5	NA
182709 Exercises to improve muscle strength	1	2	3	4	5	NA
182710 Exercises to strengthen lower abdominal muscles	1	2	3	4	5	NA
182711 Positional causes of muscle or joint pain from sitting	1	2	3	4	5	NA
182712 Positional causes of muscle or joint pain from lying	1	2	3	4	5	NA
182713 Positional causes of muscle or joint pain from lifting	1	2	3	4	5	NA
182714 Common symptoms of back injury	1	2	3	4	5	NA
182715 Personal risk activities	1	2	3	4	5	NA

3rd edition 2004; Revised 4th edition

Outcome Content References:

American Physical Therapy Association. (1996). *Taking care of your back: A physical therapist's perspective.* Washington, DC: Author.

American Physical Therapy Association. (2000). *The secret of good posture: A physical therapist's perspective.* Washington, DC: Author.

Lieber, S. J., Rudy, T. E., & Boston, R. (1999). Effects of body mechanics training on performance of repetitive lifting. *The American Journal of Occupational Therapy, 54*(2), 166-175.

McConnell, E. A. (2002). Clinical do's & don'ts. Using proper body mechanics. *Nursing 2002, 32*(15), 17.

Neal, C. (1997). The assessment of knowledge and application of proper body mechanics in the workplace. *Orthopaedic Nursing, 16*(1), 66-69.

Perry, A. G., & Potter, P. A. (1998). *Clinical nursing skills and techniques* (4th ed., pp. 877-884). St. Louis: Mosby.

Porteau-Cassard, L., Zabraniecki, L., Dromer, C., & Fournie, B. (1999). A back school program at the Toulouse-Purpan teaching hospital. Evaluation of 144 patients. *Revue Du Rhumatisme, English Edition, 66*(10), 477-483.

Richardson, C. A., Snijders, C. J., Hides, J. A., Damen, L., Pas, M. S., & Storm, J. (2002). The relation between the transversus abdominis muscles, sacroiliac joint mechanics, and low back pain. *Spine, 27*(4), 399-405.

Sorrentino, S. A. (2000). *Mosby's textbook for nursing assistants* (5th ed., pp. 242-247). St. Louis: Mosby.

Knowledge: Breastfeeding—1800

Domain-Health Knowledge & Behavior (IV)　　Care Recipient:

Class-Health Knowledge (S)　　Data Source:

Scale(s)-No knowledge to Extensive knowledge (u)

Definition: Extent of understanding conveyed about lactation and nourishment of infant through breastfeeding

OUTCOME TARGET RATING:　　Maintain at_____　　Increase to_____

Knowledge: Breastfeeding Overall Rating	No knowledge 1	Limited knowledge 2	Moderate knowledge 3	Substantial knowledge 4	Extensive knowledge 5	
INDICATORS:						
180001 Benefits of breastfeeding	1	2	3	4	5	NA
180002 Physiology of lactation	1	2	3	4	5	NA
180020 Fluid intake requirements for mother	1	2	3	4	5	NA
180003 Breastmilk composition, letdown process, foremilk versus hindmilk	1	2	3	4	5	NA
180004 Infant hunger cues	1	2	3	4	5	NA
180005 Proper technique for attaching infant to the breast	1	2	3	4	5	NA
180006 Proper infant positioning while nursing	1	2	3	4	5	NA
180007 Nutritive versus nonnutritive sucking	1	2	3	4	5	NA
180008 Evaluation of infant swallowing	1	2	3	4	5	NA
180009 Proper technique to break infant suction	1	2	3	4	5	NA
180010 Signs of adequate milk supply	1	2	3	4	5	NA
180011 Signs of well-nourished infant	1	2	3	4	5	NA
180012 Nipple evaluation	1	2	3	4	5	NA
180013 Signs of mastitis, blocked ducts, nipple trauma	1	2	3	4	5	NA
180014 Reasons for early avoidance of artificial nipples	1	2	3	4	5	NA
180021 Reasons for avoidance of water and supplements for infant	1	2	3	4	5	NA
180015 Proper breastmilk expression and storage techniques	1	2	3	4	5	NA
180016 Substances that transfer from infant through breastmilk	1	2	3	4	5	NA
180022 Relationship between breastfeeding and infant immunity	1	2	3	4	5	NA
180017 Signs of weaning readiness	1	2	3	4	5	NA
180018 Strategies to access health care services	1	2	3	4	5	NA
180023 Available support groups	1	2	3	4	5	NA

Continued

1st edition 1997; Revised 3rd edition 2004; Revised 4th edition

Outcome Content References:

Biancizzo, M. (2003). *Breastfeeding the newborn* (2nd ed.). St. Louis: Mosby.

Dowling, D., & Thanattherakul, W. (2001). Nipple confusion, alternative feeding methods, and breast-feeding supplementation: state of the science. *Newborn and Infant Nursing Reviews, 1*(4), 217-223.

Giglia, R., & Binns, C. (2006). Alcohol and lactation: A systematic review. *Nutrition & Dietetics, 63*(2), 103-116.

Lawrence, R. A., & Lawrence, R. M. (1999). *Breastfeeding: A guide for the medical profession* (5th ed.). St. Louis: Mosby.

Lovelady, C. A., Fuller, C. J., Geigerman, C. M., Hunter, C. P., & Kinsella, T. A. (2004). Immune status of physically active women during lactation. *Medicine & Science in Sports & Exercise, 36*(6), 1001-1007.

McCarter-Spaulding (2005). Medications in pregnancy and lactation. *MCN, American Journal of Maternal Child Nursing, 30*(1), 24-29.

Li, R., Rock, V. J., & Grummer-Strawn, L. (2007). Changes in public attitudes toward breastfeeding in the United States, 1999-2003. *Journal of the American Dietetic Association, 107*, 122-127.

Shrago, L., & Bocar, D. (1990). The infant's contribution to breastfeeding. *Journal of Obstetric, Gynecologic, and Neonatal Nursing, 19*(3), 209-213.

Spangler, A. (1992). *Amy Spangler's breastfeeding: A parent's guide*. Atlanta: A. Spangler Publications.

Walker, M. (1989). Functional assessment of infant breastfeeding patterns. *Birth: Issues in Perinatal Care and Education, 16*(3), 140-147.

K

Knowledge: Cancer Management—1833

Domain-Health Knowledge & Behavior (IV)
Class-Health Knowledge (S)
Scale(s)-No knowledge to Extensive knowledge (u)

Care Recipient:
Data Source:

Definition: Extent of understanding conveyed about cause, type, progress, symptoms, and treatment of cancer

OUTCOME TARGET RATING: Maintain at_____   Increase to_____

Knowledge: Cancer Management Overall Rating	No knowledge 1	Limited knowledge 2	Moderate knowledge 3	Substantial knowledge 4	Extensive knowledge 5	
INDICATORS:						
183301 Abnormal screening results	1	2	3	4	5	NA
183302 Signs and symptoms of cancer	1	2	3	4	5	NA
183303 Specific cancer diagnosis	1	2	3	4	5	NA
183304 Cause and contributing factors	1	2	3	4	5	NA
183305 Usual course of disease process	1	2	3	4	5	NA
183306 Stages of cancer	1	2	3	4	5	NA
183307 Signs and symptoms of recurrence	1	2	3	4	5	NA
183308 Available treatment options	1	2	3	4	5	NA
183309 Alternative or complementary treatments	1	2	3	4	5	NA
183310 Purpose of different treatment options	1	2	3	4	5	NA
183311 Benefits of different treatment options	1	2	3	4	5	NA
183312 Tests and procedures involved in treatment regimen	1	2	3	4	5	NA
183313 Steps in treatment regimen	1	2	3	4	5	NA
183314 Medication therapeutic effects	1	2	3	4	5	NA
183315 Medication adverse effects	1	2	3	4	5	NA
183316 Medication side effects	1	2	3	4	5	NA
183317 Potential complications of treatment	1	2	3	4	5	NA
183318 Signs and symptoms of complications of treatment	1	2	3	4	5	NA
183319 Precautions to prevent complications of treatment	1	2	3	4	5	NA
183320 Self-care responsibilities for ongoing treatment	1	2	3	4	5	NA
183321 Physical effects of cancer treatment	1	2	3	4	5	NA
183322 Effects on lifestyle	1	2	3	4	5	NA
183323 Effects on employment	1	2	3	4	5	NA

K

Continued

		No knowledge	Limited knowledge	Moderate knowledge	Substantial knowledge	Extensive knowledge	
183324	Effects on sexuality	1	2	3	4	5	NA
183325	Strategies to cope with adverse effects of disease	1	2	3	4	5	NA
183326	Survival rate	1	2	3	4	5	NA
183327	Self-care issues during recovery	1	2	3	4	5	NA
183328	Importance of positive attitude for coping with cancer	1	2	3	4	5	NA
183329	Reputable sources of cancer information	1	2	3	4	5	NA
183330	Available community resources	1	2	3	4	5	NA
183331	Available support groups	1	2	3	4	5	NA
183332	Financial resources for assistance	1	2	3	4	5	NA
183333	Health beliefs that affect adherence to treatment regimen	1	2	3	4	5	NA
183334	Benefits of disease management	1	2	3	4	5	NA

Specify cancer_____

4th edition

K

Outcome Content References:

Carlson, R. (2006, August 10). HPV vaccine, now FDA-approved, shown to protect against vaginal, vulvar intraepithelial neoplasias. *Oncology Times Meeting Reporter*, pp. 2-3.

Dein, S. (2004). Explanatory models of and attitudes towards cancer in different cultures. *The Lancet Oncology*, 5, 119-124.

Rutten, L. J. F., Arora, N. K., Bakos, A. D., Aziz, N., & Rowland, J. (2005). Information needs and sources of information among cancer patients: A systematic review of research (1980-2003). *Patient Education and Counseling*, 57, 250-261.

Shokar, N. K., Veron, S. W., & Weller, S. C. (2005). Cancer and colorectal cancer: Knowledge, beliefs, and screening preferences of a diverse patient population. *Family Medicine*, 37(5), 341-347.

Sterman, E., Gauker, S., & Krieger, J. (2003). A comprehensive approach to improving cancer pain management and patient satisfaction. *Oncology Nursing Forum*, 30(5), 857-864.

Waller, J., McCaffery, K., & Wardle, J. (2004). Measuring cancer knowledge: Comparing prompted and unprompted recall. *British Journal of Psychology*, 95, 219-234.

Knowledge: Cancer Threat Reduction—1834

Domain-Health Knowledge & Behavior (IV)
Class-Health Knowledge (S)
Scale(s)-No knowledge to Extensive knowledge (u)

Care Recipient:
Data Source:

> **Definition:** Extent of understanding conveyed about causes, prevention, and early detection of cancer

OUTCOME TARGET RATING: Maintain at_____   Increase to_____

Knowledge: Cancer Threat Reduction Overall Rating	No knowledge 1	Limited knowledge 2	Moderate knowledge 3	Substantial knowledge 4	Extensive knowledge 5	

INDICATORS:

183401	Warning signs of cancer	1	2	3	4	5	NA
183402	Cause and contributing factors	1	2	3	4	5	NA
183403	Genetic testing	1	2	3	4	5	NA
183404	Recommended cancer screenings	1	2	3	4	5	NA
183405	Cancer screening procedures	1	2	3	4	5	NA
183406	Recommended self-screenings for cancer detection	1	2	3	4	5	NA
183407	Importance of maintaining adequate sleep	1	2	3	4	5	NA
183408	Importance of regular exercise	1	2	3	4	5	NA
183409	Importance of oral screening	1	2	3	4	5	NA
183410	Diet recommendations for reducing risk	1	2	3	4	5	NA
183411	Correct use of nutritional supplements	1	2	3	4	5	NA
183412	Correct use of prescribed medication	1	2	3	4	5	NA
183413	Strategies to avoid exposure to carcinogens	1	2	3	4	5	NA
183414	Strategies to protect skin from sun exposure	1	2	3	4	5	NA
183415	Strategies to prevent cervical cancer	1	2	3	4	5	NA
183416	Strategies to manage controllable environmental risk factors	1	2	3	4	5	NA
183417	Adverse effects of tobacco use	1	2	3	4	5	NA
183418	Safe sexual practices	1	2	3	4	5	NA
183419	When to obtain assistance from a health professional	1	2	3	4	5	NA
183420	Reputable sources of cancer prevention information	1	2	3	4	5	NA

K

4th edition

Continued

Outcome Content References:

Carlson, R. (2006, August 10). HPV vaccine, now FDA-approved, shown to protect against vaginal, vulvar intraepithelial neoplasias. *Oncology Times Meeting Reporter*, pp. 2-3.

Rutten, L. J. F., Arora, N. K., Bakos, A. D., Aziz, N., & Rowland, J. (2005). Information needs and sources of information among cancer patients: A systematic review of research (1980-2003). *Patient Education and Counseling, 57,* 250-261.

Patterson, R. E., Kristal, A. R., & White, E. (1996). Do beliefs, knowledge, and perceived norms about diet and cancer predict dietary change? *American Journal of Public Health, 86*(10), 1394-1400.

Waller, J., McCaffery, K., & Wardle, J. (2004). Measuring cancer knowledge: Comparing prompted and unprompted recall. *British Journal of Psychology, 95,* 219-234.

K

Knowledge: Cardiac Disease Management—1830

Domain-Health, Knowledge, & Behavior (IV)

Class—Health Knowledge (S)

Scale(s)-No knowledge to Extensive knowledge (u)

Care Recipient:

Data Source

Definition: Extent of understanding conveyed about heart disease, its treatment, and the prevention of complications

OUTCOME TARGET RATING: Maintain at_____   Increase to_____

Knowledge: Cardiac Disease Management Overall Rating	No knowledge 1	Limited knowledge 2	Moderate knowledge 3	Substantial knowledge 4	Extensive knowledge 5	
INDICATORS:						
183001 Usual course of disease process	1	2	3	4	5	NA
183002 Signs and symptoms of early disease	1	2	3	4	5	NA
183003 Signs and symptoms of worsening disease	1	2	3	4	5	NA
183004 Benefits of disease management	1	2	3	4	5	NA
183005 Strategies to reduce risk factors	1	2	3	4	5	NA
183028 Methods to decrease treatment side effects	1	2	3	4	5	NA
183006 Importance of completing cardiac rehabilitation program	1	2	3	4	5	NA
183007 Family caregiver's role in treatment plan	1	2	3	4	5	NA
183008 Methods to measure blood pressure	1	2	3	4	5	NA
183029 Methods to monitor heart rate	1	2	3	4	5	NA
183009 Strategies to limit sodium intake	1	2	3	4	5	NA
183010 Rationale for following a low-fat, low-cholesterol diet	1	2	3	4	5	NA
183011 Strategies to increase diet adherence	1	2	3	4	5	NA
183012 Strategies to limit fluid intake	1	2	3	4	5	NA
183013 Rationale for monitoring weight	1	2	3	4	5	NA
183014 Importance of alcohol restriction	1	2	3	4	5	NA
183015 Importance of tobacco abstinence	1	2	3	4	5	NA
183030 Recommended work activity	1	2	3	4	5	NA
183031 Recommended activity level	1	2	3	4	5	NA
183032 Recommended leisure activity	1	2	3	4	5	NA
183017 Importance of regular exercise	1	2	3	4	5	NA
183018 Energy conservation techniques	1	2	3	4	5	NA

K

Continued

		No knowledge	Limited knowledge	Moderate knowledge	Substantial knowledge	Extensive knowledge	
183019	Guidelines for sexual activity	1	2	3	4	5	NA
183020	Potential sexual difficulties	1	2	3	4	5	NA
183021	Medication therapeutic effects	1	2	3	4	5	NA
183033	Medication side effects	1	2	3	4	5	NA
183034	Medication adverse effects						
183022	Strategies to manage stress	1	2	3	4	5	NA
183023	Importance of obtaining flu and pneumonia vaccines	1	2	3	4	5	NA
183035	When to obtain assistance from a health professional	1	2	3	4	5	NA
183025	Care options for assistance with medical emergencies	1	2	3	4	5	NA
183026	Importance of family learning cardiopulmonary resuscitation	1	2	3	4	5	NA
183027	Cultural influences on adherence to treatment regimen	1	2	3	4	5	NA
183036	Available support groups	1	2	3	4	5	NA
183037	Reputable sources of cardiac disease information	1	2	3	4	5	NA

3rd edition 2004; Revised 4th edition

Outcome Content References:

Alm-Roijer, C., Stagmo, M., Uden, G., & Erhardt, L. (2004). Better knowledge improves adherence to lifestyle changes and medication in patients with coronary heart disease. *European Journal of Cardiovascular Nursing, 3*(4), 321-330.

Cannon, C. P., Battler, A., Brindis, R. G., Cox, J. L., Ellis, S. G., Every, N. R., Flaherty, J. T., Harrington, R. A., Krumholz, H. M., Simoons, M. L., Van De Werf, F. J. J., & Weintraub, W. S. (2001). ACC key data elements and definitions for measuring the clinical management and outcomes of patients with acute coronary syndromes: A report of the American College of Cardiology task force on clinical data standards (acute coronary syndrome writing committee). *Journal of the American College of Cardiology, 38*, 2114-2130.

Dunbar, S. B., Jacobson, L. H., & Deaton, C. (1998). Heart failure: Strategies to enhance patient self-management. *AACN Clinical Issues: Advanced Practice in Acute & Critical Care, 9*, 244-256.

Dusseldorp, E., Van Elderan, T., Maes, S., Meulman, J, & Kraaij, V. (1999). A meta-analysis of psychoeducational programs for coronary heart disease patients. *Health Psychology, 18*, 506-519.

Hunt, S. A., Baker, D. W., Chin, M. H., Cinquegrani, M. P., Feldman, A. M., Grancis, G. S., Ganiats, T. G., Goldstein, S., Gregoratos, G., Jessup, M. L., Noble, R. J., Packer, M., Silver, M. A., & Steven, L. W. (2001). ACC/AHA guidelines for the evaluation and management of chronic heart failure in the adult: A report of the American College of Cardiology/American Heart Association Task Force on Practice Guidelines (Committee to revise the 1995 Guidelines for the Evaluation and Management of Heart Failure). *Journal of the American College of Cardiology, 38*, 2101-2113.

Johnson, J., & Pearson, V. (2000). The effects of a structured education course on stroke survivors living in the community . . . including commentary by Phipps, M. *Rehabilitation Nursing, 25*, 59-65.

Kimble, L. P., & Kunik, C. L. (2000). Knowledge and use of sublingual nitroglycerin and cardiac-related quality of life in patients with chronic stable angina. *Journal of Pain & Symptom Management, 19*(2), 109-117.

National Institutes of Health, National Heart, Lung, and Blood Institute (NHLBI), & National High Blood Pressure Education Program. (1997). *The sixth report of the Joint National Committee on Prevention, Detection, Evaluation, & Treatment of High Blood Pressure* (NIH Publication No. 98-4080). Bethesda, MD: Author.

Silcox, P. D. (2005). Congestive heart failure. In D. L. Huber (Ed.), *Disease management: A guide for case managers* (pp. 71-80). St. Louis: Saunders.

Knowledge: Child Physical Safety—1801

Domain-Health Knowledge & Behavior (IV)

Class-Health Knowledge (S)

Scale(s)-No knowledge to Extensive knowledge (u)

Care Recipient:

Data Source:

Definition: Extent of understanding conveyed about safely caring for a child from 1 year through 17 years of age

OUTCOME TARGET RATING: Maintain at_____   Increase to_____

Knowledge: Child Physical Safety Overall Rating	No knowledge 1	Limited knowledge 2	Moderate knowledge 3	Substantial knowledge 4	Extensive knowledge 5	

INDICATORS:

180101	Appropriate activities for child's developmental level	1	2	3	4	5	NA
180119	Diving hazards	1	2	3	4	5	NA
180103	Strategies to prevent drowning	1	2	3	4	5	NA
180104	Strategies to prevent electrical shock	1	2	3	4	5	NA
180105	Benefits of protective helmet	1	2	3	4	5	NA
180120	First aid techniques	1	2	3	4	5	NA
180108	Correct use of safety seats and seat belts	1	2	3	4	5	NA
180121	Age-appropriate cardiopulmonary resuscitation techniques	1	2	3	4	5	NA
180122	Heimlich maneuver	1	2	3	4	5	NA
180106	Strategies to prevent choking	1	2	3	4	5	NA
180111	Strategies to prevent farm accidents	1	2	3	4	5	NA
180123	Strategies to prevent motor vehicle accidents	1	2	3	4	5	NA
180124	Strategies to prevent cycle accidents	1	2	3	4	5	NA
180112	Strategies to prevent falls	1	2	3	4	5	NA
180113	Strategies to prevent playground accidents	1	2	3	4	5	NA
180114	Strategies to prevent burns	1	2	3	4	5	NA
180115	Correct use of smoke detectors	1	2	3	4	5	NA
180116	Proper surveillance of outdoor play	1	2	3	4	5	NA
180117	Importance of teaching stranger awareness	1	2	3	4	5	NA
180125	Strategies to prevent tobacco use	1	2	3	4	5	NA
180126	Strategies to prevent alcohol use	1	2	3	4	5	NA

K

Continued

		No knowledge	Limited knowledge	Moderate knowledge	Substantial knowledge	Extensive knowledge	
180127	Strategies to prevent recreational drug use	1	2	3	4	5	NA
180128	Strategies to prevent firearm injuries	1	2	3	4	5	NA
180129	Strategies to prevent participation in violence	1	2	3	4	5	NA
180130	Strategies to prevent medication misuse	1	2	3	4	5	NA
180131	Strategies to prevent exposure to toxic chemicals	1	2	3	4	5	NA

1st edition 1997; Revised 3rd edition 2004; Revised 4th edition

Outcome Content References:

Eichelberger, M. R., Gotschall, C. S., Feely, H. B., Harstad, P., & Bowman, L. M. (1990). Parental attitudes and knowledge of child safety. *American Journal of Diseases of Children, 144*(6), 714-720.

Gilk, D., Kronenfeld, J., & Jackson, K. (1993). Safety behaviors among parents of preschoolers. *Health Values, 17*(1), 18-25.

Grossman, D. C., & Rivera, F. P. (1992). Injury control in childhood. *Pediatric Clinics of North America, 39*(3), 471-484.

Rivera, F. P., & Howard, D. (1982). Parental knowledge of child development and injury risks. *Developmental and Behavioral Pediatrics, 3*(2), 103-105.

Wortel E., Geus, G. H., Kok, G., & van Woerkum, C. (1994). Injury control in pre-school children: A review of parental safety measures and the behavioral determinants. *Health Education Research, 9*(2), 201-213.

K

Knowledge: Conception Prevention—1821

Knowledge: Conception Prevention—1821

Domain-Health Knowledge & Behavior (IV)   Care Recipient:

Class-Health Knowledge (S)   Data Source:

Scale(s)-No knowledge to Extensive knowledge (u)

Definition: Extent of understanding conveyed about prevention of unintended pregnancy

OUTCOME TARGET RATING: Maintain at_____   Increase to_____

Knowledge: Conception Prevention Overall Rating	No knowledge 1	Limited knowledge 2	Moderate knowledge 3	Substantial knowledge 4	Extensive knowledge 5	
INDICATORS:						
182105 How conception occurs	1	2	3	4	5	NA
182106 Advantages and disadvantages of having a child	1	2	3	4	5	NA
182107 Influence of personal values on chosen contraceptive method	1	2	3	4	5	NA
182108 Periodic rhythm method	1	2	3	4	5	NA
182109 Chemical barrier methods	1	2	3	4	5	NA
182110 Hormonal therapy methods	1	2	3	4	5	NA
182111 Mechanical barrier methods	1	2	3	4	5	NA
182112 Surgical treatment options	1	2	3	4	5	NA
182101 How chosen contraceptive method works	1	2	3	4	5	NA
182102 Correct use of chosen contraceptive method	1	2	3	4	5	NA
182103 Effectiveness of chosen contraceptive method	1	2	3	4	5	NA
182104 Effect of chosen contraceptive on sexually transmitted disease transmission	1	2	3	4	5	NA

2nd edition 2000; Revised 3rd edition 2004; Revised 4th edition

Outcome Content References:

Hatcher, R. A., Trussell, J., Stewart, F., Cates, W. Jr., Stewart, G. K., Guest, F., & Kowal, D. (1998). *Contraceptive technology* (17th ed.). New York: Irvington Publishers.

Howard, M. (1991). *How to help your teenager postpone sexual involvement.* Lexington, NY: Continuum.

Miller, B., Card, J., Paikoff, R. J., & Peterson, J. (1992). *Preventing adolescent pregnancy.* Newbury Park, CA: Sage.

K

Knowledge: Congestive Heart Failure Management—1835

Domain-Health Knowledge & Behavior (IV)   Care Recipient:

Class-Health Knowledge (S)   Data Source:

Scale(s)-No knowledge to Extensive knowledge (u)

Definition: Extent of understanding conveyed about heart failure, its treatment, and the prevention of exacerbations

OUTCOME TARGET RATING: Maintain at_____   Increase to_____

Knowledge: Congestive Heart Failure Management Overall Rating	No knowledge 1	Limited knowledge 2	Moderate knowledge 3	Substantial knowledge 4	Extensive knowledge 5	
INDICATORS:						
183501 Cause and contributing factors	1	2	3	4	5	NA
183502 Signs and symptoms of early disease	1	2	3	4	5	NA
183503 Benefits of disease management	1	2	3	4	5	NA
183504 Basic actions of the heart	1	2	3	4	5	NA
183505 Signs and symptoms of congestive heart failure	1	2	3	4	5	NA
183506 Signs and symptoms of orthostatic hypotension	1	2	3	4	5	NA
183507 Signs and symptoms of anemia	1	2	3	4	5	NA
183508 Signs and symptoms of internal bleeding	1	2	3	4	5	NA
183509 Signs and symptoms of dyspnea	1	2	3	4	5	NA
183510 Signs and symptoms of tachycardia	1	2	3	4	5	NA
183511 Signs and symptoms of overexertion	1	2	3	4	5	NA
183512 Relationship of physical and emotional stress to condition	1	2	3	4	5	NA
183513 Psychosocial effect of heart failure on self	1	2	3	4	5	NA
183514 Psychosocial effect of heart failure on family	1	2	3	4	5	NA
183515 Strategies to control anxiety	1	2	3	4	5	NA
183516 Treatments to improve cardiac performance	1	2	3	4	5	NA
183517 Strategies to promote peripheral circulation	1	2	3	4	5	NA
183518 Importance of rest for disease management	1	2	3	4	5	NA
183519 Strategies to balance activity and rest	1	2	3	4	5	NA
183520 Strategies to prevent respiratory distress	1	2	3	4	5	NA

K

	No knowledge	Limited knowledge	Moderate knowledge	Substantial knowledge	Extensive knowledge	
183521	Strategies to increase resistance to infection	1	2	3	4	5	NA
183522	Pattern and type of edema	1	2	3	4	5	NA
183523	Strategies to manage dependent edema	1	2	3	4	5	NA
183524	Factors contributing to weight changes	1	2	3	4	5	NA
183525	Strategies to manage weight	1	2	3	4	5	NA
183526	Strategies to enhance diet adherence	1	2	3	4	5	NA
183527	Medication therapeutic effects	1	2	3	4	5	NA
183528	Medication side effects	1	2	3	4	5	NA
183529	Medication adverse effects	1	2	3	4	5	NA
183530	Role of diagnostic tests to disease management	1	2	3	4	5	NA
183531	Self-monitoring techniques	1	2	3	4	5	NA
183532	Effects on lifestyle	1	2	3	4	5	NA
183533	Adaptations for role performance	1	2	3	4	5	NA
183534	Effects on sexuality	1	2	3	4	5	NA
183535	Adaptations for sexual performance	1	2	3	4	5	NA
183536	Available support groups	1	2	3	4	5	NA
183537	When to obtain assistance from a health professional	1	2	3	4	5	NA

4th edition

Outcome Content References:

Bonow, R. O., Bennett, S., Casey, D. E., Ganiats, T. G., Hlatky, M. A. et al. (2005). ACC/AHA clinical performance measures for adults with chronic heart failure: A report of the American College of Cardiology/American Heart Association Task Force on Performance Measures. *Circulation, 112*, 1853-1887.

House-Fancher, M. A., & Foell, H. Y. (2004). Nursing management: Heart failure and cardiomyopathy. In S. M. Lewis, M. M. Heitkemper, & S. R. Dirksen (Eds.), *Medical-surgical nursing* (6th ed., pp. 838-860). St. Louis: Mosby.

Pina, I. L., Apstein, C. S., Balady, G. J., Belardinelli, R., Chaitman, B. R., Duscha, B. D., Fletcher, B. J., Fleg, J. L., Myers, J. N., & Sullivan, M. J. (2003). Exercise and heart failure: A statement from the American Heart Association Committee on Exercise, Rehabilitation, and Prevention. *Circulation, 107*, 1210-1225.

Silcox, P. D. (2005). Congestive heart failure. In D. L. Huber (Ed.), *Disease management: A guide for case managers* (pp. 71-80). St. Louis: Saunders.

K

Knowledge: Depression Management—1836

Domain-Health Knowledge & Behavior (IV)

Class-Health Knowledge (S)

Scale(s)-No knowledge to Extensive knowledge (u)

Care Recipient:

Data Source:

Definition: Extent of understanding conveyed about depression and interrelationships among causes, effects, and treatments

OUTCOME TARGET RATING: Maintain at_____   Increase to_____

Knowledge: Depression Management Overall Rating	No knowledge 1	Limited knowledge 2	Moderate knowledge 3	Substantial knowledge 4	Extensive knowledge 5	
INDICATORS:						
183601 Physical signs and symptoms of depression	1	2	3	4	5	NA
183602 Emotional signs and symptoms of depression	1	2	3	4	5	NA
183603 Chronic conditions that increase risk for depression	1	2	3	4	5	NA
183604 Benefits of disease management	1	2	3	4	5	NA
183605 Available treatment options	1	2	3	4	5	NA
183606 Personal treatment regimen	1	2	3	4	5	NA
183607 Relationship of treatment regimen to goals	1	2	3	4	5	NA
183608 Importance of completing treatment regimen	1	2	3	4	5	NA
183609 Personal treatment therapeutic effects	1	2	3	4	5	NA
183610 Importance of complying with treatment regimen	1	2	3	4	5	NA
183611 Importance of complying with medication regimen	1	2	3	4	5	NA
183612 Factors contributing to depression	1	2	3	4	5	NA
183613 Factors that alleviate depression	1	2	3	4	5	NA
183614 Strategies to reduce precursors of depression	1	2	3	4	5	NA
183615 Strategies to facilitate recovery	1	2	3	4	5	NA
183616 Effects of depression on daily functioning	1	2	3	4	5	NA
183617 Interrelationship of self-esteem and body image to depression	1	2	3	4	5	NA
183618 Relationship of substance use to depression	1	2	3	4	5	NA

K

		No knowledge	Limited knowledge	Moderate knowledge	Substantial knowledge	Extensive knowledge	
183619	Medication therapeutic effects	1	2	3	4	5	NA
183620	Medication side effects	1	2	3	4	5	NA
183621	Medication adverse effects	1	2	3	4	5	NA
183622	Potential medication interactions	1	2	3	4	5	NA
183623	Available support groups	1	2	3	4	5	NA
183624	Available community resources	1	2	3	4	5	NA
183625	When to obtain assistance from a health professional	1	2	3	4	5	NA

4th edition

Outcome Content References:

Blazer, D. (2002). *Depression in late life* (3rd ed.). New York: Springer.

Crowe, M., Ward, N. Dunnachie, B., & Roberts, M. (2006). Characteristics of adolescent depression. *International Journal of Mental Health Nursing, 15*, 10-18.

Eller, L. S., Corless, I., Bunch, E. H., Kemppainen, J., Holzemer, W., Nokes, K., Portillo, C., & Nicholas, P. (2005). Self-care strategies for depressive symptoms in people with HIV disease. *Journal of Advanced Nursing, 51*(2), 119-130.

Patel, V., Branch, T., Mottur-Pilson, C., & Pinard, G. (2004). Public awareness about depression: The effectiveness of a patient guideline. *International Journal of Psychiatry in Medicine, 34*(1), 1-20.

Roes, N. A. (2006). Depression 101 for addiction counselors. *Addiction Professional*, pp. 36-37.

K

Knowledge: Diabetes Management—1820

Domain-Health Knowledge & Behavior (IV)

Class-Health Knowledge (S)

Scale(s)-No knowledge to Extensive knowledge (u)

Care Recipient:

Data Source:

Definition: Extent of understanding conveyed about diabetes mellitus, its treatment, and the prevention of complications

OUTCOME TARGET RATING: Maintain at_____   Increase to_____

Knowledge: Diabetes Management Overall Rating	No knowledge 1	Limited knowledge 2	Moderate knowledge 3	Substantial knowledge 4	Extensive knowledge 5	
INDICATORS:						
182030 Cause and contributing factors	1	2	3	4	5	NA
182031 Signs and symptoms of early disease	1	2	3	4	5	NA
182002 Role of diet in blood glucose control	1	2	3	4	5	NA
182003 Prescribed meal plan	1	2	3	4	5	NA
182004 Strategies to increase diet adherence	1	2	3	4	5	NA
182005 Role of exercise in blood glucose control	1	2	3	4	5	NA
182032 Role of sleep in blood glucose control	1	2	3	4	5	NA
182006 Hyperglycemia and related symptoms	1	2	3	4	5	NA
182007 Hyperglycemia prevention	1	2	3	4	5	NA
182008 Procedures to be followed in treating hyperglycemia	1	2	3	4	5	NA
182009 Hypoglycemia and related symptoms	1	2	3	4	5	NA
182010 Hypoglycemia prevention	1	2	3	4	5	NA
182011 Procedures to be followed in treating hypoglycemia	1	2	3	4	5	NA
182012 Importance of maintaining blood glucose level within target range	1	2	3	4	5	NA
182013 Impact of acute illness on blood glucose level	1	2	3	4	5	NA
182033 How to use a monitoring device	1	2	3	4	5	NA
182015 Actions to take in response to blood glucose levels	1	2	3	4	5	NA
182016 Prescribed insulin regimen	1	2	3	4	5	NA
182034 Correct use of insulin	1	2	3	4	5	NA

K

		No knowledge	Limited knowledge	Moderate knowledge	Substantial knowledge	Extensive knowledge	
182027	Proper technique to draw up and administer insulin	1	2	3	4	5	NA
182018	Plan for rotation of injection sites	1	2	3	4	5	NA
182019	Onset, peak and duration of prescribed insulin	1	2	3	4	5	NA
182035	Proper disposal of syringes and needles	1	2	3	4	5	NA
182020	Prescribed oral medication regimen	1	2	3	4	5	NA
182036	Correct use of prescribed medication	1	2	3	4	5	NA
182037	Correct use of non-prescription medication	1	2	3	4	5	NA
182038	Proper medication storage	1	2	3	4	5	NA
182039	Medication therapeutic effects	1	2	3	4	5	NA
182040	Medication side effects	1	2	3	4	5	NA
182041	Medication adverse effects	1	2	3	4	5	NA
182042	When to obtain assistance from a health professional	1	2	3	4	5	NA
182028	Correct procedure for urine ketone testing	1	2	3	4	5	NA
182029	Importance of dilated eye exam and vision testing by an ophthalmologist	1	2	3	4	5	NA
182023	Preventive foot care practices	1	2	3	4	5	NA
182043	Reputable sources of diabetes information	1	2	3	4	5	NA
182024	Benefits of disease management	1	2	3	4	5	NA

2nd edition 2000; Revised 3rd edition 2004; Revised 4th edition

K

Outcome Content References:

Anderson, S. (1994). 7 care tips for managing patients with diabetes. *American Journal of Nursing, 94*(9), 36-38.

Boucher, J. L., Swift, C. S., Franz, M. J., Kulkami, K., Schafer, R. G., Pritchett, E., & Clark, N. G. (2007). Inpatient management of diabetes and hyperglycemia: Implications for nutrition practice and the food and nutrition professional. *Journal of the American Dietetic Association, 107*(1), 105-111.

Brody, G. (1992). Diabetic ketoacidosis and hyperosmolar hyperglycemic nonketotic coma. *Topics of Emergency Medicine, 14*(1), 12-22.

Cameron, B. L. (2002). Making diabetes management routine: How often do you and your patients screen for complications? *American Journal of Nursing, 102*(2), 26-33.

Carlson, M. (1994). Diabetic emergencies: A clinical review. *Journal of the American Academy of Physician Assistants, 7*(2), 79-86.

Clark, A. (1994). Complications and management of diabetes. *Critical Care Nursing of North America, 6*(4), 723-733.

Dalewitz, J., Khan, N., & Hershey, C. O. (2000). Barriers to control blood glucose in diabetes mellitus. *American Journal of Medical Quality, 15*(1), 16-25.

Franz, M. J. (Ed.) (2000). *A core curriculum for diabetes education* (4th ed.). Chicago, IL: American Association of Diabetes Educators.

Ibrahem, I. A. (2006). Diabetes mellitus. In D. L. Huber (Ed.), *Disease management: A guide for case managers* (pp. 81-99). St. Louis: Saunders.

Jones, T. (1994). From diabetic ketoacidosis to hyperglycemic hyperosmolar nonketotic syndrome. *Critical Care Nursing Clinics of North America, 6*(4), 703-721.

Loewen, S., & Haas, L. (1991). Complications of diabetes: Acute and chronic. *Nurse Practitioner Forum, 2*(3), 181-187.

Miller, D. K., & Fain, J. A. (2006). Diabetes self-management education. *Nursing Clinics of North America, 41*, 655-666.

Norton, R. (1995). The right mix of diet and exercise, *RN, 58*(4), 20-24.

Peragallo-Dittko, V. (1995). Diabetes 2000: Acute complications. *RN, 58*(8), 36-41.

Reising, D. L. (1995). Acute hypoglycemia: Keeping the bottom from falling out. *Nursing 25*(2), 41-48.

Knowledge: Diet—1802

Domain-Health Knowledge & Behavior (IV)

Class-Health Knowledge (S)

Scale(s)-No knowledge to Extensive knowledge (u)

Care Recipient:

Data Source:

Definition: Extent of understanding conveyed about recommended diet

OUTCOME TARGET RATING: Maintain at_____   Increase to_____

Knowledge: Diet Overall Rating	No knowledge 1	Limited knowledge 2	Moderate knowledge 3	Substantial knowledge 4	Extensive knowledge 5	
INDICATORS:						
180201 Recommended diet	1	2	3	4	5	NA
180202 Rationale for diet	1	2	3	4	5	NA
180203 Advantages of diet	1	2	3	4	5	NA
180204 Dietary goals	1	2	3	4	5	NA
180205 Relationship among diet, exercise, and weight	1	2	3	4	5	NA
180206 Food allowed in diet	1	2	3	4	5	NA
180218 Fluid allowed in diet	1	2	3	4	5	NA
180207 Food to avoid in diet	1	2	3	4	5	NA
180219 Fluid to avoid in diet	1	2	3	4	5	NA
180208 Interpretation of food labels	1	2	3	4	5	NA
180209 Guidelines for food preparation	1	2	3	4	5	NA
180220 Healthy nutritional practices	1	2	3	4	5	NA
180211 Menu planning using dietary guidelines	1	2	3	4	5	NA
180212 Strategies to change dietary habits	1	2	3	4	5	NA
180213 Diet plans for social situations	1	2	3	4	5	NA
180217 Self-monitoring techniques	1	2	3	4	5	NA
180215 Potential food and medication interactions	1	2	3	4	5	NA

Specify diet_____

1st edition 1997; Revised 3rd edition 2004; Revised 4th edition

Outcome Content References:

Bloomgarden, Z. T., Karmally, W., Metzger, J., Brothers, M., Nechemias, C., Bookman, J., Faierman, D., Ginsberg-Fellner, F., Rayfield, E., & Brown, W. V. (1987). Randomized controlled trial of diabetic patient education: Improved knowledge without improved metabolic status. *Diabetes Care, 10*(3), 263-272.

Bushnell, F. (1992). Self-care teaching for congestive heart failure patients. *Journal of Gerontological Nursing, 18*(10), 27-32.

Conn, V. S., Armer, J. M., & Hayes, K. S. (2001). Knowledge deficit. In M. Maas, K. Buckwalter, M. Hardy, T. Tripp-Reimer, M. Titler, & J. Specht (Eds.), *Nursing care of older adults: Diagnoses, outcomes & interventions* (pp. 503-515). St. Louis: Mosby.

Devins, G. M., Binik, Y. M., Mandin, H., Litourneau, P. K., Hollomby, D. J., Barre, P. E., & Prichard, S. (1990). The Kidney Disease Questionnaire: A test for measuring patient knowledge about end-stage renal disease. *Journal of Clinical Epidemiology, 43*(3), 297-307.

Garrard, J., Joynes, J. O., Mullen, L., McNeil, L., Mensing, C., Feste, C., & Etzwiler, D. D. (1987). Psychometric study of patient knowledge test. *Diabetes Care, 10*(4), 500-509.

K

Gilden, J. L., Hendryx, M., Casia, C., & Singh, S. P. (1989). The effectiveness of diabetes education programs for older patients and their spouses. *Journal of American Geriatrics Society, 37*(11), 1023-1030.

Mazzuca, S. A., Moorman, N. H., Wheeler, M. L., Norton, J. A., Fineberg, N. S., Vinicor, F., Cohen, S. J., & Clark, C. M. (1986). The diabetes education study: A controlled trial of the effects of diabetes patient education. *Diabetes Care, 9*(1), 1-10.

Redman, B. (1993). Knowledge deficit (specify). In J. M. Thompson, G. K. McFarland, J. E. Hirsch, & S. M. Tucker (Eds.), *Mosby's clinical nursing* (3rd ed., pp. 1548-1552). St. Louis: Mosby.

Scherer, Y. K., Janelli, L. M., & Schmieder, L. E. (1992). A time-series perspective of effectiveness of a health teaching program on chronic obstructive pulmonary disease. *Journal of Healthcare Education and Training, 6*(3), 7-13.

Smith, M. M., Hicks, V. L., & Heyward, V. H. (1991). Coronary disease knowledge test: Developing a valid and reliable tool. *Nurse Practitioner, 16*(4), 28, 31, 35-38.

K

Knowledge: Disease Process—1803

Domain-Health Knowledge & Behavior (IV)

Class-Health Knowledge (S)

Scale(s)-No knowledge to Extensive knowledge (u)

Care Recipient:

Data Source:

Definition: Extent of understanding conveyed about a specific disease process and prevention of complications

OUTCOME TARGET RATING: Maintain at_____   Increase to_____

Knowledge: Disease Process Overall Rating	No knowledge 1	Limited knowledge 2	Moderate knowledge 3	Substantial knowledge 4	Extensive knowledge 5	

INDICATORS:

180302	Specific disease process	1	2	3	4	5	NA
180303	Cause and contributing factors	1	2	3	4	5	NA
180304	Risk factors	1	2	3	4	5	NA
180305	Effects of disease	1	2	3	4	5	NA
180306	Signs and symptoms of disease	1	2	3	4	5	NA
180307	Usual course of disease process	1	2	3	4	5	NA
180308	Strategies to minimize disease progression	1	2	3	4	5	NA
180309	Potential complications of disease	1	2	3	4	5	NA
180310	Signs and symptoms of disease complications	1	2	3	4	5	NA
180311	Precautions to prevent complications of disease	1	2	3	4	5	NA
180313	Psychosocial effect of disease on self	1	2	3	4	5	NA
180314	Psychosocial effect of disease on family	1	2	3	4	5	NA
180315	Benefits of disease management	1	2	3	4	5	NA
180316	Available support groups	1	2	3	4	5	NA
180317	Reputable sources of disease-specific information	1	2	3	4	5	NA

Specify disease_____

1st edition 1997; Revised 3rd edition 2004; Revised 4th edition

Outcome Content References:

Bushnell, F. (1992). Self-care teaching for congestive heart failure patients. *Journal of Gerontological Nursing, 18*(10), 27-32.

Conn, V. S., Armer, J. M., & Hayes, K. S. (2001). Knowledge deficit. In M. Maas, K. Buckwalter, M. Hardy, T. Tripp-Reimer, M. Titler, & J. Specht (Eds.), *Nursing care of older adults: Diagnoses, outcomes & interventions* (pp. 503-515). St. Louis: Mosby.

Devins, G. M., Binik, Y. M., Mandin, H., Litourneau, P. K., Hollomby, D. J., Barre, P. E., & Prichard, S. (1990). The Kidney Disease Questionnaire: A test for measuring patient knowledge about end-stage renal disease. *Journal of Clinical Epidemiology, 43*(3), 297-307.

Garrard, J., Joynes, J. O., Mullen, L., McNeil, L., Mensing, C., Feste, C., & Etzwiler, D. D. (1987). Psychometric study of patient knowledge test. *Diabetes Care, 10*(4), 500-509.

Gilden, J. L., Hendryx, M., Casia, C., & Singh, S. P. (1989). The effectiveness of diabetes education programs for older patients and their spouses. *Journal of American Geriatrics Society, 37*(11), 1023-1030.

Mazzuca, S. A., Moorman, N. H., Wheeler, M. L., Norton, J. A., Fineberg, N. S., Vinicor, F., Cohen, S. J., & Clark, C. M. (1986). The diabetes education study: A controlled trial of the effects of diabetes patient education. *Diabetes Care, 9*(1), 1-10.

Redman, B. (1993). Knowledge deficit (specify). In J. M. Thompson, G. K. McFarland, J. E. Hirsch, & S. M. Tucker (Eds.), *Mosby's clinical nursing* (3rd ed., pp. 1548-1552). St. Louis: Mosby.

Scherer, Y. K., Janelli, L. M., & Schmieder, L. E. (1992). A time-series perspective of effectiveness of a health teaching program on chronic obstructive pulmonary disease. *Journal of Healthcare Education and Training, 6*(3), 7-13.

Smith, M. M., Hicks, V. L., & Heyward, V. H. (1991). Coronary Disease Knowledge Test: Developing a valid and reliable tool. *Nurse Practitioner, 16*(4), 28, 31, 35-38.

Wright, L. K. (2001). Sexual dysfunction. In M. Maas, K. Buckwalter, M. Hardy, T. Tripp-Reimer, M. Titler, & J. Specht (Eds.), *Nursing care of older adults: Diagnoses, outcomes & interventions* (pp. 733-749). St. Louis: Mosby.

K

Knowledge: Energy Conservation—1804

Domain-Health Knowledge & Behavior (IV)

Class-Health Knowledge (S)

Scale(s)-No knowledge to Extensive knowledge (u)

Care Recipient:

Data Source:

Definition: Extent of understanding conveyed about energy conservation techniques

OUTCOME TARGET RATING: Maintain at_____   Increase to_____

Knowledge: Energy Conservation Overall Rating	No knowledge 1	Limited knowledge 2	Moderate knowledge 3	Substantial knowledge 4	Extensive knowledge 5	
INDICATORS:						
180401 Recommended activity level	1	2	3	4	5	NA
180402 Activity restrictions	1	2	3	4	5	NA
180403 Appropriate activities	1	2	3	4	5	NA
180404 Factors that increase energy expenditure	1	2	3	4	5	NA
180405 Factors that decrease energy expenditure	1	2	3	4	5	NA
180406 Energy limitations	1	2	3	4	5	NA
180407 Strategies to balance activity and rest	1	2	3	4	5	NA
180416 Energy conservation techniques	1	2	3	4	5	NA
180422 Methods to monitor heart rate	1	2	3	4	5	NA
180423 Effective breathing technique	1	2	3	4	5	NA
180419 Proper body mechanics	1	2	3	4	5	NA
180420 Work simplification techniques	1	2	3	4	5	NA
180421 Correct use of assistive devices	1	2	3	4	5	NA

1st edition 1997; Revised 3rd edition 2004; Revised 4th edition

Outcome Content References:

Conn, V. S., Armer, J. M., & Hayes, K. S. (2001). Knowledge deficit. In M. Maas, K. Buckwalter, M. Hardy, T. Tripp-Reimer, M. Titler, & J. Specht (Eds.), *Nursing care of older adults: Diagnoses, outcomes & interventions* (pp. 503-515). St. Louis: Mosby.

Hart, L. K., & Freel, M. I. (1982). Fatigue. In C. M. Norris (Ed.), *Concept clarification in nursing* (pp. 251-261). Rockville, MD: Aspen.

Lubkin, I. M. (2002). *Chronic illness: Impact and interventions* (5th ed.). Boston: Jones & Bartlett.

McFarlane, E. A. (1993). Activity intolerance. In J. M. Thompson, G. K. McFarland, J. E. Hirsch, & S. M. Tucker (Eds.), *Clinical nursing* (3rd ed., pp. 1498-1500). St. Louis: Mosby.

McFarlane, E. A. (1993). High risk for activity intolerance. In J. M. Thompson, G. K. McFarland, J. E. Hirsch, & S. M. Tucker (Eds.), *Clinical nursing* (3rd ed., pp. 1497-1498). St. Louis: Mosby.

Mock, V. L. (1993). Fatigue. In J. M. Thompson, G. K. McFarland, J. E. Hirsch, & S. M. Tucker (Eds.), *Clinical nursing* (3rd ed., pp. 1504-1506). St. Louis: Mosby.

Morris, M. L. (1982). Tiredness and fatigue. In C. M. Norris (Ed.), *Concept clarification in nursing* (pp. 263-275). Rockville, MD: Aspen.

Knowledge: Fall Prevention—1828

Domain-Health Knowledge & Behavior (IV)

Class-Health Knowledge (S)

Scale(s)-No knowledge to Extensive knowledge (u)

Care Recipient:

Data Source:

Definition: Extent of understanding conveyed about prevention of falls						

OUTCOME TARGET RATING: Maintain at_____   Increase to_____

Knowledge: Fall Prevention Overall Rating	No knowledge 1	Limited knowledge 2	Moderate knowledge 3	Substantial knowledge 4	Extensive knowledge 5	
INDICATORS:						
182801 Correct use of assistive devices	1	2	3	4	5	NA
182802 Correct use of safety devices	1	2	3	4	5	NA
182803 Appropriate footwear	1	2	3	4	5	NA
182804 Correct use of grab bars	1	2	3	4	5	NA
182805 Correct use of safety gates	1	2	3	4	5	NA
182806 Correct use of window guards	1	2	3	4	5	NA
182807 Correct use of environmental lighting	1	2	3	4	5	NA
182808 When to ask for personal assistance	1	2	3	4	5	NA
182809 Use of safe transfer procedure	1	2	3	4	5	NA
182810 Reason for restraints	1	2	3	4	5	NA
182811 Exercises to reduce risk for falls	1	2	3	4	5	NA
182812 Prescribed medications that increase risk for falls	1	2	3	4	5	NA
182813 Chronic conditions that increase risk for falls	1	2	3	4	5	NA
182814 Acute illnesses that increase risk for falls	1	2	3	4	5	NA
182815 Blood pressure changes that increase risk for falls	1	2	3	4	5	NA
182816 Non-prescription medications that increase risk for falls	1	2	3	4	5	NA
182817 Strategies to safely ambulate	1	2	3	4	5	NA
182818 Importance of maintaining clear walkway	1	2	3	4	5	NA
182819 Safe use of stools and ladders	1	2	3	4	5	NA
182820 Use of rubber mats	1	2	3	4	5	NA
182821 Strategies to keep floor surfaces safe	1	2	3	4	5	NA

3rd edition 2004; Revised 4th edition

K

Continued

Outcome Content References:

Bexon, J., Echevarria, K. H., & Smith, G. B. (1999). Nursing outcome indicator: Preventing falls for elderly people. *Outcomes Management for Nursing Practice, 3*(3), 112-116.

Edwards, B. J., & Lee, S. (1998). Gait disorders and falls in a retirement home: A pilot study. *Annals of Long-Term Care, 6*(4), 140-143.

Fleck, M. M., & Forrester, D. A. (2001). The efficacy of an educational program to improve direct caregiver knowledge regarding fall prevention. *Journal for Nurses in Staff Development, 17*(1), 27-33.

Hendrich, A. L. (1996). *Falls, immobility, and restraints: A resource manual.* St. Louis: Mosby.

Malmivaara, A., Heliovaara, M., Knekt, P., Reunanen, A., & Aromaa, A. (1993). Risk factors for injurious falls leading to hospitalization or death in a cohort of 19,500 adults. *American Journal of Epidemiology, 138*(6), 384-394.

Patient information. Decreasing your risks of falls. *American Family Physician, 56*(7), 1823.

Schoenfelder, D. P., Crowell, C. M., & The Nursing Diagnosis Extension and Classification Research Team (1999). From risk for trauma to unintentional injury risk: Falls—a concept analysis. *Nursing Diagnoses, 10*(4), 149-157.

Stevens, J. A., & Olson, S. (2000). Reducing falls and resulting hip fractures among older women. *Morbidity & Mortality Weekly Report, 49*(RR-2), 1-12.

Wortel, E., & de Geus, G. H. (1993). Prevention of home related injuries of pre-school children: Safety measures taken by mothers. *Health Education Research, 8*(2), 217-231.

K

Knowledge: Fertility Promotion—1816

Domain-Health Knowledge & Behavior (IV)

Class-Health Knowledge (S)

Scale(s)-No knowledge to Extensive knowledge (u)

Care Recipient:

Data Source:

Definition: Extent of understanding conveyed about fertility testing and the conditions that affect conception

OUTCOME TARGET RATING: Maintain at_____   Increase to_____

Knowledge: Fertility Promotion Overall Rating	No knowledge 1	Limited knowledge 2	Moderate knowledge 3	Substantial knowledge 4	Extensive knowledge 5	
INDICATORS:						
181601 Effect of age	1	2	3	4	5	NA
181602 Effect of coital frequency	1	2	3	4	5	NA
181603 Effect of nutrition	1	2	3	4	5	NA
181604 Hazards of weight loss	1	2	3	4	5	NA
181606 Effect of heat on sperm count	1	2	3	4	5	NA
181607 Effect of tight clothes on sperm count	1	2	3	4	5	NA
181608 Effect of physical anomalies	1	2	3	4	5	NA
181609 Effect of pelvic surgery	1	2	3	4	5	NA
181610 Effect of pelvic infections	1	2	3	4	5	NA
181611 Influence of vaginal/uterine environment	1	2	3	4	5	NA
181612 Effect of hormone levels	1	2	3	4	5	NA
181613 Effect of thyroid function	1	2	3	4	5	NA
181614 Use of basal body temperature to predict ovulation	1	2	3	4	5	NA
181615 Symptothermal method	1	2	3	4	5	NA
181616 Ultrasonography	1	2	3	4	5	NA
181617 Influence of semen characteristics	1	2	3	4	5	NA
181618 Influence of sperm count	1	2	3	4	5	NA
181619 Postcoital test	1	2	3	4	5	NA
181620 Fertility monitoring devices	1	2	3	4	5	NA
181621 Options to reverse sterilization	1	2	3	4	5	NA
181622 Methods for semen collection	1	2	3	4	5	NA

2nd edition 2000; Revised 3rd edition 2004; Revised 4th edition

K

Outcome Content References:

Fehring, R. J. (1991). New technology in natural family planning. *Journal of Obstetric, Gynecologic, and Neonatal Nursing, 20*(3), 199-205.

Grodstein, F., Goldman, M. B., & Cramer, D. W. (1994). Infertility in women and moderate alcohol use. *American Journal of Public Health, 84*(9), 1429-1432.

Halman, L. J., Abbey, A., & Andrews, F. M. (1992). Attitudes about infertility interventions among fertile and infertile couples. *American Journal of Public Health, 82*(2), 191-194.

Rudy, E. B., & Estok, P. (1992). Professional and lay interrater reliability of urinary luteinizing hormone surges measured by OvuQuick test. *Journal of Obstetric, Gynecologic, and Neonatal Nursing, 21*(5), 407-410.

Shane, J. M. (1993). Evaluation and treatment of infertility. *Clinical Symposia, 45*(2), 2-32.

Toner, J. P., & Flood, J. T. (1993). Fertility after the age of 40. *Obstetrics and Gynecology Clinics of North America, 20*(2), 261-272.

Knowledge: Health Behavior—1805

Domain-Health Knowledge & Behavior (IV)

Class-Health Knowledge (S)

Scale(s)-No knowledge to Extensive knowledge (u)

Care Recipient:

Data Source:

Definition: Extent of understanding conveyed about the promotion and protection of health

OUTCOME TARGET RATING: Maintain at_____   Increase to_____

Knowledge: Health Behavior Overall Rating	No knowledge 1	Limited knowledge 2	Moderate knowledge 3	Substantial knowledge 4	Extensive knowledge 5	
INDICATORS:						
180501 Healthy nutritional practices	1	2	3	4	5	NA
180502 Benefits of activity and exercise	1	2	3	4	5	NA
180503 Strategies to manage stress	1	2	3	4	5	NA
180504 Normal sleep-wake patterns	1	2	3	4	5	NA
180505 Methods of family planning	1	2	3	4	5	NA
180506 Adverse health effects of tobacco use	1	2	3	4	5	NA
180507 Adverse health effects of alcohol misuse	1	2	3	4	5	NA
180508 Adverse health effects of recreational drug use	1	2	3	4	5	NA
180509 Safe use of prescribed medication	1	2	3	4	5	NA
180510 Safe use of non-prescription medication	1	2	3	4	5	NA
180511 Effect of caffeine use	1	2	3	4	5	NA
180512 Strategies to reduce the risk of accidental injury	1	2	3	4	5	NA
180513 Strategies to avoid exposure to environmental hazards	1	2	3	4	5	NA
180514 Strategies to prevent transmission of infectious disease	1	2	3	4	5	NA
180518 Health promotion services	1	2	3	4	5	NA
180519 Health protection services	1	2	3	4	5	NA
180516 Self-screening techniques	1	2	3	4	5	NA

1st edition 1997; Revised 3rd edition 2004; Revised 4th edition

Outcome Content References:

Conn, V. S., Armer, J. M., & Hayes, K. S. (2001). Knowledge deficit. In M. Maas, K. Buckwalter, M. Hardy, T. Tripp-Reimer, M. Titler, & J. Specht (Eds.), *Nursing care of older adults: Diagnoses, outcomes & interventions* (pp. 503-515). St. Louis: Mosby.

Simons-Morton, D. G., Mullen, P. D., Mains, D. A., Tabak, E. R., & Green, L. W. (1992). Characteristics of controlled studies of patient education and counseling for preventive health behaviors. *Patient Education and Counseling, 19*(2), 174-204.

Spellbring, A. M. (1991). Nursing's role in health promotion. *Nursing Clinics of North America, 16*(4), 805-814.

Tanner, E. K. W. (1991). Assessment of a health-promotive lifestyle. *Nursing Clinics of North America, 26*(4), 845-854.

U. S. Department of Health and Human Services. (1990). *Healthy People 2000. National health promotion and disease prevention objectives*. Washington, DC: Government Printing Office.

U. S. Department of Health and Human Services. (1998). *Clinician's handbook of preventive services: Put prevention into practice* (2nd ed.) Washington, DC: Government Printing Office.

Knowledge: Health Promotion—1823

Domain-Health Knowledge & Behavior (IV)

Class-Health Knowledge (S)

Scale(s)-No knowledge to Extensive knowledge (u)

Care Recipient:

Data Source:

Definition: Extent of understanding conveyed about information needed to obtain and maintain optimal health

OUTCOME TARGET RATING: Maintain at_____   Increase to_____

Knowledge: Health Promotion Overall Rating	No knowledge 1	Limited knowledge 2	Moderate knowledge 3	Substantial knowledge 4	Extensive knowledge 5	
INDICATORS:						
182308 Behaviors that promote health	1	2	3	4	5	NA
182309 Strategies to manage stress	1	2	3	4	5	NA
182310 Recommended health screenings	1	2	3	4	5	NA
182311 Recommended immunizations	1	2	3	4	5	NA
182321 Recommended self-screening for cancer detection	1	2	3	4	5	NA
182312 Reputable health care resources	1	2	3	4	5	NA
182313 Prevention and control of infection	1	2	3	4	5	NA
182314 Behaviors to prevent unintentional injuries	1	2	3	4	5	NA
182315 Behaviors to protect skin from sun exposure	1	2	3	4	5	NA
182316 Safe management of medication	1	2	3	4	5	NA
182322 Adverse health effects of alcohol misuse	1	2	3	4	5	NA
182323 Adverse health effects of tobacco use	1	2	3	4	5	NA
182324 Adverse health effects of drug use	1	2	3	4	5	NA
182318 Healthy nutritional practices	1	2	3	4	5	NA
182319 Strategies for weight management	1	2	3	4	5	NA
182320 Effective exercise routine	1	2	3	4	5	NA
182325 Relationship among diet, exercise, and weight	1	2	3	4	5	NA
182326 Strategies to avoid exposure to environmental hazards	1	2	3	4	5	NA
182327 Risk for hereditary disease	1	2	3	4	5	NA
182328 Reputable sources of information	1	2	3	4	5	NA

2nd edition 2000; Revised 3rd edition 2004; Revised 4th edition

Outcome Content References:

This is a general outcome that combines the following: Knowledge: Health Behavior, Knowledge: Health Resources, Knowledge: Personal Safety, Knowledge: Substance Use Control, Knowledge: Diet.

Knowledge: Health Resources—1806

Domain-Health Knowledge & Behavior (IV)

Class-Health Knowledge (S)

Scale(s)-No knowledge to Extensive knowledge (u)

Care Recipient:

Data Source:

Definition: Extent of understanding conveyed about relevant health care resources

OUTCOME TARGET RATING: Maintain at_____   Increase to_____

Knowledge: Health Resources Overall Rating	No knowledge 1	Limited knowledge 2	Moderate knowledge 3	Substantial knowledge 4	Extensive knowledge 5	
INDICATORS:						
180601 Reputable health care resources	1	2	3	4	5	NA
180602 When to obtain assistance from a health professional	1	2	3	4	5	NA
180603 Emergency measures	1	2	3	4	5	NA
180604 Emergency care resources	1	2	3	4	5	NA
180605 Importance of follow-up care	1	2	3	4	5	NA
180606 Plan for follow-up care	1	2	3	4	5	NA
180607 Available community resources	1	2	3	4	5	NA
180608 Strategies to access health care services	1	2	3	4	5	NA

1st edition 1997; Revised 3rd edition 2004; Revised 4th edition

Outcome Content References:

Bull, M. J. (1994). Patients' and professionals' perceptions of quality in discharge planning. *Journal of Nursing Care Quality, 8*(2), 47-61.

Conn, V. S., Armer, J. M., & Hayes, K. S. (2001). Knowledge deficit. In M. Maas, K. Buckwalter, M. Hardy, T. Tripp-Reimer, M. Titler, & J. Specht (Eds.), *Nursing care of older adults: Diagnoses, outcomes & interventions* (pp. 503-515). St. Louis: Mosby.

Redman, B. (1993). Knowledge deficit (specify). In J. M. Thompson, G. K. McFarland, J. E. Hirsch, & S. M. Tucker (Eds.), *Mosby's clinical nursing* (3rd ed., pp. 1548-1552). St. Louis: Mosby.

Wyness, M. A. (1990). Evaluation of an educational program for patients taking warfarin. *Journal of Advanced Nursing, 15*(9), 1052-1063.

Knowledge: Hypertension Management—1837

Domain-Health Knowledge & Behavior (IV)

Class-Health Knowledge (S)

Scale(s)-No knowledge to Extensive knowledge (u)

Care Recipient:

Data Source:

Definition: Extent of understanding conveyed about high blood pressure, its treatment, and the prevention of complications

OUTCOME TARGET RATING: 　　Maintain at_____　　　　Increase to_____

Knowledge: Hypertension Management Overall Rating	No knowledge 1	Limited knowledge 2	Moderate knowledge 3	Substantial knowledge 4	Extensive knowledge 5	

INDICATORS:

183701	Normal range for systolic blood pressure	1	2	3	4	5	NA
183702	Normal range for diastolic blood pressure	1	2	3	4	5	NA
183703	Target blood pressure	1	2	3	4	5	NA
183704	Methods to measure blood pressure	1	2	3	4	5	NA
183705	Potential complications of hypertension	1	2	3	4	5	NA
183706	Available treatment options	1	2	3	4	5	NA
183707	Importance of long-term treatment	1	2	3	4	5	NA
183708	Signs and symptoms of exacerbation of hypertension	1	2	3	4	5	NA
183709	Correct use of prescribed medication	1	2	3	4	5	NA
183710	Medication therapeutic effects	1	2	3	4	5	NA
183711	Medication side effects	1	2	3	4	5	NA
183712	Medication adverse effects	1	2	3	4	5	NA
183713	Importance of adherence to treatment	1	2	3	4	5	NA
183714	Importance of informing health professional of all current medication	1	2	3	4	5	NA
183715	Importance of keeping follow-up appointments	1	2	3	4	5	NA
183716	Benefits of ongoing self-monitoring	1	2	3	4	5	NA
183717	Recommended schedule for monitoring blood pressure	1	2	3	4	5	NA
183718	Benefits of weight loss	1	2	3	4	5	NA
183719	Benefits of lifestyle modifications	1	2	3	4	5	NA
183720	Strategies to manage stress	1	2	3	4	5	NA

Continued

		No knowledge	Limited knowledge	Moderate knowledge	Substantial knowledge	Extensive knowledge	
183721	Recommended diet modifications	1	2	3	4	5	NA
183722	Strategies to change dietary habits	1	2	3	4	5	NA
183723	Strategies to limit sodium intake	1	2	3	4	5	NA
183724	Strategies to enhance diet adherence	1	2	3	4	5	NA
183725	Effects of alcohol use	1	2	3	4	5	NA
183726	Importance of tobacco abstinence	1	2	3	4	5	NA
183727	Benefits of activity and exercise	1	2	3	4	5	NA
183728	Reputable sources of hypertension information	1	2	3	4	5	NA
183729	Available support groups	1	2	3	4	5	NA
183730	When to obtain assistance from a health professional	1	2	3	4	5	NA
183731	Benefits of disease management	1	2	3	4	5	NA

4th edition

K

Outcome Content References:

Baster, T., & Baster-Brooks, C. (2005). Exercise and hypertension. *Australian Family Physician, 34*(6), 419-424.

Boulware, L. E., Daumit, G. L., Frick, Minkovitz, C. S., Lawrence, R. S., & Powe, N. R. (2001). An evidence-based review of patient-centered behavioral interventions for hypertension. *American Journal of Preventive Medicine, 21*(3), 221-232.

Kaplan, N. M. (2004). Lifestyle modifications for prevention and treatment of hypertension. *The Journal of Clinical Hypertension, 6*(12), 716-719.

Knight, E. L., Bohn, R. L., Wang, P. S., Glynn, R. J., Mogun, H., & Avorn, J. (2001). Predictors of uncontrolled hypertension in ambulatory patients. *Hypertension, 38*(4), 809-814.

Morisky, D. E., Bowler, M. H., & Finlay, J. S. (1982). An educational and behavioral approach toward increasing patient activation in hypertension management. *Journal of Community Health, 7*(3), 171-182.

The National Collaborating Centre for Chronic Conditions. (2006). *Hypertension. Management of hypertension in adults in primary care: Partial update.* London: Royal College of Physicians.

Padwal, R., Campbell, N., Touyz, R. M. (2005). Applying the 2005 Canadian hypertension education program recommendations: 3. Lifestyle modifications to prevent and treat hypertension. *CMAJ, 173*(7), 749-751.

Svetkey, L. P., Erlinger, T. P., Vollmer, W. M., Feldstein, A., Cooper, L. S., Appel, L. J., Ard, J. D., Elmer, P. J., Harsha, D., & Stevens, V. J. (2005). Effect of lifestyle modifications on blood pressure by race, sex, hypertension status, and age. *Journal of Human Hypertension, 19*, 21-31.

U. S. Department of Health and Human Services. (2003). *Your guide to lowering blood pressure.* Bethesda, MD: Author.

Zernike, W., & Henderson, A. (1998). Evaluating the effectiveness of two teaching strategies for patients diagnosed with hypertension. *Journal of Clinical Nursing, 7*(1), 37-44.

Knowledge: Illness Care—1824

Domain-Health Knowledge & Behavior (IV)

Class-Health Knowledge (S)

Scale(s)-No knowledge to Extensive knowledge (u)

Care Recipient:

Data Source:

Definition: Extent of understanding conveyed about illness-related information needed to achieve and maintain optimal health

OUTCOME TARGET RATING: Maintain at_____   Increase to_____

Knowledge: Illness Care Overall Rating	No knowledge 1	Limited knowledge 2	Moderate knowledge 3	Substantial knowledge 4	Extensive knowledge 5	
INDICATORS:						
182401 Recommended diet	1	2	3	4	5	NA
182402 Specific disease process	1	2	3	4	5	NA
182403 Energy conservation techniques	1	2	3	4	5	NA
182404 Prevention and control of infection	1	2	3	4	5	NA
182405 Correct use of prescribed medication	1	2	3	4	5	NA
182406 Prescribed activity and exercise	1	2	3	4	5	NA
182407 Treatment procedure	1	2	3	4	5	NA
182408 Treatment regimen	1	2	3	4	5	NA
182409 Reputable health care resources	1	2	3	4	5	NA

2nd edition 2000; Revised 3rd edition 2004; Revised 4th edition

Outcome Content References:

This is a general outcome that combines the following: Knowledge: Diet, Knowledge: Disease Process, Knowledge: Energy Conservation, Knowledge: Medication, Knowledge: Prescribed Activity, Knowledge: Treatment Procedure, Knowledge: Treatment Regimen, Knowledge: Health Resources.

K

Knowledge: Infant Care—1819

Domain-Health Knowledge & Behavior (IV)

Class-Health Knowledge (S)

Scale(s)-No knowledge to Extensive knowledge (u)

Care Recipient:

Data Source:

Definition: Extent of understanding conveyed about caring for a baby from birth to first birthday		

OUTCOME TARGET RATING: Maintain at_____   Increase to_____

Knowledge: Infant Care Overall Rating	No knowledge 1	Limited knowledge 2	Moderate knowledge 3	Substantial knowledge 4	Extensive knowledge 5	
INDICATORS:						
181901 Normal infant characteristics	1	2	3	4	5	NA
181902 Normal growth and development	1	2	3	4	5	NA
181903 Proper holding of infant	1	2	3	4	5	NA
181904 Proper infant positioning	1	2	3	4	5	NA
181905 Infant safety practices	1	2	3	4	5	NA
181906 Swaddling	1	2	3	4	5	NA
181928 Age-appropriate cardiopulmonary resuscitation techniques	1	2	3	4	5	NA
181908 Nutritive versus nonnutritive sucking	1	2	3	4	5	NA
181909 Pros and cons of infant feeding choices	1	2	3	4	5	NA
181910 Infant feeding technique	1	2	3	4	5	NA
181911 Signs and symptoms of dehydration	1	2	3	4	5	NA
181912 Signs of jaundice	1	2	3	4	5	NA
181913 Infant bathing	1	2	3	4	5	NA
181914 Umbilical cord care	1	2	3	4	5	NA
181915 Infant diapering	1	2	3	4	5	NA
181916 Appropriate clothing for environment	1	2	3	4	5	NA
181917 Methods to measure body temperature	1	2	3	4	5	NA
181918 Infant sleep-wake patterns	1	2	3	4	5	NA
181919 Infant communication cues	1	2	3	4	5	NA
181920 Infant stimulation methods	1	2	3	4	5	NA
181921 Infant relaxation techniques	1	2	3	4	5	NA
181922 Strategies to adjust to addition of infant	1	2	3	4	5	NA
181923 Special care needs	1	2	3	4	5	NA

K

		No knowledge	Limited knowledge	Moderate knowledge	Substantial knowledge	Extensive knowledge	
181924	Considerations when choosing a childcare provider	1	2	3	4	5	NA
181926	Precautions when pets are in the household	1	2	3	4	5	NA
181925	Available community resources	1	2	3	4	5	NA
181929	Available support groups	1	2	3	4	5	NA

2nd edition 2000; Revised 3rd edition 2004; Revised 4th edition

Outcome Content References:

Association of Women's Health, Obstetricians and Neonatal Nurses. (1998). *Standards & guidelines for the professional nursing practice in the care of women and newborns* (5th ed.). Washington, DC: Author.

Nichols, F., & Humenick, S. (2000). *Childbirth education: Practice, research and theory* (2nd ed.). Philadelphia: W.B. Saunders.

Reeder, S. J., Martin, L. L., & Koniak-Griffin, D. (1997). *Maternity nursing: Family, newborn, and women's health care* (18th ed.). Philadelphia: Lippincott.

K

Knowledge: Infection Management—1842

Domain-Health Knowledge & Behavior (IV)

Class-Health Knowledge (S)

Scale(s)-No knowledge to Extensive knowledge (u)

Care Recipient:

Data Source:

> **Definition:** Extent of understanding conveyed about infection, its treatment, and the prevention of complications

OUTCOME TARGET RATING: Maintain at_____   Increase to_____

Knowledge: Infection Management Overall Rating	No knowledge 1	Limited knowledge 2	Moderate knowledge 3	Substantial knowledge 4	Extensive knowledge 5	
INDICATORS:						
184201 Mode of transmission	1	2	3	4	5	NA
184202 Factors contributing to transmission	1	2	3	4	5	NA
184203 Practices that reduce transmission	1	2	3	4	5	NA
184204 Signs and symptoms of infection	1	2	3	4	5	NA
180706 Monitoring procedures for infection	1	2	3	4	5	NA
184207 Importance of hand sanitation	1	2	3	4	5	NA
184208 Activities to increase resistance to infection	1	2	3	4	5	NA
184209 Treatment for diagnosed infection	1	2	3	4	5	NA
184210 Follow-up for diagnosed infection	1	2	3	4	5	NA
184211 Signs and symptoms of exacerbation of infection	1	2	3	4	5	NA
180712 Identification of correct name of medication	1	2	3	4	5	NA
184213 Medication side effects	1	2	3	4	5	NA
184214 Medication therapeutic effects	1	2	3	4	5	NA
184215 Medication adverse effects	1	2	3	4	5	NA
184216 Potential medication interactions	1	2	3	4	5	NA
184217 Importance of adherence to treatment	1	2	3	4	5	NA
184218 Use of probiotics in the treatment of infection	1	2	3	4	5	NA
184219 Risk of drug resistance	1	2	3	4	5	NA
184220 Importance of completing medication regimen	1	2	3	4	5	NA
184221 Influences of nutritional practices on infection	1	2	3	4	5	NA

K

		No knowledge	Limited knowledge	Moderate knowledge	Substantial knowledge	Extensive knowledge	
184222	Strategies to manage stress	1	2	3	4	5	NA
184223	Factors that affect immune response	1	2	3	4	5	NA
184224	Available support groups	1	2	3	4	5	NA
184225	Available community resources	1	2	3	4	5	NA
184226	When to obtain assistance from a health professional	1	2	3	4	5	NA

4th edition

Outcome Content References:

Centers for Disease Control and Prevention, National Center for HIV, STD, and TB Prevention & Division of Tuberculosis Elimination. (2000). *Core curriculum on tuberculosis* (4th ed.). Atlanta, GA: U.S. Department of Health and Human Services.

Conn, V. S., Armer, J. M., & Hayes, K. S. (2001). Knowledge deficit. In M. Maas, K. Buckwalter, M. Hardy, T. Tripp-Reimer, M. Titler, & J. Specht (Eds.), *Nursing care of older adults: Diagnoses, outcomes & interventions* (pp. 503-515). St. Louis: Mosby.

Joseph, A. (2006). *The impact of the environment on infections in healthcare facilities.* Princeton, NJ: Robert Wood Johnson Foundation.

National Center for Nursing Research. (1990). *HIV infection: Prevention and care.* Bethesda, MD: U. S. Department of Health and Human Services.

Rotheram-Borus, M. J., Reid, M. A., & Rosario, M. (1994). Factors mediating changes in sexual HIV risk behaviors among gay and bisexual male adolescents. *American Journal of Public Health, 84*(12), 1938-1946.

Simons-Morton, D. G., Mullen, P. D., Mains, D. A., Tabak, E. R., & Green, L. W. (1992). Characteristics of controlled studies of patient education and counseling for preventive health behaviors. *Patient Education and Counseling, 19*(2), 174-204.

Statton, P., & Alexander, N. J. (1993). Prevention of sexually transmitted infections: Physical and chemical barrier methods. *Infectious Disease Clinics of North America, 7*(4), 841-859.

Ungvarski, P. J., & Flaskerud, J. H. (1999). *HIV/AIDS: A guide to primary care management* (4th ed.). Philadelphia: W.B. Saunders.

K

Knowledge: Labor & Delivery—1817

Domain-Health Knowledge & Behavior (IV)

Class-Health Knowledge (S)

Scale(s)-No knowledge to Extensive knowledge (u)

Care Recipient:

Data Source:

Definition: Extent of understanding conveyed about labor and vaginal delivery

OUTCOME TARGET RATING: Maintain at_____   Increase to_____

Knowledge: Labor & Delivery Overall Rating	No knowledge 1	Limited knowledge 2	Moderate knowledge 3	Substantial knowledge 4	Extensive knowledge 5	

INDICATORS:

181701	Birthing options	1	2	3	4	5	NA
181702	Role of the labor coach	1	2	3	4	5	NA
181703	Signs and symptoms of labor	1	2	3	4	5	NA
181704	Stages of labor and delivery	1	2	3	4	5	NA
181705	Strategies to control pain	1	2	3	4	5	NA
181706	Effective breathing techniques	1	2	3	4	5	NA
181707	Effective relaxation techniques	1	2	3	4	5	NA
181708	Effective positioning techniques	1	2	3	4	5	NA
181709	Potential medical procedures	1	2	3	4	5	NA
181710	Potential complications of birthing	1	2	3	4	5	NA
181711	Effective pushing techniques	1	2	3	4	5	NA
181714	Delivery of infant	1	2	3	4	5	NA
181712	Delivery of placenta	1	2	3	4	5	NA

2nd edition 2000; Revised 3rd edition 2004; Revised 4th edition

Outcome Content References:

Association of Women's Health, Obstetric, and Neonatal Nurses (2004). *Core curriculum for maternal-newborn nursing.* Washington, DC: Author.

Nichols, F., & Humenick, S. (2000). *Childbirth education: Practice, research and theory* (2nd ed.). Philadelphia: W.B. Saunders.

Reeder, S. J., Martin, L. L., & Koniak-Griffin, D. (1997). *Maternity nursing: Family, newborn, and women's health care* (18th ed.). Philadelphia: Lippincott.

Knowledge: Medication—1808

Domain-Health Knowledge & Behavior (IV)

Class-Health Knowledge (S)

Scale(s)-No knowledge to Extensive knowledge (u)

Care Recipient:

Data Source:

Definition: Extent of understanding conveyed about the safe use of medication

OUTCOME TARGET RATING: Maintain at_____   Increase to_____

Knowledge: Medication Overall Rating	No knowledge 1	Limited knowledge 2	Moderate knowledge 3	Substantial knowledge 4	Extensive knowledge 5	
INDICATORS:						
180801 Importance of informing health professional of all current medication	1	2	3	4	5	NA
180802 Identification of correct name of medication	1	2	3	4	5	NA
180803 Appearance of medication	1	2	3	4	5	NA
180819 Medication therapeutic effects	1	2	3	4	5	NA
180805 Medication side effects	1	2	3	4	5	NA
180820 Medication adverse effects	1	2	3	4	5	NA
180807 Use of memory aids	1	2	3	4	5	NA
180808 Potential medication interactions	1	2	3	4	5	NA
180809 Potential interaction of medication with other agents	1	2	3	4	5	NA
180810 Correct use of prescribed medication	1	2	3	4	5	NA
180821 Correct use of non-prescription medication	1	2	3	4	5	NA
180822 Proper technique for self-injection	1	2	3	4	5	NA
180811 Self-monitoring techniques	1	2	3	4	5	NA
180812 Proper medication storage	1	2	3	4	5	NA
180815 Proper disposal of medication	1	2	3	4	5	NA
180813 Proper care of administration devices	1	2	3	4	5	NA
180823 Proper disposal of syringes and needles	1	2	3	4	5	NA
180824 Strategies to obtain required medication	1	2	3	4	5	NA
180825 Strategies to obtain required supplies	1	2	3	4	5	NA
180826 Available financial support	1	2	3	4	5	NA
180816 Required laboratory tests for monitoring medication	1	2	3	4	5	NA
180817 Importance of using medical alert identification	1	2	3	4	5	NA

Specify medication(s)_____

Continued

1st edition 1997; Revised 3rd edition 2004; Revised 4th edition

Outcome Content References:

Barry, K. (1993). Patient self-medication: An innovative approach to medication teaching. *Journal of Nursing Care Quality, 8*(1), 75-82.

Colley, C. A., & Lucas, L. M. (1993). Polypharmacy: The cure becomes the disease. *Journal of General Internal Medicine, 8(5),* 278-283.

Conn, V. S., Armer, J. M., & Hayes, K. S. (2001). Knowledge deficit. In M. Maas, K. Buckwalter, M. Hardy, T. Tripp-Reimer, M. Titler, & J. Specht (Eds.), *Nursing care of older adults: Diagnoses, outcomes & interventions* (pp. 503-515). St. Louis: Mosby.

Everitt, D. E., & Avorn, J. (1986). Drug prescribing for the elderly. *Archives of Internal Medicine, 146(12),* 2393-2396.

Kleoppel, J. W., & Henry, D. W. (1987). Teaching patients, families, and communities about their medications. In C. E. Smith (Ed.), *Patient education: Nurses in partnership with other health professionals,* (pp. 271-296). Philadelphia: W.B. Saunders.

Proos, M., Reiley, P., Eagan, J., Stengrevics, S., Castile, J., & Arian, D. (1992). A study of the effects of self-medication on patients' knowledge of and compliance with their medication regimen. *Journal of Nursing Care Quality,* (Special Report), 18-26.

Simons-Morton, D. G., Mullen, P. D., Mains, D. A., Tabak, E. R., & Green, L. W. (1992). Characteristics of controlled studies of patient education and counseling for preventive health behaviors. *Patient Education and Counseling, 19*(2), 174-204.

Togger, D. A., & Brenner, P. S. (2001). Metered dose inhalers. *American Journal of Nursing, 101*(10), 26-32, 38-39.

U. S. Department of Health and Human Services. (1990). *Healthy People 2000: National health promotion and disease prevention objectives.* Washington, DC: Government Printing Office.

U. S. Department of Health and Human Services. (1998). *Clinician's handbook of prevention services: Put prevention into practice* (2nd ed.) Washington, DC: Government Printing Office.

Waddell, D. L., Hummel, M. E., & Sumners, A. D. (2001). Three herbs you should get to know. *American Journal of Nursing, 101*(4), 48-54.

Weitzel, E. A. (2001). Risk for poisoning: Drug toxicity. In M. Maas, K. Buckwalter, M. Hardy, T. Tripp-Reimer, M. Titler, & J. Specht (Eds.), *Nursing care of older adults: Diagnoses, outcomes & interventions* (pp. 34-46). St. Louis: Mosby.

K

Knowledge: Multiple Sclerosis Management—1838

Domain-Health Knowledge & Behavior (IV)

Class-Health Knowledge (S)

Scale(s)-No knowledge to Extensive knowledge (u)

Care Recipient:

Data Source:

Definition: Extent of understanding conveyed about multiple sclerosis, its treatment, and the prevention of relapses or exacerbations

OUTCOME TARGET RATING: Maintain at_____   Increase to_____

Knowledge: Multiple Sclerosis Management Overall Rating	No knowledge 1	Limited knowledge 2	Moderate knowledge 3	Substantial knowledge 4	Extensive knowledge 5	
INDICATORS:						
183801 Signs and symptoms of multiple sclerosis	1	2	3	4	5	NA
183802 Usual course of disease process	1	2	3	4	5	NA
183803 Therapeutic effects of personal treatment regimen	1	2	3	4	5	NA
183804 Importance of rest for disease management	1	2	3	4	5	NA
183805 Relationship of fatigue to disease	1	2	3	4	5	NA
183806 Strategies to control fatigue	1	2	3	4	5	NA
183807 Factors that decrease energy expenditure	1	2	3	4	5	NA
183808 Energy conservation techniques	1	2	3	4	5	NA
183809 Strategies to manage stress	1	2	3	4	5	NA
183810 Factors that trigger relapse	1	2	3	4	5	NA
183811 Factors that trigger exacerbation	1	2	3	4	5	NA
183812 Strategies to control symptoms	1	2	3	4	5	NA
183813 Benefits of disease management	1	2	3	4	5	NA
183814 When to obtain assistance from a health professional	1	2	3	4	5	NA
183815 Medication therapeutic effects	1	2	3	4	5	NA
183816 Medication side effects	1	2	3	4	5	NA
183817 Medication adverse effects	1	2	3	4	5	NA
183818 Strategies to decrease treatment regimen side effects	1	2	3	4	5	NA
183819 Proper technique for self-injection	1	2	3	4	5	NA
183820 Potential interactions of prescribed medication with non-prescription medication	1	2	3	4	5	NA
183821 Alternative treatments	1	2	3	4	5	NA
183822 Strategies to cope with limitations	1	2	3	4	5	NA
183823 Effects of extreme heat or cold on disease	1	2	3	4	5	NA

K

Continued

		No knowledge	Limited knowledge	Moderate knowledge	Substantial knowledge	Extensive knowledge	
183824	Strategies to increase diet adherence	1	2	3	4	5	NA
183825	Strategies to increase resistance to infection	1	2	3	4	5	NA
183826	Strategies to balance activity and rest	1	2	3	4	5	NA
183827	Strategies to cope with unpredictability of disease	1	2	3	4	5	NA
183828	Strategies to enhance bladder and bowel function	1	2	3	4	5	NA
183829	Surgical treatment options	1	2	3	4	5	NA
183830	Available support groups	1	2	3	4	5	NA
183831	Available community resources	1	2	3	4	5	NA
183832	Adaptations for role performance	1	2	3	4	5	NA
183833	Reputable sources of multiple sclerosis information	1	2	3	4	5	NA

4th edition

Outcome Content References:

Denis, L., Namey, M., Costello, K., Frenette, J., Gagnon, N., Harris, C., Lowden, D., McEwan, L., Morrison, W., & Poirier, J. (2004). Long-term treatment optimization in individuals with multiple sclerosis using disease-modifying therapies: a nursing approach. *Journal of Neuroscience Nursing, 36*(1), 10-22.

Embrey, N., Lowndes, C., & Warner, R. (2003). Benchmarking best practice in relapse management of multiple sclerosis. *Nursing Standard, 17*(22), 38-42.

Jarrett, L. (2003). Attitudes to long-term care in multiple sclerosis. *Nursing Standard, 17*(17), 39-43.

Ozuna, J. M. (2004) Nursing management: Chronic neurologic problems. In S. M. Lewis, M. M. Heitkemper, & S. R. Dirksen, (Eds.) *Medical-surgical nursing: Assessment and management of clinical problems* (6th ed., pp. 1549-1580). St. Louis: Mosby .

MS Center at Washington University School of Medicine Website: http://www.neuro.wustl.edu/MS/

National Multiple Sclerosis Society. Website: http://www.nmss.org

Ward, N., & Winters, S. (2003). Results of a fatigue management programme in multiple sclerosis. *British Journal of Nursing, 12*(18), 1075-1080.

Knowledge: Ostomy Care—1829

Domain-Health Knowledge & Behavior (IV)

Class-Health Knowledge (S)

Scale(s)-No knowledge to Extensive knowledge (u)

Care Recipient:

Data Source:

Definition: Extent of understanding conveyed about maintenance of an ostomy for elimination

OUTCOME TARGET RATING: Maintain at_____   Increase to_____

Knowledge: Ostomy Care Overall Rating	No knowledge 1	Limited knowledge 2	Moderate knowledge 3	Substantial knowledge 4	Extensive knowledge 5	
INDICATORS:						
182902 Purpose of ostomy	1	2	3	4	5	NA
182901 Functioning of ostomy	1	2	3	4	5	NA
182909 Supplies required to care for ostomy	1	2	3	4	5	NA
182915 Procedure to change ostomy bag	1	2	3	4	5	NA
182908 Schedule for changing ostomy bag	1	2	3	4	5	NA
182905 How to measure stoma	1	2	3	4	5	NA
182907 Complications related to stoma	1	2	3	4	5	NA
182916 Procedure to empty ostomy bag	1	2	3	4	5	NA
182903 Skin care around ostomy	1	2	3	4	5	NA
182904 Irrigation technique	1	2	3	4	5	NA
182910 Identification of flatus-producing foods	1	2	3	4	5	NA
182911 Diet modifications	1	2	3	4	5	NA
182912 Fluid intake requirements	1	2	3	4	5	NA
182913 Odor control mechanisms	1	2	3	4	5	NA
182914 Modification of daily activities	1	2	3	4	5	NA
182917 Available support groups	1	2	3	4	5	NA

3rd edition 2004; Revised 4th edition

Outcome Content References:

Bryant, D., & Fleischer, I. (2000). Changing an ostomy appliance. *Nursing, 30*(11), 51-53.

O'Shea, H. S. (2001). Teaching the adult ostomy patient. *Journal of Wound, Ostomy, and Continence Nursing, 28*(1), 47-54.

Thompson, J. (2000). A practical ostomy guide. *RN, 63*(11), 61-68.

K

Knowledge: Pain Management—1843

Domain-Health Knowledge & Behavior (IV)

Class-Health Knowledge (S)

Scale(s)-No knowledge to Extensive knowledge (u)

Care Recipient:

Data Source:

Definition: Extent of understanding conveyed about causes, symptoms, and treatment of pain

OUTCOME TARGET RATING: Maintain at_____   Increase to_____

Knowledge: Pain Management Overall Rating	No knowledge 1	Limited knowledge 2	Moderate knowledge 3	Substantial knowledge 4	Extensive knowledge 5	

INDICATORS:

184301	Causes and contributing factors of pain	1	2	3	4	5	NA
184302	Signs and symptoms of pain	1	2	3	4	5	NA
184303	Strategies to control pain	1	2	3	4	5	NA
184304	Strategies to manage chronic pain	1	2	3	4	5	NA
184305	Prescribed medication regimen	1	2	3	4	5	NA
184306	Correct use of prescribed medication	1	2	3	4	5	NA
184307	Correct use of non-prescription medication	1	2	3	4	5	NA
184308	Safe use of prescribed medication	1	2	3	4	5	NA
184309	Safe use of non-prescription medication	1	2	3	4	5	NA
184310	Medication therapeutic effects	1	2	3	4	5	NA
184311	Medication side effects	1	2	3	4	5	NA
184312	Medication adverse effects	1	2	3	4	5	NA
184313	Potential medication interactions	1	2	3	4	5	NA
184314	Potential interaction of medication with other agents	1	2	3	4	5	NA
184315	Safety issues related to medication	1	2	3	4	5	NA
184316	Proper medication storage	1	2	3	4	5	NA
184317	Proper disposal of medication	1	2	3	4	5	NA
184318	Importance of complying with medication regimen	1	2	3	4	5	NA
184319	Importance of informing health professional of all current medication	1	2	3	4	5	NA
184320	Activity restrictions	1	2	3	4	5	NA
184321	Activity precautions	1	2	3	4	5	NA
184322	Effective positioning techniques	1	2	3	4	5	NA

K

		No knowledge	Limited knowledge	Moderate knowledge	Substantial knowledge	Extensive knowledge	
184323	Effective relaxation techniques	1	2	3	4	5	NA
184324	Effective guided imagery	1	2	3	4	5	NA
184325	Effective distraction	1	2	3	4	5	NA
184326	Effective heat/cold application	1	2	3	4	5	NA
184327	Effective electrical stimulation	1	2	3	4	5	NA
184328	Effective meditation techniques	1	2	3	4	5	NA
184329	Benefits of transcutaneous electrical nerve stimulation (TENS)	1	2	3	4	5	NA
184330	Benefits of hypnosis	1	2	3	4	5	NA
184331	Benefits of acupuncture	1	2	3	4	5	NA
184332	Benefits of biofeedback	1	2	3	4	5	NA
184333	Benefits of massage	1	2	3	4	5	NA
184334	Benefits of ongoing self-monitoring of pain	1	2	3	4	5	NA
184335	Benefits of lifestyle modifications to reduce pain	1	2	3	4	5	NA
184336	Benefits of weight loss to reduce pain	1	2	3	4	5	NA
184337	Strategies for preventive pain management	1	2	3	4	5	NA
184338	When to obtain assistance from a health professional	1	2	3	4	5	NA
184339	Available support groups	1	2	3	4	5	NA
184340	Available community resources	1	2	3	4	5	NA
184341	Reputable sources of information	1	2	3	4	5	NA

4th edition

Outcome Content References:

Barnes, S. (2001). Pain management: What do patients need to know and when do they need to know it? *Journal of PeriAnesthesia Nursing, 16*(2), 107-108.

Henrotin, Y. E., Cedraschi, C., Duplan, B., Bazin, T., & Duquesnoy, B. (2006). Information and low back pain management: A systematic review. *Spine, 31*(11), E326-E334.

Herr, K., & Kwekkeboom, K. (Eds.). (2003). Chronic pain management. *Nursing Clinics of North America, 38*, 403-560.

Sjoling, M., Nordahl, G., Olofsson, N., & Asplund, K. (2003). The impact of preoperative information on state anxiety, postoperative pain and satisfaction with pain management. *Patient Education and Counseling, 51*, 169-176.

K

Knowledge: Parenting—1826

Domain-Health Knowledge & Behavior (IV)

Class-Health Knowledge (S)

Scale(s)-No knowledge to Extensive knowledge (u)

Care Recipient:

Data Source:

Definition: Extent of understanding conveyed about provision of a nurturing and constructive environment for a child from 1 year through 17 years of age

OUTCOME TARGET RATING: Maintain at_____   Increase to_____

Knowledge: Parenting Overall Rating	No knowledge 1	Limited knowledge 2	Moderate knowledge 3	Substantial knowledge 4	Extensive knowledge 5	
INDICATORS:						
182601 Normal growth and development	1	2	3	4	5	NA
182602 Normal child behavior	1	2	3	4	5	NA
182603 Safety needs	1	2	3	4	5	NA
182604 Injury prevention	1	2	3	4	5	NA
182605 Nutrition needs	1	2	3	4	5	NA
182606 Physical care needs	1	2	3	4	5	NA
182607 Psychological needs	1	2	3	4	5	NA
182608 Emotional needs	1	2	3	4	5	NA
182609 Stimulation needs	1	2	3	4	5	NA
182610 Socialization needs	1	2	3	4	5	NA
182611 Spiritual needs	1	2	3	4	5	NA
182612 Moral guidance needs	1	2	3	4	5	NA
182613 Health supervision needs	1	2	3	4	5	NA
182614 Illness prevention	1	2	3	4	5	NA
182615 Management of common health problems	1	2	3	4	5	NA
182616 Age-appropriate expectations	1	2	3	4	5	NA
182620 Methods of discipline appropriate for developmental age	1	2	3	4	5	NA
182621 Methods of discipline appropriate for unacceptable behavior	1	2	3	4	5	NA
182618 Basic care needs	1	2	3	4	5	NA
182619 Effective communication strategies	1	2	3	4	5	NA
182622 Motor vehicle safety measures	1	2	3	4	5	NA
182623 Strategies to manage environmental risk factors	1	2	3	4	5	NA
182624 Strategies to prevent tobacco use	1	2	3	4	5	NA

K

		No knowledge	Limited knowledge	Moderate knowledge	Substantial knowledge	Extensive knowledge	
182625	Strategies to prevent alcohol use	1	2	3	4	5	NA
182626	Strategies to prevent recreational drug use	1	2	3	4	5	NA
182627	Strategies to prevent exposure to toxic chemicals	1	2	3	4	5	NA
182628	Available support groups	1	2	3	4	5	NA

3rd edition 2004; Revised 4th edition

Outcome Content References:

Craft-Rosenberg, M., & Denehy, J. (Eds.) (2001). *Nursing interventions for infants, children, and families.* Thousand Oaks, CA: Sage Publications.

Friedman, M. (1998). *Family nursing: Research, theory and practice* (4th ed.). Stamford, CT: Appleton & Lange.

Green, M., Palfrey, J. S. (Eds.). (2002). *Bright futures: Guidelines for health supervision of infants, children, and adolescents.* Arlington, VA: National Center for Education in Maternal and Child Health.

Murray, R., & Zenter, J. (1997). *Health assessment & promotion strategies through the life span* (6th ed.). Stamford, CT: Appleton & Lange.

K

Knowledge: Personal Safety—1809

Domain-Health Knowledge & Behavior (IV)

Class-Health Knowledge (S)

Scale(s)-No knowledge to Extensive knowledge (u)

Care Recipient:

Data Source:

Definition: Extent of understanding conveyed about prevention of unintentional injuries

OUTCOME TARGET RATING: Maintain at_____   Increase to_____

Knowledge: Personal Safety Overall Rating	No knowledge 1	Limited knowledge 2	Moderate knowledge 3	Substantial knowledge 4	Extensive knowledge 5	
INDICATORS:						
180901 Suffocation prevention measures	1	2	3	4	5	NA
180902 Fall prevention measures	1	2	3	4	5	NA
180903 Risk reduction strategies	1	2	3	4	5	NA
180904 Home safety measures	1	2	3	4	5	NA
180905 Water safety precautions	1	2	3	4	5	NA
180906 Fire safety measures	1	2	3	4	5	NA
180907 Burn prevention	1	2	3	4	5	NA
180908 Electrocution prevention	1	2	3	4	5	NA
180909 Poison prevention	1	2	3	4	5	NA
180910 Bicycle safety guidelines	1	2	3	4	5	NA
180911 Pedestrian safety measures	1	2	3	4	5	NA
180912 Benefits of protective helmet	1	2	3	4	5	NA
180913 Firearm safety measures	1	2	3	4	5	NA
180915 Motor vehicle safety measures	1	2	3	4	5	NA
180916 Emergency procedures	1	2	3	4	5	NA
180917 Age-specific safety risks	1	2	3	4	5	NA
180918 Personal risk behaviors	1	2	3	4	5	NA
180919 Work safety risks	1	2	3	4	5	NA
180920 Community safety risks	1	2	3	4	5	NA

1st edition 1997; Revised 3rd edition 2004; Revised 4th edition

Outcome Content References:

Conn, V. S., Armer, J. M., & Hayes, K. S. (2001). Knowledge deficit. In M. Maas, K. Buckwalter, M. Hardy, T. Tripp-Reimer, M. Titler, & J. Specht (Eds.), *Nursing care of older adults: Diagnoses, outcomes & interventions* (pp. 503-515). St. Louis: Mosby.

Simons-Morton, D. G., Mullen, P. D., Mains, D. A., Tabak, E. R., & Green, L. W. (1992). Characteristics of controlled studies of patient education and counseling for preventive health behaviors. Patient Education and Counseling, *19*(2), 174-204.

U. S. Department of Health and Human Services. (1990). *Healthy People 2000: National health promotion and disease prevention objectives.* Washington, DC: Government Printing Office.

U. S. Department of Health and Human Services. (1998). *Clinician's handbook of prevention services: Put prevention into practice* (2nd ed.) Washington, DC: Government Printing Office.

Knowledge: Postpartum Maternal Health—1818

Domain-Health Knowledge & Behavior (IV)

Class-Health Knowledge (S)

Scale(s)-No knowledge to Extensive knowledge (u)

Care Recipient:

Data Source:

> **Definition:** Extent of understanding conveyed about maternal health in the period following birth of infant

OUTCOME TARGET RATING: Maintain at_____   Increase to_____

Knowledge: Postpartum Maternal Health Overall Rating	No knowledge 1	Limited knowledge 2	Moderate knowledge 3	Substantial knowledge 4	Extensive knowledge 5	
INDICATORS:						
181801 Normal physical sensations following delivery	1	2	3	4	5	NA
181802 Routine monitoring	1	2	3	4	5	NA
181803 Normal vaginal discharge	1	2	3	4	5	NA
181804 Breast changes	1	2	3	4	5	NA
181805 Uterine involution patterns	1	2	3	4	5	NA
181806 Fundal massage	1	2	3	4	5	NA
181807 Perineal care	1	2	3	4	5	NA
181808 Episiotomy care	1	2	3	4	5	NA
181809 Cesarean section care	1	2	3	4	5	NA
181810 Coughing techniques following surgery	1	2	3	4	5	NA
181820 Recommended nutrient intake	1	2	3	4	5	NA
181821 Recommended fluid intake	1	2	3	4	5	NA
181822 Energy level changes	1	2	3	4	5	NA
181812 Strategies to balance activity and rest	1	2	3	4	5	NA
181813 Appropriate exercise	1	2	3	4	5	NA
181814 Time frame for resumption of sexual activity	1	2	3	4	5	NA
181815 Contraceptive options	1	2	3	4	5	NA
181816 Psychological changes	1	2	3	4	5	NA
181823 Postpartum body changes	1	2	3	4	5	NA
181824 Maternal role performance	1	2	3	4	5	NA
181825 Strategies to manage postpartum depression	1	2	3	4	5	NA
181826 Strategies to manage stress	1	2	3	4	5	NA
181827 Strategies to bond with infant	1	2	3	4	5	NA
181818 Available social support	1	2	3	4	5	NA
181828 When to obtain assistance from a health professional	1	2	3	4	5	NA

K

Continued

2nd edition 2000; Revised 3rd edition 2004; Revised 4th edition

Outcome Content References:

Association of Women's Health, Obstetricians and Neonatal Nurses. (1998). *Standards & guidelines for the professional nursing practice in the care of women and newborns* (5th ed.). Washington, DC: Author

Crowell, D. T. (1995). Weight change in the postpartum period. A review of the literature. *Journal of Nurse Midwifery, 40*(5), 418-423.

Nichols, F., & Humenick, S. (2000). *Childbirth education: Practice, research and theory* (2nd ed.). Philadelphia: W.B. Saunders.

Reeder, S. J., Martin, L. L., & Koniak-Griffin, D. (1997). *Maternity nursing: Family, newborn, and women's health care* (18th ed.). Philadelphia: Lippincott.

K

Knowledge: Preconception Maternal Health—1822

Domain-Health Knowledge & Behavior (IV)

Class-Health Knowledge (S)

Scale(s)-No knowledge to Extensive knowledge (u)

Care Recipient:

Data Source:

Definition: Extent of understanding conveyed about maternal health prior to conception to insure a healthy pregnancy

OUTCOME TARGET RATING: Maintain at_____   Increase to_____

Knowledge: Preconception Maternal Health Overall Rating	No knowledge 1	Limited knowledge 2	Moderate knowledge 3	Substantial knowledge 4	Extensive knowledge 5	
INDICATORS:						
182201 Factors to consider when deciding to become a parent	1	2	3	4	5	NA
182213 Usual course of pregnancy	1	2	3	4	5	NA
182203 Recommended diet	1	2	3	4	5	NA
182204 Strategies to balance activity and rest	1	2	3	4	5	NA
182214 Adverse effects of alcohol use	1	2	3	4	5	NA
182215 Adverse effects of tobacco	1	2	3	4	5	NA
182216 Adverse effects of drug use	1	2	3	4	5	NA
182206 Maternal risk factors	1	2	3	4	5	NA
182207 Environmental hazards at home that affect fetal development	1	2	3	4	5	NA
182211 Environmental hazards at work that affect fetal development	1	2	3	4	5	NA
182208 Risk for hereditary disease	1	2	3	4	5	NA
182217 Anatomic and physiological changes of pregnancy	1	2	3	4	5	NA
182212 Strategies to adjust to addition of infant	1	2	3	4	5	NA

K

2nd edition 2000; Revised 3rd edition 2004; Revised 4th edition

Outcome Content References:

Aneshensel, C. S., Becerra, R. M., Fielder, E. P., & Schuler, R. H. (1990). Onset of fertility-related events during adolescence: A prospective comparison of Mexican American and non-Hispanic White females. *American Journal of Public Health, 80*(8), 959-963.

Fehring, R. J. (1991). New technology in natural family planning. *Journal of Obstetric, Gynecologic, & Neonatal Nursing, 20*(3), 199-205.

Grodstein, F., Goldman, M. B., & Cramer, D. W. (1994). Infertility in women and moderate alcohol use. *American Journal of Public Health, 84*(9), 1429-1432.

Halman, L. J., Abbey, A., & Andrews, F. M. (1992). Attitudes about infertility interventions among fertile and infertile couples. *American Journal of Public Health, 82*(2), 191-194.

Rudy, E. B., & Estok, P. (1992). Professional and lay interrater reliability of urinary luteinizing hormone surges measured by OvuQuik test. *Journal of Obstetric, Gynecologic, & Neonatal Nursing, 21*(5), 407-411.

Shane, J. M. (1993). Evaluation and treatment of infertility. *Clinical Symposia, 45*(2), 2-32.

Summers, L. (1993). Preconception care: An opportunity to maximize health in pregnancy. *Journal of Nurse Midwifery, 38*(4), 188-198.

Toner, J. P., & Flood, J. T. (1993). Fertility after the age of 40. *Obstetrics & Gynecology Clinics of North America, 20*(2), 261-272.

Knowledge: Pregnancy—1810

Domain-Health Knowledge & Behavior (IV)
Class-Health Knowledge (S)
Scale(s)-No knowledge to Extensive knowledge (u)

Care Recipient:
Data Source:

Definition: Extent of understanding conveyed about promotion of a healthy pregnancy and prevention of complications

OUTCOME TARGET RATING:　　Maintain at_____　　　Increase to_____

Knowledge: Pregnancy Overall Rating	No knowledge 1	Limited knowledge 2	Moderate knowledge 3	Substantial knowledge 4	Extensive knowledge 5	
INDICATORS:						
181026　Importance of frequent prenatal care	1	2	3	4	5	NA
181027　Importance of prenatal education	1	2	3	4	5	NA
181028　Importance of frequent visits	1	2	3	4	5	NA
181003　Warning signs of pregnancy complications	1	2	3	4	5	NA
181004　Major fetal developmental milestones	1	2	3	4	5	NA
181029　Fetal movement pattern	1	2	3	4	5	NA
181005　Anatomic and physiological changes of pregnancy	1	2	3	4	5	NA
181006　Psychological changes associated with pregnancy	1	2	3	4	5	NA
181030　Emotional changes associated with pregnancy	1	2	3	4	5	NA
181007　Strategies to balance activity and rest	1	2	3	4	5	NA
181008　Proper body mechanics	1	2	3	4	5	NA
181009　Benefits of activity and exercise	1	2	3	4	5	NA
181010　Healthy nutritional practices	1	2	3	4	5	NA
181011　Healthy weight gain pattern	1	2	3	4	5	NA
181031　Correct use of nutritional supplements	1	2	3	4	5	NA
181032　Correct use of medication	1	2	3	4	5	NA
181033　Correct use of non-prescription medication	1	2	3	4	5	NA
181013　Importance of dental care	1	2	3	4	5	NA
181014　Appropriate self-care for discomforts of pregnancy	1	2	3	4	5	NA
181015　Safe sexual practices	1	2	3	4	5	NA
181016　Correct use of motor vehicle safety devices	1	2	3	4	5	NA

K

		No knowledge	Limited knowledge	Moderate knowledge	Substantial knowledge	Extensive knowledge	
181034	Birthing options	1	2	3	4	5	NA
181018	Signs and symptoms of labor	1	2	3	4	5	NA
181019	Effective labor techniques	1	2	3	4	5	NA
181020	Strategies to prevent infection	1	2	3	4	5	NA
181035	Signs of potential domestic abuse	1	2	3	4	5	NA
181021	Strategies to escape domestic abuse	1	2	3	4	5	NA
181022	Strategies to adjust to addition of infant	1	2	3	4	5	NA
181023	Environmental hazards	1	2	3	4	5	NA
181024	Teratogenic agents	1	2	3	4	5	NA
181036	Effects of smoking on fetus	1	2	3	4	5	NA
181037	Effects of alcohol use on fetus	1	2	3	4	5	NA
181038	Effects of illicit drug use on fetus	1	2	3	4	5	NA

2nd edition 2000; Revised 3rd edition 2004; Revised 4th edition

Outcome Content References:

Association of Women's Health, Obstetric, and Neonatal Nurses (2004). *Core curriculum for maternal-newborn nursing.* Washington, DC: Author.

Bell, R., & O'Neill, M. (1994). Exercise and pregnancy: A review. *Birth, 21*(2), 85-95.

Freda, M. C., Andersen, H. F., Dawes, K., & Merkatz, I. R. (1993). What pregnant women want to know: A comparison of client and provider perceptions. *Journal of Obstetric, Gynecologic, and Neonatal Nursing, 22*(3), 237.

Kearney, M. H., Murphy, S., Irwin, K., & Rosenbaum, M. (1995). Salvaging self: A grounded theory of pregnancy on crack cocaine. *Nursing Research, 44*(4), 208-213.

Lowdermilk, D. L., & Perry, S. E. (2004). *Maternity & women's health care* (8th ed.). St. Louis: Mosby.

McFarlane, J., Parker, B., & Soeken, K. (1996). Abuse during pregnancy: Associations with maternal health and infant birth weight. *Nursing Research, 45*(1), 37-42.

Olds, S. B., London, M. L., & Ladewig, P. W. (1996). *Maternal-newborn nursing: A family-centered approach* (5th ed.). Menlo Park, CA: Addison-Wesley.

K

Knowledge: Pregnancy & Postpartum Sexual Functioning—1839

Domain-Health Knowledge & Behavior (IV)

Class-Health Knowledge (S)

Scale(s)-No knowledge to Extensive knowledge (u)

Care Recipient:

Data Source:

Definition: Extent of understanding conveyed about sexual function during pregnancy and postpartum

OUTCOME TARGET RATING: Maintain at_____   Increase to_____

Knowledge: Pregnancy & Postpartum Sexual Functioning Overall Rating	No knowledge 1	Limited knowledge 2	Moderate knowledge 3	Substantial knowledge 4	Extensive knowledge 5	
INDICATORS:						
183901 Non-pregnant anatomy	1	2	3	4	5	NA
183902 Normal changes in body image	1	2	3	4	5	NA
183903 Physiology of female sexual functioning	1	2	3	4	5	NA
183904 Anatomic and physiological changes of pregnancy	1	2	3	4	5	NA
183905 Psychological changes associated with pregnancy	1	2	3	4	5	NA
183906 Emotional changes associated with pregnancy	1	2	3	4	5	NA
183907 Anatomic and physiological changes of postpartum	1	2	3	4	5	NA
183908 Psychological changes associated with postpartum	1	2	3	4	5	NA
183909 Emotional changes associated with postpartum	1	2	3	4	5	NA
183910 Potential changes in sexual desire and response	1	2	3	4	5	NA
183911 Intercourse restrictions during pregnancy	1	2	3	4	5	NA
183912 Intercourse restrictions during postpartum	1	2	3	4	5	NA
183913 Modification of coital position to prevent injury	1	2	3	4	5	NA
183914 Modification of coital position to prevent discomfort	1	2	3	4	5	NA
183915 Modification of sexual activity for mutual satisfaction	1	2	3	4	5	NA
183916 Use of vaginal water-based lubricant	1	2	3	4	5	NA
183917 Safe sexual practices	1	2	3	4	5	NA
183918 Strategies to prevent sexually transmitted diseases	1	2	3	4	5	NA

K

		No knowledge	Limited knowledge	Moderate knowledge	Substantial knowledge	Extensive knowledge	
183919	Importance of contraception or abstinence during early postpartum	1	2	3	4	5	NA
183920	Societal influences on personal sexual behavior	1	2	3	4	5	NA
183921	Cultural influences on personal sexual behavior	1	2	3	4	5	NA

4th edition

Outcome Content References:

Lowdermilk, D. L., & Perry, S. E. (2004). *Maternity & women's health care* (8th ed.). St. Louis: Mosby.

Matthey, S., Morgan, M., Healey, L., Barnett, B., Kavanagh, D. J., & Howie, P. (2002). Postpartum issue for expectant mothers and fathers. *JOGNN: Journal of Obstetric, Gynecologic, & Neonatal Nursing, 31*(4), 428-435.

Olds, S. B., London, M. L., Ladewig, P. W., & Davidson, M. R. (2004). *Maternal-newborn nursing & women's health care* (7th ed.). Upper Saddle River, NJ: Prentice Hall.

K

Knowledge: Prescribed Activity—1811

Domain-Health Knowledge & Behavior (IV)

Class-Health Knowledge (S)

Scale(s)-No knowledge to Extensive knowledge (u)

Care Recipient:

Data Source:

Definition: Extent of understanding conveyed about prescribed activity and exercise

OUTCOME TARGET RATING: Maintain at_____   Increase to_____

Knowledge: Prescribed Activity Overall Rating	No knowledge 1	Limited knowledge 2	Moderate knowledge 3	Substantial knowledge 4	Extensive knowledge 5	
INDICATORS:						
181101 Prescribed activity and exercise	1	2	3	4	5	NA
181102 Purpose of activity	1	2	3	4	5	NA
181103 Expected effects of activity	1	2	3	4	5	NA
181104 Activity restrictions	1	2	3	4	5	NA
181105 Activity precautions	1	2	3	4	5	NA
181116 Strategies to safely ambulate	1	2	3	4	5	NA
181117 Appropriate footwear	1	2	3	4	5	NA
181106 Factors that decrease the ability to perform activity	1	2	3	4	5	NA
181107 Strategies to gradually increase activity	1	2	3	4	5	NA
181118 Methods to monitor heart rate	1	2	3	4	5	NA
181119 Methods to monitor respiratory rate	1	2	3	4	5	NA
181111 Realistic exercise routine	1	2	3	4	5	NA
181110 Obstacles to implementing exercise routine	1	2	3	4	5	NA
181112 Proper performance of exercise	1	2	3	4	5	NA
181120 Benefits of activity and exercise	1	2	3	4	5	NA

1st edition 1997; Revised 3rd edition 2004; Revised 4th edition

Outcome Content References:

Bushnell, F. (1992). Self-care teaching for congestive heart failure patients. *Journal of Gerontological Nursing, 18*(10), 27-32.

Conn, V. S., Armer, J. M., & Hayes, K. S. (2001). Knowledge deficit. In M. Maas, K. Buckwalter, M. Hardy, T. Tripp-Reimer, M. Titler, & J. Specht (Eds.), *Nursing care of older adults: Diagnoses, outcomes & interventions* (pp. 503-515). St. Louis: Mosby.

Devins, G. M., Binik, Y. M., Mandin, H., Litourneau, P. K., Hollomby, D. J., Barre, P. E., & Prichard, S. (1990). The Kidney Disease Questionnaire: A test for measuring patient knowledge about end-stage renal disease. *Journal of Clinical Epidemiology, 43*(3), 297-307.

Garrard, J., Joynes, J. O., Mullen, L., McNeil, L., Mensing, C., Feste, C., & Etzwiler, D. D. (1987). Psychometric study of patient knowledge test. *Diabetes Care, 10*(4), 500-509.

Gilden, J. L., Hendryx, M., Casia, C., & Singh, S. P. (1989). The effectiveness of diabetes education programs for older patients and their spouses. *Journal of American Geriatrics Society, 37*(11), 1023-1030.

Mazzuca S. A., Moorman, N. H., Wheeler, M. L., Norton, J. A., Fineberg, N. S., Vinicor, F., Cohen, S. J., & Clark, C. M. (1986). The diabetes education study: A controlled trial of the effects of diabetes patient education. *Diabetes Care, 9*(1), 1-10.

Redman, B. (1993). Knowledge deficit (specify). In J. M. Thompson, G. K. McFarland, J. E. Hirsch, & S. M. Tucker (Eds.), *Mosby's clinical nursing* (3rd ed., pp. 1548-1552). St. Louis: Mosby.

Scherer, Y. K., Janelli, L. M., & Schmieder, L. E. (1992). A time-series perspective of effectiveness of a health teaching program on chronic obstructive pulmonary disease. *Journal of Healthcare Education and Training, 6*(3), 7-13.

Smith, M. M., Hicks, V. L., & Heyward, V. H. (1991). Coronary Disease Knowledge Test: Developing a valid and reliable tool. *Nurse Practitioner, 16*(4), 28, 31, 35-38.

K

Knowledge: Preterm Infant Care—1840

Domain-Health Knowledge & Behavior (IV)

Class-Health Knowledge (S)

Scale(s)-No knowledge to Extensive knowledge (u)

Care Recipient:

Data Source:

Definition: Extent of understanding conveyed about the care of a premature infant born 24 to 37 weeks (term) gestation

OUTCOME TARGET RATING: Maintain at_____   Increase to_____

Knowledge: Preterm Infant Care Overall Rating	No knowledge 1	Limited knowledge 2	Moderate knowledge 3	Substantial knowledge 4	Extensive knowledge 5	
INDICATORS:						
184001 Cause and contributing factors for prematurity	1	2	3	4	5	NA
184002 Premature infant characteristics	1	2	3	4	5	NA
184003 Major developmental milestones	1	2	3	4	5	NA
184004 Proper infant positioning	1	2	3	4	5	NA
184005 Infant sleep-wake pattern	1	2	3	4	5	NA
184006 Respiratory needs	1	2	3	4	5	NA
184007 Thermoregulation needs	1	2	3	4	5	NA
184008 Skin care needs	1	2	3	4	5	NA
184009 Physiologic monitoring needs	1	2	3	4	5	NA
184010 Hydration monitoring needs	1	2	3	4	5	NA
184011 Glucose monitoring needs	1	2	3	4	5	NA
184012 Pain management strategies	1	2	3	4	5	NA
184013 Prescribed medication	1	2	3	4	5	NA
184014 Diagnostic imaging tests	1	2	3	4	5	NA
184015 Laboratory tests	1	2	3	4	5	NA
184016 Nutritional needs	1	2	3	4	5	NA
184017 Importance of environmental control	1	2	3	4	5	NA
184018 Importance of kangaroo care	1	2	3	4	5	NA
184019 Neonatal intensive care routine	1	2	3	4	5	NA
184020 Parenting strategies in the hospital	1	2	3	4	5	NA
184021 Strategies to enhance bonding	1	2	3	4	5	NA
184022 Strategies to adjust to addition of infant	1	2	3	4	5	NA
184023 Strategies to enhance sibling support	1	2	3	4	5	NA
184024 Available support groups	1	2	3	4	5	NA
184025 Reputable sources of information	1	2	3	4	5	NA
184026 Financial resources for assistance	1	2	3	4	5	NA
184027 Discharge planning	1	2	3	4	5	NA

4th edition

K

Outcome Content References:

Merenstein, G. B. (2002). *Handbook of neonatal intensive care* (5th ed.). Mosby: St. Louis.

Zaichkin, J. (1996). *Newborn intensive care: What every parent needs to know*. Petaluma, CA: NICU Inc.

Knowledge: Sexual Functioning—1815

Domain-Health Knowledge & Behavior (IV)

Class-Health Knowledge (S)

Scale(s)-No knowledge to Extensive knowledge (u)

Care Recipient:

Data Source:

> **Definition:** Extent of understanding conveyed about sexual development and responsible sexual practices

OUTCOME TARGET RATING: Maintain at_____   Increase to_____

Knowledge: Sexual Functioning Overall Rating	No knowledge 1	Limited knowledge 2	Moderate knowledge 3	Substantial knowledge 4	Extensive knowledge 5	

INDICATORS:

181501	Sexual anatomy	1	2	3	4	5	NA
181502	Function of sexual anatomy	1	2	3	4	5	NA
181503	Physical changes with puberty	1	2	3	4	5	NA
181504	Emotional changes with puberty	1	2	3	4	5	NA
181505	Reproduction	1	2	3	4	5	NA
181506	Physical changes with aging	1	2	3	4	5	NA
181507	Emotional changes with aging	1	2	3	4	5	NA
181508	Societal influences on personal sexual behavior	1	2	3	4	5	NA
181509	Safe sexual practices	1	2	3	4	5	NA
181510	Effective contraception	1	2	3	4	5	NA
181511	Strategies to prevent sexually transmitted diseases	1	2	3	4	5	NA

2nd edition 2000; Revised 3rd edition 2004; Revised 4th edition

Outcome Content References:

Howard, M. (1991). *How to help your teenager postpone sexual involvement.* Lexington, NY: Continuum Publishing Co.

Nass, G., Libby, R., & Fischer, M. P. (1989). *Sexual choices: An introduction to human sexuality* (2nd ed.). Monterey, CA: Wadsworth Health Sciences.

Neinstein, L. S. (2002). *Adolescent health care: A practical guide.* Philadelphia: Lippincott Williams & Wilkins.

Tuttle, B. (1984). Adult sexual response. In L. P. Higgins & J. W. Hawkins (Eds.), *Human sexuality across the life span: Implications for nursing practice* (pp. 39-76). Monterey, CA: Wadsworth Health Sciences Division.

Wright, L. K. (2001). Altered sexuality patterns. In M. Maas, K. Buckwalter, M. Hardy, T. Tripp-Reimer, M. Titler, & J. Specht (Eds.), *Nursing care of older adults: Diagnoses, outcomes & interventions* (pp. 750-761). St. Louis: Mosby.

Knowledge: Substance Use Control—1812

Domain-Health Knowledge & Behavior (IV)

Class-Health Knowledge (S)

Scale(s)-No knowledge to Extensive knowledge (u)

Care Recipient:

Data Source:

Definition: Extent of understanding conveyed about controlling the use of addictive drugs, toxic chemicals, tobacco, or alcohol

OUTCOME TARGET RATING: Maintain at_____   Increase to_____

Knowledge: Substance Use Control Overall Rating	No knowledge 1	Limited knowledge 2	Moderate knowledge 3	Substantial knowledge 4	Extensive knowledge 5	
INDICATORS:						
181201 Personal risk for substance misuse	1	2	3	4	5	NA
181202 Adverse health effects of substance use	1	2	3	4	5	NA
181203 Benefits of eliminating substance use	1	2	3	4	5	NA
181205 Social consequences of substance use	1	2	3	4	5	NA
181206 Personal responsibility to manage substance misuse	1	2	3	4	5	NA
181207 Threats to substance use control	1	2	3	4	5	NA
181208 Support for substance use control	1	2	3	4	5	NA
181209 Strategies to prevent substance use	1	2	3	4	5	NA
181210 Strategies to manage substance use	1	2	3	4	5	NA
181211 Benefits of ongoing self-monitoring	1	2	3	4	5	NA
181212 Potential for relapse in efforts to control substance use	1	2	3	4	5	NA
181213 Strategies to prevent relapses in substance use	1	2	3	4	5	NA
181214 Signs of dependence during substance withdrawal	1	2	3	4	5	NA
181216 Signs and symptoms of substance withdrawal	1	2	3	4	5	NA
181217 Available support groups	1	2	3	4	5	NA

Specify substance_____

1st edition 1997; Revised 3rd edition 2004; Revised 4th edition

Outcome Content References:

Eells, M. A. W. (1991). Strategies for promotion of avoiding harmful substances. *Nursing Clinics of North America, 26*(40), 915-927.

Hall, J. A., & Williams, J. K. (2005). Substance abuse. In D. L. Huber (Ed.), *Disease management: A guide for case managers* (pp. 187-202). St. Louis: Saunders.

Simons-Morton, D. G., Mullen, P. D., Mains, D. A., Tabak, E. R., & Green, L. W. (1992). Characteristics of controlled studies of patient education and counseling for preventive health behaviors. *Patient Education and Counseling, 19*(2), 174-204.

Tanner, E. K. (1991). Assessment of a health-promotive lifestyle. *Nursing Clinics of North America, 26*(4), 845-854.

U. S. Department of Health and Human Services. (1990). *Healthy People 2000, National health promotion and disease prevention objectives*. Washington, DC: Government Printing Office.

U. S. Department of Health and Human Services. (1998). *Clinician's handbook of prevention services: Put prevention into practice* (2nd ed.) Washington, DC: Government Printing Office.

Knowledge: Treatment Procedure—1814

Domain-Health Knowledge & Behavior (IV)

Class-Health Knowledge (S)

Scale(s)-No knowledge to Extensive knowledge (u)

Care Recipient:

Data Source:

> **Definition:** Extent of understanding conveyed about a procedure required as part of a treatment regimen

OUTCOME TARGET RATING: Maintain at_____   Increase to_____

Knowledge: Treatment Procedure Overall Rating	No knowledge 1	Limited knowledge 2	Moderate knowledge 3	Substantial knowledge 4	Extensive knowledge 5	
INDICATORS:						
181401 Treatment procedure	1	2	3	4	5	NA
181402 Purpose of procedure	1	2	3	4	5	NA
181403 Steps in procedure	1	2	3	4	5	NA
181405 Precautions related to procedure	1	2	3	4	5	NA
181406 Restrictions related to procedure	1	2	3	4	5	NA
181404 Correct use of equipment	1	2	3	4	5	NA
181407 Proper care of equipment	1	2	3	4	5	NA
181409 Appropriate action for complications	1	2	3	4	5	NA
181410 Treatment side effects	1	2	3	4	5	NA
181412 Contraindications for procedure	1	2	3	4	5	NA

Specify procedure _____

1st edition 1997; Revised 3rd edition 2004; Revised 4th edition

Outcome Content References:

Conn, V. S., Armer, J. M., & Hayes, K. S. (2001). Knowledge deficit. In M. Maas, K. Buckwalter, M. Hardy, T. Tripp-Reimer, M. Titler, & J. Specht (Eds.), *Nursing care of older adults: Diagnoses, outcomes & interventions* (pp. 503-515). St. Louis: Mosby.

Redman, B. K. (2001). *The practice of patient education* (9th ed.). St. Louis: Mosby.

Roe, B. H. (1990). Study of the effects of education on the management of urine drainage systems by patients and carers. *Journal of Advanced Nursing, 15*(5), 517-524.

Sarisley, C. (1987). Designing a teaching program for outpatient antibiotic therapy. *Journal of Nursing Staff Development, 3*(3), 128-135.

Smith, C. E. (1987). *Patient education: Nurses in partnership with other health professionals.* Orlando, FL: Gruen & Stratton.

Togger, D. A., & Brenner, P. S. (2001). Metered dose inhalers. *American Journal of Nursing, 101*(10), 26-32, 38-39.

Knowledge: Treatment Regimen—1813

Domain-Health Knowledge & Behavior (IV)   Care Recipient:

Class-Health Knowledge (S)   Data Source:

Scale(s)-No knowledge to Extensive knowledge (u)

Definition: Extent of understanding conveyed about a specific treatment regimen

OUTCOME TARGET RATING: Maintain at_____   Increase to_____

Knowledge: Treatment Regimen Overall Rating	No knowledge 1	Limited knowledge 2	Moderate knowledge 3	Substantial knowledge 4	Extensive knowledge 5	
INDICATORS:						
181310 Specific disease process	1	2	3	4	5	NA
181301 Rationale for treatment	1	2	3	4	5	NA
181302 Self-care responsibilities for ongoing treatment	1	2	3	4	5	NA
181303 Self-care responsibilities for emergency situations	1	2	3	4	5	NA
181315 Self-monitoring techniques	1	2	3	4	5	NA
181304 Expected effects of treatment	1	2	3	4	5	NA
181305 Prescribed diet	1	2	3	4	5	NA
181306 Prescribed medication regimen	1	2	3	4	5	NA
181307 Prescribed activity	1	2	3	4	5	NA
181308 Prescribed exercise	1	2	3	4	5	NA
181309 Prescribed procedure	1	2	3	4	5	NA
181316 Benefits of disease management	1	2	3	4	5	NA

1st edition 1997; Revised 2nd edition 2000; Revised 3rd edition 2004; Revised 4th edition

Outcome Content References:

Bushnell, F. (1992). Self-care teaching for congestive heart failure patients. *Journal of Gerontological Nursing, 18*(10), 27-32.

Conn, V. S., Armer, J. M., & Hayes, K. S. (2001). Knowledge deficit. In M. Maas, K. Buckwalter, M. Hardy, T. Tripp-Reimer, M. Titler, & J. Specht (Eds.), *Nursing care of older adults: Diagnoses, outcomes & interventions* (pp. 503-515). St. Louis: Mosby.

Devins, G. M., Binik, Y. M., Mandin, H., Litourneau, P. K., Hollomby, D. J., Barre, P. E., & Prichard, S. (1990). The Kidney Disease Questionnaire: A test for measuring patient knowledge about end-stage renal disease. *Journal of Clinical Epidemiology, 43*(3), 297-307.

Garrard, J., Joynes, J. O., Mullen, L., McNeil, L., Mensing, C., Feste, C., & Etzwiler, D. D. (1987). Psychometric study of patient knowledge test. *Diabetes Care, 10*(4), 500-509.

Gilden, J. L., Hendryx, M., Casia, C., & Singh, S. P. (1989). The effectiveness of diabetes education programs for older patients and their spouses. *Journal of American Geriatrics Society, 37*(11), 1023-1030.

Mazzuca, S. A., Moorman, N. H., Wheeler, M. L., Norton, J. A., Fineberg, N. S., Vinicor, F., Cohen, S. J., & Clark, C. M. (1986). The diabetes education study: A controlled trial of the effects of diabetes patient education. *Diabetes Care, 9*(1), 1-10.

Redman, B. (1993). Knowledge deficit (specify). In J. M. Thompson, G. K. McFarland, J. E. Hirsch, & S. M. Tucker (Eds.), *Mosby's clinical nursing* (3rd ed., pp. 1548-1552). St. Louis: Mosby.

Scherer, Y. K., Janelli, L. M., & Schmieder, L. E. (1992). A time-series perspective of effectiveness of a health teaching program on chronic obstructive pulmonary disease. *Journal of Healthcare Education & Training, 6*(3), 7-13.

Smith, M. M., Hicks, V. L., & Heyward, V. H. (1991). Coronary Disease Knowledge Test: Developing a valid and reliable tool. *Nurse Practitioner, 16*(4), 28, 31, 35-38.

Zwygart-Stauffacher, M. (2001). Ineffective management of therapeutic regimen. In M. Maas, K. Buckwalter, M. Hardy, T. Tripp-Reimer, M. Titler, & J. Specht (Eds.), *Nursing care of older adults: Diagnoses, outcomes & interventions* (pp. 86-92). St. Louis: Mosby.

K

Knowledge: Weight Management—1841

Domain-Health Knowledge & Behavior (IV)   Care Recipient:

Class-Health Knowledge (S)   Data Source:

Scale(s)-No knowledge to Extensive knowledge (u)

Definition: Extent of understanding conveyed about the promotion and maintenance of optimal body weight and fat percentage congruent with height, frame, gender, and age

OUTCOME TARGET RATING: Maintain at_____   Increase to_____

Knowledge: Weight Management Overall Rating	No knowledge 1	Limited knowledge 2	Moderate knowledge 3	Substantial knowledge 4	Extensive knowledge 5	
INDICATORS:						
184101 Optimal personal weight	1	2	3	4	5	NA
184102 Optimal body mass index (BMI)	1	2	3	4	5	NA
184103 Strategies to reach optimal weight	1	2	3	4	5	NA
184104 Strategies to maintain optimal weight	1	2	3	4	5	NA
184105 Relationship among diet, exercise, and weight	1	2	3	4	5	NA
184106 Health risks related to overweight	1	2	3	4	5	NA
184107 Health risks related to underweight	1	2	3	4	5	NA
184108 Appetite versus hunger	1	2	3	4	5	NA
184109 Healthy nutritional practices	1	2	3	4	5	NA
184110 Optimum fluid intake	1	2	3	4	5	NA
184111 Strategies to modify food intake	1	2	3	4	5	NA
184112 Food cravings that trigger unhealthy eating	1	2	3	4	5	NA
184113 Emotional states that trigger unhealthy eating	1	2	3	4	5	NA
184114 Benefits of activity and exercise	1	2	3	4	5	NA
184115 Exercise strategies for maintaining optimal weight	1	2	3	4	5	NA
184116 Obstacles to implementing exercise routine	1	2	3	4	5	NA
184117 Strategies to modify behavior	1	2	3	4	5	NA
184118 Lifestyle changes to promote optimal weight	1	2	3	4	5	NA
184119 Benefits of prescribed weight loss medication	1	2	3	4	5	NA
184120 Potential dangers of non-prescription medication	1	2	3	4	5	NA

K

		No knowledge	Limited knowledge	Moderate knowledge	Substantial knowledge	Extensive knowledge	
184121	Surgical treatment options for weight loss	1	2	3	4	5	NA
184122	Benefits of hypnosis	1	2	3	4	5	NA
184123	Benefits of alternative therapies	1	2	3	4	5	NA
184124	Benefits of social support	1	2	3	4	5	NA
184125	Risks associated with treatment options	1	2	3	4	5	NA
184126	Available support groups	1	2	3	4	5	NA
184127	Available community resources	1	2	3	4	5	NA
184128	Reputable sources of information	1	2	3	4	5	NA
184129	Self-monitoring techniques	1	2	3	4	5	NA
184130	When to obtain assistance from a health professional	1	2	3	4	5	NA

4th edition

Outcome Content References:

Dennis, K. E. (2004). Weight management in women. *Nursing Clinics of North America, 39*(1), 231-241.

Huether, S., & McCance, K. (Eds.). (2002). *Pathophysiology: the biologic basis for disease in adults and children* (4th ed.). St. Louis: Mosby.

Lewis, S., Heitkemper, M., & Dirksen, S. (Eds.). (2004). *Medical-surgical nursing: Assessment and management of clinical problems* (6th ed., pp. 991-1000). St. Louis: Mosby.

National Heart, Lung and Blood Institute. (2005). *Aim for a healthy weight* (NIH Publication No. 05-5213). Bethesda, MD: U. S. Department of Health and Human Services.

National Heart, Lung and Blood Institute and the North American Association for the Study of Obesity. (2000). *The practical guide to the identification, evaluation, and treatment of overweight and obesity in adults* (NIH Publication No. 00-4084). Bethesda, MD: U.S. Department of Health and Human Services.

K

Leisure Participation—1604

Domain-Health Knowledge & Behavior (IV)

Class-Health Behavior (Q)

Scale(s)-Never demonstrated to Consistently demonstrated (m)

Care Recipient:

Data Source:

Definition: Use of relaxing, interesting, and enjoyable activities to promote well-being

OUTCOME TARGET RATING: Maintain at_____   Increase to_____

Leisure Participation Overall Rating	Never demonstrated 1	Rarely demonstrated 2	Sometimes demonstrated 3	Often demonstrated 4	Consistently demonstrated 5	

INDICATORS:

160401	Participates in activities other than regular work	1	2	3	4	5	NA
160410	Participates in high physical demand leisure activities	1	2	3	4	5	NA
160411	Participates in low physical demand leisure activities	1	2	3	4	5	NA
160412	Selects leisure activities of interest	1	2	3	4	5	NA
160402	Expresses satisfaction with leisure activities	1	2	3	4	5	NA
160403	Uses appropriate social interaction skills	1	2	3	4	5	NA
160404	Feels relaxed from leisure activities	1	2	3	4	5	NA
160413	Enjoys leisure activities	1	2	3	4	5	NA
160405	Exhibits creativity through leisure activities	1	2	3	4	5	NA
160407	Identifies recreational options	1	2	3	4	5	NA

1st edition 1997; Revised 3rd edition 2004; Revised 4th edition

Outcome Content References:

Ansello, E. F. (1985). *The activity coordinator as environmental press.* New York: The Haworth Press.

+Drummond, A. E. R., & Walker, M. F. (1994). The Nottingham Leisure Questionnaire for stroke patients. *British Journal of Occupational Therapy, 57*(11), 414-418.

Everard, K. M., Lach, H. W., Fisher, E. B., & Baum, M. C. (2000). Relationship of activity and social support to the functional health of older adults. *Journal of Gerontology. Series B, Psychological Sciences and Social Sciences, 55*(4), P208-P212.

Godin, G., Jobin, J., & Bouillon, J. (1986). Assessment of leisure time exercise behavior by self-report: A concurrent validity study. *Canadian Journal of Public Health, 77*(5), 359-362.

Gordon, M. D. (1987). Pediatric recreational therapy after thermal injury. *Journal of Burn Rehabilitation, 8*(4), 336-340.

Johnson, S. W., McSweeney, M., & Webster, R. E. (1989). Leisure: How to promote inpatient motivation after discharge. *Journal of Psychosocial Nursing, 27*(9), 29-31.

Jongbloed, L., & Morgan, D. (1991). An investigation of involvement in leisure activities after a stroke. *The American Journal of Occupational Therapy, 45*(5), 420-427.

Klein, M. M. (1985). The therapeutics of recreation. *Physical Occupational Therapy Pediatrics, 4*(3), 9-11.

Peterson, C. A., & Stumbo, N. J. (1999). *Therapeutic recreation program design: Principles and procedures* (3rd ed.). San Francisco: Benjamin Cummings.

Rantz, M. J., & Popejoy, L. (2001). Diversional activity deficit. In M. Maas, K. Buckwalter, M. Hardy, T. Tripp-Reimer, M. Titler, & J. Specht (Eds.), *Nursing care of older adults: Diagnoses, outcomes & interventions* (pp. 385-396). St. Louis: Mosby.

L

Loneliness Severity—1203

Domain-Psychosocial Health (III)

Class-Psychological Well-Being (M)

Scale(s)-Severe to None (n)

Care Recipient:

Data Source:

Definition: Severity of emotional, social, or existential isolation response						

OUTCOME TARGET RATING: Maintain at_____   Increase to_____

Loneliness Severity Overall Rating	Severe 1	Substantial 2	Moderate 3	Mild 4	None 5	
INDICATORS:						
120301 Sense of unfounded dread	1	2	3	4	5	NA
120302 Sense of desperation	1	2	3	4	5	NA
120303 Sense of extreme restlessness	1	2	3	4	5	NA
120304 Sense of hopelessness	1	2	3	4	5	NA
120305 Sense of not belonging	1	2	3	4	5	NA
120306 Sense of loss due to separation from another	1	2	3	4	5	NA
120307 Sense of social isolation	1	2	3	4	5	NA
120308 Sense of not being understood	1	2	3	4	5	NA
120309 Sense of being excluded	1	2	3	4	5	NA
120310 Sense that time seems endless	1	2	3	4	5	NA
120311 Difficulty in planning	1	2	3	4	5	NA
120312 Difficulty in establishing contact with others	1	2	3	4	5	NA
120313 Difficulty overcoming separateness	1	2	3	4	5	NA
120314 Difficulty in effecting a mutual relationship	1	2	3	4	5	NA
120315 Mood fluctuations	1	2	3	4	5	NA
120316 Impaired concentration	1	2	3	4	5	NA
120317 Non-assertiveness	1	2	3	4	5	NA
120318 Difficulty making decisions	1	2	3	4	5	NA
120328 Unhealthy eating pattern	1	2	3	4	5	NA
120320 Sleep disturbance	1	2	3	4	5	NA
120321 Headaches	1	2	3	4	5	NA
120322 Nausea	1	2	3	4	5	NA
120323 Decreased activity level	1	2	3	4	5	NA
120324 Pain	1	2	3	4	5	NA
120325 Spiritual discomfort	1	2	3	4	5	NA
120327 Depression	1	2	3	4	5	NA

1st edition 1997; Revised 3rd edition 2004; Revised 4th edition

Continued

L

Outcome Content References:

Copel, L. C. (1988). Loneliness: A conceptual model. *Journal of Psychosocial Nursing, 26*(1), 14-19.

Ellison, C. W. (1978). Loneliness: A social-developmental analysis. *Journal of Psychology and Theology, 6*(1), 3-17.

Peplau, H. E. (1955). Loneliness. *American Journal of Nursing, 55*(12), 1476-1481.

Peplau, L. A., & Pearlman, D. (Eds.). (1982). *Loneliness: A sourcebook of current theory, research, and therapy*. New York: John Wiley.

+Russell, D., Peplau, L. A., & Cutrona, C. E. (1980). The revised UCLA Loneliness Scale: Concurrent and discriminant validity evidence. *Journal of Personality and Social Psychology, 39*(3), 472-480.

+Russell, D., Peplau, L. A., & Ferguson, M. (1978). Develoing a measure of loneliness. *Journal of Personality Assessment, 42*(3), 290-294.

Weiss, R. S. (Ed.). (1973). *Loneliness: The experience of emotional and social isolation*. Cambridge, MA: The MIT Press.

West, D. A., Kellner, R., & Moore-West, M. (1986). The effects of loneliness: A review of the literature. *Comparative Psychiatry, 27*(4), 351-363.

L

Maternal Status: Antepartum—2509

Domain-Family Health (VI)   Care Recipient:

Class-Family Member Health Status (Z)   Data Source:

Scale(s)-Severe deviation from normal range to No deviation from normal range (b) and Severe to None (n)

Definition: Extent to which maternal well-being is within normal limits from conception to the onset of labor

OUTCOME TARGET RATING: Maintain at_____   Increase to_____

Maternal Status: Antepartum Overall Rating	Severe deviation from normal range 1	Substantial deviation from normal range 2	Moderate deviation from normal range 3	Mild deviation from normal range 4	No deviation from normal range 5	
INDICATORS:						
250901 Emotional attachment to fetus	1	2	3	4	5	NA
250902 Coping with discomforts of pregnancy	1	2	3	4	5	NA
250903 Mood lability	1	2	3	4	5	NA
250904 Weight change	1	2	3	4	5	NA
250907 Cognitive status	1	2	3	4	5	NA
250908 Visual acuity	1	2	3	4	5	NA
250910 Neurological reflexes	1	2	3	4	5	NA
250916 Blood pressure	1	2	3	4	5	NA
250917 Radial pulse rate	1	2	3	4	5	NA
250926 Apical heart rate	1	2	3	4	5	NA
250929 Respiratory rate	1	2	3	4	5	NA
250918 Body temperature	1	2	3	4	5	NA
250919 Urine protein	1	2	3	4	5	NA
250920 Urine glucose	1	2	3	4	5	NA
250921 Blood glucose	1	2	3	4	5	NA
250922 Hemoglobin	1	2	3	4	5	NA
250923 Liver enzymes	1	2	3	4	5	NA
250924 Blood count	1	2	3	4	5	NA
	Severe	Substantial	Moderate	Mild	None	
250905 Edema	1	2	3	4	5	NA
250906 Headache	1	2	3	4	5	NA
250909 Seizure activity	1	2	3	4	5	NA
250911 Nausea	1	2	3	4	5	NA
250928 Vomiting	1	2	3	4	5	NA
250912 Abdominal pain	1	2	3	4	5	NA
250913 Epigastric pain	1	2	3	4	5	NA
250914 Vaginal bleeding	1	2	3	4	5	NA
250915 Vaginal discharge	1	2	3	4	5	NA
250927 Heartburn	1	2	3	4	5	NA

M

Continued

2nd edition 2000; Revised 3rd edition 2004; Revised 4th edition

Outcome Content References:

Armour, K. (2004). Using surveillance to improve maternal and fetal outcomes: Antepartum maternal-fetal assessment. *AWHONN Lifelines, 8*(3), 232-240.

Association of Women's Health, Obstetricians and Neonatal Nurses. (1998). *Standards & guidelines for the professional nursing practice in the care of women and newborns* (5th ed.). Washington, DC: Author.

Association of Women's Health, Obstetric and Neonatal Nurses. (1998). *Clinical competencies and educational guide: Limited ultrasound examinations in obstetric and gynecologic/infertility settings.* Washington, DC: Author.

Chez, B. F., Skurnick, J. H., Chez, R. A., Verklan, M. T., Biggs, S., & Hage, M. L. (1990). Interpretations of nonstress tests by obstetric nurses. *Journal of Obstetric, Gynecologic, and Neonatal Nursing, 19*(3), 227-232.

Givens, S. R., & Moore, M. L. (1995). Status report on maternal and child health indicators. *Journal of Perinatal and Neonatal Nursing, 9*(1), 8-18.

Lowdermilk, D. L., & Perry, S. E. (2003). *Maternity nursing* (6th ed.). St. Louis: Mosby.

Nichols, F., & Humenick, S. (2000). *Childbirth education: Practice, research and theory* (2nd ed.). Philadelphia: W.B. Saunders.

Nurses Association of the American College of Obstetricians and Gynecologists. (1991). *NAACOBG standards for the nursing care of women and newborns* (4th ed.). Washington, DC: Author.

Reeder, S. J., Martin, L. L., & Koniak-Griffin, D. (1997). *Maternity nursing: Family, newborn, and women's health care* (18th ed.). Philadelphia: J.B. Lippincott.

M

Maternal Status: Intrapartum—2510

Domain-Family Health (VI)
Class-Family Member Health Status (Z)
Scale(s)-Severe deviation from normal range to No deviation from normal range (b) and Severe to None (n)

Care Recipient:
Data Source:

Definition: Extent to which maternal well-being is within normal limits from onset of labor to delivery

OUTCOME TARGET RATING: Maintain at_____   Increase to_____

Maternal Status: Intrapartum Overall Rating	Severe deviation from normal range 1	Substantial deviation from normal range 2	Moderate deviation from normal range 3	Mild deviation from normal range 4	No deviation from normal range 5	
INDICATORS:						
251001 Coping with discomforts of labor	1	2	3	4	5	NA
251003 Use of techniques to facilitate labor	1	2	3	4	5	NA
251004 Uterine contraction frequency	1	2	3	4	5	NA
251005 Uterine contraction duration	1	2	3	4	5	NA
251006 Uterine contraction intensity	1	2	3	4	5	NA
251007 Progression of cervical dilation	1	2	3	4	5	NA
251009 Blood pressure	1	2	3	4	5	NA
251010 Radial pulse rate	1	2	3	4	5	NA
251021 Apical heart rate	1	2	3	4	5	NA
251011 Blood glucose	1	2	3	4	5	NA
251012 Body temperature	1	2	3	4	5	NA
251013 Urine output	1	2	3	4	5	NA
251014 Visual acuity	1	2	3	4	5	NA
251015 Cognitive status	1	2	3	4	5	NA
251016 Neurological reflexes	1	2	3	4	5	NA
	Severe	**Substantial**	**Moderate**	**Mild**	**None**	
251008 Vaginal bleeding	1	2	3	4	5	NA
251017 Seizure activity	1	2	3	4	5	NA
251018 Headache	1	2	3	4	5	NA
251019 Epigastric pain	1	2	3	4	5	NA
251022 Pain with contractions	1	2	3	4	5	NA
251023 Back pain	1	2	3	4	5	NA
251024 Nausea	1	2	3	4	5	NA
251025 Vomiting	1	2	3	4	5	NA

2nd edition 2000; Revised 3rd edition 2004

Outcome Content References:

Dickason, E. J., Schultz, M. O., & Silverman, B. L. (1994). *Maternal-infant nursing care* (3rd ed.). St. Louis: Mosby.
Hodnett, E. (1996). Nursing support of the laboring woman. *Journal of Obstetric and Neonatal Nursing, 25*(3), 257-263.
Lowe, N. K. (1996). The pain and discomfort of labor and birth. *Journal of Obstetric and Neonatal Nursing, 25*(1), 82-92.
Mattson, S. (Ed.). (2000). *Core curriculum for maternal-newborn nursing* (2nd ed.). Philadelphia: W.B. Saunders.

M

Maternal Status: Postpartum—2511

Domain-Family Health (VI)

Class-Family Member Health Status (Z)

Scale(s)-Severe deviation from normal range to No deviation from normal range (b) and Severe to None (n)

Care Recipient:

Data Source:

Definition: Extent to which maternal well-being is within normal limits from delivery of placenta to completion of involution

OUTCOME TARGET RATING: Maintain at_____   Increase to_____

Maternal Status: Postpartum Overall Rating	Severe deviation from normal range 1	Substantial deviation from normal range 2	Moderate deviation from normal range 3	Mild deviation from normal range 4	No deviation from normal range 5	

INDICATORS:

251101	Mood equilibrium	1	2	3	4	5	NA
251102	Comfort	1	2	3	4	5	NA
251103	Blood pressure	1	2	3	4	5	NA
251104	Apical heart rate	1	2	3	4	5	NA
251123	Radial pulse rate	1	2	3	4	5	NA
251105	Peripheral circulation	1	2	3	4	5	NA
251106	Uterine fundal height	1	2	3	4	5	NA
251107	Lochia amount	1	2	3	4	5	NA
251124	Lochia color	1	2	3	4	5	NA
251108	Breast fullness	1	2	3	4	5	NA
251109	Breast comfort	1	2	3	4	5	NA
251110	Perineal healing	1	2	3	4	5	NA
251111	Incisional healing	1	2	3	4	5	NA
251112	Body temperature	1	2	3	4	5	NA
251114	Urinary elimination	1	2	3	4	5	NA
251115	Bowel elimination	1	2	3	4	5	NA
251116	Food and fluid intake	1	2	3	4	5	NA
251117	Physical activity	1	2	3	4	5	NA
251118	Endurance	1	2	3	4	5	NA
251119	Liver enzymes	1	2	3	4	5	NA
251120	Hemoglobin	1	2	3	4	5	NA
251121	White blood count	1	2	3	4	5	NA

		Severe	Substantial	Moderate	Mild	None	
251113	Infection	1	2	3	4	5	NA
251125	Incisional pain	1	2	3	4	5	NA
251126	Fatigue	1	2	3	4	5	NA
251127	Vaginal bleeding	1	2	3	4	5	NA
251128	Depression	1	2	3	4	5	NA

2nd edition 2000; Revised 3rd edition 2004

M

Outcome Content References:

Association of Women's Health, Obstetricians and Neonatal Nurses. (1998). *Standards & guidelines for the professional nursing practice in the care of women and newborns* (5th ed.). Washington, DC: Author.

Beck, C. T. (1992). The lived experience of postpartum depression: A phenomenological study. *Nursing Research, 41*(3), 166-170.

Bond, L. (1993). Physiological changes. In S. Mattson & J. E. Smith (Eds.), *AWHONN: Core Curriculum for maternal newborn nursing*. Philadelphia: W.B. Saunders.

Nichols, F., & Humenick, S. (2000). *Childbirth education: Practice, research and theory* (2nd ed.). Philadelphia: W.B. Saunders.

Reeder, S. J., Martin, L. L., & Koniak-Griffin, D. (1997). *Maternity nursing: Family, newborn, and women's health care* (18th ed.). Philadelphia: J.B. Lippincott.

M

Mechanical Ventilation Response: Adult—0411

Domain-Physiologic Health (II)   Care Recipient:

Class-Cardiopulmonary (E)   Data Source:

Scale(s)-Severe deviation from normal range to No deviation from normal range (b) and Severe to None (n)

Definition: Alveolar exchange and tissue perfusion are effectively supported by mechanical ventilation

OUTCOME TARGET RATING: Maintain at_____   Increase to_____

Mechanical Ventilation Response: Adult Overall Rating	Severe deviation from normal range 1	Substantial deviation from normal range 2	Moderate deviation from normal range 3	Mild deviation from normal range 4	No deviation from normal range 5	
INDICATORS:						
041102 Respiratory rate	1	2	3	4	5	NA
041103 Respiratory rhythm	1	2	3	4	5	NA
041104 Depth of inspiration	1	2	3	4	5	NA
041126 Inspiratory capacity	1	2	3	4	5	NA
041106 Tidal volume	1	2	3	4	5	NA
041107 Vital capacity	1	2	3	4	5	NA
041108 FiO_2 (fraction of inspired oxygen) meets oxygen demand	1	2	3	4	5	NA
041109 PaO_2 (partial pressure of oxygen in arterial blood)	1	2	3	4	5	NA
041110 $PaCO_2$ (partial pressure of carbon dioxide in arterial blood)	1	2	3	4	5	NA
041111 Arterial pH	1	2	3	4	5	NA
041112 Oxygen saturation	1	2	3	4	5	NA
041113 Peripheral tissue perfusion	1	2	3	4	5	NA
041114 End tidal carbon dioxide	1	2	3	4	5	NA
041115 Pulmonary function tests	1	2	3	4	5	NA
041116 Chest x-ray findings	1	2	3	4	5	NA
041117 Ventilation perfusion balance	1	2	3	4	5	NA

	Severe	Substantial	Moderate	Mild	None	
041122 Asymmetrical chest wall movement	1	2	3	4	5	NA
041123 Asymmetrical chest wall expansion	1	2	3	4	5	NA
041124 Difficulty breathing with ventilator	1	2	3	4	5	NA
041126 Adventitious breath sounds	1	2	3	4	5	NA
041137 Atelectasis	1	2	3	4	5	NA

M

		Severe	Substantial	Moderate	Mild	None	
041125	Anxiety	1	2	3	4	5	NA
041128	Restlessness	1	2	3	4	5	NA
041129	Impaired skin integrity at tracheostomy site	1	2	3	4	5	NA
041130	Hypoxia	1	2	3	4	5	NA
041131	Pulmonary infection	1	2	3	4	5	NA
041132	Respiratory secretions	1	2	3	4	5	NA
041133	Difficulty communicating needs	1	2	3	4	5	NA

Type and mode of ventilation_____

3rd edition 2004; Revised 4th edition

Outcome Content References:

Abel, M. (2001). Fast track protocol for patients undergoing cardiopulmonary bypass. Fast track protocol—Anesthesiology Department Website, Mayo Medical Center: http://anesthesia.mayo.edu/DIVISIONS/cvt/Procedures/FastTrack-Protoco.htm

Bickley, L. S., & Hoekelman, R. A. (1998). *Bates' guide to physical examination and history taking* (7th ed.). Philadelphia: Lippincott Williams & Wilkins.

Chlan, L. (2000). Music therapy as a nursing intervention for patients supported by mechanical ventilation. *AACN Clinical Issues, 11*(1), 128-138.

Coates, L. (2000). Care of the ventilated patient. *Nursing Standard, 14*(28), 60.

Hanneman, S., (1999). Protocols for practice, applying research at the bedside. *Critical Care Nurse, 9*(5), 86-89.

Henderson, N. (1999). Mechanical ventilation. *Nursing Standard, 13*(44), 49-54.

Kelly-Heidenthal, P., & O'Connor, M. (1994). Nursing assessment of portable AP chest x-rays. *Dimensions of Critical Care Nursing, 13*(3), 127-132.

Smeltzer, S. C., & Bare, B. G. (2004). *Brunner & Suddarth's textbook of medical surgical nursing* (10th ed.). Philadelphia: Lippincott Williams & Wilkins.

M

Mechanical Ventilation Weaning Response: Adult—0412

Domain-Physiologic Health (II)　　　　　　　　　　　*Care Recipient:*

Class-Cardiopulmonary (E)　　　　　　　　　　　　*Data Source:*

Scale(s)-Severe deviation from normal range to No deviation from normal range (b) and Severe to None (n)

Definition: Respiratory and psychological adjustment to progressive removal of mechanical ventilation

OUTCOME TARGET RATING:　　Maintain at_____　　　Increase to_____

Mechanical Ventilation Weaning Response: Adult Overall Rating	Severe deviation from normal range 1	Substantial deviation from normal range 2	Moderate deviation from normal range 3	Mild deviation from normal range 4	No deviation from normal range 5	
INDICATORS:						
041202 Spontaneous respiratory rate	1	2	3	4	5	NA
041203 Spontaneous respiratory rhythm	1	2	3	4	5	NA
041204 Spontaneous respiratory depth	1	2	3	4	5	NA
041205 Apical heart rate	1	2	3	4	5	NA
041208 PaO$_2$ (partial pressure of oxygen in arterial blood)	1	2	3	4	5	NA
041209 PaCO$_2$ (partial pressure of carbon dioxide in arterial blood)	1	2	3	4	5	NA
041210 Arterial pH	1	2	3	4	5	NA
041211 Oxygen saturation	1	2	3	4	5	NA
041212 Vital capacity	1	2	3	4	5	NA
041213 Tidal volume	1	2	3	4	5	NA
041214 Minute ventilation <10 L/minute	1	2	3	4	5	NA
041215 Positive end-expiratory pressure	1	2	3	4	5	NA
041219 Chest x-ray findings	1	2	3	4	5	NA
041220 Ventilation perfusion balance	1	2	3	4	5	NA
	Severe	Substantial	Moderate	Mild	None	
041223 Difficulty breathing on own	1	2	3	4	5	NA
041224 Respiratory secretions	1	2	3	4	5	NA
041225 Anxiety	1	2	3	4	5	NA
041226 Fear	1	2	3	4	5	NA
041227 Impaired gag reflex	1	2	3	4	5	NA
041228 Impaired cough reflex	1	2	3	4	5	NA
041229 Impaired drive to breathe	1	2	3	4	5	NA

M

		Severe	Substantial	Moderate	Mild	None	
041230	Adventitious breath sounds	1	2	3	4	5	NA
041231	Asymmetrical chest wall movement	1	2	3	4	5	NA
041232	Asymmetrical chest wall expansion	1	2	3	4	5	NA
041233	Atelectasis	1	2	3	4	5	NA
041234	Restlessness	1	2	3	4	5	NA
041235	Discomfort	1	2	3	4	5	NA
041236	Difficulty communicating needs	1	2	3	4	5	NA

3rd edition 2004; Revised 4th edition

Outcome Content References:

Abel, M. (2001). Fast track protocol for patients undergoing cardiopulmonary bypass. Fast track protocol—Anesthesiology Department Website, Mayo Medical Center: http://anesthesia.mayo.edu/DIVISIONS/cvt/Procedures/FastTrack-Protoco.htm

Burns, S. M., Fahey, S. A., Barton, D. M., & Clack, D. (1991). Weaning from mechanical ventilation: A method for assessment and intervention. *AACN Clinical Issues for Critical Care Nurses, 2*(3), 372-387.

Chlan, L. (2000). Music therapy as a nursing intervention for patients supported by mechanical ventilation. *AACN Clinical Issues, 11*(1), 128-138.

Coates, L. (2000). Care of the ventilated patient. *Nursing Standard, 14*(28), 60.

Hanneman, S. (1999). Protocols for practice, applying research at the bedside. *Critical Care Nurse, 9*(5), 86-89.

Henderson, N. (1999). Mechanical ventilation. *Nursing Standard, 13*(44), 49-54.

Kelly-Heidenthal, P., & O'Connor, M., (1994). Nursing assessment of portable AP chest x-rays. *Dimensions of Critical Care Nursing, 13*(3), 127-132.

Morganroth, M. L., Morganroth, J. l., Nett, L. M., & Petty, T. L. (1984). Criteria for weaning from prolonged mechanical ventilation. *Archives of Internal Medicine, 144*(5), 1012-1016.

Smeltzer, S. C., & Bare, B. G. (2004). *Brunner & Suddarth's textbook of medical surgical nursing* (10th ed.). Philadelphia: Lippincott Williams & Wilkins.

Urban, N., Greenlee, K., Krumberger, J., & Winkelman, C. (1995). *Guidelines for critical care nursing.* St. Louis: Mosby.

Yang, K. L., & Tobin, M. J. (1991). A prospective study of indexes predicting the outcome trials of weaning a patient from mechanical ventilation. *New England Journal of Medicine, 324*(21), 1445-1450.

M

Medication Response—2301

Domain-Physiologic Health (II)

Class-Therapeutic Response (a)

Scale(s)-Severely compromised to Not compromised (a) and Severe to None (n)

Care Recipient:

Data Source:

Definition: Therapeutic and adverse effects of prescribed medication

OUTCOME TARGET RATING: Maintain at_____   Increase to_____

Medication Response Overall Rating	Severely compromised 1	Substantially compromised 2	Moderately compromised 3	Mildly compromised 4	Not compromised 5	
INDICATORS:						
230101 Expected therapeutic effects	1	2	3	4	5	NA
230102 Expected change in blood chemistries	1	2	3	4	5	NA
230103 Expected change in symptoms	1	2	3	4	5	NA
230111 Maintenance of expected blood levels	1	2	3	4	5	NA
230112 Expected behavioral response	1	2	3	4	5	NA
	Severe	Substantial	Moderate	Mild	None	
230105 Allergic reaction	1	2	3	4	5	NA
230106 Adverse effects	1	2	3	4	5	NA
230107 Medication interactions	1	2	3	4	5	NA
230108 Medication tolerance	1	2	3	4	5	NA
230113 Adverse behavioral effects	1	2	3	4	5	NA

Specify medication_____

2nd edition 2000; Revised 3rd edition 2004; Revised 4th edition

Outcome Content References:

Arnold, G. J. (1998). Clinical recognition of adverse drug reactions: Obstacles and opportunities for the nursing profession. *Journal of Nursing Care Quality, 13*(2), 45-55.

Hodgson, B. B., & Kizior, R. J. (2003). *Saunders nursing drug book 2003* (3rd ed.). Philadelphia: W.B. Saunders.

Katzung, B. G. (Ed.). (2000). *Basic and clinical pharmacology* (8th ed.). Norwalk, CT: Appleton & Lange.

Shannon, M. T., Wilson, B. A., & Stang, C. L. (1995). *Drugs and nursing implications* (8th ed.). Norwalk, CT: Appleton & Lange, Springhouse. (1998). *Nurse practitioner's drug handbook* (2nd ed.). Springhouse, PA: Author.

Memory—0908

Domain-Physiologic Health (II)   Care Recipient:

Class-Neurocognitive (J)   Data Source:

Scale(s)-Severely compromised to Not compromised (a)

Definition: Ability to cognitively retrieve and report previously stored information

OUTCOME TARGET RATING: Maintain at_____   Increase to_____

Memory Overall Rating	Severely compromised 1	Substantially compromised 2	Moderately compromised 3	Mildly compromised 4	Not compromised 5	
INDICATORS:						
090801 Recalls immediate information accurately	1	2	3	4	5	NA
090802 Recalls recent information accurately	1	2	3	4	5	NA
090803 Recalls remote information accurately	1	2	3	4	5	NA

1st edition 1997; Revised 3rd edition 2004

Outcome Content References:

Abraham, I., & Reel, S. (1993). Cognitive nursing interventions with long-term residents: Effects on neurocognitive dimensions. *Archives of Psychiatric Nursing, 6*(6), 356-365.

Agostinelli, B., Demers, K., Garrigan, D., & Waszynski, C. (1994). Targeted interventions: Use of the Mini-Mental State Exam. *Journal of Gerontological Nursing, 20*(8), 15-23.

Dellasega, C. (1992). Home health nurses' assessments of cognition. *Applied Nursing Research, 5*(3), 127-133.

Foreman, M., Theis, S., & Anderson, M. A. (1993). Adverse events in the hospitalized elderly. *Clinical Nursing Research, 2*(3), 360-370.

Gerdner, L. A., & Hall, G. R. (2001). Chronic confusion. In M. Maas, K. Buckwalter, M. Hardy, T. Tripp-Reimer, M. Titler, & J. Specht (Eds.), *Nursing care of older adults: Diagnoses, outcomes & interventions* (pp. 421-441). St. Louis: Mosby.

Mason, P. (1989). Cognitive assessment parameters and tools for the critically injured adult. *Critical Care Nursing Clinics of North America, 1*(1), 45-53.

+Pfeiffer, E. (1975). A short portable mental status questionnaire for the assessment of organic brain deficit in elderly patients. *American Geriatrics Society, 23*(10), 433-441.

Strub, R. L., & Black, F. W. (2000). *The mental status examination in neurology* (4th ed.). Philadelphia: F.A. Davis.

M

Mobility—0208

Domain-Functional Health (I)

Class-Mobility (C)

Scale(s)-Severely compromised to Not compromised (a)

Care Recipient:

Data Source:

Definition: Ability to move purposefully in own environment independently with or without assistive device

OUTCOME TARGET RATING: Maintain at_____   Increase to_____

Mobility Overall Rating	Severely compromised 1	Substantially compromised 2	Moderately compromised 3	Mildly compromised 4	Not compromised 5	
INDICATORS:						
020801 Balance	1	2	3	4	5	NA
020809 Coordination	1	2	3	4	5	NA
020810 Gait	1	2	3	4	5	NA
020803 Muscle movement	1	2	3	4	5	NA
020804 Joint movement	1	2	3	4	5	NA
020802 Body positioning performance	1	2	3	4	5	NA
020805 Transfer performance	1	2	3	4	5	NA
020811 Running	1	2	3	4	5	NA
020812 Jumping	1	2	3	4	5	NA
020813 Crawling	1	2	3	4	5	NA
020806 Walking	1	2	3	4	5	NA
020814 Moves with ease	1	2	3	4	5	NA

1st edition 1997; Revised 3rd edition 2004

Outcome Content References:

Maas, M. L., & Specht, J. P. (2001). Impaired physical mobility. In M. Maas, K. Buckwalter, M. Hardy, T. Tripp-Reimer, M. Titler, & J. Specht (Eds.), *Nursing care of older adults: Diagnoses, outcomes & interventions* (pp. 337-365). St. Louis: Mosby.

+Podsiadlo, D., & Richardson, S. (1991). The timed "Up & Go": A test of basic functional mobility for frail elderly persons. *Journal of the American Geriatrics Society, 39*(2), 142-148.

Rukenstein, L. Z., Wieland, D., & Bernakei, R. (Eds.). (1995). *Geriatric assessment technology: The state of the art.* New York: Springer.

Mood Equilibrium—1204

Domain-Psychosocial Health (III)

Class-Psychological Well-Being (M)

Care Recipient:

Data Source:

Scale(s)-Never demonstrated to Consistently demonstrated (m) and Consistently demonstrated to Never demonstrated (t)

Definition: Appropriate adjustment of prevailing emotional tone in response to circumstances

OUTCOME TARGET RATING: Maintain at_____   Increase to_____

Mood Equilibrium Overall Rating	Never demonstrated 1	Rarely demonstrated 2	Sometimes demonstrated 3	Often demonstrated 4	Consistently demonstrated 5	
INDICATORS:						
120401 Exhibits affect that fits situation	1	2	3	4	5	NA
120402 Exhibits non-labile mood	1	2	3	4	5	NA
120403 Exhibits impulse control	1	2	3	4	5	NA
120404 Reports adequate sleep	1	2	3	4	5	NA
120405 Exhibits concentration	1	2	3	4	5	NA
120406 Speaks at moderate pace	1	2	3	4	5	NA
120423 Maintains personal grooming and hygiene	1	2	3	4	5	NA
120411 Wears appropriate clothing for situation	1	2	3	4	5	NA
120412 Maintains stable weight	1	2	3	4	5	NA
120413 Exhibits normal appetite	1	2	3	4	5	NA
120424 Reports compliance with medication regimen	1	2	3	4	5	NA
120425 Reports compliance with treatment regimen	1	2	3	4	5	NA
120415 Shows interest in surroundings	1	2	3	4	5	NA
120417 Exhibits stable energy level	1	2	3	4	5	NA
120418 Accomplishes daily tasks	1	2	3	4	5	NA

	Consistently demonstrated	Often demonstrated	Sometimes demonstrated	Rarely demonstrated	Never demonstrated	
120407 Flight of ideas	1	2	3	4	5	NA
120408 Grandiosity	1	2	3	4	5	NA
120409 Euphoria	1	2	3	4	5	NA
120416 Suicide ideation	1	2	3	4	5	NA
120420 Depression	1	2	3	4	5	NA
120421 Lethargy	1	2	3	4	5	NA
120422 Hyperactivity	1	2	3	4	5	NA

1st edition 1997; Revised 3rd edition 2004; Revised 4th edition

M

Continued

Outcome Content References:

George, L. K., Blazer, D. B., Hughes, D. C., & Fowler N. (1989). Social support and the outcome of major depression. *British Journal of Psychiatry, 154*, 478-485.

Keitner, G. I., & Miller, I. W. (1990). Family functioning and major depression: An overview. *American Journal of Psychiatry, 147*(9), 1128-1137.

Maynard, C. K. (1993). Comparison of effectiveness of group interventions for depression in women. *Archives of Psychiatric Nursing, 7*(5), 277-283.

Maynard, C. (1993). Psychoeducational approach to depression in women. *Journal of Psychosocial Nursing and Mental Health Services, 31*(12), 9-14.

Piven, M. L., & Buckwalter, K. C. (2001). Depression. In M. Maas, K. Buckwalter, M. Hardy, T. Tripp-Reimer, M. Titler, & J. Specht (Eds.), *Nursing care of older adults: Diagnoses, outcomes & interventions* (pp. 521-542). St. Louis: Mosby.

Porth, C. M. (2002). *Pathophysiology: Concepts of altered health states* (6th ed.). Philadelphia: Lippincott Williams & Wilkins.

Stuart, G. W., & Laraia, M. T. (2001). *Principles and practice of psychiatric nursing* (7th ed.). St. Louis: Mosby.

+Underwood, B., & Froming, W. J. (1980). The Mood Survey: A personality measure of happy and sad moods. *Journal of Personality Assessment, 44*(4), 404-413.

M

Motivation—1209

Domain-Psychosocial Health (III)

Class-Psychological Well-Being (M)

Scale(s)-Never demonstrated to Consistently demonstrated (m)

Care Recipient:

Data Source:

Definition: Inner urge that moves or prompts an individual to positive action(s)

OUTCOME TARGET RATING: Maintain at_____   Increase to_____

Motivation Overall Rating	Never demonstrated 1	Rarely demonstrated 2	Sometimes demonstrated 3	Often demonstrated 4	Consistently demonstrated 5	
INDICATORS:						
120901 Plans for the future	1	2	3	4	5	NA
120902 Develops an action plan	1	2	3	4	5	NA
120903 Obtains resources as needed	1	2	3	4	5	NA
120904 Obtains support as needed	1	2	3	4	5	NA
120905 Self-initiates goal-directed behavior	1	2	3	4	5	NA
120906 Seeks new experiences	1	2	3	4	5	NA
120907 Maintains positive self-esteem	1	2	3	4	5	NA
120908 Welcomes opportunity to make contributions	1	2	3	4	5	NA
120916 Maintains flexibility	1	2	3	4	5	NA
120910 Expresses belief in ability to perform action	1	2	3	4	5	NA
120911 Expresses that performance will lead to desired outcome	1	2	3	4	5	NA
120912 Completes tasks	1	2	3	4	5	NA
120913 Accepts responsibility for actions	1	2	3	4	5	NA
120917 Anticipates intrinsic reward	1	2	3	4	5	NA
120918 Anticipates extrinsic reward	1	2	3	4	5	NA
120915 Expresses intent to act	1	2	3	4	5	NA

3rd edition 2004; Revised 4th edition

Outcome Content References:

Ellis, J. R., & Hartley, C. L. (1999). *Managing and coordinating nursing care* (3rd ed.). Philadelphia: Lippincott Williams & Wilkins.

Glickstein, J. (1990). Motivation in geriatric rehabilitation. *Focus on Geriatric Care and Rehabilitation, 3*(8), 1-3.

Mali, P. (1978). *Improving total productivity: MBO strategies for business, government, and not-for-profit organizations.* New York: Wiley.

Marriner-Tomey, A. (1996). *Guide to nursing management and leadership* (5th ed.). St. Louis: Mosby.

Resnick, B. (1998). Motivating older adults to perform functional activities. *Journal of Gerontological Nursing, 24*(11), 23-20.

Resnick, B., Zimmerman, S. I., Magaziner, J., & Adelman, A. (1998). Use of the apathy evaluation scale as a measure of motivation in elderly people. *Rehabilitation Nursing, 23*(3), 141-147.

Vroom, V. (1964). *Work and motivation.* New York: Wiley.

M

Multiple Sclerosis Self-Management—1631

Domain-Health Knowledge & Behavior (IV)

Class-Health Behavior (Q)

Scale(s)-Never demonstrated to Consistently demonstrated (m)

Care Recipient:

Data Source:

Definition: Personal actions to manage multiple sclerosis and prevent disease progression

OUTCOME TARGET RATING: Maintain at_____   Increase to_____

Multiple Sclerosis Self-Management Overall Rating	Never demonstrated 1	Rarely demonstrated 2	Sometimes demonstrated 3	Often demonstrated 4	Consistently demonstrated 5	
INDICATORS:						
163101 Accepts health care provider's diagnoses	1	2	3	4	5	NA
163102 Seeks information about methods to maintain musculoskeletal health	1	2	3	4	5	NA
163103 Participates in health care decision-making process	1	2	3	4	5	NA
163104 Performs treatment regimen as prescribed	1	2	3	4	5	NA
163105 Identifies symptoms of disease progression	1	2	3	4	5	NA
163106 Identifies ways to cope with functional changes	1	2	3	4	5	NA
163107 Monitors symptom onset	1	2	3	4	5	NA
163108 Monitors symptom persistence	1	2	3	4	5	NA
163109 Monitors symptom severity	1	2	3	4	5	NA
163110 Monitors symptom frequency	1	2	3	4	5	NA
163111 Reports symptoms of worsening disease	1	2	3	4	5	NA
163112 Reports signs and symptoms of mood changes	1	2	3	4	5	NA
163113 Obtains health care when warning signs occur	1	2	3	4	5	NA
163114 Uses symptom relief measures	1	2	3	4	5	NA
163115 Obtains required medication	1	2	3	4	5	NA
163116 Uses medication as prescribed	1	2	3	4	5	NA
163117 Monitors prescribed medication therapeutic effects	1	2	3	4	5	NA
163118 Monitors medication side effects	1	2	3	4	5	NA

		Never demonstrated	Rarely demonstrated	Sometimes demonstrated	Often demonstrated	Consistently demonstrated	
163119	Uses correct procedure for injection administration	1	2	3	4	5	NA
163120	Rotates injection sites	1	2	3	4	5	NA
163121	Stores medications correctly	1	2	3	4	5	NA
163122	Uses preventative measures to reduce medication side effects	1	2	3	4	5	NA
163123	Follows recommended diet	1	2	3	4	5	NA
163124	Uses strategies to control fatigue	1	2	3	4	5	NA
163125	Balances activity and rest	1	2	3	4	5	NA
163126	Participates in recommended exercise routine	1	2	3	4	5	NA
163127	Uses energy conservation techniques	1	2	3	4	5	NA
163128	Adjusts life routine for optimal health	1	2	3	4	5	NA
163129	Uses stress management techniques	1	2	3	4	5	NA
163130	Uses alternative treatment techniques	1	2	3	4	5	NA
163131	Obtains flu and pneumonia immunizations	1	2	3	4	5	NA
163132	Obtains liver function tests	1	2	3	4	5	NA
163133	Uses strategies to enhance bladder function	1	2	3	4	5	NA
163134	Uses strategies to enhance bowel function	1	2	3	4	5	NA
163135	Avoids extremes of temperatures	1	2	3	4	5	NA
163136	Keeps appointments with health professional	1	2	3	4	5	NA
163137	Maintains plan for medical emergencies	1	2	3	4	5	NA
163138	Uses community resources as needed	1	2	3	4	5	NA

4th edition

Outcome Content References:

Denis, L., Namey, M., Costello, K., Frenette, J., Gagnon, N., Harris, C., Lowden, D., McEwan, L., Morrison, W., & Poirier, J. (2004). Long-term treatment optimization in individuals with multiple sclerosis using disease-modifying therapies: a nursing approach. *Journal of Neuroscience Nursing, 36*(1), 10-22.

Embrey, N., Lowndes, C., & Warner, R. (2003). Benchmarking best practice in relapse management of multiple sclerosis. *Nursing Standard, 17*(22), 38-42.

Jarrett, L. (2003). Attitudes to long-term care in multiple sclerosis. *Nursing Standard, 17*(17), 39-43.

MS Center at Washington University School of Medicine Website: http://www.neuro.wustl.edu/MS/

National Multiple Sclerosis Society. Website: http://www.nmss.org

Ozuna, J. M. (2004). Nursing management: Chronic neurologic problems. In S. M. Lewis, M. M. Heitkemper, & S. R. Dirksen, *Medical-surgical nursing: Assessment and management of clinical problems* (6th ed., pp. 1549-1580). St. Louis: Mosby.

Ward, N., & Winters S. (2003). Multiple sclerosis. Results of a fatigue management programme in multiple sclerosis. *British Journal of Nursing, 12*(18), 1075-80.

M

Nausea & Vomiting Control—1618

Domain-Health, Knowledge & Behavior (IV)

Class-Health Behavior (Q)

Scale-Never demonstrated to Consistently demonstrated (m)

Care Recipient:

Data Source:

Definition: Personal actions to control nausea, retching, and vomiting symptoms

OUTCOME TARGET RATING: Maintain at_____   Increase to_____

Nausea & Vomiting Control Overall Rating	Never demonstrated 1	Rarely demonstrated 2	Sometimes demonstrated 3	Often demonstrated 4	Consistently demonstrated 5	
INDICATORS:						
161801 Recognizes onset of nausea	1	2	3	4	5	NA
161802 Describes causal factors	1	2	3	4	5	NA
161803 Recognizes precipitating stimuli	1	2	3	4	5	NA
161804 Uses diary to monitor symptoms over time	1	2	3	4	5	NA
161805 Uses preventive measures	1	2	3	4	5	NA
161806 Avoids causal factors when possible	1	2	3	4	5	NA
161807 Avoids disagreeable odors	1	2	3	4	5	NA
161808 Uses antiemetic medication as recommended	1	2	3	4	5	NA
161809 Reports failure of antiemetic treatment	1	2	3	4	5	NA
161810 Reports bothersome side effects from antiemetics	1	2	3	4	5	NA
161811 Reports uncontrolled symptoms to health professional	1	2	3	4	5	NA
161812 Reports nausea, retching, and vomiting controlled	1	2	3	4	5	NA

3rd edition 2004

Outcome Content References:

Brown, J. K., & Hogan, C. M. (1990). Chemotherapy. In S. L. Groenwald, M. H. Frogge, M. Goodman, & C. H. Yarbro (Eds.), *Cancer nursing: Principles and practice* (pp. 230-283). Sudbury, MA: Jones and Bartlett.

Engstrom, C., Hernandez, I., Haywood, J., & Lilenbaum, R. (1999). The efficacy and cost effectiveness of new antiemetic guidelines. *Oncology Nursing Forum, 26*(9), 1453-1458.

Houston, D. (1997). Supportive therapies for cancer chemotherapy patients and the role of the oncology nurse. *Cancer Nursing, 20*(6), 409-413.

Nolte, J. J., Berkery, R., Pizzo, B., Baltzer, L., Grossano, D., Lucarelli, C. D., & Kris, M. G. (1998). Assuring the optimal use of serotonin antagonist antiemetics: The process for development and implementation of institutional antiemetic guidelines at Memorial Sloan-Kettering Cancer Center. *Journal of Clinical Oncology, 16*(2), 771-778.

Rhodes, V. A., McDaniel, R. W., Simms, S. G., & Johnson, M. (1995). Nurses' perceptions of antiemetic effectiveness. *Oncology Nursing Forum, 22*(8), 1243-1252.

Wickham, R. (1999). Nausea and vomiting. In C. H. Yarbro, M. H. Frogge, & M. Goodman (Eds.), *Cancer symptom management* (pp. 228-263). Sudbury, MA: Jones and Bartlett.

N

Nausea & Vomiting: Disruptive Effects—2106

Domain-Perceived Health (V)

Class-Symptom Status (V)

Scale(s)-Severe to None (n)

Care Recipient:

Data Source:

Definition: Severity of observed or reported disruptive effects of nausea, retching, and vomiting on daily functioning

OUTCOME TARGET RATING: Maintain at_____   Increase to_____

Nausea & Vomiting: Disruptive Effects Overall Rating	Severe 1	Substantial 2	Moderate 3	Mild 4	None 5	
INDICATORS:						
210601 Decreased fluid intake	1	2	3	4	5	NA
210602 Decreased food intake	1	2	3	4	5	NA
210603 Decreased urine output	1	2	3	4	5	NA
210604 Altered fluid balance	1	2	3	4	5	NA
210605 Altered serum electrolytes	1	2	3	4	5	NA
210606 Altered acid/base balance	1	2	3	4	5	NA
210607 Altered nutritional status	1	2	3	4	5	NA
210608 Weight loss	1	2	3	4	5	NA
210609 Malaise	1	2	3	4	5	NA
210610 Lethargy	1	2	3	4	5	NA
210611 Intolerance of movement	1	2	3	4	5	NA
210612 Impaired physical activity	1	2	3	4	5	NA
210613 Interrupted sleep	1	2	3	4	5	NA
210614 Withdrawal from interpersonal relationships	1	2	3	4	5	NA
210615 Impaired role performance	1	2	3	4	5	NA
210616 Impaired work performance	1	2	3	4	5	NA
210617 Interference with leisure activities	1	2	3	4	5	NA
210618 Interference with activities of daily living (ADLs)	1	2	3	4	5	NA
210619 Anxiety	1	2	3	4	5	NA
210620 Depression	1	2	3	4	5	NA
210621 Emotional stress	1	2	3	4	5	NA
210622 Helplessness	1	2	3	4	5	NA
210623 Side effects from antiemetic medication	1	2	3	4	5	NA
210624 Treatment delays due to symptom severity	1	2	3	4	5	NA

N

3rd edition 2004

Continued

Outcome Content References:

Cotanch, P. H. (1988). Measuring nausea and vomiting. In M. Frank-Stromborg (Ed.), *Instruments for clinical nursing research* (pp. 313-321). Norwalk, CT: Appleton & Lange.

Engelking, C., Wickham, R., & Iwamoto, R. (1996). Cancer-related gastrointestinal symptoms: Dilemmas in assessment and management. *Developments in Supportive Cancer Care, 1*(1), 3-10.

Ezzone, S., Baker, C., Rosselet, R., & Terepka, E. (1998). Music as an adjunct to antiemetic therapy. *Oncology Nursing Forum, 25*(9), 1551-1556.

Low, K. G. (1996). Nausea and vomiting in pregnancy: A review of the research. *Journal of Gender, Culture, and Health, 1*(3), 151-172.

Rhodes, V. A., & McDaniel, R. W. (1997). Measuring nausea, vomiting, and retching. In M. Frank-Stromborg & S. J. Olsen (Eds.), *Instruments for Clinical Health-Care Research* (2nd ed., pp. 509-517). Sudbury, MA: Jones and Bartlett.

Wickham, R. (1999). Nausea and vomiting. In C. H. Yarbro, M. H. Frogge, & M. Goodman (Eds.), *Cancer symptom management* (pp. 228-263). Sudbury, MA: Jones and Bartlett.

N

Nausea & Vomiting Severity—2107

Domain-Perceived Health (V)
Class-Symptom Status (V)
Scale(s)-Severe to None (n)

Care Recipient:
Data Source:

Definition: Severity of nausea, retching, and vomiting symptoms

OUTCOME TARGET RATING: Maintain at_____   Increase to_____

Nausea & Vomiting Severity Overall Rating	Severe 1	Substantial 2	Moderate 3	Mild 4	None 5	
INDICATORS:						
210701 Frequency of nausea	1	2	3	4	5	NA
210702 Intensity of nausea	1	2	3	4	5	NA
210703 Distress of nausea	1	2	3	4	5	NA
210704 Frequency of retching	1	2	3	4	5	NA
210705 Intensity of retching	1	2	3	4	5	NA
210706 Distress of retching	1	2	3	4	5	NA
210707 Frequency of vomiting	1	2	3	4	5	NA
210708 Intensity of vomiting	1	2	3	4	5	NA
210709 Distress of vomiting	1	2	3	4	5	NA
210710 Excessive secretion of saliva	1	2	3	4	5	NA
210711 Alteration in taste	1	2	3	4	5	NA
210712 Intolerance of odors	1	2	3	4	5	NA
210713 Weight loss	1	2	3	4	5	NA
210714 Heartburn	1	2	3	4	5	NA
210715 Gastric pain	1	2	3	4	5	NA
210716 Projectile vomiting	1	2	3	4	5	NA
210717 Blood in emesis	1	2	3	4	5	NA
210718 Coffee ground emesis	1	2	3	4	5	NA
210719 Fecal odor of emesis	1	2	3	4	5	NA

Duration of nausea: ____(hours) ____(days) ____(months)

Amount of emesis _____(ml)

3rd edition 2004

Outcome Content References:

Cotanch, P. H. (1988). Measuring nausea and vomiting. In M. Frank-Stromborg (Ed.), *Instruments for clinical nursing research* (pp. 313-321). Norwalk, CT: Appleton & Lange.

Engstrom, C., Hernandez, I., Haywood, J., & Lilenbaum, R. (1999). The efficacy and cost effectiveness of new antiemetic guidelines. *Oncology Nursing Forum, 26*(9), 1453-1458.

Rhodes, V. A., & McDaniel, R. W. (1997). Measuring nausea, vomiting, and retching. In M. Frank-Stromborg & S. J. Olsen (Eds.), *Instruments for clinical health-care research* (2nd ed., pp. 509-517). Sudbury, MA: Jones and Bartlett.

Rhodes, V. A., & McDaniel, R. W. (1999). The index of nausea, vomiting, and retching: A new format of the index of nausea and vomiting. *Oncology Nursing Forum, 26*(5), 889-894.

Wickham, R. (1999). Nausea and vomiting. In C. H. Yarbro, M. H. Frogge, & M. Goodman (Eds.), *Cancer symptom management* (pp. 228-263). Sudbury, MA: Jones and Bartlett.

N

Neglect Cessation—2513

Domain-Family Health (VI)

Class-Family Member Health Status (Z)

Scale(s)-None to Extensive (i)

Care Recipient:

Data Source:

Definition: Evidence that the victim is no longer receiving substandard care

OUTCOME TARGET RATING: Maintain at_____   Increase to_____

Neglect Cessation Overall Rating	None 1	Limited 2	Moderate 3	Substantial 4	Extensive 5	

INDICATORS:

		None 1	Limited 2	Moderate 3	Substantial 4	Extensive 5	
251301	Evidence that physical neglect has ceased	1	2	3	4	5	NA
251302	Evidence that emotional neglect has ceased	1	2	3	4	5	NA
251303	Evidence that financial neglect has ceased	1	2	3	4	5	NA
251304	Evidence that spiritual neglect has ceased	1	2	3	4	5	NA
251305	Evidence that health care neglect has ceased	1	2	3	4	5	NA

3rd edition 2004

Outcome Content References:

Aber, J. L., Allen, J. P., Carlson, V., & Cicchetti, D. (1990). The effects of maltreatment on development during early childhood: Recent studies and their theoretical, clinical, and policy implications. In D. Cicchetti & V. Carlson (Eds.), *Child maltreatment: Theory and research on the causes and consequences of child abuse and neglect* (pp. 579-619). New York: Cambridge University Press.

Cicchetti, D., & Carlson, V. (Eds.). (1989). *Child maltreatment: Theory and research on the causes and consequences of child abuse and neglect.* New York: Cambridge University Press.

Cowen, P. S. (2001). Elder mistreatment. In M. Maas, K. Buckwalter, M. Hardy, T. Tripp-Reimer, M. Titler, & J. Specht (Eds.), *Nursing care of older adults: Diagnoses, outcomes & interventions* (pp. 93-114). St. Louis: Mosby.

Fulmer, T., & Ashley, J. (1989). Clinical indicators of elder neglect. *Applied Nursing Research, 2*(4), 161-167.

Hudson, M. F., & Johnson, T. F. (1986). Elder neglect and abuse: A review of the literature [Monograph]. *Annual Review of Nursing Research, 6,* 81-134.

Lobo, M. L., Barnard, K. E., & Coombs, J. B. (1992). Failure to thrive: A parent-infant interaction perspective. *Journal of Pediatric Nursing, 7*(4), 251-261.

Olds, D. L., Henderson, C. R., Chamberlin, R., & Tatelbaum R. (1986). Preventing child abuse and neglect: A randomized trial of nurse home visitation. *Pediatrics, 78*(1), 65-78.

Silverman, J., & Hudson, M. F. (2000). Elder mistreatment: A guide for medical professionals. *North Carolina Medical Journal, 61*(5), 291-296.

Weinman, M. L., Schreiber, N. B., & Robinson, M. (1992). Adolescent mothers: Were there any gains in a parent education program? *Family and Community Health, 15*(3), 1-10.

Young, L. (1981). *Physical child neglect.* Chicago: The National Committee for Prevention of Child Abuse.

N

Neglect Recovery—2512

Domain-Family Health (VI)

Class-Family Member Health Status (Z)

Scale(s)-None to Extensive (i) and Extensive to None (h)

Care Recipient:

Data Source:

> **Definition:** Extent of physical, emotional, and spiritual healing following the cessation of substandard care

OUTCOME TARGET RATING: Maintain at_____   Increase to_____

Neglect Recovery Overall Rating	None 1	Limited 2	Moderate 3	Substantial 4	Extensive 5	
INDICATORS:						
251201 Maintenance of personal hygiene	1	2	3	4	5	NA
251205 Appropriate clothing for weather	1	2	3	4	5	NA
251206 Cleanliness of living environment	1	2	3	4	5	NA
251207 Safety of living environment	1	2	3	4	5	NA
251209 Provision of supervision required	1	2	3	4	5	NA
251210 Demonstration of interest in life	1	2	3	4	5	NA
251211 Expressions of pride in self	1	2	3	4	5	NA
251212 Expressions of hope	1	2	3	4	5	NA
251213 Timely meeting of emotional needs	1	2	3	4	5	NA
251214 Provision of appropriate health care	1	2	3	4	5	NA
251215 Provision of recommended diet	1	2	3	4	5	NA
251216 Provision of medication regimen	1	2	3	4	5	NA
251217 Use of appropriate equipment or appliance	1	2	3	4	5	NA
251220 Normal development	1	2	3	4	5	NA
251218 Normal growth	1	2	3	4	5	NA
251219 Provision of cognitive stimulation	1	2	3	4	5	NA
251221 Expectations of responsibilities reasonable for age	1	2	3	4	5	NA
251224 Consistency of behavior with social norms	1	2	3	4	5	NA

	Extensive	Substantial	Moderate	Limited	None	
251202 Hunger	1	2	3	4	5	NA
251208 Skin breakdown	1	2	3	4	5	NA
251223 Substance abuse	1	2	3	4	5	NA

Continued

		Extensive	Substantial	Moderate	Limited	None	
251227	Fatigue	1	2	3	4	5	NA
251228	Malnutrition	1	2	3	4	5	NA
251229	Dehydration	1	2	3	4	5	NA
251230	Inappropriate attention-seeking behavior	1	2	3	4	5	NA

1st edition 1997, Revised 3rd edition 2004; Revised 4th edition

Outcome Content References:

Aber, J. L., Allen, J. P., Carlson, V., & Cicchetti, D. (1990). The effects of maltreatment on development during early childhood: Recent studies and their theoretical, clinical, and policy implications. In D. Cicchetti & V. Carlson (Eds.), *Child maltreatment: Theory and research on the causes and consequences of child abuse and neglect* (pp. 579-619). New York: Cambridge University Press.

Cicchetti, D., & Carlson, V. (Eds.). (1989). *Child maltreatment: Theory and research on the causes and consequences of child abuse and neglect.* New York: Cambridge University Press.

Cowen, P. S. (2001). Elder mistreatment. In M. Maas, K. Buckwalter, M. Hardy, T. Tripp-Reimer, M. Titler, & J. Specht (Eds.), *Nursing care of older adults: Diagnoses, outcomes & interventions* (pp. 93-114). St. Louis: Mosby.

Fulmer, T., & Ashley, J. (1989). Clinical indicators of elder neglect. *Applied Nursing Research, 2*(4), 161-167.

Fulmer, T., & Paveza, G. (1998). Neglect in the elderly patient. *Nursing Clinics of North America, 33*(3), 457-466.

Hudson, M. F., & Johnson, T. F. (1986). Elder neglect and abuse: A review of the literature [Monograph]. *Annual Review of Nursing Research, 6*, 81-134.

Lobo, M. L., Barnard, K. E., & Coombs, J. B. (1992). Failure to thrive: A parent-infant interaction perspective. *Journal of Pediatric Nursing, 7*(4), 251-261.

Olds, D. L., Henderson, C. R., Chamberlin, R., & Tatelbaum R. (1986). Preventing child abuse and neglect: A randomized trial of nurse home visitation. *Pediatrics, 78*(1), 65-78.

Polansky, N. A., Halley, C., & Polansky, N. F. (1977). *Profile of neglect: A survey of the state of knowledge.* Washington, DC: U.S. Department of Health, Education, and Welfare.

Weinman, M. L., Schreiber, N. B., & Robinson, M. (1992). Adolescent mothers: Were there any gains in a parent education program? *Family and Community Health, 15*(3), 1-10.

Young, L. (1981). *Physical child neglect.* Chicago: The National Committee for Prevention of Child Abuse.

N

Neurological Status—0909

Domain-Physiologic Health (II)

Class-Neurocognitive (J)

Scale(s)-Severely compromised to Not compromised (a) and Severe to None (n)

Care Recipient:

Data Source:

Definition: Ability of the peripheral and central nervous system to receive, process, and respond to internal and external stimuli

OUTCOME TARGET RATING: Maintain at_____   Increase to_____

Neurological Status Overall Rating	Severely compromised 1	Substantially compromised 2	Moderately compromised 3	Mildly compromised 4	Not compromised 5	
INDICATORS:						
090901 Consciousness	1	2	3	4	5	NA
090902 Central motor control	1	2	3	4	5	NA
090903 Cranial sensory and motor function	1	2	3	4	5	NA
090904 Spinal sensory and motor function	1	2	3	4	5	NA
090905 Autonomic function	1	2	3	4	5	NA
090906 Intracranial pressure	1	2	3	4	5	NA
090907 Communication appropriate to situation	1	2	3	4	5	NA
090908 Pupil size	1	2	3	4	5	NA
090909 Pupil reactivity	1	2	3	4	5	NA
090910 Eye movement pattern	1	2	3	4	5	NA
090911 Breathing pattern	1	2	3	4	5	NA
090913 Sleep-rest pattern	1	2	3	4	5	NA
090917 Blood pressure	1	2	3	4	5	NA
090918 Pulse pressure	1	2	3	4	5	NA
090919 Respiratory rate	1	2	3	4	5	NA
090920 Hyperthermia	1	2	3	4	5	NA
090921 Apical heart rate	1	2	3	4	5	NA
090922 Radial pulse rate	1	2	3	4	5	NA
090923 Cognitive orientation	1	2	3	4	5	NA
090924 Cognitive status	1	2	3	4	5	NA
	Severe	Substantial	Moderate	Mild	None	
090914 Seizure activity	1	2	3	4	5	NA
090915 Headaches	1	2	3	4	5	NA

1st edition 1997; Revised 3rd edition 2004

Continued

Outcome Content References:

American Nurses' Association Council on Medical-Surgical Nursing Practice and American Association of Neuroscience Nurses. (1986). *Neuroscience nursing practice: process and outcome criteria for selected diagnoses*. Washington, DC: Government Printing Office.

Hickey, J. V. (2002). *The clinical practice of neurological and neurosurgical nursing* (5th ed.). Philadelphia: Lippincott Williams & Wilkins.

Mitchell, P. H., Hodges, L. C., Muwaswes, M., & Walleck, C. A. (Eds.). (1988). *AANN's neuroscience nursing: Phenomena and practice*. Norwalk, CT: Appleton & Lange.

Riess, P. C. (1995). *Validity and reliability of the Riess Intracranial Aneurysm Assessment Tool and the Glasgow Coma Scale in the aneurysm population*. Master's thesis, The University of Iowa, Iowa City.

Smeltzer, S. C., & Bare, B. G. (Eds.). (2003). *Brunner and Suddarth's textbook of medical-surgical nursing* (10th ed.). Philadelphia: Lippincott Williams & Wilkins.

+Teasdale, G., & Jennett, B. (1974). Assessment of coma and impaired consciousness: A practical scale. *Lancet, 2*, 81-84.

N

Neurological Status: Autonomic—0910

Domain-Physiologic Health (II)

Class-Neurocognitive (J)

Scale(s)-Severely compromised to Not compromised (a) and Severe to None (n)

Care Recipient:

Data Source:

Definition: Ability of the autonomic nervous system to coordinate visceral and homeostatic function

OUTCOME TARGET RATING: Maintain at_____   Increase to_____

Neurological Status: Autonomic Overall Rating	Severely compromised 1	Substantially compromised 2	Moderately compromised 3	Mildly compromised 4	Not compromised 5	
INDICATORS:						
091001 Apical heart rate	1	2	3	4	5	NA
091020 Radial pulse rate	1	2	3	4	5	NA
091002 Systolic blood pressure	1	2	3	4	5	NA
091003 Diastolic blood pressure	1	2	3	4	5	NA
091004 Cardiac pump effectiveness	1	2	3	4	5	NA
091005 Vasodilatation response	1	2	3	4	5	NA
091006 Vasoconstriction response	1	2	3	4	5	NA
091007 Perspiration response pattern	1	2	3	4	5	NA
091008 Goose bumps response pattern	1	2	3	4	5	NA
091009 Bowel elimination pattern	1	2	3	4	5	NA
091010 Intestinal motility	1	2	3	4	5	NA
091011 Urinary elimination pattern	1	2	3	4	5	NA
091021 Pupil reactivity	1	2	3	4	5	NA
091013 Thermoregulation	1	2	3	4	5	NA
091014 Peripheral tissue perfusion	1	2	3	4	5	NA
091015 Sexual organ response	1	2	3	4	5	NA
	Severe	**Substantial**	**Moderate**	**Mild**	**None**	
091016 Bronchospasms	1	2	3	4	5	NA
091017 Intestinal spasms	1	2	3	4	5	NA
091018 Bladder spasms	1	2	3	4	5	NA
091022 Headaches	1	2	3	4	5	NA
091023 Dilated pupils	1	2	3	4	5	NA
091024 Constricted pupils	1	2	3	4	5	NA
091025 Hyperthermia	1	2	3	4	5	NA
091026 Dysreflexia	1	2	3	4	5	NA

1st edition 1997; Revised 3rd edition 2004

Outcome Content References:

McCance, K. L., & Huether, S. E. (2002). *Pathophysiology: The biologic basis for disease in adults and children* (4th ed.). St. Louis: Mosby.
Smeltzer, S. C., & Bare, B. G. (Eds.). (2003). *Brunner and Suddarth's textbook of medical-surgical nursing* (10th ed.). Philadelphia: Lippincott Williams & Wilkins.

N

Neurological Status: Central Motor Control—0911

Domain-Physiologic Health (II)

Class-Neurocognitive (J)

Scale(s)-Severely compromised to Not compromised (a) and Severe to None (n)

Care Recipient:

Data Source:

Definition: Ability of the central nervous system to coordinate skeletal muscle activity for body movement

OUTCOME TARGET RATING: Maintain at_____   Increase to_____

Neurological Status: Central Motor Control Overall Rating	Severely compromised 1	Substantially compromised 2	Moderately compromised 3	Mildly compromised 4	Not compromised 5	
INDICATORS:						
091101 Balance	1	2	3	4	5	NA
091103 Maintenance of posture	1	2	3	4	5	NA
091104 Infantile reflexes (automatisms)	1	2	3	4	5	NA
091105 Babinski's reflex	1	2	3	4	5	NA
091106 Deep tendon reflexes	1	2	3	4	5	NA
091112 Purposeful movement on command	1	2	3	4	5	NA
	Severe	**Substantial**	**Moderate**	**Mild**	**None**	
091113 Gait abnormalities	1	2	3	4	5	NA
091107 Spasticity	1	2	3	4	5	NA
091108 Involuntary movements	1	2	3	4	5	NA
091109 Nystagmus	1	2	3	4	5	NA
091110 Seizure activity	1	2	3	4	5	NA

1st edition 1997; Revised 3rd edition 2004

Outcome Content References:

American Nurses' Association Council on Medical-Surgical Nursing Practice and American Association of Neuroscience Nurses. (1986). *Neuroscience nursing practice: Process and outcome criteria for selected diagnoses.* Washington, DC: Government Printing Office.

Bickley, L. (2002). *Bates' guide to physical examination and history taking* (8th ed.). Philadelphia: Lippincott Williams & Wilkins.

Hickey, J. V. (2002). *The clinical practice of neurological and neurosurgical nursing* (5th ed.). Philadelphia: Lippincott Williams & Wilkins.

Mitchell, P. H., Hodges, L. C., Muwaswes, M., & Walleck, C. A. (Eds.). (1988). *AANN's neuroscience nursing: Phenomena and practice.* Norwalk, CT: Appleton & Lange.

Smeltzer, S. C., & Bare, B. G. (Eds.). (2003). *Brunner and Suddarth's textbook of medical-surgical nursing* (10th ed.). Philadelphia: Lippincott Williams & Wilkins.

Neurological Status: Consciousness—0912

Domain-Physiologic Health (II)

Class-Neurocognitive (J)

Scale(s)-Severely compromised to Not compromised (a) and Severe to None (n)

Care Recipient:

Data Source:

Definition: Arousal, orientation, and attention to the environment

OUTCOME TARGET RATING: Maintain at_____   Increase to_____

Neurological Status: Consciousness Overall Rating	Severely compromised 1	Substantially compromised 2	Moderately compromised 3	Mildly compromised 4	Not compromised 5	
INDICATORS:						
091201 Opens eyes to external stimuli	1	2	3	4	5	NA
091202 Cognitive orientation	1	2	3	4	5	NA
091203 Communication appropriate to situation	1	2	3	4	5	NA
091204 Obeys commands	1	2	3	4	5	NA
091205 Motor responses to noxious stimuli	1	2	3	4	5	NA
091206 Attends to environmental stimuli	1	2	3	4	5	NA
	Severe	**Substantial**	**Moderate**	**Mild**	**None**	
091207 Seizure activity	1	2	3	4	5	NA
091209 Abnormal flexion	1	2	3	4	5	NA
091210 Abnormal extension	1	2	3	4	5	NA
091211 Stupor	1	2	3	4	5	NA
091212 Trance state	1	2	3	4	5	NA
091213 Delirium	1	2	3	4	5	NA
091214 Coma	1	2	3	4	5	NA

Glasgow Coma Scale score_____

1st edition 1997; Revised 3rd edition 2004; Revised 4th edition

N

Outcome Content References:

American Nurses' Association Council on Medical-Surgical Nursing Practice and American Association of Neuroscience Nurses. (1986). *Neuroscience nursing practice: process and outcome criteria for selected diagnoses.* Washington, DC: Government Printing Office.

Hickey, J. V. (2002). *The clinical practice of neurological and neurosurgical nursing* (5th ed.). Philadelphia: Lippincott Williams & Wilkins.

Mitchell, P. H., Hodges, L. C., Muwaswes, M., & Walleck, C. A. (Eds.). (1988). *AANN's neuroscience nursing: Phenomena and practice.* Norwalk, CT: Appleton & Lange.

Riess, P. C. (1995). *Validity and reliability of the Riess Intracranial Aneurysm Assessment Tool and the Glasgow Coma Scale in the aneurysm population.* Master's thesis, The University of Iowa: Iowa City.

Smeltzer, S. C., & Bare, B. G. (Eds.). (2003). *Brunner and Suddarth's textbook of medical-surgical nursing* (10th ed.). Philadelphia: Lippincott Williams & Wilkins.

Neurological Status: Cranial Sensory/Motor Function—0913

Domain-Physiologic Health (II)
Class-Neurocognitive (J)
Scale(s)-Severely compromised to Not compromised (a) and Severe to None (n)

Care Recipient:
Data Source:

Definition: Ability of the cranial nerves to convey sensory and motor impulses

OUTCOME TARGET RATING: Maintain at_____   Increase to_____

Neurological Status: Cranial Sensory/Motor Function Overall Rating	Severely compromised 1	Substantially compromised 2	Moderately compromised 3	Mildly compromised 4	Not compromised 5	
INDICATORS:						
091301 Olfaction	1	2	3	4	5	NA
091302 Vision	1	2	3	4	5	NA
091303 Corneal reflex	1	2	3	4	5	NA
091304 Taste	1	2	3	4	5	NA
091305 Hearing	1	2	3	4	5	NA
091317 Speech	1	2	3	4	5	NA
091306 Facial sensation	1	2	3	4	5	NA
091307 Facial muscle movement	1	2	3	4	5	NA
091318 Facial symmetry	1	2	3	4	5	NA
091319 Bilateral muscle strength	1	2	3	4	5	NA
091308 Swallowing	1	2	3	4	5	NA
091309 Gag reflex	1	2	3	4	5	NA
091310 Tongue movement	1	2	3	4	5	NA
091312 Purposeful head movement	1	2	3	4	5	NA
091320 Purposeful shoulder movement	1	2	3	4	5	NA

	Severe	Substantial	Moderate	Mild	None	
091314 Dizziness	1	2	3	4	5	NA
091315 Pronator drift	1	2	3	4	5	NA
091321 Involuntary head movement	1	2	3	4	5	NA
091322 Involuntary facial movement	1	2	3	4	5	NA
091323 Tics	1	2	3	4	5	NA
091324 Hoarseness	1	2	3	4	5	NA
091325 Nasal tone to voice	1	2	3	4	5	NA
091326 Unilateral facial paralysis	1	2	3	4	5	NA

1st edition 1997; Revised 3rd edition 2004

Outcome Content References:

Bickley, L. (2002). *Bates' guide to physical examination and history taking* (8th ed.). Philadelphia: Lippincott Williams & Wilkins.

McCance, K. L., & Huether, S. E. (2002). *Pathophysiology: The biologic basis for disease in adults and children* (4th ed.). St. Louis: Mosby.

Riess, P. C. (1995). *Validity and reliability of the Riess Intracranial Aneurysm Assessment Tool and the Glasgow Coma Scale in the aneurysm population.* Master's thesis, The University of Iowa: Iowa City.

Smeltzer, S. C., & Bare, B. G. (Eds.). (2003). *Brunner and Suddarth's textbook of medical-surgical nursing* (10th ed.). Philadelphia: Lippincott Williams & Wilkins.

Neurological Status: Peripheral—0917

Domain-Physiologic Health (II)   Care Recipient:

Class-Neurocognitive (J)   Data Source:

Scale(s)-Severely compromised to Not compromised (a) and Severe to None (n)

Definition: Ability of the peripheral nervous system to transmit impulses to and from the central nervous system

OUTCOME TARGET RATING: Maintain at_____   Increase to_____

Neurological Status: Peripheral Overall Rating	Severely compromised 1	Substantially compromised 2	Moderately compromised 3	Mildly compromised 4	Not compromised 5	
INDICATORS:						
091701 Sensation in upper right extremity	1	2	3	4	5	NA
091702 Sensation in upper left extremity	1	2	3	4	5	NA
091703 Sensation in lower right extremity	1	2	3	4	5	NA
091704 Sensation in lower left extremity	1	2	3	4	5	NA
091705 Sensation equal bilaterally	1	2	3	4	5	NA
091706 Motor function in upper right extremity	1	2	3	4	5	NA
091707 Motor function in upper left extremity	1	2	3	4	5	NA
091708 Motor function in lower right extremity	1	2	3	4	5	NA
091709 Motor function in lower left extremity	1	2	3	4	5	NA
091710 Motor function equal bilaterally	1	2	3	4	5	NA
091711 Skin color in upper right extremity	1	2	3	4	5	NA
091712 Skin color in upper left extremity	1	2	3	4	5	NA
091713 Skin color in lower right extremity	1	2	3	4	5	NA
091714 Skin color in lower left extremity	1	2	3	4	5	NA
091715 Proprioception in upper right extremity	1	2	3	4	5	NA
091716 Proprioception in upper left extremity	1	2	3	4	5	NA
091717 Proprioception in lower right extremity	1	2	3	4	5	NA
091718 Proprioception in lower left extremity	1	2	3	4	5	NA
091719 Proprioception equal bilaterally	1	2	3	4	5	NA

N

Continued

		Severely compromised	Substantially compromised	Moderately compromised	Mildly compromised	Not compromised	
091720	Hot/cold discrimination in upper right extremity	1	2	3	4	5	NA
091721	Hot/cold discrimination in upper left extremity	1	2	3	4	5	NA
091722	Hot/cold discrimination in lower right extremity	1	2	3	4	5	NA
091723	Hot/cold discrimination in lower left extremity	1	2	3	4	5	NA
091724	Hot/cold discrimination equal bilaterally	1	2	3	4	5	NA
091725	Muscle tone in upper right extremity	1	2	3	4	5	NA
091726	Muscle tone in upper left extremity	1	2	3	4	5	NA
091727	Muscle tone in lower right extremity	1	2	3	4	5	NA
091728	Muscle tone in lower left extremity	1	2	3	4	5	NA
091729	Muscle tone equal bilaterally	1	2	3	4	5	NA
		Severe	**Substantial**	**Moderate**	**Mild**	**None**	
091730	Hyperesthesia in upper right extremity	1	2	3	4	5	NA
091731	Hyperesthesia in upper left extremity	1	2	3	4	5	NA
091732	Hyperesthesia in lower right extremity	1	2	3	4	5	NA
091733	Hyperesthesia in lower left extremity	1	2	3	4	5	NA
091734	Hypoesthesia in upper right extremity	1	2	3	4	5	NA
091735	Hypoesthesia in upper left extremity	1	2	3	4	5	NA
091736	Hypoesthesia in lower right extremity	1	2	3	4	5	NA
091737	Hypoesthesia in lower left extremity	1	2	3	4	5	NA
091738	Pain in upper right extremity	1	2	3	4	5	NA
091739	Pain in upper left extremity	1	2	3	4	5	NA
091740	Pain in lower right extremity	1	2	3	4	5	NA
091741	Pain in lower left extremity	1	2	3	4	5	NA
091742	Paresthesia in upper right extremity	1	2	3	4	5	NA
091743	Paresthesia in upper left extremity	1	2	3	4	5	NA
091744	Paresthesia in lower right extremity	1	2	3	4	5	NA
091745	Paresthesia in lower left extremity	1	2	3	4	5	NA

N

4th edition

Outcome Content References:

Huether, S. E., & McCance, K. L. (2000). *Understanding pathophysiology* (2nd ed., p. 344). St Louis: Mosby.

Kidd, P. S., & Wagner, K. D. (2001). *High acuity nursing* (3rd ed., pp. 638-639). Upper Saddle River, NJ: Prentice Hall.

Swearingen, P. L. (Ed.). (2003). *Manual of medical-surgical nursing care: Nursing interventions & collaborative management* (5th ed., pp. 207). St. Louis: Mosby.

N

Neurological Status: Spinal Sensory/Motor Function—0914

Domain-Physiologic Health (II)

Class-Neurocognitive (J)

Scale(s)-Severely compromised to Not compromised (a) and Severe to None (n)

Care Recipient:

Data Source:

Definition: Ability of the spinal nerves to convey sensory and motor impulses

OUTCOME TARGET RATING: Maintain at_____   Increase to_____

Neurological Status: Spinal Sensory Motor/Function Overall Rating	Severely compromised 1	Substantially compromised 2	Moderately compromised 3	Mildly compromised 4	Not compromised 5	
INDICATORS:						
091401 Head and shoulder movement	1	2	3	4	5	NA
091402 Autonomic function	1	2	3	4	5	NA
091403 Deep tendon reflexes	1	2	3	4	5	NA
091404 Upper body skin sensation	1	2	3	4	5	NA
091409 Lower body skin sensation	1	2	3	4	5	NA
091405 Upper body strength	1	2	3	4	5	NA
091410 Lower body strength	1	2	3	4	5	NA
	Severe	**Substantial**	**Moderate**	**Mild**	**None**	
091406 Flaccidity	1	2	3	4	5	NA
091407 Pronator drift	1	2	3	4	5	NA
091411 Involuntary movement	1	2	3	4	5	NA
091412 Fasciculation	1	2	3	4	5	NA

1st edition 1997; Revised 3rd edition 2004

Outcome Content References:

Bickley, L. (2002). *Bates' guide to physical examination and history taking* (8th ed.). Philadelphia: Lippincott Williams & Wilkins.

Riess, P. C. (1995). *Validity and reliability of the Riess Intracranial Aneurysm Assessment Tool and the Glasgow Coma Scale in the aneurysm population.* Master's thesis, The University of Iowa: Iowa City.

Smeltzer, S. C., & Bare, B. G. (Eds.). (2003). *Brunner and Suddarth's textbook of medical-surgical nursing* (10th ed.). Philadelphia: Lippincott Williams & Wilkins.

Newborn Adaptation—0118

Domain-Functional Health (I)

Class-Growth & Development (B)

Scale(s)-Severe deviation from normal range to No deviation from normal range (b)

Care Recipient:

Data Source:

Definition: Adaptive response to the extrauterine environment by a physiologically mature newborn during the first 28 days

OUTCOME TARGET RATING: Maintain at_____   Increase to_____

Newborn Adaptation Overall Rating	Severe deviation from normal range 1	Substantial deviation from normal range 2	Moderate deviation from normal range 3	Mild deviation from normal range 4	No deviation from normal range 5	
INDICATORS:						
011801 Apgar score	1	2	3	4	5	NA
011802 Gestational age index	1	2	3	4	5	NA
011803 Apical heart rate (100-160 bpm)	1	2	3	4	5	NA
011804 Respiratory rate (30-60)	1	2	3	4	5	NA
011805 Blood pressure ratio of arm to leg	1	2	3	4	5	NA
011806 Oxygen saturation <90%	1	2	3	4	5	NA
011807 Thermoregulation	1	2	3	4	5	NA
011808 Skin color	1	2	3	4	5	NA
011809 Eyes clear	1	2	3	4	5	NA
011810 Cord drying	1	2	3	4	5	NA
011811 Weight	1	2	3	4	5	NA
011812 Feeding tolerance	1	2	3	4	5	NA
011813 Suck reflex	1	2	3	4	5	NA
011814 Muscle tone	1	2	3	4	5	NA
011815 Smooth, synchronous movement	1	2	3	4	5	NA
011816 Attentiveness to stimuli	1	2	3	4	5	NA
011817 Response to stimuli	1	2	3	4	5	NA
011818 Sustained alertness during interaction	1	2	3	4	5	NA
011819 Interaction with caregiver	1	2	3	4	5	NA
011820 Self-consolability	1	2	3	4	5	NA
011821 Blood glucose	1	2	3	4	5	NA
011822 Coombs test	1	2	3	4	5	NA
011823 Bilirubin level	1	2	3	4	5	NA
011824 Bowel elimination	1	2	3	4	5	NA
011825 Urinary elimination	1	2	3	4	5	NA

2nd edition 2000; Revised 3rd edition 2004

N

Continued

Outcome Content References:

American Academy of Pediatrics & The American College of Obstetricians and Gynecologists. (1997). *Guidelines for perinatal care* (4th ed.). Washington, DC: American College of Obstetricians and Gynecologists.

Association of Women's Health, Obstetricians and Neonatal Nurses. (1998). *Standards & guidelines for the professional nursing practice in the care of women and newborns* (5th ed.). Washington, DC: Author

AWHONN Voice. (1996). Clinical commentary: Physiologic assessment of the healthy newborn. *Journal of Obstetric, Gynecologic, and Neonatal Nursing, 4*(6), 5-6.

Committee on Fetus and Newborn. (1993). Routine evaluation of blood pressure, hematocrit, and glucose in newborns. *Pediatrics, 92*(3), 474-476.

Murray, S. S., McKinney, E. S., & Gorrie, T. M. (2002). *Foundations of maternal-newborn nursing* (3rd ed.). Philadelphia: W.B. Saunders.

Simpson, K. R., & Creehan, P. A. (2001). *AWHONN's perinatal nursing* (2nd ed.). Philadelphia: Lippincott Williams & Wilkins.

N

Nutritional Status—1004

Domain-Physiologic Health (II)   Care Recipient:

Class-Digestion & Nutrition (K)   Data Source:

Scale(s)-Severe deviation from normal range to No deviation from normal range (b)

Definition: Extent to which nutrients are available to meet metabolic needs

OUTCOME TARGET RATING: Maintain at_____   Increase to_____

Nutritional Status Overall Rating	Severe deviation from normal range 1	Substantial deviation from normal range 2	Moderate deviation from normal range 3	Mild deviation from normal range 4	No deviation from normal range 5	
INDICATORS:						
100401 Nutrient intake	1	2	3	4	5	NA
100402 Food intake	1	2	3	4	5	NA
100408 Fluid intake	1	2	3	4	5	NA
100403 Energy	1	2	3	4	5	NA
100405 Weight/height ratio	1	2	3	4	5	NA
100409 Hematocrit	1	2	3	4	5	NA
100410 Muscle tone	1	2	3	4	5	NA
100411 Hydration	1	2	3	4	5	NA

1st edition 1997; Revised 3rd edition 2004

Outcome Content References:

Chang, B. L., Uman, G. C., Linn, L. S., Ware, J. E., & Kane, R. L. (1985). Adherence to healthcare regimens among elderly women. *Nursing Research, 34*(1), 27-31.

Collinsworth, R., & Boyle, K. (1989). Nutritional assessment of the elderly. *Journal of Gerontological Nursing, 15*(12), 17-21.

Curtas, S., Chapman, G., & Meguid, M. (1989). Evaluation of nutritional status. *Nursing Clinics of North America, 24*(2), 301-313.

Folsom, A. R., Kaye, S. A., Sellers, T. A., Hang, C. P., Cerhan, J. R., Potter, J. D., & Prineas, R. J. (1993). Body fat distribution and five year risk of death in older women. *Journal of the American Medical Association, 269*(4), 483-487.

Gianino, S., & St. John, R. E. (1993). Nutritional assessment of the patient in the intensive care unit. *Critical Care Nursing Clinics of North America, 5*(1), 1-16.

+Guigoz, Y., Vallas, B., & Garry, P. J. (1996). Mini Nutritional Assessment: A practical assessment tool for grading the nutritional state of elderly patients. *Facts and Research in Gerontology, 4*(Suppl. 2), 15-59.

Tandy, L., & Malan, S. (2001). Impaired swallowing. In M. Maas, K. Buckwalter, M. Hardy, T. Tripp-Reimer, M. Titler, & J. Specht (Eds.), *Nursing care of older adults: Diagnoses, outcomes & interventions* (pp. 158-171). St. Louis: Mosby.

Wakefield, B. (2001). Altered nutrition: Less than body requirements. In M. Maas, K. Buckwalter, M. Hardy, T. Tripp-Reimer, M. Titler, & J. Specht (Eds.), *Nursing care of older adults: Diagnoses, outcomes & interventions* (pp. 145-157). St. Louis: Mosby.

N

Nutritional Status: Biochemical Measures—1005

Domain-Physiologic Health (II)

Class-Digestion & Nutrition (K)

Scale(s)-Severe deviation from normal range to No deviation from normal range (b)

Care Recipient:

Data Source:

Definition: Body fluid components and chemical indices of nutritional status

OUTCOME TARGET RATING: Maintain at_____   Increase to_____

Nutritional Status: Biochemical Measures Overall Rating	Severe deviation from normal range 1	Substantial deviation from normal range 2	Moderate deviation from normal range 3	Mild deviation from normal range 4	No deviation from normal range 5	
INDICATORS:						
100501 Serum albumin	1	2	3	4	5	NA
100502 Serum prealbumin	1	2	3	4	5	NA
100514 Serum creatinine	1	2	3	4	5	NA
100503 Hematocrit	1	2	3	4	5	NA
100504 Hemoglobin	1	2	3	4	5	NA
100510 Serum transferrin	1	2	3	4	5	NA
100505 Total iron binding capacity	1	2	3	4	5	NA
100506 Lymphocyte count	1	2	3	4	5	NA
100507 Blood glucose	1	2	3	4	5	NA
100508 Blood cholesterol	1	2	3	4	5	NA
100509 Blood triglycerides	1	2	3	4	5	NA
100511 24-hour urinary creatinine	1	2	3	4	5	NA
100512 Urinary urea nitrogen	1	2	3	4	5	NA

1st edition 1997; Revised 3rd edition 2004

Outcome Content References:

Chang, B. L., Uman, G. C., Linn, L. S., Ware, J. E., & Kane, R. L. (1985). Adherence to healthcare regimens among elderly women. *Nursing Research, 34*(1), 27-31.

Collinsworth, R., & Boyle, K. (1989). Nutritional assessment of the elderly. *Journal of Gerontological Nursing, 15*(12), 17-21.

Curtas, S., Chapman, G., & Meguid, M. (1989). Evaluation of nutritional status. *Nursing Clinics of North America, 24*(2), 301-313.

Folsom, A. R., Kaye, S. A., Sellers, T. A., Hang, C. P., Cerhan, J. R., Potter, J. D., & Prineas, R. J. (1993). Body fat distribution and five year risk of death in older women. *Journal of the American Medical Association, 269*(4), 483-487.

Gianino, S., & St. John, R. E. (1993). Nutritional assessment of the patient in the intensive care unit. *Critical Care Nursing Clinics of North America, 5*(1), 1-16.

N

Nutritional Status: Energy—1007

Domain-Physiologic Health (II)   Care Recipient:

Class-Digestion & Nutrition (K)   Data Source:

Scale(s)-Severe deviation from normal range to No deviation from normal range (b)

Definition: Extent to which nutrients and oxygen provide cellular energy

OUTCOME TARGET RATING: Maintain at_____   Increase to_____

Nutritional Status: Energy Overall Rating	Severe deviation from normal range 1	Substantial deviation from normal range 2	Moderate deviation from normal range 3	Mild deviation from normal range 4	No deviation from normal range 5	
INDICATORS:						
100701 Stamina	1	2	3	4	5	NA
100702 Endurance	1	2	3	4	5	NA
100703 Hand grip strength	1	2	3	4	5	NA
100708 Muscle tone	1	2	3	4	5	NA
100704 Tissue healing	1	2	3	4	5	NA
100705 Infection resistance	1	2	3	4	5	NA
100706 Growth (children)	1	2	3	4	5	NA

1st edition 1997; Revised 3rd edition 2004

Outcome Content References:

Chang, B. L., Uman, G. C., Linn, L. S., Ware, J. E., & Kane, R. L. (1985). Adherence to healthcare regimens among elderly women. *Nursing Research, 34*(1), 27-31.

Collinsworth, R., & Boyle, K. (1989). Nutritional assessment of the elderly. *Journal of Gerontological Nursing, 15*(12), 17-21.

Curtas, S., Chapman, G., & Meguid, M. (1989). Evaluation of nutritional status. *Nursing Clinics of North America, 24*(2), 301-313.

+Dartmouth Primary Care Cooperative Information Project. (1987). *COOP Charts.* Hanover, NH: Department of Community and Family Medicine, Dartmouth Medical School.

Folsom, A. R., Kaye, S. A., Sellers, T. A., Hang, C. P., Cerhan, J. R., Potter, J. D., & Prineas, R. J. (1993). Body fat distribution and 5 year risk of death in older women. *Journal of the American Medical Association, 269*(4), 483-487.

Gianino, S., & St. John, R. E. (1993). Nutritional assessment of the patient in the intensive care unit. *Critical Care Nursing Clinics of North America, 5*(1), 1-16.

N

Nutritional Status: Food & Fluid Intake—1008

Domain-Physiologic Health (II)

Class-Digestion & Nutrition (K)

Scale(s)-Not adequate to Totally adequate (f)

Care Recipient:

Data Source:

Definition: Amount of food and fluid taken into the body over a 24-hour period

OUTCOME TARGET RATING: Maintain at_____   Increase to_____

Nutritional Status: Food & Fluid Intake Overall Rating	Not adequate 1	Slightly adequate 2	Moderately adequate 3	Substantially adequate 4	Totally adequate 5	

INDICATORS:

100801	Oral food intake	1	2	3	4	5	NA
100802	Tube feeding intake	1	2	3	4	5	NA
100803	Oral fluid intake	1	2	3	4	5	NA
100804	Intravenous fluid intake	1	2	3	4	5	NA
100805	Parenteral nutrition intake	1	2	3	4	5	NA

1st edition 1997; Revised 3rd edition 2004

Outcome Content References:

Champagne, M. T., & Ashley, M. L. (1989). Nutritional support in the critically ill elderly patient. *Critical Care Nursing Quarterly, 12*(1), 15-25.

Coyle, E. F. (2004). Fluid and fuel intake during exercise. *Journal of Sports Sciences, 22*, 39-55.

Duggal, A., & Lawrence, R. M. (2001). Aspects of food refusal in the elderly: The "hunger strike." *International Journal of Eating Disorders, 30*(2), 213-216.

Gianino, S., & St. John, R. E. (1993). Nutritional assessment of the patient in the intensive care unit. *Critical Care Nursing Clinics of North America, 5*(1), 1-16.

Keithley, J. K., & Kohn, C. L. (1990). Managing nutritional problems in people with AIDS. *Oncology Nursing Forum, 17*(1), 23-27.

N

Nutritional Status: Nutrient Intake—1009

Domain-Physiologic Health (II)

Class-Digestion & Nutrition (K)

Scale(s)-Not adequate to Totally adequate (f)

Care Recipient:

Data Source:

Definition: Nutrient intake to meet metabolic needs

OUTCOME TARGET RATING: Maintain at_____   Increase to_____

Nutritional Status: Nutrient Intake Overall Rating	Not adequate 1	Slightly adequate 2	Moderately adequate 3	Substantially adequate 4	Totally adequate 5	
INDICATORS:						
100901 Caloric intake	1	2	3	4	5	NA
100902 Protein intake	1	2	3	4	5	NA
100903 Fat intake	1	2	3	4	5	NA
100904 Carbohydrate intake	1	2	3	4	5	NA
100910 Fiber intake	1	2	3	4	5	NA
100905 Vitamin intake	1	2	3	4	5	NA
100906 Mineral intake	1	2	3	4	5	NA
100907 Iron intake	1	2	3	4	5	NA
100908 Calcium intake	1	2	3	4	5	NA
100911 Sodium intake	1	2	3	4	5	NA

1st edition 1997; Revised 3rd edition 2004; Revised 4th edition

N

Outcome Content References:

Champagne, M. T., & Ashley, M. L. (1989). Nutritional support in the critically ill elderly patient. *Critical Care Nursing Quarterly, 12*(1), 15-25.

Coyle, E. F. (2004). Fluid and fuel intake during exercise. *Journal of Sports Sciences, 22,* 39-55.

Gianino, S., & St. John, R. E. (1993). Nutritional assessment of the patient in the intensive care unit. *Critical Care Nursing Clinics of North America, 5*(1), 1-16.

Keithley, J. K., & Kohn, C. L. (1990). Managing nutritional problems in people with AIDS. *Oncology Nursing Forum, 17*(1), 23-27.

Oral Hygiene—1100

Domain-Physiologic Health (II)   *Care Recipient:*

Class-Tissue Integrity (L)   *Data Source:*

Scale(s)-Severely compromised to Not compromised (a) and Severe to None (n)

Definition: Condition of the mouth, teeth, gums, and tongue

OUTCOME TARGET RATING: Maintain at_____   Increase to_____

Oral Hygiene Overall Rating	Severely compromised 1	Substantially compromised 2	Moderately compromised 3	Mildly compromised 4	Not compromised 5	
INDICATORS:						
110001 Cleanliness of mouth	1	2	3	4	5	NA
110002 Cleanliness of teeth	1	2	3	4	5	NA
110003 Cleanliness of gums	1	2	3	4	5	NA
110004 Cleanliness of tongue	1	2	3	4	5	NA
110005 Cleanliness of dentures	1	2	3	4	5	NA
110006 Cleanliness of dental appliances	1	2	3	4	5	NA
110007 Fit of dentures	1	2	3	4	5	NA
110008 Fit of dental appliances	1	2	3	4	5	NA
110009 Moistness of lips	1	2	3	4	5	NA
110010 Moisture of oral mucosa and tongue	1	2	3	4	5	NA
110011 Color of mucous membranes	1	2	3	4	5	NA
110012 Oral mucosa integrity	1	2	3	4	5	NA
110013 Tongue integrity	1	2	3	4	5	NA
110014 Gum integrity	1	2	3	4	5	NA

	Severe	Substantial	Moderate	Mild	None	
110017 Halitosis	1	2	3	4	5	NA
110018 Bleeding	1	2	3	4	5	NA
110021 Pain	1	2	3	4	5	NA
110022 Oral mucosa lesions	1	2	3	4	5	NA
110023 Dental caries	1	2	3	4	5	NA
110024 Gingivitis	1	2	3	4	5	NA
110025 Periodontal disease	1	2	3	4	5	NA

Dental Prosthesis YES / NO

1st edition 1997; Revised 3rd edition 2004; Revised 4th edition

Outcome Content References:

Fischman, S. (1993). Self-care: Practical periodontal care in today's practice. *International Dental Journal, 43,* 179-183.

Jones, J. A. (1989). Integrating the oral examination into clinical practice. *Hospital Practice, 24*(10A), 23-24, 26-27, 30.

+Kayser-Jones, J., Bird, W. F., Paul, S. M., Long, L., & Schell, E. S. (1995). An instrument to assess the oral health status of nursing home residents. *The Gerontologist, 35*(6), 814-824.

Matteson, M. A., McConnell E. S., & Linton, A. D. (1997). *Gerontological nursing: Concepts & practice* (2nd ed.). Philadelphia: W.B. Saunders.

Raybould, T. P., Carpenter, A. D., Ferretti, G. A., Brown, A. T., Lillich, T. T., & Henslee, J. (1994). Emergence of gram-negative bacilli in the mouths of bone marrow transplant recipients using chlorhexidine mouth rinse. *Oncology Nursing Forum, 21*(4), 691-696.

Richardson, A. (1987). A process standard for oral care. *Nursing Times, 83*(32), 38-40.

Speedie, G. (1983). Nursology of mouth care: Preventing, comforting and seeking activities related to mouth care. *Journal of Advanced Nursing, 8*(1), 33-40.

Ostomy Self-Care—1615

Domain-Health Knowledge & Behavior (IV)

Class-Health Behavior (Q)

Scale(s)-Never demonstrated to Consistently demonstrated (m)

Care Recipient:

Data Source:

Definition: Personal actions to maintain ostomy for elimination

OUTCOME TARGET RATIING: Maintain at_____   Increase to_____

Ostomy Self-Care Overall Rating		Never demonstrated 1	Rarely demonstrated 2	Sometimes demonstrated 3	Often demonstrated 4	Consistently demonstrated 5	
161501	Describes functioning of ostomy	1	2	3	4	5	NA
161502	Describes purpose of ostomy	1	2	3	4	5	NA
161503	Appears comfortable viewing stoma	1	2	3	4	5	NA
161504	Measures stoma for proper appliance fit	1	2	3	4	5	NA
161520	Maintains skin care around ostomy	1	2	3	4	5	NA
161521	Uses correct irrigation technique	1	2	3	4	5	NA
161507	Empties ostomy bag	1	2	3	4	5	NA
161508	Changes ostomy bag	1	2	3	4	5	NA
161509	Monitors for complications related to stoma	1	2	3	4	5	NA
161510	Monitors amount and consistency of stool	1	2	3	4	5	NA
161511	Follows schedule for changing ostomy bag	1	2	3	4	5	NA
161512	Obtains ostomy supplies	1	2	3	4	5	NA
161513	Avoids flatus-producing food and drink	1	2	3	4	5	NA
161514	Maintains adequate fluid intake	1	2	3	4	5	NA
161515	Follows recommended diet	1	2	3	4	5	NA
161516	Avoids odor-producing foods	1	2	3	4	5	NA
161522	Modifies daily activities to optimize self-care	1	2	3	4	5	NA
161523	Obtains assistance from a health professional	1	2	3	4	5	NA
161519	Expresses acceptance of ostomy	1	2	3	4	5	NA

3rd edition 2004; Revised 4th edition

Continued

Outcome Content References:

Bryant, D., & Fleischer, I. (2000). Changing an ostomy appliance. *Nursing, 30*(11), 51-53.

Lee, J. (2001). Nurse prescribing in practice: Patient choice in stoma care. *British Journal of Community Nursing, 6*(1), 33-34, 36-37.

Martins, M. L., & Cardoso, M. (2001). Group participative education for persons with an ostomy. *World Council of Enterostomal Therapists Journal, 21*(4), 8-17.

Metcalf, C. (1999). Clinical stoma care: Empowering patients through teaching practical skills. *British Journal of Nursing, 8*(9), 593-600.

Sage, S. J. (1991). Nephrostomy dressing change procedure. *Ostomy Wound Management, 32*, 32-33, 35-36.

Secord, C., Jackman, M., Wright, L., & Winton, S. (2001). Adjusting to life with an ostomy. *Canadian Nurse, 97*(1), 29-32.

Thompson, J. (2000). A practical ostomy guide. *RN, 63*(11), 61-68.

O

Pain: Adverse Psychological Response—1306

Domain-Perceived Health (V)

Class-Symptom Status (V)

Scale(s)-Severe to None (n)

Care Recipient:

Data Source:

Definition: Severity of observed or reported adverse cognitive and emotional responses to physical pain

OUTCOME TARGET RATING: Maintain at_____   Increase to_____

Pain: Adverse Psychological Response Overall Rating	Severe 1	Substantial 2	Moderate 3	Mild 4	None 5	
INDICATORS:						
130601 Slowing of thought processes	1	2	3	4	5	NA
130602 Memory impairment	1	2	3	4	5	NA
130603 Interference with concentration	1	2	3	4	5	NA
130604 Indecision	1	2	3	4	5	NA
130605 Pain distress	1	2	3	4	5	NA
130606 Concern about tolerating the pain	1	2	3	4	5	NA
130607 Concern about burdening others	1	2	3	4	5	NA
130608 Concern about abandonment	1	2	3	4	5	NA
130609 Depression	1	2	3	4	5	NA
130610 Anxiety	1	2	3	4	5	NA
130611 Sadness	1	2	3	4	5	NA
130612 Helplessness	1	2	3	4	5	NA
130613 Hopelessness	1	2	3	4	5	NA
130614 Worthlessness	1	2	3	4	5	NA
130615 Sense of isolation	1	2	3	4	5	NA
130616 Fear of procedures and equipment	1	2	3	4	5	NA
130617 Fear of unbearable pain	1	2	3	4	5	NA
130618 Annoyance with disruptive effects of pain	1	2	3	4	5	NA
130619 Suicidal thoughts	1	2	3	4	5	NA
130620 Pessimistic thoughts	1	2	3	4	5	NA
130621 Bitterness toward others	1	2	3	4	5	NA
130622 Anger over disabling effects of pain	1	2	3	4	5	NA

2nd edition 2000; Revised 3rd edition 2004

Outcome Content References:

Copp, L. A. (1974). The spectrum of suffering. *American Journal of Nursing, 74*(3), 491-495.

Kalfoss, M. H. (1992). The assessment of psychological distress. *Scandinavian Journal of Caring Science, 6*(1), 23-28.

Price, D. D., & Harkins, S. W. (1992). Psychophysical approaches to pain measurement and assessment. In D. C. Turk & R. Melzack (Eds.), *Handbook of pain assessment* (pp. 111-134). New York: The Guilford Press.

Puntillo, K. A., & Wilkie, D. J. (1991). Assessment of pain in the critically ill. In K. A. Puntillo (Ed.), *Pain in the critically ill* (pp. 45-64). Gaithersburg, MD: Aspen.

Pain Control—1605

Domain-Health Knowledge & Behavior (IV)

Class-Health Behavior (Q)

Scale(s)-Never demonstrated to Consistently demonstrated (m)

Care Recipient:

Data Source:

Definition: Personal actions to control pain

OUTCOME TARGET RATING: Maintain at_____   Increase to_____

Pain Control Overall Rating	Never demonstrated 1	Rarely demonstrated 2	Sometimes demonstrated 3	Often demonstrated 4	Consistently demonstrated 5	
INDICATORS:						
160502 Recognizes pain onset	1	2	3	4	5	NA
160501 Describes causal factors	1	2	3	4	5	NA
160510 Uses diary to monitor symptoms over time	1	2	3	4	5	NA
160503 Uses preventive measures	1	2	3	4	5	NA
160504 Uses non-analgesic relief measures	1	2	3	4	5	NA
160505 Uses analgesics as recommended	1	2	3	4	5	NA
160513 Reports changes in pain symptoms to health professional	1	2	3	4	5	NA
160507 Reports uncontrolled symptoms to health professional	1	2	3	4	5	NA
160508 Uses available resources	1	2	3	4	5	NA
160509 Recognizes associated symptoms of pain	1	2	3	4	5	NA
160511 Reports pain controlled	1	2	3	4	5	NA

1st edition 1997; Revised 2nd edition 2000; Revised 3rd edition 2004

Outcome Content References:

Howe, C. J. (1993). A new standard of care for pediatric pain management. *American Journal of Maternal Child Nursing, 18*(6), 325-329.

+Hurley, A. C., Volicer, B. J., Hanrahan, P. A., Houde, S., & Volicer, L. (1992). Assessment of discomfort in advanced Alzheimer's patients. *Research in Nursing and Health, 15*(5), 369-377.

Mobily, P., & Herr, K. A. (2001). Pain. In M. Maas, K. Buckwalter, M. Hardy, T. Tripp-Reimer, M. Titler, & J. Specht (Eds.), *Nursing care of older adults: Diagnoses, outcomes & interventions* (pp. 455-475). St. Louis: Mosby.

Puntillo, K., & Weiss, S. J. (1994). Pain: Its mediators and associated morbidity in critically ill cardiovascular surgical patients. *Nursing Research, 43*(1), 31-36.

Sherbourne, C. D. (1992). Pain measures. In A. L. Stewart & J. E. Ware, Jr. (Eds.), *Measuring functioning and well-being* (pp. 220-234). Durham, NC: Duke University Press.

+Walker, S. N., Sechrist, K. R., & Pender, N. J. (1995). *The health-promoting lifestyle profile II.* Omaha, NE: University of Nebraska at Omaha.

+Walker, S. N., Sechrist, K. R., & Pender, N. J. (1987). The health-promoting lifestyle profile: Development and psychometric characteristics. *Nursing Research, 36*(2), 76-81.

Pain: Disruptive Effects—2101

Domain-Perceived Health (V)

Class-Symptom Status (V)

Scale(s)-Severe to None (n) and Severely compromised to Not compromised (a)

Care Recipient:

Data Source:

Definition: Severity of observed or reported disruptive effects of chronic pain on daily functioning

OUTCOME TARGET RATING: Maintain at_____   Increase to_____

Pain: Disruptive Effects Overall Rating	Severe 1	Substantial 2	Moderate 3	Mild 4	None 5	
INDICATORS:						
210101 Disruption of interpersonal relationships	1	2	3	4	5	NA
210102 Impaired role performance	1	2	3	4	5	NA
210108 Impaired concentration	1	2	3	4	5	NA
210110 Impaired mood	1	2	3	4	5	NA
210111 Lack of patience	1	2	3	4	5	NA
210112 Interrupted sleep	1	2	3	4	5	NA
210119 Disruption of routine	1	2	3	4	5	NA
210113 Impaired physical mobility	1	2	3	4	5	NA
210114 Impaired self-care	1	2	3	4	5	NA
210115 Loss of appetite	1	2	3	4	5	NA
210117 Impaired urinary elimination	1	2	3	4	5	NA
210120 Impaired bowel elimination	1	2	3	4	5	NA
210123 Absenteeism from work	1	2	3	4	5	NA
210124 Absenteeism from school	1	2	3	4	5	NA
210122 Difficulty maintaining employment	1	2	3	4	5	NA

	Severely compromised	Substantially compromised	Moderately compromised	Mildly compromised	Not compromised	
210103 Play activities	1	2	3	4	5	NA
210104 Leisure activities	1	2	3	4	5	NA
210125 Work productivity	1	2	3	4	5	NA
210126 School productivity	1	2	3	4	5	NA
210106 Life enjoyment	1	2	3	4	5	NA
210107 Sense of control	1	2	3	4	5	NA
210109 Sense of hope	1	2	3	4	5	NA

1st edition 1997; Revised 3rd edition 2004; Revised 4th edition

Outcome Content References:

Howe, C. J. (1993). A new standard of care for pediatric pain management. *American Journal of Maternal Child Nursing, 18*(6), 325-329.

Continued

Mobily, P., & Herr, K. A. (2001). Pain. In M. Maas, K. Buckwalter, M. Hardy, T. Tripp-Reimer, M. Titler, & J. Specht (Eds.), *Nursing care of older adults: Diagnoses, outcomes & interventions* (pp. 455-475). St. Louis: Mosby.

Puntillo, K., & Weiss, S. J. (1994). Pain: Its mediators and associated mobility in critically ill cardiovascular surgical patients. *Nursing Research, 43*(1), 31-36.

Sherbourne, C. D. (1992). Pain measures. In A. L. Stewart & J. E. Ware, Jr. (Eds.), *Measuring functioning and well-being* (pp. 220-234). Durham, NC: Duke University Press.

+Von Korff, M., Ormel, J., Keefe, F. J., & Dworkin, S. F. (1992). Grading the severity of chronic pain. *Pain, 50*(2), 133-149.

P

Pain Level—2102

Domain-Perceived Health (V)

Class-Symptom Status (V)

Care Recipient:

Data Source:

Scale(s)-Severe to None (n) and Severe deviation from normal range to No deviation from normal range (b)

Definition: Severity of observed or reported pain

OUTCOME TARGET RATING: Maintain at_____   Increase to_____

Pain Level Overall Rating	Severe 1	Substantial 2	Moderate 3	Mild 4	None 5	
INDICATORS:						
210201 Reported pain	1	2	3	4	5	NA
210204 Length of pain episodes	1	2	3	4	5	NA
210221 Rubbing affected area	1	2	3	4	5	NA
210217 Moaning and crying	1	2	3	4	5	NA
210206 Facial expressions of pain	1	2	3	4	5	NA
210208 Restlessness	1	2	3	4	5	NA
210222 Agitation	1	2	3	4	5	NA
210223 Irritability	1	2	3	4	5	NA
210224 Wincing	1	2	3	4	5	NA
210225 Tearing	1	2	3	4	5	NA
210226 Diaphoresis	1	2	3	4	5	NA
210218 Pacing	1	2	3	4	5	NA
210219 Narrowed focus	1	2	3	4	5	NA
210209 Muscle tension	1	2	3	4	5	NA
210215 Loss of appetite	1	2	3	4	5	NA
210227 Nausea	1	2	3	4	5	NA
210228 Food intolerance	1	2	3	4	5	NA

	Severe deviation from normal range	Substantial deviation from normal range	Moderate deviation from normal range	Mild deviation from normal range	No deviation from normal range	
210210 Respiratory rate	1	2	3	4	5	NA
210211 Apical heart rate	1	2	3	4	5	NA
210220 Radial pulse rate	1	2	3	4	5	NA
210212 Blood pressure	1	2	3	4	5	NA
210214 Perspiration	1	2	3	4	5	NA

Site of pain _____

1st edition 1997; Revised 3rd edition 2004; Revised 4th edition

Outcome Content References:

Herr, K., Coyne, P. J., Key, T., Manworren, R., McCaffery, M., Merkel, S., Pelosi-Kelly, J., & Wild, L. (2006). Pain assessment in the nonverbal patient: Position statement with clinical practice recommendations. *Pain Management Nursing, 7*(2), 44-52.

Howe, C. J. (1993). A new standard of care for pediatric pain management. *American Journal of Maternal Child Nursing, 18*(6), 325-329.

Continued

P

+Hurley, A. C., Volicer, B. J., Hanrahan, P. A., Houde, S., & Volicer, L. (1992). Assessment of discomfort in advanced Alzheimer's patients. *Research in Nursing and Health, 15*(5), 369-377.

Mayer, D. M., Torma, L., Byock, I., & Norris, K. (2001). Speaking the language of pain. *American Journal of Nursing, 101*(2), 44-50.

Melzack, R. (1975). The McGill Pain Questionnaire: Major properties and scoring methods. *Pain, 30*(1), 277-299.

Merkel, S. (2002). Pain assessment in infants and young children: The Finger Span Scale. *American Journal of Nursing, 102*(11), 55-56.

Mobily, P., & Herr, K. A. (2001). Pain. In M. Maas, K. Buckwalter, M. Hardy, T. Tripp-Reimer, M. Titler, & J. Specht (Eds.), *Nursing care of older adults: Diagnoses, outcomes & interventions* (pp. 455-475). St. Louis: Mosby.

Puntillo, K., & Weiss, S. J. (1994). Pain: Its mediators and associated morbidity in critically ill cardiovascular surgical patients. *Nursing Research, 43*(1), 31-36.

Sherbourne, C. D. (1992). Pain measures. In A. L. Stewart, & J. E. Ware, Jr. (Eds.), *Measuring functioning and well-being* (pp. 220-234). Durham, NC: Duke University Press.

+Wong, D., & Baker, C. M. (1988). Pain in children: Comparison of assessment scales. *Pediatric Nursing, 14*(1), 9-17.

P

Parent-Infant Attachment—1500

Domain-Psychosocial Health (III)
Class-Social Interaction (P)
Scale(s)-Never demonstrated to Consistently demonstrated (m)

Care Recipient:
Data Source:

Definition: Parent and infant behaviors that demonstrate an enduring affectionate bond

OUTCOME TARGET RATING: Maintain at_____   Increase to_____

Parent-Infant Attachment Overall Rating	Never demonstrated 1	Rarely demonstrated 2	Sometimes demonstrated 3	Often demonstrated 4	Consistently demonstrated 5	

INDICATORS:

150001	Practices healthy behaviors during pregnancy	1	2	3	4	5	NA
150002	Assigns specific attributes to fetus	1	2	3	4	5	NA
150003	Prepares for infant prior to birth	1	2	3	4	5	NA
150004	Verbalizes positive feelings toward infant	1	2	3	4	5	NA
150005	Holds infant close	1	2	3	4	5	NA
150006	Touches, strokes, pats infant	1	2	3	4	5	NA
150007	Kisses infant	1	2	3	4	5	NA
150008	Smiles at infant	1	2	3	4	5	NA
150009	Visits nursery	1	2	3	4	5	NA
150011	Uses en face position	1	2	3	4	5	NA
150012	Uses eye contact	1	2	3	4	5	NA
150013	Vocalizes to infant	1	2	3	4	5	NA
150014	Plays with infant	1	2	3	4	5	NA
150015	Responds to infant cues	1	2	3	4	5	NA
150016	Consoles infant	1	2	3	4	5	NA
150024	Holds infant for feeding	1	2	3	4	5	NA
150018	Keeps infant dry, clean, and warm	1	2	3	4	5	NA
150019	Infant looks at parent	1	2	3	4	5	NA
150020	Infant responds to parent's cues	1	2	3	4	5	NA
150021	Infant seeks proximity with parent	1	2	3	4	5	NA

Specify parent _____

1st edition 1997; Revised 3rd edition 2004; Revised 4th edition

Outcome Content References:

Ainsworth, M. S., & Wittig, B. A. (1969). Attachment and exploratory behavior of one-year-olds in a strange situation. In B. M. Foss (Ed.), *Determinants of infant behavior* (pp. 111-133). London: Methuen.

Kennell, J., Jerauld, R., Wolfe, H., Chesler, D., Kreger, N. C., McAlpine, W., Steffa, M., & Klaus, M. H. (1974). Maternal behavior one year after early and extended post-partum contact. *Developmental Medicine and Child Neurology, 16*(2), 172-279.

Koniak-Griffin, D. (1988). The relationship between social support, self-esteem, and maternal-fetal attachment in adolescents. *Research in Nursing and Health, 11*(4), 269-278.

+Müller, M. (1994). A questionnaire to measure mother-to-infant attachment. *Journal of Nursing Measurements, 2*(2), 129-141.

Norr, K. F., Roberts, J. E., & Freese, U. (1989). Early postpartum rooming-in and maternal attachment behaviors in a group of medically indigent primiparas. *Journal of Nurse-Midwifery, 34*(2), 85-91.

Parenting: Adolescent Physical Safety—2902

Domain-Family Health (VI)

Class-Parenting (d)

Scale(s)-Never demonstrated to Consistently demonstrated (m)

Care Recipient:

Data Source:

Definition: Parental actions to prevent physical injury in an adolescent from 12 years through 17 years of age

OUTCOME TARGET RATING: Maintain at_____   Increase to_____

Parenting: Adolescent Physical Safety Overall Rating	Never demonstrated 1	Rarely demonstrated 2	Sometimes demonstrated 3	Often demonstrated 4	Consistently demonstrated 5	

INDICATORS:

290201	Uses strategies to protect from sun exposure	1	2	3	4	5	NA
290226	Encourages appropriate clothing for activity	1	2	3	4	5	NA
290203	Maintains warning devices	1	2	3	4	5	NA
290204	Practices family fire escape plan	1	2	3	4	5	NA
290205	Maintains smoke-free environment	1	2	3	4	5	NA
290206	Monitors use of sport and recreational equipment	1	2	3	4	5	NA
290207	Uses strategies to encourage use of protective gear during high-risk activities	1	2	3	4	5	NA
290208	Uses strategies to encourage seat belt use	1	2	3	4	5	NA
290209	Uses strategies to encourage safe driving	1	2	3	4	5	NA
290210	Uses strategies to prevent water accidents	1	2	3	4	5	NA
290211	Uses strategies to prevent firearm injuries	1	2	3	4	5	NA
290212	Uses strategies to prevent participation in violence	1	2	3	4	5	NA
290213	Uses strategies to prevent tobacco use	1	2	3	4	5	NA
290214	Uses strategies to prevent alcohol use	1	2	3	4	5	NA
290215	Uses strategies to prevent recreational drug use	1	2	3	4	5	NA
290216	Uses strategies to prevent medication misuse	1	2	3	4	5	NA
290217	Uses strategies to prevent exposure to toxic chemicals	1	2	3	4	5	NA

P

	Never demonstrated	Rarely demonstrated	Sometimes demonstrated	Often demonstrated	Consistently demonstrated	
290218	Uses strategies to prevent exposure to excessive noise	1	2	3	4	5	NA
290228	Uses strategies to postpone sexual activity	1	2	3	4	5	NA
290220	Uses strategies to prevent high-risk sexual activity	1	2	3	4	5	NA
290229	Uses strategies to prevent communicable diseases	1	2	3	4	5	NA
290222	Protects from physical abuse	1	2	3	4	5	NA
290223	Protects from sexual abuse	1	2	3	4	5	NA
290224	Monitors for warning signs of self-harm	1	2	3	4	5	NA
290227	Obtains training to prepare for emergencies	1	2	3	4	5	NA

3rd edition 2004; Revised 4th edition

Outcome Content References:

Bernardo, L., Garnder, J. J., & Seibel, K. (2001). Playground injuries in children: A review and Pennsylvania trauma center experience. *Journal of the Society of Pediatrics Nurses, 6*(1), 11-20.

Gresham, L. S., Zirkle, D. L., Tolchin, S., Jones, C., Maroufi, A., & Miranda, J. (2001). Partnering for injury prevention: Evaluation of a curriculum-based intervention program among elementary school children. *Journal of Pediatric Nursing, 16*(2), 79-87.

Hall-Long, B. A., Schell, K., & Corrigan, V. (2001). Youth safety education and injury prevention program. *Pediatric Nursing, 27*(2), 141-148.

Polivka, B. J., & Ryan-Wenger, N. (1999). Health promotion and injury prevention behaviors of elementary school children. *Pediatric Nursing, 25*(2), 127-134.

P

Parenting: Early/Middle Childhood Physical Safety—2901

Domain-Family Health (VI) Care Recipient:

Class-Parenting (d) Data Source:

Scale(s)-Never demonstrated to Consistently demonstrated (m)

Definition: Parental actions to avoid physical injury of a child from 3 years through 11 years of age

OUTCOME TARGET RATING: Maintain at_____ Increase to_____

Parenting: Early/Middle Childhood Physical Safety Overall Rating	Never demonstrated 1	Rarely demonstrated 2	Sometimes demonstrated 3	Often demonstrated 4	Consistently demonstrated 5	

INDICATORS:

290101	Selects safe, age-appropriate toys	1	2	3	4	5	NA
290102	Provides supervision around pets and animals	1	2	3	4	5	NA
290103	Provides supervision around water	1	2	3	4	5	NA
290104	Avoids leaving child in motor vehicle unsupervised	1	2	3	4	5	NA
290105	Monitors proper use of car seat/seat belt	1	2	3	4	5	NA
290106	Supervises selection of weather-appropriate clothing	1	2	3	4	5	NA
290107	Protects from sun exposure	1	2	3	4	5	NA
290108	Maintains environment to prevent harmful falls	1	2	3	4	5	NA
290109	Maintains environment to prevent burns, electrical shock, and chemical exposure	1	2	3	4	5	NA
290110	Maintains environment to prevent poisoning	1	2	3	4	5	NA
290111	Practices family fire escape plan	1	2	3	4	5	NA
290112	Keeps medication out of reach	1	2	3	4	5	NA
290113	Maintains warning devices	1	2	3	4	5	NA
290114	Locks or removes doors from unused appliances	1	2	3	4	5	NA
290115	Maintains smoke-free environment	1	2	3	4	5	NA
290116	Insures home playground equipment meets safety guidelines	1	2	3	4	5	NA
290117	Provides supervision while on playground equipment	1	2	3	4	5	NA

P

		Never demonstrated	Rarely demonstrated	Sometimes demonstrated	Often demonstrated	Consistently demonstrated	
290118	Selects appropriate clothing for activity	1	2	3	4	5	NA
290119	Uses strategies to encourage use of protective helmet	1	2	3	4	5	NA
290120	Uses strategies to encourage use of protective gear during high-risk activities	1	2	3	4	5	NA
290121	Eliminates access to firearms	1	2	3	4	5	NA
290122	Protects from exposure to violence	1	2	3	4	5	NA
290123	Monitors use of sport and recreational equipment	1	2	3	4	5	NA
290124	Uses strategies to prevent tobacco use	1	2	3	4	5	NA
290125	Uses strategies to prevent alcohol use	1	2	3	4	5	NA
290126	Uses strategies to prevent recreational drug use	1	2	3	4	5	NA
290127	Uses strategies to prevent medication misuse	1	2	3	4	5	NA
290128	Uses strategies to prevent exposure to toxic chemicals	1	2	3	4	5	NA
290129	Uses strategies to prevent exposure to excessive noise	1	2	3	4	5	NA
290130	Uses strategies to prevent precocious sexual behavior	1	2	3	4	5	NA
290131	Protects from physical abuse	1	2	3	4	5	NA
290132	Protects from sexual abuse	1	2	3	4	5	NA
290134	Obtains training to prepare for emergencies	1	2	3	4	5	NA

3rd edition 2004; Revised 4th edition

Outcome Content References:

Bernardo, L., Garnder, J. J., & Seibel, K. (2001). Playground injuries in children: A review and Pennsylvania trauma center experience. *Journal of the Society of Pediatrics Nurses*, *6*(1), 11-20.

Gresham, L. S., Zirkle, D. L., Tolchin, S., Jones, C., Maroufi, A., & Miranda, J. (2001). Partnering for injury prevention: Evaluation of a curriculum-based intervention program among elementary school children. *Journal of Pediatric Nursing*, *16*(2), 79-87.

Hall-Long, B. A., Schell, K., & Corrigan, V. (2001). Youth safety education and injury prevention program. *Pediatric Nursing*, *27*(2), 141-148.

Polivka, B. J., & Ryan-Wenger, N. (1999). Health promotion and injury prevention behaviors of elementary school children. *Pediatric Nursing*, *25*(2), 127-134.

U.S. Consumer Product Safety Commission. (1997). *Handbook for public playground safety*. Washington, D.C.: Author.

P

Parenting: Infant/Toddler Physical Safety—2900

Domain-Family Health (VI)

Class-Parenting (d)

Scale(s)-Never demonstrated to Consistently demonstrated (m)

Care Recipient:

Data Source:

Definition: Parental actions to avoid physical injury of a child from birth through 2 years of age

OUTCOME TARGET RATING: Maintain at_____   Increase to_____

Parenting: Infant/Toddler Physical Safety Overall Rating	Never demonstrated 1	Rarely demonstrated 2	Sometimes demonstrated 3	Often demonstrated 4	Consistently demonstrated 5	

INDICATORS:

290001	Handles infant/toddler properly	1	2	3	4	5	NA
290002	Uses crib that meets safety regulations	1	2	3	4	5	NA
290003	Positions on back for sleep	1	2	3	4	5	NA
290004	Selects safe, age-appropriate toys	1	2	3	4	5	NA
290005	Keeps sharp-pointed objects out of reach	1	2	3	4	5	NA
290006	Selects foods that prevent choking	1	2	3	4	5	NA
290007	Stores formula/breastmilk safely	1	2	3	4	5	NA
290008	Provides constant supervision around pets and animals	1	2	3	4	5	NA
290009	Provides constant supervision around water	1	2	3	4	5	NA
290010	Avoids leaving infant/toddler in motor vehicle unsupervised	1	2	3	4	5	NA
290011	Uses car seat appropriately	1	2	3	4	5	NA
290012	Selects weather-appropriate clothing	1	2	3	4	5	NA
290013	Protects from sun exposure	1	2	3	4	5	NA
290014	Maintains environment to prevent suffocation	1	2	3	4	5	NA
290015	Maintains environment to prevent harmful falls	1	2	3	4	5	NA
290016	Maintains environment to prevent burns, electrical shock, and chemical exposure	1	2	3	4	5	NA
290017	Maintains environment to prevent poisoning	1	2	3	4	5	NA
290018	Keeps medication out of reach	1	2	3	4	5	NA

P

		Never demonstrated	Rarely demonstrated	Sometimes demonstrated	Often demonstrated	Consistently demonstrated	
290019	Maintains smoke-free environment	1	2	3	4	5	NA
290020	Uses strategies to prevent exposure to excessive noise	1	2	3	4	5	NA
290021	Maintains warning devices	1	2	3	4	5	NA
290028	Obtains training to prepare for emergencies	1	2	3	4	5	NA
290023	Insures home playground equipment meets safety guidelines	1	2	3	4	5	NA
290024	Provides supervision while on playground equipment	1	2	3	4	5	NA
290025	Insures that infant/toddler wears helmet properly	1	2	3	4	5	NA
290026	Protects from physical abuse	1	2	3	4	5	NA
290027	Protects from sexual abuse	1	2	3	4	5	NA

3rd edition 2004; Revised 4th edition

Outcome Content References:

Kendrick, D., & Marsh, P. (1998). Babywalkers: Prevalence of use and relationship with other safety practices. *Injury Prevention, 4*(4), 295-298.

Kotch, J., Dufort, V. M., Stewart, P., Fieberg, J., McMurray, M., O'Brien, S., Ngui, E. M., & Brennan, M. (1997). Injuries among children in home and out-of-home care. *Injury Prevention, 3*(4), 267-271.

McBrien, M. (1997). Regency home care pediatric checklist. *Home Care Manager, 1*(2), 17.

Murphy, J. (1999). Pediatric occupant care safety: Clinical implications based on recent literature. *Pediatric Nursing, 25*(2), 137-144, 147-148.

O-Dea, T., Saly, G., & Holte, J. (1998). Safety investigation: Interaction of infant radiant warmers and bilirubin phototherapy lights in the regulation of temperature of newborn infants. *Biomedical Instrument Technology, 32*(4), 355-369.

Showers, J. (1992). "Don't shake the baby": The effectiveness of a prevention program. *Child Abuse & Neglect, 16*(1), 11-18.

Thompson, R., & Emslie, A. (2000). Young children and the risk of accidental injury: Running an audit at nine months. *Community Practitioner, 73*(10), 799-800.

U.S. Consumer Product Safety Commission. (1997). *Handbook for public playground safety*. Washington, D.C.: Author.

Wong, D., Hockenberry-Eaton, M., Wilson, D., Winkelstein, M. L., & Schwartz, P. (2001). *Wong's essentials of pediatric nursing* (6th ed). St. Louis: Mosby.

P

Parenting Performance—2211

Domain-Family Health (VI)

Class-Parenting (d)

Scale(s)-Never demonstrated to Consistently demonstrated (m)

Care Recipient:

Data Source:

Definition: Parental actions to provide a child a nurturing and constructive physical, emotional, and social environment

OUTCOME TARGET RATING: Maintain at_____   Increase to_____

Parenting Performance Overall Rating	Never demonstrated 1	Rarely demonstrated 2	Sometimes demonstrated 3	Often demonstrated 4	Consistently demonstrated 5	

INDICATORS:

221101	Provides for child's physical needs	1	2	3	4	5	NA
221122	Provides age-appropriate nutrition	1	2	3	4	5	NA
221102	Eliminates controllable environmental hazards	1	2	3	4	5	NA
221130	Provides preventative health care	1	2	3	4	5	NA
221131	Provides episodic health care	1	2	3	4	5	NA
221123	Provides structure for child	1	2	3	4	5	NA
221104	Stimulates cognitive development	1	2	3	4	5	NA
221105	Stimulates social development	1	2	3	4	5	NA
221106	Stimulates emotional growth	1	2	3	4	5	NA
221107	Stimulates spiritual growth	1	2	3	4	5	NA
221124	Stimulates moral growth	1	2	3	4	5	NA
221125	Imparts values that promote functioning in society	1	2	3	4	5	NA
221126	Provides appropriate supervision for child	1	2	3	4	5	NA
221127	Selects appropriate supplemental caregiver	1	2	3	4	5	NA
221128	Monitors supplemental caregiver	1	2	3	4	5	NA
221108	Uses community resources	1	2	3	4	5	NA
221110	Uses interactions appropriate for child's temperament	1	2	3	4	5	NA
221111	Uses behavior management	1	2	3	4	5	NA
221112	Uses age-appropriate discipline	1	2	3	4	5	NA
221113	Provides for child's special needs	1	2	3	4	5	NA
221114	Interacts positively with child	1	2	3	4	5	NA

P

	Never demonstrated	Rarely demonstrated	Sometimes demonstrated	Often demonstrated	Consistently demonstrated	
221115 Empathizes with child	1	2	3	4	5	NA
221129 Maintains open communication	1	2	3	4	5	NA
221116 Verbalizes positive attributes of child	1	2	3	4	5	NA
221117 Exhibits a loving relationship	1	2	3	4	5	NA
221118 Expresses realistic expectations of parental role	1	2	3	4	5	NA
221119 Expresses satisfaction with parental role	1	2	3	4	5	NA
221120 Expresses positive self-esteem	1	2	3	4	5	NA

1st edition 1997; Revised 3rd edition 2004; Revised 4th edition

Outcome Content References:

Causby, V., Nixon, C., & Bright, J. M. (1991). Influences on adolescent mother-infant interactions. *Adolescence, 26*(103), 619-630.

+Clarke, M., & Hornick, J. (1984). The development of the Nurturance Inventory: An instrument for assessing parenting practices. *Child Psychiatry & Human Development, 15*(1), 49-63.

Fulton, A. M., Murphy, K. R., & Anderson, S. L. (1991). Increasing adolescent mothers' knowledge of child development: An intervention program. *Adolescence, 26*(101), 73-81.

Greaves, P., Glik, D. C., Kronenfeld, J. J., & Jackson, K. (1994). Determinants of controllable in-home child safety hazards. *Health Education Research, 9*(3), 307-315.

Mercer, R. T., & Ferketich, S. L. (1994). Predictors of maternal role competence by risk status. *Nursing Research, 43*(1), 38-43.

Ohashi, J. P. (1992). Maternal role satisfaction: A new approach to assessing parenting. *Scholarly Inquiry for Nursing Practice: An International Journal, 6*(2), 135-149.

Reece, S. M. (1995). Stress and maternal adaptation in first-time mothers more than 35 years old. *Applied Nursing Research, 8*(2), 61-66.

Thompson, P. J., Powell, M. J., Patterson, R. J., & Ellerbee, S. M. (1995). Adolescent parenting: Outcomes and maternal perceptions. *Journal of Obstetric, Gynecologic, and Neonatal Nursing, 24*(8), 713-718.

P

Parenting: Psychosocial Safety—1901

Domain-Family Health (VI)

Class-Parenting (d)

Scale(s)-Never demonstrated to Consistently demonstrated (m)

Care Recipient:

Data Source:

Definition: Parental actions to protect a child from social contacts that might cause harm or injury

OUTCOME TARGET RATING: Maintain at_____   Increase to_____

Parenting: Psychosocial Safety Overall Rating	Never demonstrated 1	Rarely demonstrated 2	Sometimes demonstrated 3	Often demonstrated 4	Consistently demonstrated 5	

INDICATORS:

190101	Monitors playmates	1	2	3	4	5	NA
190102	Monitors social contacts	1	2	3	4	5	NA
190115	Fosters open communication	1	2	3	4	5	NA
190104	Selects appropriate supplemental caregiver	1	2	3	4	5	NA
190103	Monitors supplemental caregiver	1	2	3	4	5	NA
190105	Recognizes risk for abuse	1	2	3	4	5	NA
190106	Uses strategies to eliminate risk for abuse	1	2	3	4	5	NA
190107	Actions to eliminate abuse	1	2	3	4	5	NA
190109	Provides required level of supervision	1	2	3	4	5	NA
190112	Uses strategies to prevent high-risk social behavior	1	2	3	4	5	NA
190113	Prevents gang participation	1	2	3	4	5	NA
190116	Fosters mutually interactive communication about sex	1	2	3	4	5	NA
190117	Sets clear rules for behavior	1	2	3	4	5	NA
190119	Maintains structure in child's life	1	2	3	4	5	NA
190120	Maintains daily routine in child's life	1	2	3	4	5	NA

1st edition 1997; Revised 3rd edition 2004; Revised 4th edition

Outcome Content References:

Glick, D., Kronenfeld, J., & Jackson, K. (1993). Safety behaviors among parents of preschoolers. *Health Values, 17*(1), 18-27.

Howell, J. C., & Lynch, J. P. (2000). Youth gangs in schools. *YGS Bulletin.* Washington, DC: U.S. Department of Justice, Office of Justice Programs, Office of Juvenile Justice and Delinquency Prevention.

Jackson, C., & Foshee, V. A. (1998). Violence-related behaviors of adolescents: Relations with responsive and demanding parenting. *Journal of Adolescent Research, 13*(3), 343-359.

Jensen, L. R., Williams, S. D., Thurman, D. J., & Keller, P. A. (1992). Submersion injuries for children less than 5 years in urban Utah. *Western Journal of Medicine, 157*(6), 641-644.

Quan, L., Gore, E. J., Wentz, K., Allen, J., & Novack, A. H. (1989). Ten year study of pediatric drownings and near-drownings in King County, Washington: Lessons in injury prevention. *Pediatrics, 83*(6), 1035-1040.

Rosenthal, D. A., Feldman, S. S., & Edwards, D. (1998). Mum's the word: Mother's perspectives on communication about sexuality with adolescents. *Journal of Adolescence, 21*(6), 727-743.

Walker, M., Schmidt, L., & Lunghofer, L. (1993). Youth gangs. In M. I. Singer, L. T. Singer, & T. M. Anglin (Eds.), *Handbook for screening adolescents at psychosocial risk* (pp. 504-522). New York: Lexington Books.

P

Participation in Health Care Decisions—1606

Domain-Health Knowledge & Behavior (IV)

Class-Health Behavior (Q)

Scale(s)-Never demonstrated to Consistently demonstrated (m)

Care Recipient:

Data Source:

Definition: Personal involvement in selecting and evaluating health care options to achieve desired outcome

OUTCOME TARGET RATING:　Maintain at_____　Increase to_____

Participation in Health Care Decisions Overall Rating	Never demonstrated 1	Rarely demonstrated 2	Sometimes demonstrated 3	Often demonstrated 4	Consistently demonstrated 5	

INDICATORS:

160601	Claims decision-making responsibility	1	2	3	4	5	NA
160602	Exhibits self-direction in decision making	1	2	3	4	5	NA
160603	Seeks reputable information	1	2	3	4	5	NA
160604	Defines available options	1	2	3	4	5	NA
160605	Specifies health outcome preferences	1	2	3	4	5	NA
160606	Identifies health outcome priorities	1	2	3	4	5	NA
160607	Identifies barriers to desired outcome achievement	1	2	3	4	5	NA
160608	Uses problem-solving techniques to achieve desired outcomes	1	2	3	4	5	NA
160609	States intent to act on decision	1	2	3	4	5	NA
160610	Identifies available support for achieving desired outcomes	1	2	3	4	5	NA
160611	Seeks health care services to meet desired outcomes	1	2	3	4	5	NA
160612	Negotiates for care preferences	1	2	3	4	5	NA
160613	Monitors barriers to outcome achievement	1	2	3	4	5	NA
160614	Identifies level of outcome achievement	1	2	3	4	5	NA
160615	Evaluates satisfaction with care outcomes	1	2	3	4	5	NA

1st edition 1997; Revised 3rd edition 2004

Outcome Content References:

Conn, V., Taylor, S., & Casey, B. (1992). Cardiac rehabilitation program participation and outcomes after myocardial infarction. *Rehabilitation Nursing, 17*(2), 58-62.

+Ende, J., Kazis, L., Ash, A., & Moskowitz, M. A. (1989). Measuring patient's desire for autonomy: Decision making and information-seeking preferences among medical patients. *Journal of General Internal Medicine, 4*(1), 23-30.

Hegyvary, S. T. (1993). Patient care outcomes related to management of symptoms. In J. J. Fitzpatrick & J. J. Stevenson (Eds.), *Annual review of nursing research* (Vol. 11, pp. 145-168). New York: Springer.

Weiler, K., & Moorhead, S. A. (2001). Self-determination. In M. Maas, K. Buckwalter, M. Hardy, T. Tripp-Reimer, M. Titler, & J. Specht (Eds.), *Nursing care of older adults: Diagnoses, outcomes & interventions* (pp. 706-718). St. Louis: Mosby.

P

Personal Autonomy—1614

Domain-Health, Knowledge & Behavior (IV)

Class-Health Behavior (Q)

Scale(s)-Never demonstrated to Consistently demonstrated (m)

Care Recipient:

Data Source:

Definition: Personal actions of a competent individual to exercise governance in life decisions

OUTCOME TARGET RATING: Maintain at_____   Increase to_____

Personal Autonomy Overall Rating	Never demonstrated 1	Rarely demonstrated 2	Sometimes demonstrated 3	Often demonstrated 4	Consistently demonstrated 5	
INDICATORS:						
161401 Makes informed life decisions	1	2	3	4	5	NA
161402 Considers other opinions when making choices	1	2	3	4	5	NA
161403 Expresses independence with decision-making process	1	2	3	4	5	NA
161404 Makes decisions free from undue pressure by parents	1	2	3	4	5	NA
161405 Makes decisions free from undue pressure by spouse	1	2	3	4	5	NA
161406 Makes decisions free from undue pressure by children	1	2	3	4	5	NA
161407 Makes decisions free from undue pressure by extended family	1	2	3	4	5	NA
161408 Makes decisions free from undue pressure by friends	1	2	3	4	5	NA
161409 Makes decisions free from undue pressure by health provider	1	2	3	4	5	NA
161410 Asserts personal preferences	1	2	3	4	5	NA
161411 Participates in health care decisions	1	2	3	4	5	NA
161412 Expresses satisfaction with life choices	1	2	3	4	5	NA

3rd edition 2004

Outcome Content References:

Aveyard, H. (2000). Is there a concept of autonomy that can usefully inform nursing practice? *Journal of Advanced Nursing,* 32(2), 352-358.

Brennan, M. (1997). A concept analysis of consent. *Journal of Advanced Nursing, 25*(3), 477-484.

Dworkin, G. (1988). *The theory and practice of autonomy.* Cambridge: Cambridge University Press.

Valimaki, M., & Leino-Kilpi, H. (1998). Preconditions for and consequences of self-determination: The psychiatric patient's point of view. *Journal of Advanced Nursing, 27(1),* 204-212.

Wiens, A. G. (1993). Patient autonomy: A theoretical framework for nursing. *Journal of Professional Nursing, 9*(2), 95-103.

P

Personal Health Status—2006

Domain-Perceived Health (V)

Class-Health & Life Quality (U)

Scale-Severely compromised to Not compromised (a)

Care Recipient:

Data Source:

Definition: Overall physical, psychological, social, and spiritual functioning of an adult 18 years or older

OUTCOME TARGET RATING: Maintain at_____   Increase to_____

Personal Health Status Overall Rating	Severely compromised 1	Substantially compromised 2	Moderately compromised 3	Mildly compromised 4	Not compromised 5	
INDICATORS:						
200601 Physical fitness	1	2	3	4	5	NA
200602 Mobility level	1	2	3	4	5	NA
200603 Energy level	1	2	3	4	5	NA
200604 Comfort level	1	2	3	4	5	NA
200605 Performance of activities of daily living	1	2	3	4	5	NA
200606 Performance of instrumental activities of daily living	1	2	3	4	5	NA
200607 Resistance to infection	1	2	3	4	5	NA
200608 Tissue healing	1	2	3	4	5	NA
200609 Sleep-rest pattern	1	2	3	4	5	NA
200610 Gastrointestinal function	1	2	3	4	5	NA
200611 Cardiac function	1	2	3	4	5	NA
200612 Peripheral tissue perfusion	1	2	3	4	5	NA
200613 Neurologic function	1	2	3	4	5	NA
200614 Pulmonary function	1	2	3	4	5	NA
200615 Kidney function	1	2	3	4	5	NA
200626 Sensory function	1	2	3	4	5	NA
200627 Sexual function	1	2	3	4	5	NA
200628 Endocrine function	1	2	3	4	5	NA
200616 Weight	1	2	3	4	5	NA
200617 Nutritional status	1	2	3	4	5	NA
200618 Cognitive status	1	2	3	4	5	NA
200619 Mental health	1	2	3	4	5	NA
200629 Symptom control	1	2	3	4	5	NA
200630 Pain control	1	2	3	4	5	NA
200620 Mood equilibrium	1	2	3	4	5	NA
200621 Spiritual life	1	2	3	4	5	NA
200622 Ability to cope	1	2	3	4	5	NA

P

Continued

		Severely compromised	Substantially compromised	Moderately compromised	Mildly compromised	Not compromised	
200623	Adjustment to chronic conditions	1	2	3	4	5	NA
200631	Ability to communicate	1	2	3	4	5	NA
200624	Ability to express emotions	1	2	3	4	5	NA
200625	Social relationships	1	2	3	4	5	NA

3rd edition 2004; Revised 4th edition

Outcome Content References:

Bergner, M., Bobbit, R. A., Carter, W. B., & Gilson, B. S. (1981). The sickness impact profile: Development and final revision of a health status measure. *Medical Care, 19*(8), 787-805.

Kline, N. W. (1988). *Psychophysiological process of stress in people with a chronic physical illness*. Doctoral dissertation. The University of Michigan, Ann Arbor, MI.

Mossberg, K., & McFarland, C. (2001). A patient-oriented health status measure in outpatient rehabilitation. *American Journal of Physical Medicine & Rehabilitation, 80*(12), 896-902.

Radosevich, D., & Pruit, M. (1995). *Twelve-item Health Status Questionnaire*. Bloomington, MN: Health Outcomes Institute.

Ware, J. E., & Sherbourne, C. D. (1992). The MOS 36-item short-form health survey (SF-36). I. Conceptual framework and item selection. *Medical Care, 30*(6), 473-483.

P

Personal Resiliency—1309

Domain-Psychosocial Health (III)

Class-Psychosocial Adaptation (N)

Scale(s)-Never demonstrated to Consistently demonstrated (m)

Care Recipient:

Data Source:

Definition: Positive adaptation and function of an individual following significant adversity or crisis

OUTCOME TARGET RATING: Maintain at_____   Increase to_____

Personal Resiliency Overall Rating	Never demonstrated 1	Rarely demonstrated 2	Sometimes demonstrated 3	Often demonstrated 4	Consistently demonstrated 5	
INDICATORS:						
130901 Verbalizes positive outlook	1	2	3	4	5	NA
130902 Uses effective coping strategies	1	2	3	4	5	NA
130903 Expresses emotions	1	2	3	4	5	NA
130904 Clarifies ambiguous communication	1	2	3	4	5	NA
130905 Communicates clearly and appropriately for age	1	2	3	4	5	NA
130906 Exhibits positive mood	1	2	3	4	5	NA
130907 Exhibits positive self-esteem	1	2	3	4	5	NA
130908 Expresses comfort with solitude	1	2	3	4	5	NA
130909 Expresses self-efficacy	1	2	3	4	5	NA
130910 Takes responsibility for own actions	1	2	3	4	5	NA
130911 Verbalizes an enhanced sense of control	1	2	3	4	5	NA
130912 Seeks emotional support	1	2	3	4	5	NA
130913 Weighs alternatives to problem-solving	1	2	3	4	5	NA
130914 Adapts to adversities as challenges	1	2	3	4	5	NA
130915 Proposes practical, constructive solutions for disputes	1	2	3	4	5	NA
130916 Makes progress toward goals	1	2	3	4	5	NA
130917 Uses strategies to promote safety	1	2	3	4	5	NA
130918 Uses strategies to avoid violent situations	1	2	3	4	5	NA
130919 Avoids drug misuse	1	2	3	4	5	NA
130920 Avoids alcohol misuse	1	2	3	4	5	NA
130921 Removes self from abusive relationships	1	2	3	4	5	NA

P

Continued

		Never demonstrated	Rarely demonstrated	Sometimes demonstrated	Often demonstrated	Consistently demonstrated	
130922	Practices safe sex	1	2	3	4	5	NA
130923	Refrains from harming others	1	2	3	4	5	NA
130924	Identifies role models	1	2	3	4	5	NA
130925	Identifies available community resources	1	2	3	4	5	NA
130926	Uses available community resources	1	2	3	4	5	NA
130927	Uses available support groups	1	2	3	4	5	NA
130928	Participates in employment	1	2	3	4	5	NA
130929	Participates in curricular school activities	1	2	3	4	5	NA
130930	Participates in extracurricular school activities	1	2	3	4	5	NA
130931	Participates in community activities	1	2	3	4	5	NA
130932	Participates in leisure activities	1	2	3	4	5	NA
130933	Uses educational and vocational resources	1	2	3	4	5	NA
130934	Verbalizes readiness to learn	1	2	3	4	5	NA

4th edition

Outcome Content References:

Fergus, S., & Zimmerman, M. A. (2005). Adolescent resilience: A framework for understanding healthy development in the face of risk. *Annual Review of Public Health, 26*(1), 399-419.

Gorman, C., Dale, S. S., Grossman, W., Klarreich, K., McDowell, J., & Whitaker, L. (2005). The importance of resilience. *Time, 165*(3), A52-A55.

Luthar, S. S., & Cicchetti, D. (2000). The construct of resilience: A critical evaluation and guidelines for future work. *Child Development, 71*(3), 543-562.

Luthar, S. S., & Cicchetti, D. (2000). The construct of resilience: Implications for interventions and social policies. *Development and Psychopathology, 12*(4), 857-885.

Masten, A. S. (2001). Ordinary magic. Resilience processes in development. *American Psychologist, 56*(3), 227-238.

Masten, A. S., Hubbard, J. J., Gest, S. D., Tellegen, A., Garmezy, N., & Ramirez, M. (1999). Competence in the context of adversity: Pathways to resilience and maladaptation from childhood to late adolescence. *Development and Psychopathology, 11*(1), 143-169.

Rogers, S. K., Muir, K., & Evenson, C. R. (2003). Signs of resilience: Assets that support deaf adults' success in bridging the deaf and hearing worlds. *American Annuals of the Deaf, 148*(3), 222-232.

Sinclair, V. G., & Wallston, K. A. (2004). The development and psychometric evaluation of the brief resilient coping scale. *Assessment, 11*(1), 94-101.

P

Personal Safety Behavior—1911

Domain-Health Knowledge & Behavior (IV)
Class-Risk Control & Safety (T)
Scale(s)-Never demonstrated to Consistently demonstrated (m)

Care Recipient:
Data Source:

Definition: Personal actions that prevent physical injury to self

OUTCOME TARGET RATING: Maintain at_____   Increase to_____

Personal Safety Behavior Overall Rating	Never demonstrated 1	Rarely demonstrated 2	Sometimes demonstrated 3	Often demonstrated 4	Consistently demonstrated 5	
INDICATORS:						
191102 Stores food to minimize spoilage	1	2	3	4	5	NA
191103 Prepares food to minimize contamination	1	2	3	4	5	NA
191104 Uses protective helmet and gear during high-risk activities	1	2	3	4	5	NA
191105 Uses seat belt appropriately	1	2	3	4	5	NA
191106 Selects appropriate clothing for activity	1	2	3	4	5	NA
191127 Uses strategies to protect from sun exposure	1	2	3	4	5	NA
191128 Uses proper body mechanics	1	2	3	4	5	NA
191107 Uses assistive devices correctly	1	2	3	4	5	NA
191108 Practices safe leisure activities	1	2	3	4	5	NA
191109 Practices safe sexual behaviors	1	2	3	4	5	NA
191110 Uses tools correctly	1	2	3	4	5	NA
191111 Uses machinery correctly	1	2	3	4	5	NA
191113 Avoids recreational drug use	1	2	3	4	5	NA
191129 Follows medication precautions	1	2	3	4	5	NA
191117 Avoids tobacco use	1	2	3	4	5	NA
191123 Avoids smoking in bed	1	2	3	4	5	NA
191124 Uses precautions with flammable material	1	2	3	4	5	NA
191118 Avoids alcohol misuse	1	2	3	4	5	NA
191125 Avoids operating motor vehicle when using alcohol	1	2	3	4	5	NA
191130 Avoids operating motor vehicle when using substances that impair function	1	2	3	4	5	NA
191131 Uses strategies to prevent communicable diseases	1	2	3	4	5	NA
191119 Avoids high-risk behaviors	1	2	3	4	5	NA
191120 Observes speed limits/rules of the road	1	2	3	4	5	NA
191126 Protects self from injury	1	2	3	4	5	NA

P

Continued

1st edition 1997; Revised 3rd edition 2004; Revised 4th edition

Outcome Content References:

+Hettler, B. (1982). Wellness promotion and risk reduction on a university campus. In M. Faber & A. Reinhardt (Eds.), *Promoting health through risk reduction.* New York: Macmillan.

Sorock, G. S. (1988). Falls among the elderly: Epidemiology and prevention. *American Journal of Preventive Medicine, 4*(5), 252-255.

Weitzel, E. (2001). Unilateral neglect. In M. Maas, K. Buckwalter, M. Hardy, T. Tripp-Reimer, M. Titler, & J. Specht (Eds.), *Nursing care of older adults: Diagnoses, outcomes & interventions* (pp. 492-502). St. Louis: Mosby.

P

Personal Well-Being—2002

Domain-Perceived Health (V)   Care Recipient:

Class-Health & Life Quality (U)   Data Source:

Scale(s)-Not at all satisfied to Completely satisfied (s)

Definition: Extent of positive perception of one's health status

OUTCOME TARGET RATING: Maintain at_____   Increase to_____

Personal Well-Being Overall Rating	Not at all satisfied 1	Somewhat satisfied 2	Moderately satisfied 3	Very satisfied 4	Completely satisfied 5	
INDICATORS:						
200201 Performance of activities of daily living	1	2	3	4	5	NA
200212 Performance of usual roles	1	2	3	4	5	NA
200202 Psychological health	1	2	3	4	5	NA
200203 Social relationships	1	2	3	4	5	NA
200204 Spiritual life	1	2	3	4	5	NA
200205 Physical health	1	2	3	4	5	NA
200206 Cognitive status	1	2	3	4	5	NA
200207 Ability to cope	1	2	3	4	5	NA
200208 Ability to relax	1	2	3	4	5	NA
200209 Level of happiness	1	2	3	4	5	NA
200210 Ability to express emotions	1	2	3	4	5	NA
200213 Ability to control activities	1	2	3	4	5	NA
200214 Opportunities for health care choice(s)	1	2	3	4	5	NA

1st edition 1997; Revised 3rd edition 2004; Revised 4th edition

P

Outcome Content References:

Davidhizar, R. E., & Giger, J. N. (2001). Powerlessness. In M. Maas, K. Buckwalter, M. Hardy, T. Tripp-Reimer, M. Titler, & J. Specht (Eds.), *Nursing care of older adults: Diagnoses, outcomes & interventions* (pp. 562-570). St. Louis: Mosby.

+Dupuy, H. (1984). The Psychological General Well-Being (PCWB) Index. In N. K. Wenger, M. E. Mattson, C. D. Furberg, & J. Elinson (Eds.), *Assessment of quality of life in clinical trials of cardiovascular therapies* (pp. 170-183, 353-356). Greenwich, CT: Le Jacq Publishing.

Ferrell, B., Grant, M., Schmidt, G. M., Rhiner, M., Whitehead, C. P., & Forman, S. J. (1992). The meaning of quality of life for bone marrow transplant survivors. Part 1. *Cancer Nursing, 15*(3), 153-160.

Ferrell, B. R., Dow, K. H., Leigh, S., Ly, J., & Gulasekaram, P. (1995). Quality of life in long-term cancer survivors. *Oncology Nursing Forum, 22*(6), 915-922.

Kozier, B., Erb, G., & Blais, K. (1992). *Concepts and issues in nursing practice* (2nd ed.). Redwood City, CA: Addison-Wesley Nursing.

+Revicki, D. A., Leidy, N. K., & Howland, L. (1996). Evaluating the psychometric characteristics of the Psychological General Well-Being Index with a new response scale. *Quality of Life Research, 5*(4), 419-425.

Stewart, A., Ware, J., Jr., Sherbourne, C., & Wells, K. (1992). Psychological distress/well-being and cognitive functioning measures. In A. Stewart & J. Ware, Jr. (Eds.), *Measuring functioning and well-being: The medical outcomes study approach* (pp. 102-142). Durham, NC: Duke University Press.

Waterman, J. D., Blegen, M., Clinton, P., & Specht, J. P. (2001). Social isolation. In M. Maas, K. Buckwalter, M. Hardy, T. Tripp-Reimer, M. Titler, & J. Specht (Eds.), *Nursing care of older adults: Diagnoses, outcomes & interventions* (pp. 651-663). St. Louis: Mosby.

Whedon, M., & Ferrell, B. R. (1994). Quality of life in adult bone marrow transplant patients: Beyond the first year. *Seminars in Oncology Nursing, 10*(1), 42-57.

Physical Aging—0113

Domain-Functional Health (I)

Class-Growth & Development (B)

Scale(s)-Severe deviation from normal range to No deviation from normal range (b)

Care Recipient:

Data Source:

Definition: Normal physical changes that occur with the natural aging process

OUTCOME TARGET RATING: Maintain at_____   Increase to_____

Physical Aging Overall Rating	Severe deviation from normal range 1	Substantial deviation from normal range 2	Moderate deviation from normal range 3	Mild deviation from normal range 4	No deviation from normal range 5	
INDICATORS:						
011318 Memory	1	2	3	4	5	NA
011319 Cognitive status	1	2	3	4	5	NA
011301 Mean body mass	1	2	3	4	5	NA
011302 Bone density	1	2	3	4	5	NA
011303 Cardiac output	1	2	3	4	5	NA
011304 Vital capacity	1	2	3	4	5	NA
011305 Blood pressure	1	2	3	4	5	NA
011306 Skin elasticity	1	2	3	4	5	NA
011307 Muscle strength	1	2	3	4	5	NA
011320 Joint mobility	1	2	3	4	5	NA
011321 Sensory acuity	1	2	3	4	5	NA
011322 Bladder muscle tone	1	2	3	4	5	NA
011323 Resistance to infection	1	2	3	4	5	NA
011308 Hearing acuity	1	2	3	4	5	NA
011309 Visual acuity	1	2	3	4	5	NA
011310 Olfactory acuity	1	2	3	4	5	NA
011311 Taste acuity	1	2	3	4	5	NA
011312 Basal metabolic rate	1	2	3	4	5	NA
011313 Fat distribution pattern	1	2	3	4	5	NA
011314 Hair distribution pattern	1	2	3	4	5	NA
011315 Menstrual pattern	1	2	3	4	5	NA
011316 Sexual functioning	1	2	3	4	5	NA

1st edition 1997; Revised 3rd edition 2004

Outcome Content References:

Bemben, M. G., & McCalip, G. A. (1999). Strength and power relationships as a function of age. *Journal of Strength & Conditioning Research, 13*(4), 330-338.

Kennedy-Malone, L., Fletcher, K. R., & Plank, L. M. (Eds.). (2000). *Management guidelines for gerontological nurse practitioners* (pp. 3-24, 536-553). Philadelphia: F.A. Davis.

McWhorter, J. W., & Schuerman, S. E. (2002). Balance and aging. *Orthopaedic Physical Therapy Clinics of North America, 11*(1), 111-130.

Rice, F. P. (2001). *Human development: A life-span approach.* Upper Saddle River, NJ: Prentice Hall.

Schuster, C., & Ashburn, S. (1992). *The process of human development: A holistic approach* (3rd ed.). Philadelphia: J.B. Lippincott.

Wong, A. M., Lin, Y., Chou, S., Tang, F., & Wong, P. (2001). Coordination exercise and postural stability in elderly people: Effect of Tai Chi Chuan. *Archives of Physical Medicine & Rehabilitation, 82*(5), 608-612.

Physical Fitness—2004

Domain-Perceived Health (V)

Class-Health & Life Quality (U)

Scale(s)-Severely compromised to Not compromised (a)

Care Recipient:

Data Source:

Definition: Performance of physical activities with vigor

OUTCOME TARGET RATING: Maintain at_____ Increase to_____

Physical Fitness Overall Rating		Severely compromised 1	Substantially compromised 2	Moderately compromised 3	Mildly compromised 4	Not compromised 5	
INDICATORS:							
200401	Muscle strength	1	2	3	4	5	NA
200402	Muscle endurance	1	2	3	4	5	NA
200403	Joint flexibility	1	2	3	4	5	NA
200404	Performance of physical activities	1	2	3	4	5	NA
200405	Performance of routine exercise	1	2	3	4	5	NA
200406	Cardiovascular function	1	2	3	4	5	NA
200407	Respiratory function	1	2	3	4	5	NA
200408	Aerobic fitness	1	2	3	4	5	NA
200409	Body mass index	1	2	3	4	5	NA
200410	Waist to hip ratio	1	2	3	4	5	NA
200411	Blood pressure	1	2	3	4	5	NA
200412	Target heart rate during exercise	1	2	3	4	5	NA
200414	Resting heart rate	1	2	3	4	5	NA

2nd edition 2000; Revised 3rd edition 2004

Outcome Content References:

American College of Sports Medicine. (2000). *Guidelines for exercise testing and prescription* (6th ed.). Baltimore: Williams & Wilkins.

Brown, M., Sinacore, D. R., Ehsani, A. A., Binder, E. F., Holloszy, J. O., & Kohrt, W. M. (2000). Low-intensity exercise as a modifier of physical frailty in older adults. *Archives of Physical Medicine & Rehabilitation, 81*(7), 960-965.

Cauderay, M., Narring, F., & Michaud, P. (2000). A cross-sectional survey assessing physical fitness of 9-to 19-year old girls and boys in Switzerland. *Pediatric Exercise Science, 12*(4), 398-412.

NIH Consensus Development Panel on Physical Activity and Cardiovascular Health. (1996). Physical activity and cardiovascular health. *Journal of the American Medical Association, 276*(3), 241-246.

Haskell, W. L., Lee, I., Pate, R. R., Powell, K. E., Blair, S. N., Franklin, B. A., Macera, C. A., Health, G. W., Thompson, P. D., & Bauman, A. (2007). Physical activity and public health. Updated recommendation for adults from the American College of Sports Medicine and American Heart Association.

U.S. Department of Health and Human Services. (2000). *Healthy People 2010.* Washington, DC: Government Printing Office.

U.S. Department of Health and Human Services. (1991). *Healthy People 2000: National health promotion and disease prevention objectives.* (DHHS Pub No (PHS) 91-50012). Washington, DC: Government Printing Office.

P

Physical Injury Severity—1913

Domain-Health Knowledge & Behavior (IV)

Class-Risk Control & Safety (T)

Scale(s)-Severe to None (n)

Care Recipient:

Data Source:

Definition: Severity of injuries from accidents and trauma						

OUTCOME TARGET RATING: Maintain at_____   Increase to_____

Physical Injury Severity Overall Rating	Severe 1	Substantial 2	Moderate 3	Mild 4	None 5	
INDICATORS:						
191301 Skin abrasions	1	2	3	4	5	NA
191302 Bruises	1	2	3	4	5	NA
191303 Lacerations	1	2	3	4	5	NA
191304 Burns	1	2	3	4	5	NA
191305 Extremity sprains	1	2	3	4	5	NA
191306 Back sprains	1	2	3	4	5	NA
191307 Extremity fractures	1	2	3	4	5	NA
191308 Pelvic fractures	1	2	3	4	5	NA
191309 Hip fractures	1	2	3	4	5	NA
191310 Spinal fractures	1	2	3	4	5	NA
191311 Cranial fractures	1	2	3	4	5	NA
191312 Facial fractures	1	2	3	4	5	NA
191313 Dental injuries	1	2	3	4	5	NA
191314 Open head injuries	1	2	3	4	5	NA
191315 Closed head injuries	1	2	3	4	5	NA
191316 Impaired mobility	1	2	3	4	5	NA
191319 Impaired cognition	1	2	3	4	5	NA
191320 Decreased level of consciousness	1	2	3	4	5	NA

1st edition 1997; Revised 3rd edition 2004; Revised 4th edition

Outcome Content References:

Lawrence, J. I., & Maher, P. L. (1992). An interdisciplinary falls consult team: A collaborative approach to patient falls. *Journal of Nursing Care Quality, 6*(3), 21-29.

Llewellyn, J., Martin, B., Shekleton, M., & Firlit, S. (1988). Analysis of falls in the acute surgical and cardiovascular surgical patient. *Applied Nursing Research, 1*(3), 116-121.

+Maas, M., Swanson, E., Buckwalter, K. C., Specht, J. P., Tripp-Reimer, T., Lenth, R., Tranel, D., Reed, D., Broffit, B., Brenneman, D., Peters, J., Rose, D., Kelley, L., Schutte, D. L., & Sun, C. (1999). *Final report: Nursing Interventions for Alzheimer's: Family Role Trials* (NINR R01-NRO1689). Rockville, MD: National Institutes of Health.

P

Physical Maturation: Female—0114

Domain-Functional Health (I)

Class-Growth & Development (B)

Scale(s)-Severe deviation from normal range to No deviation from normal range (b)

Care Recipient:

Data Source:

> **Definition:** Normal physical changes in the female that occur with the transition from childhood to adulthood

OUTCOME TARGET RATING: Maintain at_____   Increase to_____

Physical Maturation: Female Overall Rating	Severe deviation from normal range 1	Substantial deviation from normal range 2	Moderate deviation from normal range 3	Mild deviation from normal range 4	No deviation from normal range 5	
INDICATORS:						
011401 Growth spurt between 9.5-14.5 years of age	1	2	3	4	5	NA
011402 Bone closure	1	2	3	4	5	NA
011403 Voice changes	1	2	3	4	5	NA
011404 Adult hair distribution	1	2	3	4	5	NA
011405 Breast development	1	2	3	4	5	NA
011406 Menstruation onset	1	2	3	4	5	NA
011407 Increased muscle mass	1	2	3	4	5	NA
011408 Decreased body fat	1	2	3	4	5	NA
011409 Increased sebaceous secretions	1	2	3	4	5	NA
011410 Increased perspiration	1	2	3	4	5	NA

1st edition 1997; Revised 3rd edition 2004

P

Outcome Content References:

Hockenberry, M. J., Wilson, D., Winkelstein, M. L., & Kline, N. E. (2003). *Wong's nursing care of infants and children* (7th ed.). St. Louis: Mosby.

Rice, F. P. (2001). *Human development: A life-span approach.* Upper Saddle River, NJ: Prentice Hall.

Schuster, C., & Ashburn, S. (1992). *The process of human development: A holistic approach* (3rd ed.). Philadelphia: J.B. Lippincott.

Physical Maturation: Male—0115

Domain-Functional Health (I)

Class-Growth & Development (B)

Scale(s)-Severe deviation from normal range to No deviation from normal range (b)

Care Recipient:

Data Source:

Definition: Normal physical changes in the male that occur with the transition from childhood to adulthood

OUTCOME TARGET RATING: Maintain at_____ Increase to_____

Physical Maturation: Male Overall Rating	Severe deviation from normal range 1	Substantial deviation from normal range 2	Moderate deviation from normal range 3	Mild deviation from normal range 4	No deviation from normal range 5	
011501 Growth spurt between 10.5-16 years of age	1	2	3	4	5	NA
011502 Bone closure	1	2	3	4	5	NA
011503 Voice changes	1	2	3	4	5	NA
011504 Adult hair distribution	1	2	3	4	5	NA
011505 Testicular descent	1	2	3	4	5	NA
011506 Penis enlargement	1	2	3	4	5	NA
011507 First ejaculation of sperm (wet dream)	1	2	3	4	5	NA
011508 Increased muscle mass	1	2	3	4	5	NA
011509 Decreased body fat	1	2	3	4	5	NA
011510 Increased sebaceous secretions	1	2	3	4	5	NA
011511 Increased perspiration	1	2	3	4	5	NA

1st edition 1997; Revised 3rd edition 2004

Outcome Content References:

Hockenberry, M. J., Wilson, D., Winkelstein, M. L., & Kline, N. E. (2003). *Wong's nursing care of infants and children* (7th ed.). St. Louis: Mosby.

Rice, F. P. (2001). *Human development: A life-span approach.* Upper Saddle River, NJ: Prentice Hall.

Schuster, C., & Ashburn, S. (1992). *The process of human development: A holistic approach* (3rd ed.). Philadelphia: J.B. Lippincott.

P

Play Participation—0116

Domain-Functional Health (I)

Class-Growth & Development (B)

Scale(s)-Never demonstrated to Consistently demonstrated (m)

Care Recipient:

Data Source:

Definition: Use of activities by a child from 1 year through 11 years of age to promote enjoyment, entertainment, and development

OUTCOME TARGET RATING: Maintain at_____   Increase to_____

Play Participation Overall Rating	Never demonstrated 1	Rarely demonstrated 2	Sometimes demonstrated 3	Often demonstrated 4	Consistently demonstrated 5	
INDICATORS:						
011601 Participates in play activities	1	2	3	4	5	NA
011610 Expresses satisfaction with play activities	1	2	3	4	5	NA
011603 Enjoys play activities	1	2	3	4	5	NA
011604 Uses social skills during play activities	1	2	3	4	5	NA
011605 Uses physical skills during play activities	1	2	3	4	5	NA
011606 Uses imagination during play activities	1	2	3	4	5	NA
011607 Expresses emotions during play activities	1	2	3	4	5	NA
011608 Uses role playing	1	2	3	4	5	NA

1st edition 1997; Revised 3rd edition 2004

Outcome Content References:

Gillis, A. J. (1989). The effect of play on immobilized children in hospital. *International Journal of Nursing Studies, 26*(3), 261-269.

Gray, E. (1989). The emotional and play needs of the dying child. *Issues in Comprehensive Pediatric Nursing, 12*(2/3), 207-224.

Jack, L. W. (1987). Using play in psychiatric rehabilitation. *Journal of Psychosocial Nursing, 25*(7), 17-20.

Post, C. (1990). Play therapy with an abused child: A case study. *Journal of Child and Adolescent Psychiatric and Mental Health Nursing, 2*(2), 48-51.

P

Postpartum Maternal Health Behavior—1624

Domain-Health Knowledge & Behavior (IV)

Class-Health Behavior (Q)

Scale(s)-Never demonstrated to Consistently demonstrated (m)

Care Recipient:

Data Source:

Definition: Personal actions to promote health of a mother in the period following birth of infant

OUTCOME TARGET RATING: Maintain at_____   Increase to_____

Postpartum Maternal Health Behavior Overall Rating	Never demonstrated 1	Rarely demonstrated 2	Sometimes demonstrated 3	Often demonstrated 4	Consistently demonstrated 5	

INDICATORS:

162401	Adapts to maternal role	1	2	3	4	5	NA
162402	Bonds with infant	1	2	3	4	5	NA
162403	Checks uterine fundus	1	2	3	4	5	NA
162404	Monitors lochia changes	1	2	3	4	5	NA
162405	Maintains perineum care	1	2	3	4	5	NA
162406	Maintains care of surgical incision	1	2	3	4	5	NA
162407	Maintains care of episiotomy	1	2	3	4	5	NA
162408	Monitors discomfort from episiotomy	1	2	3	4	5	NA
162409	Monitors for signs and symptoms of infection	1	2	3	4	5	NA
162410	Monitors for signs of postpartum depression	1	2	3	4	5	NA
162411	Monitors for nipple tenderness	1	2	3	4	5	NA
162412	Monitors breasts for engorgement	1	2	3	4	5	NA
162413	Monitors for stress incontinence	1	2	3	4	5	NA
162414	Monitors for development of new health problems	1	2	3	4	5	NA
162415	Uses water-based vaginal lubricant	1	2	3	4	5	NA
162416	Obtains health care when warning signs occur	1	2	3	4	5	NA
162417	Uses effective pain management strategies	1	2	3	4	5	NA
162418	Uses stress management techniques	1	2	3	4	5	NA
162419	Monitors anxiety level	1	2	3	4	5	NA
162420	Monitors comfort status	1	2	3	4	5	NA
162421	Maintains adequate nutrient intake	1	2	3	4	5	NA

P

		Never demonstrated	Rarely demonstrated	Sometimes demonstrated	Often demonstrated	Consistently demonstrated	
162422	Maintains adequate fluid intake	1	2	3	4	5	NA
162423	Participates in regular exercise	1	2	3	4	5	NA
162424	Performs pelvic floor exercises	1	2	3	4	5	NA
162425	Balances activity and rest	1	2	3	4	5	NA
162426	Monitors sleep patterns	1	2	3	4	5	NA
162427	Uses strategies to obtain needed sleep	1	2	3	4	5	NA
162428	Obtains assistance from health professional for depression as needed	1	2	3	4	5	NA
162429	Discusses options for birth control with health professional	1	2	3	4	5	NA
162430	Follows recommendations for sexual activity restrictions	1	2	3	4	5	NA
162431	Obtains assistance from health professional as needed	1	2	3	4	5	NA
162432	Uses family support	1	2	3	4	5	NA
162433	Uses available support groups	1	2	3	4	5	NA
162434	Participates in postpartum checkups	1	2	3	4	5	NA

4th edition

Outcome Content References:

Borders, N. (2006). After the afterbirth: A critical review of postpartum health relative to method of delivery. *American College of Nurse-Midwives, 51*(4), 242-248.

Geoghegan, A. H. (2006). Not just an option: Postpartum depression screening becomes law in the State of New Jersey. *Nursing Spectrum—New York & New Jersey Edition, 18A*(20), 8-9.

Piejko, E. (2006). The postpartum visit: Why wait 6 weeks? *Australian Family Physician, 35*(9), 674-678.

Wisner, K. L., Chambers, C., & Sit, D. Y. (2006). Postpartum depression: A major public health problem. *Journal of the American Medical Association, 296*(21), 2616-2618.

P

Post-Procedure Recovery—2303

Domain-Physiologic Health (II)

Class-Therapeutic Response (a)

Scale(s)-Severe deviation from normal range to No deviation from normal range (b) and Severe to None (n)

Care Recipient:

Data Source:

Definition: Extent to which an individual returns to baseline function following a procedure(s) requiring anesthesia or sedation

OUTCOME TARGET RATING: Maintain at_____   Increase to_____

Post-Procedure Recovery Overall Rating	Severe deviation from normal range 1	Substantial deviation from normal range 2	Moderate deviation from normal range 3	Mild deviation from normal range 4	No deviation from normal range 5	
INDICATORS:						
230301 Patent airway	1	2	3	4	5	NA
230302 Spontaneous respirations	1	2	3	4	5	NA
230303 Respiratory rate	1	2	3	4	5	NA
230304 Depth of inspiration	1	2	3	4	5	NA
230305 Forceful cough	1	2	3	4	5	NA
230306 O$_2$ saturation 92%-94% room air	1	2	3	4	5	NA
230307 Systolic blood pressure within 20 mm Hg of baseline	1	2	3	4	5	NA
230308 Aldrete score	1	2	3	4	5	NA
230309 Gag reflex	1	2	3	4	5	NA
230310 Swallowing ability	1	2	3	4	5	NA
230311 Retains oral fluids	1	2	3	4	5	NA
230312 Answers questions	1	2	3	4	5	NA
230313 Fully awake	1	2	3	4	5	NA
230314 Moves extremities on command	1	2	3	4	5	NA
230315 Ambulation tolerance	1	2	3	4	5	NA
230316 Thermoregulation	1	2	3	4	5	NA
230317 Urine output	1	2	3	4	5	NA
230318 Voiding	1	2	3	4	5	NA
230325 Fluid balance	1	2	3	4	5	NA
230326 Electrolyte and acid/base balance	1	2	3	4	5	NA
230327 Wound tissue perfusion	1	2	3	4	5	NA
	Severe	Substantial	Moderate	Mild	None	
230319 Drainage from tube/drain	1	2	3	4	5	NA
230320 Drainage on dressing	1	2	3	4	5	NA
230321 Nausea	1	2	3	4	5	NA
230322 Vomiting	1	2	3	4	5	NA
230323 Shivering	1	2	3	4	5	NA
230324 Pain	1	2	3	4	5	NA

P

3rd edition 2004; Revised 4th edition

Outcome Content References:

Aldrete, J. A. (1998). Modifications to the postanesthesia score for use in ambulatory surgery. *Journal of PeriAnesthesia Nursing, 13*(3), 148-155.

Aldrete J. A., & Kroulik, D. (1970). A postanesthetic recovery score. *Anesthesia & Analgesia, 49*(6), 924-934.

Cohen, S. E., Hamilton, C. L., Riley, E. T., Walker, D. S., Macario, A., & Halpern, J. W. (1998). Obstetric postanesthesia care unit stays: Reevaluation of discharge criteria after regional anesthesia. *Anesthesiology, 89*(6), 1559-1565.

Craney, J. M., & Gorman, L. N. (1997). Conscious sedation and implantable devices. Safe and effective sedation during pacemaker and implantable cardioverter defibrillator placement. *Critical Care Nursing Clinics of North America, 9*(3), 325-334.

Gross, J. B., Bailey, P. L., Caplan, R. A., Connes, R. T., Cote, B. S., Kapur, P. A., Zerwas, J. M., & Zuccaro, G. (1996). Practice guidelines for sedation and analgesia by non-anesthesiologists. *Anesthesiology, 84*(2), 459-471.

Joint Commission on Accreditation of Healthcare Organizations. (2001). *Comprehensive accreditation manual for hospitals: The official handbook*. Oakbrook Terrace, IL: Author.

Piper, S. N., Suttner, S. W., Schmidt, C. C., Maleck, W. H., Kumle, B., & Boldt, J. (1999). Nefopam and clonidine in the prevention of post anesthetic shivering. *Anaesthesia, 54*(7), 695-699.

P

Prenatal Health Behavior—1607

Domain-Health Knowledge & Behavior (IV)

Class-Health Behavior (Q)

Scale(s)-Never demonstrated to Consistently demonstrated (m)

Care Recipient:

Data Source:

Definition: Personal actions to promote a healthy pregnancy and a healthy newborn

OUTCOME TARGET RATING: Maintain at_____   Increase to_____

Prenatal Health Behavior Overall Rating	Never demonstrated 1	Rarely demonstrated 2	Sometimes demonstrated 3	Often demonstrated 4	Consistently demonstrated 5	
INDICATORS:						
160701 Maintains healthy preconceptual state	1	2	3	4	5	NA
160702 Uses proper body mechanics	1	2	3	4	5	NA
160703 Keeps appointments for prenatal care	1	2	3	4	5	NA
160704 Maintains healthy weight gain pattern	1	2	3	4	5	NA
160705 Receives proper dental care	1	2	3	4	5	NA
160706 Uses motor vehicle safety devices correctly	1	2	3	4	5	NA
160707 Attends childbirth education classes	1	2	3	4	5	NA
160709 Participates in regular exercise	1	2	3	4	5	NA
160710 Maintains adequate nutrient intake for pregnancy	1	2	3	4	5	NA
160711 Practices safe sex	1	2	3	4	5	NA
160721 Uses medication as prescribed	1	2	3	4	5	NA
160712 Consults health professional about non-prescription medication use	1	2	3	4	5	NA
160713 Avoids environmental hazards	1	2	3	4	5	NA
160714 Avoids exposure to infectious diseases	1	2	3	4	5	NA
160715 Avoids recreational drug use	1	2	3	4	5	NA
160716 Avoids alcohol use	1	2	3	4	5	NA
160717 Avoids tobacco use	1	2	3	4	5	NA
160718 Avoids teratogenic agents	1	2	3	4	5	NA
160719 Avoids abusive situations	1	2	3	4	5	NA

2nd edition 2000; Revised 3rd edition 2004

Outcome Content References:

Bell, R., & O'Neill M. (1994). Exercise and pregnancy: A review. *Birth, 21*(2), 85-95.

Crowell, D. T. (1995). Weight change in the postpartum period. A review of the literature. *Journal of Nurse Midwifery, 40*(5), 418-423.

Freda, M. C., Andersen, H. F., Damus, K., & Merkatz, I. R. (1993). What pregnant women want to know: A comparison of client and provider perceptions. *Journal of Obstetric, Gynecologic, and Neonatal Nursing, 22*(3), 237.

Kearney, M. H., Murphy, S., Irwin, K., & Rosenbaum, M. (1995). Salvaging self: A grounded theory of pregnancy on crack cocaine. *Nursing Research, 44*(4), 208-213.

McFarlane, J., Parker, B., & Soeken, K. (1996). Abuse during pregnancy: Associations with maternal health and infant birth weight. *Nursing Research, 45*(1), 37-42.

Olds, S., London, M. L., & Ladewig, P. W. (1996). *Maternal-newborn nursing: A family-centered approach* (5th ed.). Menlo Park, CA: Addison-Wesley.

Shapiro, H. R. (1993). Prenatal education in the work place. *AWHONNS Clinical Issues in Perinatal & Women's Health Nursing, 4*(1), 113-121.

Summers, L. (1993). Preconception care: An opportunity to maximize health in pregnancy. *Journal of Nurse Midwifery, 38*(4), 188-198.

P

Pre-Procedure Readiness—1921

Domain-Health Knowledge & Behavior (IV)

Class-Risk Control & Safety (T)

Scale(s)-Not adequate to Totally adequate (f)

Care Recipient:

Data Source:

Definition: Readiness of a patient to safely undergo a procedure requiring anesthesia or sedation

OUTCOME TARGET RATING: Maintain at_____ Increase to_____

Pre-Procedure Readiness Overall Rating	Not adequate 1	Slightly adequate 2	Moderately adequate 3	Substantially adequate 4	Totally adequate 5	
INDICATORS:						
192101 Knowledge of procedure	1	2	3	4	5	NA
192102 Knowledge of pre-procedure routines	1	2	3	4	5	NA
192103 Knowledge of post-procedure routines	1	2	3	4	5	NA
192104 Knowledge of potential risks and complications	1	2	3	4	5	NA
192105 Identification of changes in health status	1	2	3	4	5	NA
192106 Identification of past adverse reaction to anesthetics	1	2	3	4	5	NA
192107 Bowel prep status	1	2	3	4	5	NA
192108 Intake restriction status	1	2	3	4	5	NA
192109 Completion of skin prep	1	2	3	4	5	NA
192110 Knowledge of identification routines	1	2	3	4	5	NA
192111 Participation in marking procedural site	1	2	3	4	5	NA
192112 Completion of required lab work	1	2	3	4	5	NA
192113 Completion of required physical exam	1	2	3	4	5	NA
192114 Provision of signed consent	1	2	3	4	5	NA
192115 Reported personal preparation for procedure	1	2	3	4	5	NA
192116 Modification of regimen	1	2	3	4	5	NA
192117 Reported changes in medication required for procedure	1	2	3	4	5	NA
192118 Discussion of concerns about procedure	1	2	3	4	5	NA
192119 Discussion of questions prior to procedure	1	2	3	4	5	NA
192120 Participation in pre-procedure checklist	1	2	3	4	5	NA

P

4th edition

Outcome Content References:

American Organization of Perioperative Nurses. (2006). *Standards, recommended practices and guidelines*. Denver: Author.

Barnes, S. (2001). Preparing for surgery: Providing the details. *Journal of PeriAnesthesia Nursing, 16*(1), 31-32.

Saufl, N. Mm (2004). Universal protocol for preventing wrong site, wrong procedure, wrong person surgery. *Journal of PeriAnesthesia Nursing, 19*(5), 348-351.

Smeltzer, S. C., & Bare, B. G. (2004). *Brunner & Suddarth's textbook of medical surgical nursing* (10th ed.). Philadelphia: Lippincott Williams & Wilkins.

P

Preterm Infant Organization—0117

Domain-Functional Health (I)
Class-Growth & Development (B)
Scale(s)-Severely compromised to Not compromised (a)

Care Recipient:
Data Source:

Definition: Extrauterine integration of physiologic and behavioral function by the infant born 24 to 37 (term) weeks gestation

OUTCOME TARGET RATING: Maintain at_____   Increase to_____

Preterm Infant Organization Overall Rating	Severely compromised 1	Substantially compromised 2	Moderately compromised 3	Mildly compromised 4	Not compromised 5	
INDICATORS:						
011701 Apical heart rate (120-160 bpm)	1	2	3	4	5	NA
011702 Gestational age index	1	2	3	4	5	NA
011703 Respiratory rate (30-60)	1	2	3	4	5	NA
011704 Oxygen saturation >85%	1	2	3	4	5	NA
011705 Thermoregulation	1	2	3	4	5	NA
011706 Skin color	1	2	3	4	5	NA
011707 Feeding tolerance	1	2	3	4	5	NA
011708 Relaxed muscle tone	1	2	3	4	5	NA
011709 Smooth synchronous movement	1	2	3	4	5	NA
011710 Flexed posture	1	2	3	4	5	NA
011711 Hands brought to mouth	1	2	3	4	5	NA
011712 Deep sleep	1	2	3	4	5	NA
011713 Light sleep	1	2	3	4	5	NA
011714 Quiet-alert	1	2	3	4	5	NA
011715 Active-alert	1	2	3	4	5	NA
011716 Attentiveness to stimuli	1	2	3	4	5	NA
011717 Response to stimuli	1	2	3	4	5	NA
011718 Appropriate time-out signals	1	2	3	4	5	NA
011719 Sustained alertness during interaction	1	2	3	4	5	NA
011720 Interaction with caregiver	1	2	3	4	5	NA
011721 Self-consolability	1	2	3	4	5	NA

2nd edition 2000; Revised 3rd edition 2004

Outcome Content References

Blackburn, S. T., &. VanderBerg, K. A. (1993). Assessment and management of neurodevelopmental behavior development. In C. Kenner, A. Bueggenmeyer, & L. P. Gunderson (Eds.), *Comprehensive neonatal nursing* (pp. 1094-1121). Philadelphia: W.B. Saunders.

D'Apolito, K. (1991). What is an organized infant? *Neonatal Network, 2*(1), 23-29.

Deacon, J., & O'Neill, P. (Eds.). (1999). *Core curriculum for neonatal intensive care nursing* (2nd ed.). Philadelphia: W.B. Saunders.

Jorgensen, K. M. (1993). *Developmental care of the preterm infant*. South Weymouth, MA: Children's Medical Ventures.

Mattson, S., & Smith, J. E. (Eds.). (2000). *Core curriculum for maternal-newborn nursing* (2nd ed.). Philadelphia: W.B. Saunders.

McGrath, J. M., & Conliffe-Torres, S. (1996). Integrating family centered developmental assessment and interventions with routine cares in the neonatal intensive care unit. *Nursing Clinics of North America, 31*(2), 367-385.

National Association of Neonatal Nurses. (1993). *Infant developmental care guidelines*. Petaluma, CA: Author.

P

Psychomotor Energy—0006

Domain-Functional Health (I)

Class-Energy Maintenance (A)

Scale(s)-Never demonstrated to Consistently demonstrated (m) and Consistently demonstrated to Never demonstrated (t)

Care Recipient:

Data Source:

Definition: Personal drive and energy to maintain activities of daily living, nutrition, and personal safety

OUTCOME TARGET RATING: Maintain at_____   Increase to_____

Psychomotor Energy Overall Rating	Never demonstrated 1	Rarely demonstrated 2	Sometimes demonstrated 3	Often demonstrated 4	Consistently demonstrated 5	

INDICATORS:

000601	Exhibits affect that fits situation	1	2	3	4	5	NA
000602	Exhibits concentration	1	2	3	4	5	NA
000603	Maintains personal grooming and hygiene	1	2	3	4	5	NA
000604	Exhibits normal appetite	1	2	3	4	5	NA
000613	Complies with medication regimen	1	2	3	4	5	NA
000614	Complies with therapeutic regimen	1	2	3	4	5	NA
000606	Shows interest in surroundings	1	2	3	4	5	NA
000608	Exhibits stable energy level	1	2	3	4	5	NA
000609	Exhibits ability to accomplish daily tasks	1	2	3	4	5	NA

		Consistently demonstrated	Often demonstrated	Sometimes demonstrated	Rarely demonstrated	Never demonstrated	
000607	Suicide ideation	1	2	3	4	5	NA
000611	Lethargy	1	2	3	4	5	NA
000612	Depression	1	2	3	4	5	NA

2nd edition 2000; Revised 3rd edition 2004; Revised 4th edition

Outcome Content References:

American Psychiatric Association. (2000). *Diagnostic and statistical manual of mental disorders* (4th ed., text revision). Washington, DC: Author.

Lieberman, H. R. (2006). Mental energy: Assessing the cognitive. *Nutrition Reviews, 64*(7), 57–59.

P

Psychosocial Adjustment: Life Change—1305

Domain-Psychosocial Health (III)   Care Recipient:

Class-Psychosocial Adaptation (N)   Data Source:

Scale(s)-Never demonstrated to Consistently demonstrated (m)

Definition: Adaptive psychosocial response of an individual to a significant life change

OUTCOME TARGET RATING: Maintain at_____   Increase to_____

Psychosocial Adjustment: Life Change Overall Rating	Never demonstrated 1	Rarely demonstrated 2	Sometimes demonstrated 3	Often demonstrated 4	Consistently demonstrated 5	
INDICATORS:						
130501 Sets realistic goals	1	2	3	4	5	NA
130502 Maintains self-esteem	1	2	3	4	5	NA
130503 Maintains productivity	1	2	3	4	5	NA
130504 Reports feeling useful	1	2	3	4	5	NA
130505 Verbalizes optimism about present	1	2	3	4	5	NA
130506 Verbalizes optimism about future	1	2	3	4	5	NA
130507 Reports feeling empowered	1	2	3	4	5	NA
130508 Identifies multiple coping strategies	1	2	3	4	5	NA
130509 Uses effective coping strategies	1	2	3	4	5	NA
130510 Uses effective financial management strategies	1	2	3	4	5	NA
130513 Uses available social support	1	2	3	4	5	NA
130514 Participates in leisure activities	1	2	3	4	5	NA
130511 Expresses satisfaction with living arrangements	1	2	3	4	5	NA
130512 Reports feeling socially engaged	1	2	3	4	5	NA

1st edition 1997; Revised 3rd edition 2004

Outcome Content References:

Hernan, J. A. (1984). Exploding aging myths through retirement counseling. *Journal of Gerontological Nursing, 10*(4), 31-33.

Johnson, R. A. (2001). Relocation stress syndrome. In M. Maas, K. Buckwalter, M. Hardy, T. Tripp-Reimer, M. Titler, & J. Specht (Eds.), *Nursing care of older adults: Diagnoses, outcomes & interventions* (pp. 619-630). St. Louis: Mosby.

+Liang, J. (1984). Dimensions of the Life Satisfaction Index A: A structural formulation. *Journal of Gerontology, 39*(5), 613-622.

+Neugarten, B. L., Havighurst, R. J., & Tobin, S. (1961). The measurement of life satisfaction. *Journal of Gerontology, 16*, 134-143.

Neuhs, H. P. (1991). Ready for retirement? *Geriatric Nursing, 12*(5), 240-241.

Rosenkoetter, M. M. (1985). Is your older client ready for a role change after retirement? *Journal of Gerontological Nursing, 11*(9), 21-24.

Tincher, B. J. V. (1992). Retirement: Perspectives and theory. *Physical & Occupational Therapy in Geriatrics, 11*(1), 55-62.

P

Quality of Life—2000

Domain-Perceived Health (V)
Class-Health & Life Quality (U)
Scale(s)-Not at all satisfied to Completely satisfied (s)

Care Recipient:
Data Source:

Definition: Extent of positive perception of current life circumstances

OUTCOME TARGET RATING: Maintain at_____   Increase to_____

Quality of Life Overall Rating	Not at all satisfied 1	Somewhat satisfied 2	Moderately satisfied 3	Very satisfied 4	Completely satisfied 5	
INDICATORS:						
200001 Health status	1	2	3	4	5	NA
200002 Social circumstances	1	2	3	4	5	NA
200003 Environmental circumstances	1	2	3	4	5	NA
200013 Privacy	1	2	3	4	5	NA
200014 Dignity	1	2	3	4	5	NA
200015 Autonomy	1	2	3	4	5	NA
200004 Economic status	1	2	3	4	5	NA
200005 Education level	1	2	3	4	5	NA
200006 Occupation	1	2	3	4	5	NA
200007 Close relationships	1	2	3	4	5	NA
200008 Achievement of life goals	1	2	3	4	5	NA
200009 Ability to cope	1	2	3	4	5	NA
200010 Self-concept	1	2	3	4	5	NA
200011 Pervasive mood	1	2	3	4	5	NA
200016 Independence in activities of daily living	1	2	3	4	5	NA

Q

1st edition 1997; Revised 3rd edition 2004; Revised 4th edition

Outcome Content References:

Andrews, F., & Withey, S. (1976). *Social indicators of well-being: Americans' perceptions of life quality.* New York: Plenum Press.

Davidhizar, R. E., & Giger, J. N. (2001). Powerlessness. In M. Maas, K. Buckwalter, M. Hardy, T. Tripp-Reimer, M. Titler, & J. Specht (Eds.), *Nursing care of older adults: Diagnoses, outcomes & interventions* (pp. 562-570). St. Louis: Mosby.

+Diener, E., Emmons, R. A., Larsen, R. J., & Griffin, S. (1985). The Satisfaction with Life Scale. *Journal of Personality Assessment, 49*(1), 71-75.

Gill, L., & Flenstein, A. R. (1994). A critical appraisal of the quality of quality-of-life measurements. *Journal of the American Medical Association, 272*(8), 619-626.

Padilla, G., Ferrell, B., Grant, M., & Rhiner, M. (1990). Defining the content domain of quality of life for cancer patients with pain. *Cancer Nursing, 13*(2), 108-115.

Ragsdale, D., Kotarba, J., & Morrow, J. (1992). Quality of life of hospitalized persons with AIDS. *Image—The Journal of Nursing Scholarship, 24*(4), 259-265.

Stewart, A., Ware, J., Sherbourne, C., & Wells, K. (1992). Psychological distress/well-being and cognitive functioning measures. In A. Stewart & J. Ware, Jr. (Eds.), *Measuring functioning and well-being: The medical outcomes study approach* (pp. 102-142). Durham, NC: Duke University Press.

Respiratory Status—0415

Domain-Physiologic Health (II)   *Care Recipient:*

Class-Cardiopulmonary (E)   *Data Source:*

Scale(s)-Severe deviation from normal range to No deviation from normal range (b) and Severe to None (n)

Definition: Movement of air in and out of the lungs and exchange of carbon dioxide and oxygen at the alveolar level

OUTCOME TARGET RATING: Maintain at_____   Increase to_____

Respiratory Status Overall Rating	Severe deviation from normal range 1	Substantial deviation from normal range 2	Moderate deviation from normal range 3	Mild deviation from normal range 4	No deviation from normal range 5	
INDICATORS:						
041501 Respiratory rate	1	2	3	4	5	NA
041502 Respiratory rhythm	1	2	3	4	5	NA
041503 Depth of inspiration	1	2	3	4	5	NA
041504 Auscultated breath sounds	1	2	3	4	5	NA
041505 Tidal volume	1	2	3	4	5	NA
041506 Achievement of expected incentive spirometer	1	2	3	4	5	NA
041507 Vital capacity	1	2	3	4	5	NA
041508 Oxygen saturation	1	2	3	4	5	NA
041509 Pulmonary function tests	1	2	3	4	5	NA

	Severe	Substantial	Moderate	Mild	None	
041510 Accessory muscle use	1	2	3	4	5	NA
041511 Chest retraction	1	2	3	4	5	NA
041512 Pursed lips breathing	1	2	3	4	5	NA
041513 Cyanosis	1	2	3	4	5	NA
041514 Dyspnea at rest	1	2	3	4	5	NA
041515 Dyspnea with mild exertion	1	2	3	4	5	NA
041516 Restlessness	1	2	3	4	5	NA
041517 Somnolence	1	2	3	4	5	NA
041518 Diaphoresis	1	2	3	4	5	NA
041519 Impaired cognition	1	2	3	4	5	NA
041520 Accumulation of sputum	1	2	3	4	5	NA
041521 Atelectasis	1	2	3	4	5	NA
041522 Adventitious breath sounds	1	2	3	4	5	NA

R

Continued

		Severe	Substantial	Moderate	Mild	None	
041523	Impaired expiration	1	2	3	4	5	NA
041524	Gasping	1	2	3	4	5	NA
041525	Agonal respirations	1	2	3	4	5	NA
041526	Grunting	1	2	3	4	5	NA
041527	Clubbing of fingers	1	2	3	4	5	NA
041528	Nasal flaring	1	2	3	4	5	NA
041529	Restlessness	1	2	3	4	5	NA
041530	Fever	1	2	3	4	5	NA
041531	Coughing	1	2	3	4	5	NA

4th edition

Outcome Content References:

Bailey, P. H., Colella, T., & Mossey, S. (2004). COPD-intuition or template: Nurse's stories of acute exacerbations of chronic obstructive pulmonary disease. *Journal of Clinical Nursing, 13*, 756-764.

Booker, R. (2005). A spirometer in primary care—as essential as a stethoscope. *Primary Health Care, 15*(5), 33-36.

Loeb, M., McArther, M., Peeling, R. W., Petric, M., & Simor, A. E. (2000). Surveillance for outbreaks of respiratory tract infections in nursing homes. *Canadian Medical Association Journal, 162*(8), 1133-1137.

Mintz, M. L. (2006). *Disorders of the respiratory tract: Common challenges in primary care.* Totowa, NJ: Humana Press.

Smeltzer, S. C., & Bare, B. G. (2004). *Brunner & Suddarth's textbook of medical surgical nursing* (10th ed.). Philadelphia: Lippincott Williams & Wilkins.

R

Respiratory Status: Airway Patency—0410

Domain-Physiologic Health (II)　　　　　　　　　*Care Recipient:*

Class-Cardiopulmonary (E)　　　　　　　　　　*Data Source:*

Scale(s)-Severe deviation from normal range to No deviation from normal range (b) and Severe to None (n)

Definition: Open, clear tracheobronchial passages for air exchange

OUTCOME TARGET RATING:　　　Maintain at_____　　　　Increase to_____

Respiratory Status: Airway Patency Overall Rating	Severe deviation from normal range 1	Substantial deviation from normal range 2	Moderate deviation from normal range 3	Mild deviation from normal range 4	No deviation from normal range 5	
INDICATORS:						
041004　Respiratory rate	1	2	3	4	5	NA
041005　Respiratory rhythm	1	2	3	4	5	NA
041011　Depth of inspiration	1	2	3	4	5	NA
041012　Ability to clear secretions	1	2	3	4	5	NA

	Severe	Substantial	Moderate	Mild	None	
041002　Anxiety	1	2	3	4	5	NA
041011　Fear	1	2	3	4	5	NA
041003　Choking	1	2	3	4	5	NA
041007　Adventitious breath sounds	1	2	3	4	5	NA
041013　Nasal flaring	1	2	3	4	5	NA
041014　Gasping	1	2	3	4	5	NA
041015　Dyspnea at rest	1	2	3	4	5	NA
041016　Dyspnea with mild exertion	1	2	3	4	5	NA
041018　Accessory muscle use	1	2	3	4	5	NA
041019　Coughing	1	2	3	4	5	NA
041020　Accumulation of sputum	1	2	3	4	5	NA
041021　Agonal respirations	1	2	3	4	5	NA

2nd edition 2000; Revised 3rd edition 2004; Revised 4th edition

R

Outcome Content References:

Clochesy, J. M., Brey, C., Cardin, S., Whittaker, A. A., & Rudy, E. B. (1996). *Critical care nursing* (2nd ed.). Philadelphia: W.B. Saunders.

Lewis, S. M., Collier, I. C., Heitkermper, M. M., & Dirksen, S. R. (2000). *Medical-surgical nursing: Assessment & management of clinical problems* (5th ed.). St. Louis: Mosby.

McCance, K. L., & Huether, S. E. (2002). *Pathophysiology: The biologic basis for disease in adults and children* (4th ed.). St. Louis: Mosby.

Smeltzer, S. C., & Bare, B. G. (2004). *Brunner & Suddarth's textbook of medical surgical nursing* (10th ed.). Philadelphia: Lippincott Williams & Wilkins.

Respiratory Status: Gas Exchange—0402

Domain-Physiologic Health (II)

Class-Cardiopulmonary (E)

Scale(s)-Severe deviation from normal range to No deviation from normal range (b) and Severe to None (n)

Care Recipient:

Data Source:

Definition: Alveolar exchange of carbon dioxide and oxygen to maintain arterial blood gas concentrations

OUTCOME TARGET RATING: Maintain at_____   Increase to_____

Respiratory Status: Gas Exchange Overall Rating	Severe deviation from normal range 1	Substantial deviation from normal range 2	Moderate deviation from normal range 3	Mild deviation from normal range 4	No deviation from normal range 5	
INDICATORS:						
040208 Partial pressure of oxygen in arterial blood (PaO$_2$)	1	2	3	4	5	NA
040209 Partial pressure of carbon dioxide in arterial blood (PaCO$_2$)	1	2	3	4	5	NA
040210 Arterial pH	1	2	3	4	5	NA
040211 Oxygen saturation	1	2	3	4	5	NA
040212 End tidal carbon dioxide	1	2	3	4	5	NA
040213 Chest x-ray findings	1	2	3	4	5	NA
040214 Ventilation perfusion balance	1	2	3	4	5	NA

	Severe	Substantial	Moderate	Mild	None	
040203 Dyspnea at rest	1	2	3	4	5	NA
040204 Dyspnea with mild exertion	1	2	3	4	5	NA
040205 Restlessness	1	2	3	4	5	NA
040206 Cyanosis	1	2	3	4	5	NA
040207 Somnolence	1	2	3	4	5	NA
040216 Impaired cognition	1	2	3	4	5	NA

1st edition 1997; Revised 2nd edition 2000; Revised 3rd edition 2004; Revised 4th edition

Outcome Content References:

Ahrens, T. (1993). Changing perspectives in the assessment of oxygenation. *Critical Care Nurse, 13*(4), 78-83.

Berry, B. E., & Pinard, A. E. (2002). Assessing tissue oxygenation. *Critical Care Nurse, 22*(3), 22-36.

Hayden, R. (1992). What keeps oxygenation on track? *American Journal of Nursing, 92*(12), 32-40.

Janson-Bjerklie, S. (1993). Predicting the outcomes of living with asthma. *Research in Nursing and Health, 16*(4), 241-249.

McCarty, K., & Wilkins, R. (1990). Synopsis of clinical findings in respiratory disorders. In R. Wilkins, R. L. Sheldon, & S. J. Krider (Eds.), *Clinical assessment in respiratory care* (2nd ed., pp. 294-302). St. Louis: Mosby.

Morton, P. (1989). Respiratory systems. In P. Morton (Ed.), *Health assessment in nursing* (pp. 243-281). Springhouse, PA: Springhouse.

Patrick, M. (1991). *Medical-surgical nursing: Pathophysiological concepts* (2nd ed.). Philadelphia: J.B. Lippincott.

Potter, P., & Perry, A. (1991). *Oxygenation: Basic nursing theory and practice.* St. Louis: Mosby.

Smeltzer, S. C., & Bare, B. G. (2004). *Brunner & Suddarth's textbook of medical surgical nursing* (10th ed.). Philadelphia: Lippincott Williams & Wilkins.

R

Respiratory Status: Ventilation—0403

Domain-Physiologic Health (II)   *Care Recipient:*

Class-Cardiopulmonary (E)   *Data Source:*

Scale(s)-Severe deviation from normal range to No deviation from normal range (b) and Severe to None (n)

Definition: Movement of air in and out of the lungs

OUTCOME TARGET RATING: Maintain at_____   Increase to_____

Respiratory Status: Ventilation Overall Rating	Severe deviation from normal range 1	Substantial deviation from normal range 2	Moderate deviation from normal range 3	Mild deviation from normal range 4	No deviation from normal range 5	
INDICATORS:						
040301	Respiratory rate	1	2	3	4	5	NA
040302	Respiratory rhythm	1	2	3	4	5	NA
040303	Depth of inspiration	1	2	3	4	5	NA
040318	Percussed sounds	1	2	3	4	5	NA
040324	Tidal volume	1	2	3	4	5	NA
040325	Vital capacity	1	2	3	4	5	NA
040326	Chest x-ray findings	1	2	3	4	5	NA
040327	Pulmonary function tests	1	2	3	4	5	NA

		Severe	Substantial	Moderate	Mild	None	
040309	Accessory muscle use	1	2	3	4	5	NA
040310	Adventitious breath sounds	1	2	3	4	5	NA
040311	Chest retraction	1	2	3	4	5	NA
040312	Pursed lips breathing	1	2	3	4	5	NA
040313	Dyspnea at rest	1	2	3	4	5	NA
040314	Dyspnea with exertion	1	2	3	4	5	NA
040315	Orthopnea	1	2	3	4	5	NA
040317	Tactile fremitus	1	2	3	4	5	NA
040329	Asymmetrical chest expansion	1	2	3	4	5	NA
040330	Impaired vocalization	1	2	3	4	5	NA
040331	Accumulation of sputum	1	2	3	4	5	NA
040332	Impaired expiration	1	2	3	4	5	NA
040333	Distorted voice sounds on auscultation	1	2	3	4	5	NA
040334	Atelectasis	1	2	3	4	5	NA

Continued

R

1st edition 1997; Revised 3rd edition 2004; Revised 4th edition

Outcome Content References:

Ahrens, T. (1993). Changing perspectives in the assessment of oxygenation. *Critical Care Nurse, 13*(4), 78-83.

+Guyatt, G. H., Berman, L. B., Townsend, M., Pugsley, S. O., & Chambers, L. W. (1987). A measure of quality of life for clinical trials in chronic lung disease. *Thorax, 42*(10), 773-778.

Hayden, R. (1992). What keeps oxygenation on track? *American Journal of Nursing, 92*(12), 32-40.

Janson-Bjerklie, S. (1993). Predicting the outcomes of living with asthma. *Research in Nursing and Health, 16*(4), 241-249.

Morton, P. (1989). Respiratory systems. In P. Morton (Ed.), *Health assessment in nursing* (pp. 243-281). Springhouse, PA: Springhouse.

Patrick, M. (1991). *Medical-surgical nursing: Pathophysiological concepts* (2nd ed.). Philadelphia: J.B. Lippincott.

Potter, P., & Perry, A. (1991). *Oxygenation: Basic nursing theory and practice.* St. Louis: Mosby.

Smeltzer, S. C., & Bare, B. G. (2004). *Brunner & Suddarth's textbook of medical surgical nursing* (10th ed.). Philadelphia: Lippincott Williams & Wilkins.

Wakefield, B. (2001). Ineffective breathing pattern. In M. Maas, K. Buckwalter, M. Hardy, T. Tripp-Reimer, M. Titler, & J. Specht (Eds.), *Nursing care of older adults: Diagnoses, outcomes & interventions* (pp. 313-323). St. Louis: Mosby.

Wilkins, R., & Sheldon, R. (2005). *Clinical assessment in respiratory care* (5th ed.). St. Louis: Mosby.

R

Rest—0003

Domain-Functional Health (I)

Class-Energy Maintenance (A)

Scale(s)-Severely compromised to Not compromised (a)

Care Recipient:

Data Source:

Definition: Quantity and pattern of diminished activity for mental and physical rejuvenation

OUTCOME TARGET RATING: Maintain at_____   Increase to_____

Rest Overall Rating	Severely compromised 1	Substantially compromised 2	Moderately compromised 3	Mildly compromised 4	Not compromised 5	
INDICATORS:						
000301 Amount of rest	1	2	3	4	5	NA
000302 Rest pattern	1	2	3	4	5	NA
000303 Rest quality	1	2	3	4	5	NA
000304 Physically rested	1	2	3	4	5	NA
000305 Mentally rested	1	2	3	4	5	NA
000308 Emotionally rested	1	2	3	4	5	NA
000309 Energy restored after rest	1	2	3	4	5	NA
000310 Rested appearance	1	2	3	4	5	NA

1st edition 1997; Revised 3rd edition 2004; Revised 4th edition

Outcome Content References:

Brown, D. R., Morgan, W. P., & Raglin, J. S. (1993). Effects of exercise and rest on the state anxiety and blood pressure of physically challenged college students. *Journal of Sports Medicine and Physical Fitness, 33*(3), 300-305.

Ellis, J. R., & Nowlis, E. A. (1994). *Providing nursing care within the nursing process* (5th ed.). Philadelphia: J.B. Lippincott.

+Lee, K. A., Hicks, G., & Nino-Murcia, G. (1991). Validity and reliability of a scale to assess fatigue. *Psychiatry Research, 36*(3), 291-298.

Potter, P. A., & Perry, A. G. (2001). *Fundamentals of nursing* (5th ed.). St. Louis: Mosby.

Smeltzer, S. C., & Bare, B. G. (Eds.). (2003). *Brunner and Suddarth's textbook of medical-surgical nursing* (10th ed.). Philadelphia: Lippincott Williams & Wilkins.

R

Risk Control—1902

Domain-Health Knowledge & Behavior (IV)

Class-Risk Control & Safety (T)

Scale(s)-Never demonstrated to Consistently demonstrated (m)

Care Recipient:

Data Source:

Definition: Personal actions to prevent, eliminate, or reduce modifiable health threats

OUTCOME TARGET RATING: Maintain at_____   Increase to_____

Risk Control Overall Rating	Never demonstrated 1	Rarely demonstrated 2	Sometimes demonstrated 3	Often demonstrated 4	Consistently demonstrated 5	
INDICATORS:						
190201 Acknowledges risk factors	1	2	3	4	5	NA
190202 Monitors environmental risk factors	1	2	3	4	5	NA
190203 Monitors personal behavior risk factors	1	2	3	4	5	NA
190204 Develops effective risk control strategies	1	2	3	4	5	NA
190205 Adjusts risk control strategies	1	2	3	4	5	NA
190206 Commits to risk control strategies	1	2	3	4	5	NA
190207 Follows selected risk control strategies	1	2	3	4	5	NA
190208 Modifies lifestyle to reduce risk	1	2	3	4	5	NA
190209 Avoids exposure to health threats	1	2	3	4	5	NA
190210 Participates in screening for associated health problems	1	2	3	4	5	NA
190211 Participates in screening for identified risks	1	2	3	4	5	NA
190212 Obtains recommended immunizations	1	2	3	4	5	NA
190213 Uses health care services congruent with needs	1	2	3	4	5	NA
190214 Uses personal support systems to reduce risk	1	2	3	4	5	NA
190215 Uses community resources to reduce risk	1	2	3	4	5	NA

R

		Never demonstrated	Rarely demonstrated	Sometimes demonstrated	Often demonstrated	Consistently demonstrated	
190216	Recognizes changes in health status	1	2	3	4	5	NA
190217	Monitors health status changes	1	2	3	4	5	NA

1st edition 1997; Revised 3rd edition 2004

Outcome Content References:

+Hettler, B. (1982). Wellness promotion and risk reduction on a university campus. In M. Faber & A. Reinhardt (Eds.), *Promoting health through risk reduction*. New York: Macmillan.

Nease, R. (1994). Risk attitudes in gambles involving length of life: Aspirations, variations, and ruminations. *Medical Decision Making, 14*(2), 210-213.

Perez-Stable, E., Marin, G., & Marin, B. (1994). Behavioral risk factors: A comparison of Latinos and non-Latino whites in San Francisco. *American Journal of Public Health, 84*(6), 971-976.

Rost, K., Burnam, M., & Smith, G. (1993). Development of screeners for depressive disorders and substance abuse history. *Medical Care, 31*(3), 189-200.

Ryan, P. (1983). Altered health maintenance. In J. M. Thompston, et al. (Eds.), *Mosby's clinical nursing* (3rd ed., pp. 1425-1427). St. Louis: Mosby.

Simons-Morton, D. G., Mullen, P. D., Mains, D. A., Tabak, E. R., & Green, L. W. (1992). Characteristics of controlled studies of patient education and counseling for preventive health behaviors. *Patient Education and Counseling, 19*(2), 174-204.

Tandy, L., & Malan, S. (2001). Impaired swallowing. In M. Maas, K. Buckwalter, M. Hardy, T. Tripp-Reimer, M. Titler, & J. Specht (Eds.), *Nursing care of older adults: Diagnoses, outcomes & interventions* (pp. 158-171). St. Louis: Mosby.

U.S. Department of Health and Human Services. (1998). *Clinician's handbook of preventive services: Put prevention into practice* (2nd ed.). Washington, DC: Government Printing Office.

R

Risk Control: Alcohol Use—1903

Domain-Health Knowledge & Behavior (IV)

Class-Risk Control & Safety (T)

Scale(s)-Never demonstrated to Consistently demonstrated (m)

Care Recipient:

Data Source:

Definition: Personal actions to prevent, eliminate, or reduce alcohol use that poses a threat to health

OUTCOME TARGET RATING: Maintain at_____   Increase to_____

Risk Control: Alcohol Use Overall Rating	Never demonstrated 1	Rarely demonstrated 2	Sometimes demonstrated 3	Often demonstrated 4	Consistently demonstrated 5	
INDICATORS:						
190301 Acknowledges risk for alcohol misuse	1	2	3	4	5	NA
190302 Acknowledges personal consequences associated with alcohol misuse	1	2	3	4	5	NA
190303 Monitors environment for factors encouraging alcohol misuse	1	2	3	4	5	NA
190304 Monitors personal alcohol use patterns	1	2	3	4	5	NA
190305 Develops effective alcohol control strategies	1	2	3	4	5	NA
190306 Adjusts alcohol use control strategies	1	2	3	4	5	NA
190307 Commits to alcohol use control strategies	1	2	3	4	5	NA
190308 Follows selected alcohol use control strategies	1	2	3	4	5	NA
190309 Participates in screening for associated health problems	1	2	3	4	5	NA
190310 Uses health care services congruent with needs	1	2	3	4	5	NA
190311 Uses personal support systems to control alcohol misuse	1	2	3	4	5	NA
190312 Uses support group to control alcohol misuse	1	2	3	4	5	NA

R

	Never demonstrated	Rarely demonstrated	Sometimes demonstrated	Often demonstrated	Consistently demonstrated	
190313 Uses community resources to control alcohol misuse	1	2	3	4	5	NA
190314 Recognizes changes in general health status	1	2	3	4	5	NA
190315 Monitors health status changes	1	2	3	4	5	NA
190316 Controls alcohol intake	1	2	3	4	5	NA

1st edition 1997; Revised 3rd edition 2004

Outcome Content References:

+MacNeil, G. (1991). A short-form scale to measure alcohol abuse. *Research on Social Work Practice, 1*(1), 68-75.

McCuster, J., Stoddard, A. M., Zapka, J. G., & Lewis, B. F. (1993). Behavioral outcomes of AIDS educational interventions for drug users in short term treatment, *American Journal of Public Health, 83*(10), 1463-1466.

Simons-Morton, D. G., Mullen, P. D., Mains, D. A., Tabek, E. R., & Green, L. W. (1992). Characteristics of controlled studies of patient education and counseling for preventive health behaviors. *Patient Education and Counseling, 19*(2), 174-204.

Talashek, M. L., Gerace, L. M., & Starr, K. L. (1994). The substance abuse pandemic: Determinants to guide interventions. *Public Health Nursing, 11*(2), 131-139.

U.S. Department of Health and Human Services. (1998). *Clinician's handbook of preventive services: Put prevention into practice* (2nd ed.). Washington, DC: Government Printing Office.

R

Risk Control: Cancer—1917

Domain-Health Knowledge & Behavior (IV)

Class-Risk Control & Safety (T)

Scale(s)-Never demonstrated to Consistently demonstrated (m)

Care Recipient:

Data Source:

Definition: Personal actions to detect or reduce the threat of cancer

OUTCOME TARGET RATING: Maintain at_____   Increase to_____

Risk Control: Cancer Overall Rating	Never demonstrated 1	Rarely demonstrated 2	Sometimes demonstrated 3	Often demonstrated 4	Consistently demonstrated 5	
INDICATORS:						
191701 Seeks current information about cancer prevention	1	2	3	4	5	NA
191702 Avoids exposure to carcinogens	1	2	3	4	5	NA
191703 Protects self from carcinogens	1	2	3	4	5	NA
191710 Eliminates tobacco use	1	2	3	4	5	NA
191704 Modifies environment to eliminate exposure to carcinogens	1	2	3	4	5	NA
191705 Follows dietary recommendations for reducing risk	1	2	3	4	5	NA
191706 Performs recommended self-assessments for cancer detection	1	2	3	4	5	NA
191707 Participates in recommended cancer screening	1	2	3	4	5	NA
191711 Obtains recommended vaccinations	1	2	3	4	5	NA
191712 Obtains health care services following abnormal screening results	1	2	3	4	5	NA

2nd edition 2000; Revised 3rd edition 2004; Revised 4th edition

Outcome Content References:

American Nurses Association. (1994). *Clinicians handbook of preventive services*. Waldorf, MD: American Nurses Publishing.

Machia, J. (2001). Breast cancer: Risk, prevention, & tamoxifen. *American Journal of Nursing, 101*(4), 26-36.

U.S. Department of Health and Human Services. (1998). *Clinician's handbook of preventive services: Put prevention into practice* (2nd ed.). Washington, DC: Government Printing Office.

U.S. Preventive Services Task Force. (1996). *Guide to clinical preventive services* (2nd ed.). Baltimore: Williams & Wilkins.

R

Risk Control: Cardiovascular Health—1914

Domain-Health Knowledge & Behavior (IV)   *Care Recipient:*

Class-Risk Control & Safety (T)   *Data Source:*

Scale(s)-Never demonstrated to Consistently demonstrated (m)

Definition: Personal actions to eliminate or reduce threats to cardiovascular health

OUTCOME TARGET RATING: Maintain at_____   Increase to_____

Risk Control: Cardiovascular Health Overall Rating	Never demonstrated 1	Rarely demonstrated 2	Sometimes demonstrated 3	Often demonstrated 4	Consistently demonstrated 5	

INDICATORS:

191401	Acknowledges risk for cardiovascular disease	1	2	3	4	5	NA
191402	Acknowledges ability to change behavior	1	2	3	4	5	NA
191403	Avoids tobacco use	1	2	3	4	5	NA
191404	Monitors blood pressure	1	2	3	4	5	NA
191405	Monitors radial pulse rate	1	2	3	4	5	NA
191406	Uses stress management techniques	1	2	3	4	5	NA
191407	Uses effective weight control strategies	1	2	3	4	5	NA
191408	Follows recommended diet	1	2	3	4	5	NA
191409	Uses health care services congruent with need	1	2	3	4	5	NA
191410	Follows non-prescription medication precautions	1	2	3	4	5	NA
191411	Seeks information about methods to maintain cardiovascular health	1	2	3	4	5	NA
191412	Monitors effects of stimulants	1	2	3	4	5	NA
191413	Participates in screening for cholesterol	1	2	3	4	5	NA
191414	Uses medication as prescribed	1	2	3	4	5	NA
191415	Participates in regular exercise	1	2	3	4	5	NA

R

Continued

		Never demonstrated	Rarely demonstrated	Sometimes demonstrated	Often demonstrated	Consistently demonstrated	
191416	Participates in aerobic exercise	1	2	3	4	5	NA

2nd edition 2000; Revised 3rd edition 2004

Outcome Content References:

Gomel, M., Oldenburg, B., Simpson, J. M., & Owen, N. (1993). Work-site cardiovascular risk reduction: A randomized trial of health risk assessment, education, counseling, and incentives. *American Journal of Public Health, 83*(9), 1231-1238.

Wenger, N. K., Froelicher, E. S., Smith, L. K., et al. (1995). *Cardiac rehabilitation,* Clinical practice guideline No. 17 (AHCPR Publication No. 96-0672). Rockville, MD: U.S. Department of Health and Human Services. Public Health Services, Agency for Health Care Policy and Research and the National Heart, Lung, and Blood Institute.

Winkleby, M. A., Flora, J. A., & Kraemer, H. C. (1994). A community-based heart disease intervention: Predictors of change. *American Journal of Public Health, 84*(5), 767-771.

R

Risk Control: Drug Use—1904

Domain-Health Knowledge & Behavior (IV)

Class-Risk Control & Safety (T)

Scale(s)-Never demonstrated to Consistently demonstrated (m)

Care Recipient:

Data Source:

Definition: Personal actions to prevent, eliminate, or reduce drug use that poses a threat to health

OUTCOME TARGET RATING: Maintain at_____   Increase to_____

Risk Control: Drug Use Overall Rating	Never demonstrated 1	Rarely demonstrated 2	Sometimes demonstrated 3	Often demonstrated 4	Consistently demonstrated 5	

INDICATORS:

190401	Acknowledges risk for drug misuse	1	2	3	4	5	NA
190402	Acknowledges consequences of drug misuse	1	2	3	4	5	NA
190403	Monitors environment for factors encouraging drug misuse	1	2	3	4	5	NA
190404	Monitors personal drug use pattern	1	2	3	4	5	NA
190405	Develops effective drug use control strategies	1	2	3	4	5	NA
190406	Adjusts drug use control strategies	1	2	3	4	5	NA
190407	Commits to drug use control strategies	1	2	3	4	5	NA
190408	Follows selected drug use control strategies	1	2	3	4	5	NA
190409	Participates in screening for associated health problems	1	2	3	4	5	NA
190410	Uses health care services congruent with need	1	2	3	4	5	NA
190411	Uses personal support systems to control drug misuse	1	2	3	4	5	NA
190412	Uses support group to control drug misuse	1	2	3	4	5	NA
190413	Uses community resources to control drug misuse	1	2	3	4	5	NA
190414	Recognizes changes in general health status	1	2	3	4	5	NA

R

Continued

	Never demonstrated	Rarely demonstrated	Sometimes demonstrated	Often demonstrated	Consistently demonstrated	
190415 Monitors health status changes	1	2	3	4	5	NA
190416 Eliminates adverse drug use	1	2	3	4	5	NA

1st edition 1997; Revised 3rd edition 2004

Outcome Content References:

Brown, N. K. (2000). Clinical judgments of high-risk behavior during recovery. *Journal of Psychoactive Drugs, 32*(3), 299-304.

McCuster, J., Stoddard, A. M., Zapka, J. G., & Lewis, B. F. (1993). Behavioral outcomes of AIDS educational interventions for drug users in short term treatment. *American Journal of Public Health, 83*(10), 1463-1466.

Simons-Morton, D. G., Mullen, P. D., Mains, D. A., Tabek, E. R., & Green, L. W. (1992). Characteristics of controlled studies of patient education and counseling for preventive health behaviors. *Patient Education and Counseling, 19*(2), 174-204.

+Skinner, H. A. (1982). The drug abuse screening test. *Addictive Behaviors, 7*(4), 363-371.

Talashek, M. L., Gerace, L. M., & Starr, K. L. (1994). The substance abuse pandemic: Determinants to guide interventions. *Public Health Nursing, 11*(2), 131-139.

U.S. Department of Health and Human Services. (1998). *Clinician's handbook of preventive services: Put prevention into practice* (2nd ed.). Washington, DC: Government Printing Office.

Weitzel, E. A. (2001). Risk for poisoning: Drug toxicity. In M. Maas, K. Buckwalter, M. Hardy, T. Tripp-Reimer, M. Titler, & J. Specht (Eds.), *Nursing care of older adults: Diagnoses, outcomes & interventions* (pp. 34-46). St. Louis: Mosby.

R

Risk Control: Hearing Impairment—1915

Domain-Health Knowledge & Behavior (IV)   *Care Recipient:*

Class-Risk Control & Safety (T)   *Data Source:*

Scale(s)-Never demonstrated to Consistently demonstrated (m)

Definition: Personal actions to prevent, eliminate, or reduce threats to hearing function

OUTCOME TARGET RATING: Maintain at_____   Increase to_____

Risk Control: Hearing Impairment Overall Rating	Never demonstrated 1	Rarely demonstrated 2	Sometimes demonstrated 3	Often demonstrated 4	Consistently demonstrated 5	
INDICATORS:						
191501 Monitors symptoms of hearing deterioration	1	2	3	4	5	NA
191502 Protects eardrum integrity	1	2	3	4	5	NA
191503 Avoids trauma to the ear	1	2	3	4	5	NA
191504 Reduces noise exposure	1	2	3	4	5	NA
191505 Maintains normal amount of cerumen	1	2	3	4	5	NA
191506 Manages ear infections	1	2	3	4	5	NA
191507 Uses hearing protective devices	1	2	3	4	5	NA
191508 Obtains periodic ear examinations	1	2	3	4	5	NA
191509 Obtains periodic hearing tests	1	2	3	4	5	NA
191510 Uses ear medication as prescribed	1	2	3	4	5	NA
191511 Avoids placing objects in ear	1	2	3	4	5	NA

2nd edition 2000; Revised 3rd edition 2004

Outcome Content References:

Burrell, L. O. (Ed.). (1992). *Adult nursing in hospital and community settings*. Norwalk, CT: Appleton & Lange.

Phipps, W. J., Monahan, F. D., Sands J. K., Marek, J., & Neighbors, M. (Eds.). (2003). *Medical-surgical nursing: Concepts and clinical practice* (7th ed). St. Louis: Mosby.

Smeltzer, S. C., & Bare, B. G. (Eds.). (2003). *Brunner and Suddarth's textbook of medical-surgical nursing* (10th ed.). Philadelphia: Lippincott Williams & Wilkins.

U.S. Department of Health and Human Services. (1998). *Clinician's handbook of preventive services: Put prevention into practice* (2nd ed.). Washington, DC: Government Printing Office.

R

Risk Control: Hyperthermia—1922

Domain-Health Knowledge & Behavior (IV)

Class-Risk Control & Safety (T)

Scale(s)-Never demonstrated to Consistently demonstrated (m)

Care Recipient:

Data Source:

Definition: Personal actions to prevent, detect, or reduce the threat of high body temperature

OUTCOME TARGET RATING:　　Maintain at＿＿＿＿＿　　　　Increase to＿＿＿＿＿

Risk Control: Hyperthermia Overall Rating	Never demonstrated 1	Rarely demonstrated 2	Sometimes demonstrated 3	Often demonstrated 4	Consistently demonstrated 5	
INDICATORS:						
192201 Acknowledges personal risk	1	2	3	4	5	NA
192202 Identifies signs and symptoms of hyperthermia	1	2	3	4	5	NA
192203 Acknowledges health conditions that accelerate heat production	1	2	3	4	5	NA
192204 Acknowledges environmental factors that increase body temperature	1	2	3	4	5	NA
192205 Acknowledges risk of being in a car during warm weather	1	2	3	4	5	NA
192206 Acknowledges relationship of age to body temperature	1	2	3	4	5	NA
192207 Modifies living environment to control body temperature	1	2	3	4	5	NA
192208 Modifies fluid intake as appropriate	1	2	3	4	5	NA
192209 Modifies physical activity to control body temperature	1	2	3	4	5	NA
192210 Wears appropriate clothing	1	2	3	4	5	NA
192211 Maintains intact skin integument	1	2	3	4	5	NA
192212 Participates in screening for health problems that increase risk	1	2	3	4	5	NA
192213 Performs self-protective actions to control body temperature	1	2	3	4	5	NA

R

		Never demonstrated	Rarely demonstrated	Sometimes demonstrated	Often demonstrated	Consistently demonstrated	
192214	Identifies prescribed medication effects on body temperature	1	2	3	4	5	NA
192215	Avoids strenuous activities to reduce risk	1	2	3	4	5	NA
192216	Avoids alcohol consumption	1	2	3	4	5	NA
192217	Uses community shelters to reduce risk	1	2	3	4	5	NA
192218	Performs outdoor activities at coolest part of day	1	2	3	4	5	NA
192219	Allows for acclimatization to warmer temperature when traveling	1	2	3	4	5	NA

4th edition

Outcome Content References:

Ballester, J. M., & Harchelroad, F. P. (1999). Hyperthermia: How to recognize and prevent heat-related illnesses. *Geriatrics, 54*(7), 20-24.

DeVaul, R. (2003). Heat stress precautions. *Occupational Health & Safety, 72*(5), 86-88.

Elliott, F. (2006). Take stock to stop heat stress. *Occupational Health & Safety, 75*(5), 98-99.

McLaren, C., Null, J., & Quinn, J. (2005). Heat stress from enclosed vehicles: Moderate ambient temperatures cause significant temperature rise in enclosed vehicles. *Pediatrics, 116*, 109-112.

Nixdorf-Miller, A., & Hunsaker, D. M. Hunsaker, J. C. III, (2006). Hypothermia and hyperthermia medicolegal investigation of morbidity and mortality from exposure to environmental temperature extremes. *Archives of Pathologic Laboratory Medicine, 130*(9), 1297-1304.

Potter, P. A., & Perry, A. G. (2002). Vital signs. In *Basic nursing* (5th ed.). St. Louis: Mosby.

Wood, L. (2004). Heat resistant: How to identify the rationale with which to support the frequency and type of health monitoring of employees, in relation to heat exposure in their working roles. *Occupational Health, 56*(7), 25-30.

R

Risk Control: Hypothermia—1923

Domain-Health Knowledge & Behavior (IV)

Class-Risk Control & Safety (T)

Scale(s)-Never demonstrated to Consistently demonstrated (m)

Care Recipient:

Data Source:

Definition: Personal actions to prevent, detect, or reduce the threat of low body temperature

OUTCOME TARGET RATING: Maintain at_____   Increase to_____

Risk Control: Hypothermia Overall Rating	Never demonstrated 1	Rarely demonstrated 2	Sometimes demonstrated 3	Often demonstrated 4	Consistently demonstrated 5	
INDICATORS:						
192301 Acknowledges personal risk of hypothermia	1	2	3	4	5	NA
192302 Identifies signs and symptoms of hypothermia	1	2	3	4	5	NA
192303 Acknowledges health conditions that decrease heat production	1	2	3	4	5	NA
192304 Acknowledges conditions that jeopardize ability to conserve heat	1	2	3	4	5	NA
192305 Acknowledges health conditions that promote heat loss	1	2	3	4	5	NA
192306 Acknowledges environmental factors that decrease body temperature	1	2	3	4	5	NA
192307 Acknowledges relationship of age to body temperature	1	2	3	4	5	NA
192308 Modifies living environment to promote heat conservation	1	2	3	4	5	NA
192309 Modifies physical activity to control body temperature	1	2	3	4	5	NA
192310 Maintains emergency cold weather supplies in vehicle	1	2	3	4	5	NA
192311 Maintains intact skin integument	1	2	3	4	5	NA

R

		Never demonstrated	Rarely demonstrated	Sometimes demonstrated	Often demonstrated	Consistently demonstrated	
192312	Participates in screening for health problems that increase risk	1	2	3	4	5	NA
192313	Performs self-protective actions to control body temperature	1	2	3	4	5	NA
192314	Modifies fluid intake as appropriate	1	2	3	4	5	NA
192315	Wears appropriate clothing	1	2	3	4	5	NA
192316	Performs outdoor activities at warmest part of day	1	2	3	4	5	NA
192317	Identifies prescribed medication effects on temperature	1	2	3	4	5	NA
192318	Allows for acclimatization to colder temperature when traveling	1	2	3	4	5	NA

4th edition

Outcome Content References:

Cuddy, M. (2004). The effects of drugs on thermoregulation. *Advanced Practice in Acute Clinical Care, 15*(2), 238-253.

Elliott, F. (2005). Do the prep work. *Occupational Health & Safety, 74*(11), 68, 70.

Keresztes, P. A., & Brick, K. (2006). Therapeutic hypothermia after cardiac arrest. *Dimensions of Critical Care Nursing, 25*(2), 71-76.

Neno, R. (2005). Hypothermia: Assessment, treatment and prevention. *Nursing Standard, 19*(20), 47-52.

Nixdorf-Miller, A., & Hunsaker, D. M. Hunsaker, J. C. III, (2006). Hypothermia and hyperthermia medicolegal investigation of morbidity and mortality from exposure to environmental temperature extremes. *Archives of Pathologic Laboratory Medicine, 130*(9), 1297-1304.

Potter, P. A., & Perry, A. G. (2002). Vital signs. In *Basic nursing* (5th ed.). St. Louis: Mosby.

R

Risk Control: Infectious Process—1924

Domain-Health Knowledge & Behavior (IV)

Class-Risk Control & Safety (T)

Scale(s)-Never demonstrated to Consistently demonstrated (m)

Care Recipient:

Data Source:

Definition: Personal actions to prevent, eliminate, or reduce the threat of infection

OUTCOME TARGET RATING: Maintain at_____ Increase to_____

Risk Control: Infectious Process Overall Rating	Never demonstrated 1	Rarely demonstrated 2	Sometimes demonstrated 3	Often demonstrated 4	Consistently demonstrated 5	
INDICATORS:						
192401 Acknowledges personal risk for infection	1	2	3	4	5	NA
192402 Acknowledges personal consequences associated with infection	1	2	3	4	5	NA
192403 Acknowledges behaviors associated with risk for infection	1	2	3	4	5	NA
192404 Identifies infection risk in everyday situations	1	2	3	4	5	NA
192405 Identifies personal signs and symptoms that indicate potential risk	1	2	3	4	5	NA
192406 Seeks validation of perceived infection risk	1	2	3	4	5	NA
192407 Identifies strategies to protect self from others with infection	1	2	3	4	5	NA
192408 Monitors personal behaviors for factors associated with infection risk	1	2	3	4	5	NA
192409 Monitors environment for factors associated with infection risk	1	2	3	4	5	NA
192410 Monitors time of infectious disease incubation period	1	2	3	4	5	NA
192411 Maintains a clean environment	1	2	3	4	5	NA

R

		Never demonstrated	Rarely demonstrated	Sometimes demonstrated	Often demonstrated	Consistently demonstrated	
192412	Uses strategies to disinfect supplies	1	2	3	4	5	NA
192413	Develops effective infection control strategies	1	2	3	4	5	NA
192414	Uses universal precautions	1	2	3	4	5	NA
192415	Practices hand sanitization	1	2	3	4	5	NA
192416	Practices infection control strategies	1	2	3	4	5	NA
192417	Adjusts infection control strategies as needed	1	2	3	4	5	NA
192418	Practices actions to promote rest	1	2	3	4	5	NA
192419	Practices actions to promote fluid intake	1	2	3	4	5	NA
192420	Monitors changes in general health status	1	2	3	4	5	NA
192421	Takes immediate actions to reduce risk	1	2	3	4	5	NA
192422	Obtains recommended immunizations	1	2	3	4	5	NA
192423	Uses reputable sources of information	1	2	3	4	5	NA
192424	Uses health care services congruent with need	1	2	3	4	5	NA

4th edition

Outcome Content References:

Carruthers, S. (2003). The ins and outs of injection in Western Australia. *Journal of Substance Use, 8,* 11-18.

Grundmann, H., Aires-de-Sousa, M., Boyce, J., & Tiemersma, E. (2006). Emergence and resurgence of methicillin-resistant *Staphylococcus aureus* as a public-health threat. *Lancet, 368,* 874-885.

Krein, S. L., Olmsted, R. N., Hofer, T. P., Kowalski, C., Forman, J., Banaszak, J., & Saint, S. (2006). Translating infection prevention evidence into practice using quantitative and qualitative research. *American Journal of Infection Control, 34,* 507-512.

Nichol, K. L., & Treanor, J. J. (2006). Vaccines for seasonal and pandemic influenza. *Journal of Infectious Diseases, 194*(Suppl. 2), S111-S118.

Veenema, T. G., & Toke, J. (2006). Early detection and surveillance for biopreparedness and emerging infectious diseases. *Online Journal of Issues in Nursing, 11*(1), Manuscript 2.

R

Risk Control: Sexually Transmitted Diseases (STD)—1905

Domain-Health Knowledge & Behavior (IV)

Class-Risk Control & Safety (T)

Scale(s)-Never demonstrated to Consistently demonstrated (m)

Care Recipient:

Data Source:

Definition: Personal actions to prevent, eliminate, or reduce behaviors associated with sexually transmitted disease

OUTCOME TARGET RATING: Maintain at_____   Increase to_____

Risk Control: Sexually Transmitted Diseases (STD) Overall Rating	Never demonstrated 1	Rarely demonstrated 2	Sometimes demonstrated 3	Often demonstrated 4	Consistently demonstrated 5	

INDICATORS:

190501	Acknowledges individual risk for sexually transmitted disease	1	2	3	4	5	NA
190502	Acknowledges personal consequences associated with sexually transmitted disease	1	2	3	4	5	NA
190503	Monitors contacts for sexually transmitted disease exposure risks	1	2	3	4	5	NA
190504	Monitors personal behaviors for sexually transmitted disease exposure risk	1	2	3	4	5	NA
190505	Develops effective strategies to reduce sexually transmitted disease exposure	1	2	3	4	5	NA
190506	Adjusts exposure control strategies	1	2	3	4	5	NA
190507	Commits to exposure control strategies	1	2	3	4	5	NA
190508	Follows selected exposure control strategies	1	2	3	4	5	NA
190509	Inquires of partner's sexually transmitted disease status before sexual activity	1	2	3	4	5	NA
190510	Uses methods to control sexually transmitted disease transmission	1	2	3	4	5	NA

R

		Never demonstrated	Rarely demonstrated	Sometimes demonstrated	Often demonstrated	Consistently demonstrated	
190511	Recognizes sexually transmitted disease signs and symptoms	1	2	3	4	5	NA
190512	Participates in screening for sexually transmitted disease	1	2	3	4	5	NA
190513	Participates in screening for associated health problems	1	2	3	4	5	NA
190514	Uses community health care services for sexually transmitted disease treatment	1	2	3	4	5	NA
190515	Complies with treatment for sexually transmitted disease	1	2	3	4	5	NA
190516	Notifies sexual partner(s) in event of sexually transmitted disease infection	1	2	3	4	5	NA
190517	Maintains absence of sexually transmitted disease	1	2	3	4	5	NA

1st edition 1997; Revised 3rd edition 2004

R

Outcome Content References:

+Card, J. J. (Ed.). (1993). *Handbook of adolescent sexuality and pregnancy: Research and evaluation instruments.* Thousand Oaks, CA: Sage.

Marston, C., & King, E. (2006). Factors that shape young people's sexual behaviour: A systematic review. *Lancet, 386,* 1581-1586.

Miller, K. E., & Graves, J. C. (2000). Update on the prevention and treatment of sexually transmitted diseases. *American Family Physician, 61*(2), 379-386.

Panel on Clinical Practices for Treatment of HIV Infection. (2002). Guidelines for the use of antiretroviral agents in HIV-infected adults and adolescents. Washington, D.C.: U,S: Department of Health and Human Services.

Rotheram-Borus, M. J., Reid, M. A., & Rosario, M. (1994). Factors mediating changes in sexual HIV risk behaviors among gay and bisexual male adolescents. *American Journal of Public Health, 84*(12), 1938-1946.

Simons-Morton, D. G., Mullen, P. D., Mains, D. A., Tabak, E. R., & Green, L. W. (1992). Characteristics of controlled studies of patient education and counseling for preventive health behaviors. *Patient Education and Counseling, 19*(2), 174-204.

U.S. Department of Health and Human Services. (1998). *Clinician's handbook of preventive services: Put prevention into practice* (2nd ed.). Washington, DC: Government Printing Office.

Risk Control: Sun Exposure—1925

Domain-Health Knowledge & Behavior (IV)

Class-Risk Control & Safety (T)

Scale(s)-Never demonstrated to Consistently demonstrated (m)

Care Recipient:

Data Source:

Definition: Personal actions to prevent or reduce threats to the skin and eyes from sun exposure

OUTCOME TARGET RATING: Maintain at_____   Increase to_____

Risk Control: Sun Exposure Overall Rating	Never demonstrated 1	Rarely demonstrated 2	Sometimes demonstrated 3	Often demonstrated 4	Consistently demonstrated 5	
INDICATORS:						
192501 Acknowledges personal risk of sun exposure	1	2	3	4	5	NA
192502 Selects sunscreen with recommended sun protection factor (SPF) or greater	1	2	3	4	5	NA
192503 Applies appropriate amount of sunscreen	1	2	3	4	5	NA
192504 Reapplies sunscreen as needed	1	2	3	4	5	NA
192505 Avoids sun exposure between 10 a.m. and 3 p.m.	1	2	3	4	5	NA
192506 Monitors length of sun exposure	1	2	3	4	5	NA
192507 Seeks outdoor activities in the shade	1	2	3	4	5	NA
192508 Wears appropriate clothing to protect skin	1	2	3	4	5	NA
192509 Wears hat with 4-inch brim to protect head and face	1	2	3	4	5	NA
192510 Uses ointment to protect lips	1	2	3	4	5	NA
192511 Wears ultraviolet (UV) protection glasses when outdoors	1	2	3	4	5	NA
192512 Avoids use of ultraviolet (UV) devices	1	2	3	4	5	NA
192513 Follows recommendations for regular skin inspection	1	2	3	4	5	NA

R

		Never demonstrated	Rarely demonstrated	Sometimes demonstrated	Often demonstrated	Consistently demonstrated	
192514	Checks medication side effects for photosensitivity	1	2	3	4	5	NA
192515	Uses reliable resources on sun protection	1	2	3	4	5	NA

4th edition

Outcome Content References:

Castanedo-Cazares, J. P., Lepe, V., Torres-Alvarez, B., & Moncada, B. (2003). A simple measure for applying sunscreen while on holidays. *Dermatology Online Journal, 9*(3), 23. Retrieved September 20, 2005, from http://dermatology.cdlib.org/93/letters/sunscreen/castanedo.html

Centers for Disease Control and Prevention. (April 26, 2002). Guidelines for school programs to prevent skin cancer. *MMWR Morbidity and Mortality Reports: Recommendations and Reports, 51*(RR04), 1-15. Retrieved September 20, 2005, from http://www.cdc.gov/mmwr/preview/mmwrhtml/rr5104a1.htm

Geller, A., Rutsch, L., Kenausis, K., & Zhang, Z. (2003). Evaluation of the SunWise school program. *Journal of School Nursing, 19*(2), 93-99.

Hatmaker, G. (2003). Development of a skin cancer prevention program. *Journal of School Nursing, 19*(2), 89-92.

Livingston, P. M., White, V., Hayman, J., & Dobbinson, S. (2003). Sun exposure and sun protection behaviours among Australian adolescents: Trends over time. *Preventive Medicine, 37*, 577-584.

Scarlett, W. L. (2003). Ultraviolet radiation: Sun exposure, tanning beds, and vitamin D levels. *Journal of the American Osteopathic Association, 103*(8), 371-375.

R

Risk Control: Tobacco Use—1906

Domain-Health Knowledge & Behavior (IV)

Class-Risk Control & Safety (T)

Scale(s)-Never demonstrated to Consistently demonstrated (m)

Care Recipient:

Data Source:

Definition: Personal actions to prevent tobacco use

OUTCOME TARGET RATING: Maintain at_____   Increase to_____

Risk Control: Tobacco Use Overall Rating	Never demonstrated 1	Rarely demonstrated 2	Sometimes demonstrated 3	Often demonstrated 4	Consistently demonstrated 5	
INDICATORS:						
190601 Acknowledges risk for tobacco use	1	2	3	4	5	NA
190619 Acknowledges personal benefits associated with tobacco use	1	2	3	4	5	NA
190602 Acknowledges personal consequences associated with tobacco use	1	2	3	4	5	NA
190603 Monitors environment for factors encouraging tobacco use	1	2	3	4	5	NA
190620 Acknowledges consequences of peer pressure	1	2	3	4	5	NA
190610 Uses health care services congruent with needs	1	2	3	4	5	NA
190612 Uses personal support systems to prevent tobacco use	1	2	3	4	5	NA
190613 Uses support group to prevent tobacco use	1	2	3	4	5	NA
190615 Monitors health status changes	1	2	3	4	5	NA
190618 Recognizes changes in general health status	1	2	3	4	5	NA
190621 Uses strategies to prevent tobacco use around peers	1	2	3	4	5	NA
190622 Recognizes social influences to engage in tobacco use	1	2	3	4	5	NA

R

		Never demonstrated	Rarely demonstrated	Sometimes demonstrated	Often demonstrated	Consistently demonstrated	
190623	Recognizes cultural influences to engage in tobacco use	1	2	3	4	5	NA
190624	Participates in physical activity	1	2	3	4	5	NA
190625	Avoids social situations that encourage tobacco use	1	2	3	4	5	NA
190626	Uses reputable sources of information	1	2	3	4	5	NA
190614	Uses community resources to prevent tobacco use	1	2	3	4	5	NA

1st edition 1997; Revised 3rd edition 2004; Revised 4th edition

Outcome Content References:

+Fagerstrom, K. O. (1978). Measuring degree of physical dependence in tobacco smoking with reference to individualization of treatment. *Addiction Behavior, 3*, 235-241.

Hirdes, J. P., & Maxwell, M. A. (1994). Smoking cessation and quality of life outcomes among older adults in the Campbell's survey on well-being. *Canadian Journal of Public Health, 85*(2), 99-102.

Simons-Morton, D. G., Mullen, P. D., Mains, D. A., Tabak, E. R., & Green, L. W. (1992). Characteristics of controlled studies of patient education and counseling for preventive health behaviors. *Patient Education and Counseling, 19*(2), 174-204.

Sussman, S., Dent, C. W., Stacy, A. W., Sun, P., Craig, S., Simon, T. R., Burton, D., & Flay, B. R. (1993). Project towards no tobacco use: 1-year behavioral outcomes, *American Journal of Public Health, 83*(9), 1245-1250.

Talashek, M. L., Gerace, L. M., & Starr, K. L. (1994). The substance abuse pandemic: Determinants to guide interventions. *Public Health Nursing, 11*(2), 131-139.

U.S. Department of Health and Human Services. (1998). *Clinician's handbook of preventive services: Put prevention into practice* (2nd ed.). Washington: DC: Government Printing Office.

U.S. Department of Health and Human Services. (1996). *Smoking cessation* (AHCPR Publication No. 96-0692). Rockville, MD: Public Health Service Agency for Health Care Policy and Research.

Winsor, R. A., Lowe, J. B., Perkins, L. L., Smith-Yoder, D., Artz, L., Crawford, M., Amburgy, K., & Boyd, N. R. (1993). Health education for pregnant smokers: Its behavioral impact and cost benefit. *American Journal of Public Health, 83*(2), 201-206.

R

Risk Control: Unintended Pregnancy—1907

Domain-Health Knowledge & Behavior (IV)

Class-Risk Control & Safety (T)

Scale(s)-Never demonstrated to Consistently demonstrated (m)

Care Recipient:

Data Source:

Definition: Personal actions to prevent or reduce the possibility of unintended pregnancy

OUTCOME TARGET RATING: Maintain at_____   Increase to_____

Risk Control: Unintended Pregnancy Overall Rating	Never demonstrated 1	Rarely demonstrated 2	Sometimes demonstrated 3	Often demonstrated 4	Consistently demonstrated 5	
INDICATORS:						
190701 Acknowledges risk for unintended pregnancy	1	2	3	4	5	NA
190703 Describes personal consequences associated with unintended pregnancy	1	2	3	4	5	NA
190705 Understands physiological processes of conception	1	2	3	4	5	NA
190706 Develops effective pregnancy prevention strategies	1	2	3	4	5	NA
190707 Adjusts pregnancy prevention strategies	1	2	3	4	5	NA
190708 Commits to pregnancy prevention strategies	1	2	3	4	5	NA
190709 Follows selected pregnancy prevention strategies	1	2	3	4	5	NA
190710 Uses support system to enhance prevention strategies	1	2	3	4	5	NA
190711 Uses available community resources	1	2	3	4	5	NA
190712 Identifies appropriate contraceptive method for self	1	2	3	4	5	NA
190713 Obtains contraceptive supplies and devices	1	2	3	4	5	NA

R

		Never demonstrated	Rarely demonstrated	Sometimes demonstrated	Often demonstrated	Consistently demonstrated	
190714	Uses contraceptive methods correctly	1	2	3	4	5	NA
190715	Uses health care services congruent with need	1	2	3	4	5	NA

1st edition 1997; Revised 3rd edition 2004

Outcome Content References:

+Card, J. J. (Ed.). (1993). *Handbook of adolescent sexuality and pregnancy: Research and evaluation instruments.* Thousand Oaks, CA: Sage.

Simons-Morton, D. G., Mullen, P. D., Mains, D. A., Tabak, E. R., & Green, L. W. (1992). Characteristics of controlled studies of patient education and counseling for preventive health behaviors. *Patient Education and Counseling, 19*(2), 174-204.

U.S. Department of Health and Human Services. (1998). *Clinician's handbook of preventive services: Put prevention into practice* (2nd ed.). Washington, DC: Government Printing Office.

R

Risk Control: Visual Impairment—1916

Domain-Health Knowledge & Behavior (IV)

Class-Risk Control & Safety (T)

Scale(s)-Never demonstrated to Consistently demonstrated (m)

Care Recipient:

Data Source:

Definition: Personal actions to prevent, eliminate, or reduce threats to visual function

OUTCOME TARGET RATING: Maintain at_____   Increase to_____

Risk Control: Visual Impairment Overall Rating	Never demonstrated 1	Rarely demonstrated 2	Sometimes demonstrated 3	Often demonstrated 4	Consistently demonstrated 5	
INDICATORS:						
191601 Monitors symptoms of vision deterioration	1	2	3	4	5	NA
191602 Monitors environment for eye hazards	1	2	3	4	5	NA
191603 Avoids trauma to the eye	1	2	3	4	5	NA
191604 Uses adequate lighting for activity being performed	1	2	3	4	5	NA
191605 Takes breaks from activity causing eye strain	1	2	3	4	5	NA
191606 Monitors symptoms of eye disease	1	2	3	4	5	NA
191607 Uses eye medication as prescribed	1	2	3	4	5	NA
191608 Uses devices to protect eyes	1	2	3	4	5	NA
191609 Obtains eye exams	1	2	3	4	5	NA
191611 Obtains glaucoma screening	1	2	3	4	5	NA
191612 Obtains macular degeneration screening	1	2	3	4	5	NA

2nd edition 2000; Revised 3rd edition 2004

Outcome Content References:

Burrell, L. O. (Ed.). (1992). *Adult nursing in hospital and community settings.* Norwalk, CT: Appleton & Lange.

Cataract Management Guideline Panel. (1993). *Cataracts in adults: Management of functional impairment,* Clinical practice guideline No. 4 (AHCPR Publication No. 93-0542). Rockville, MD: U.S. Department of Health and Human Services. Public Health Services, Agency for Health Care Policy and Research.

Phipps, W. J., Monahan, F. D., Sands J. K., Marek, J., & Neighbors, M. (Eds.). (2003). *Medical-surgical nursing: Concepts and clinical practice* (7th ed.). St. Louis: Mosby.

Smeltzer, S. C., & Bare, B. G. (Eds.). (2003). *Brunner and Suddarth's textbook of medical-surgical nursing* (10th ed.). Philadelphia: Lippincott Williams & Wilkins.

U.S. Department of Health and Human Services. (1998). *Clinician's handbook of preventive services: Put prevention into practice* (2nd ed.). Washington, DC: Government Printing Office.

Risk Detection—1908

Domain-Health Knowledge & Behavior (IV)

Class-Risk Control & Safety (T)

Scale(s)-Never demonstrated to Consistently demonstrated (m)

Care Recipient:

Data Source:

Definition: Personal actions to identify personal health threats					

OUTCOME TARGET RATING: Maintain at_____   Increase to_____

Risk Detection Overall Rating	Never demonstrated 1	Rarely demonstrated 2	Sometimes demonstrated 3	Often demonstrated 4	Consistently demonstrated 5

INDICATORS:

190801	Recognizes signs and symptoms that indicate risks	1	2	3	4	5	NA
190802	Identifies potential health risks	1	2	3	4	5	NA
190803	Seeks validation of perceived risks	1	2	3	4	5	NA
190804	Performs self-examinations at recommended intervals	1	2	3	4	5	NA
190805	Participates in screening at recommended intervals	1	2	3	4	5	NA
190806	Acquires knowledge of family history	1	2	3	4	5	NA
190807	Maintains updated knowledge of family history	1	2	3	4	5	NA
190808	Maintains updated knowledge of personal history	1	2	3	4	5	NA
190809	Uses resources to stay informed about personal risks	1	2	3	4	5	NA
190810	Uses health care services congruent with need	1	2	3	4	5	NA
190812	Obtains information about changes in health recommendations	1	2	3	4	5	NA

1st edition 1997; Revised 3rd edition 2004

R

Outcome Content References:

Bamberg, R., Acton, R. T., Goodson, L., Go, R., Struempler, B., & Roseman, J. M. (1989). The effect of risk assessment in conjunction with health promotion education on compliance with preventive behaviors. *Journal of Allied Health, 18*(1), 271-281.

+Hettler, B. (1982). Wellness promotion and risk reduction on a university campus. In M. Faber & A. Reinhardt (Eds.), *Promoting health through risk reduction* (pp. 207-238). New York: Macmillan.

Sickle Cell Disease Guideline Panel. (1993). *Sickle Cell Disease: Screening, diagnosis, management, and counseling in newborn and infants,* Clinical practice guideline No. 6 (AHCPR Publication No. 93-0562). Rockville, MD: U.S. Department of Health and Human Services. Public Health Services, Agency for Health Care Policy and Research.

Simons-Morton, D. G., Mullen, P. D., Mains, D. A., Tabak, E. R., & Green, L. W. (1992). Characteristics of controlled studies of patient education and counseling for preventive health behaviors. *Patient Education and Counseling, 19*(2), 174-204.

U.S. Department of Health and Human Services. (1998). *Clinician's handbook of preventive services: Put prevention into practice* (2nd ed.). Washington, DC: Government Printing Office.

R

Role Performance—1501

Domain-Psychosocial Health (III)

Class-Social Interaction (P)

Scale(s)-Not adequate to Totally adequate (f)

Care Recipient:

Data Source:

Definition: Congruence of an individual's role behavior with role expectations

OUTCOME TARGET RATING: Maintain at_____   Increase to_____

Role Performance Overall Rating	Not adequate 1	Slightly adequate 2	Moderately adequate 3	Substantially adequate 4	Totally adequate 5	
INDICATORS:						
150107 Description of role changes with illness or disability	1	2	3	4	5	NA
150108 Description of role changes with elderly dependents	1	2	3	4	5	NA
150109 Description of role changes with new family member	1	2	3	4	5	NA
150110 Description of role changes when family member leaves home	1	2	3	4	5	NA
150111 Reported strategies for role change(s)	1	2	3	4	5	NA
150101 Performance of role expectations	1	2	3	4	5	NA
150102 Knowledge of role transition periods	1	2	3	4	5	NA
150103 Performance of family role behaviors	1	2	3	4	5	NA
150115 Performance of parental role behaviors	1	2	3	4	5	NA
150113 Performance of intimate role behaviors	1	2	3	4	5	NA
150104 Performance of community role behaviors	1	2	3	4	5	NA
150105 Performance of work role behaviors	1	2	3	4	5	NA
150106 Performance of friendship role behaviors	1	2	3	4	5	NA
150112 Reported comfort with role expectations	1	2	3	4	5	NA
150116 Reported comfort with role change(s)	1	2	3	4	5	NA

1st edition 1997; Revised 3rd edition 2004

Outcome Content References:

Knutson, A. L. (1965). *The individual, society, and health behavior*. New York: Sage.

Moorhead, S. A. (1985). Role supplementation. In G. M. Bulechek, & J. C. McCloskey (Eds.), *Nursing interventions: Treatments for nursing diagnoses* (pp. 152-159). Philadelphia: W.B. Saunders.

+Weissman, M. M., & Bothwell, S. (1976). Assessment of social adjustment by patient self-report. *Archives of General Psychiatry*, 33(9), 1111-1115.

R

Safe Home Environment—1910

Domain-Health Knowledge & Behavior (IV)

Class-Risk Control & Safety (T)

Scale(s)-Not adequate to Totally adequate (f)

Care Recipient:

Data Source:

Definition: Physical arrangements to minimize environmental factors that might cause physical harm or injury in the home

OUTCOME TARGET RATING: Maintain at_____   Increase to_____

Safe Home Environment Overall Rating	Not adequate 1	Slightly adequate 2	Moderately adequate 3	Substantially adequate 4	Totally adequate 5	

INDICATORS:

191026	Building maintenance	1	2	3	4	5	NA
191027	Provision of exterior lighting	1	2	3	4	5	NA
191028	Provision of interior lighting	1	2	3	4	5	NA
191029	Availability of clean water	1	2	3	4	5	NA
191030	Cleanliness of dwelling	1	2	3	4	5	NA
191031	Elimination of rodents and insects	1	2	3	4	5	NA
191032	Space to move safely in dwelling	1	2	3	4	5	NA
191033	Locks on windows	1	2	3	4	5	NA
191034	Locks on doors	1	2	3	4	5	NA
191002	Placement of handrails	1	2	3	4	5	NA
191023	Carbon monoxide detector maintenance	1	2	3	4	5	NA
191003	Smoke detector maintenance	1	2	3	4	5	NA
191004	Use of personal alarm system	1	2	3	4	5	NA
191005	Provision of accessible telephone	1	2	3	4	5	NA
191006	Placement of appropriate hazard warning labels	1	2	3	4	5	NA
191024	Safe storage of medication	1	2	3	4	5	NA
191007	Proper disposal of medication	1	2	3	4	5	NA
191008	Provision of assistive devices in accessible location	1	2	3	4	5	NA
191009	Provision of equipment that meets safety standards	1	2	3	4	5	NA
191010	Safe storage of firearms	1	2	3	4	5	NA
191011	Safe storage of hazardous materials	1	2	3	4	5	NA
191012	Safe disposal of hazardous materials	1	2	3	4	5	NA

S

	Not adequate	Slightly adequate	Moderately adequate	Substantially adequate	Totally adequate	
191025	Safe storage of matches/lighters	1	2	3	4	5	NA
191034	Elimination of toxic fumes	1	2	3	4	5	NA
191035	Elimination of tobacco smoke	1	2	3	4	5	NA
191013	Arrangement of furniture to reduce risks	1	2	3	4	5	NA
191014	Provision of safe play area	1	2	3	4	5	NA
191015	Removal of doors from unused appliances	1	2	3	4	5	NA
191016	Correction of lead hazard risks	1	2	3	4	5	NA
191017	Provision of safe age-appropriate toys	1	2	3	4	5	NA
191018	Use of electrical outlet covers	1	2	3	4	5	NA
191019	Room temperature regulation	1	2	3	4	5	NA
191020	Elimination of harmful noise levels	1	2	3	4	5	NA
191021	Placement of window guards	1	2	3	4	5	NA

1st edition 1997; Revised 3rd edition 2004; Revised 4th edition

Outcome Content References:

Black, S. (2002). Safe home. *Nursing Standard, 16*(25), 16-17.

Halperin, S. F., Bass, J. L., & Mehta, K. A., (1983). Knowledge of accident prevention among parents of young children in nine Massachusetts towns. *Public Health Reports, 98*(6), 548-552.

Head, B. J. (2001). Impaired home maintenance management. In M. Maas, K. Buckwalter, M. Hardy, T. Tripp-Reimer, M. Titler, & J. Specht (Eds.), *Nursing care of older adults: Diagnoses, outcomes & interventions* (pp. 64-74). St. Louis: Mosby.

Mayhew, M. S. (1991). Strategies for promoting safety and preventing injury. *Nursing Clinics of North America, 26*(1), 885-893.

+Tymchuk, A. J. (1997). Home dangers and precautions: Interview/observation. *The UCLA Parent/Child Health & Wellness Project.*

Wasserman, R. C., Dameron, D. O., Brozicevic, M. M., & Aronson, R. A. (1989). Injury hazards in home day care. *The Journal of Pediatrics, 114*(4), 591-593.

Weitzel, E. (2001). Unilateral neglect. In M. Maas, K. Buckwalter, M. Hardy, T. Tripp-Reimer, M. Titler, & J. Specht (Eds.), *Nursing care of older adults: Diagnoses, outcomes & interventions* (pp. 492-502). St. Louis: Mosby.

S

Safe Wandering—1926

Domain-Health Knowledge & Behavior (IV)   *Care Recipient:*

Class-Risk Control & Safety (T)   *Data Source:*

Scale(s)-Never demonstrated to Consistently demonstrated (m) and Consistently demonstrated to Never demonstrated (t)

Definition: Safe, socially acceptable moving about without apparent purpose in an individual with cognitive impairment

OUTCOME TARGET RATING: Maintain at_____   Increase to_____

Safe Wandering Overall Rating	Never demonstrated 1	Rarely demonstrated 2	Sometimes demonstrated 3	Often demonstrated 4	Consistently demonstrated 5	
INDICATORS:						
192601 Moves about without harming self	1	2	3	4	5	NA
192602 Moves about without harming others	1	2	3	4	5	NA
192603 Sits for more than 5 minutes at a time	1	2	3	4	5	NA
192604 Paces a given route	1	2	3	4	5	NA
192605 Appears content in environment	1	2	3	4	5	NA
192606 Remains in secure area when unaccompanied	1	2	3	4	5	NA
192607 Moves about only in own and public space	1	2	3	4	5	NA
192608 Uses own toileting facilities	1	2	3	4	5	NA
192609 Performs purposeful activities	1	2	3	4	5	NA
192610 Locates landmarks in familiar setting	1	2	3	4	5	NA
192611 Can be redirected from unsafe activities	1	2	3	4	5	NA
192612 Distracts easily	1	2	3	4	5	NA
192613 Dresses appropriately	1	2	3	4	5	NA

	Consistently demonstrated	Often demonstrated	Sometimes demonstrated	Rarely demonstrated	Never demonstrated	
192614 Falls	1	2	3	4	5	NA
192615 Appears agitated	1	2	3	4	5	NA
192616 Bumps into obstacles while moving	1	2	3	4	5	NA

S

		Consistently demonstrated	Often demonstrated	Sometimes demonstrated	Rarely demonstrated	Never demonstrated	
192617	States wants to go home	1	2	3	4	5	NA
192618	Attempts to elope from secure area	1	2	3	4	5	NA
192619	Gets lost in secure area	1	2	3	4	5	NA
192620	Invades others' space	1	2	3	4	5	NA
192621	Upsets others in environment	1	2	3	4	5	NA
192622	Disrupts group activities	1	2	3	4	5	NA

4th edition

Outcome Content References:

Algase, D. L., Beattie, E. R. A., Song, J. A., Milke, D., Duffield, C., & Cowan, B. (2004). Validation of the Algase Wandering Scale (Version 2) in a cross cultural sample. *Aging & Mental Health, 8*(2), 133-142.

Algase, D. L., Son, G., Beattie, E., Song, J., Leitsch, S., & Yao, L. (2004). The interrelatedness of wandering and wayfinding in a community sample of persons with dementia. *Dementia and Geriatric Cognitive Disorders, 17*(3), 231-239.

Aud, M. A. (2004). Dangerous wandering: Elopements of older adults with dementia from long-term care facilities. *American Journal of Alzheimer's Disease and Other Dementias, 19*(6), 361-368.

Kelley, L. S., Buckwalter, K. C., & Maas, M. L. (1999). Access to health care resources for family caregivers of elderly persons with dementia. *Nursing Outlook, 47*(1), 8-14.

Kiely, D. K., Morris, J. N., & Algase, D. L. (2000). Resident characteristics associated with wandering in nursing homes. *International Journal of Geriatric Psychiatry, 15*(11),1013-1020.

Maas, M., Reed, D., Park, M., Specht, J., Schutte, D., Kelley, L., Buckwalter, K., & Tripp-Reimer, T. (2004). Outcomes of family involvement in care intervention for caregivers of individuals with dementia. *Nursing Research, 53*(2), 76-86.

Williams-Burgess, C., Ugeriza, D., & Gabbai, M. (1996). Agitation in older persons with dementia: A research synthesis. *Online Journal of Knowledge Synthesis for Nursing, E3*(1), 97.

S

Seizure Control—1620

Domain-Health Knowledge & Behavior (IV)

Class-Health Behavior (Q)

Scale(s)-Never demonstrated to Consistently demonstrated (m)

Care Recipient:

Data Source:

Definition: Personal actions to reduce or minimize the occurrence of seizure episodes

OUTCOME TARGET RATING: Maintain at_____   Increase to_____

Seizure Control Overall Rating	Never demonstrated 1	Rarely demonstrated 2	Sometimes demonstrated 3	Often demonstrated 4	Consistently demonstrated 5	
INDICATORS:						
162001 Describes precipitating seizure factors	1	2	3	4	5	NA
162002 Uses medication as prescribed	1	2	3	4	5	NA
162016 Obtains needed medication	1	2	3	4	5	NA
162004 Contacts health professional when medication side effects occur	1	2	3	4	5	NA
162006 Avoids seizure triggers/risk factors	1	2	3	4	5	NA
162017 Obtains medical attention immediately if seizure frequency increases	1	2	3	4	5	NA
162008 Uses effective stress reduction techniques to decrease seizure activity	1	2	3	4	5	NA
162109 Maintains positive attitude toward seizure disorder	1	2	3	4	5	NA
162010 Maintains role performance	1	2	3	4	5	NA
162011 Maintains social relationships	1	2	3	4	5	NA
162012 Maintains sleep-wake pattern	1	2	3	4	5	NA
162013 Follows prescribed physical exercise program	1	2	3	4	5	NA
162015 Implements safety practices in environment	1	2	3	4	5	NA

3rd edition 2004; Revised 4th edition

Outcome Content References:

Dilorio, C., Faherty, B., & Manteuffel, B. (1993). Learning needs of persons with epilepsy: A comparison of perceptions of persons with epilepsy, nurses and physicians. *Journal of Neuroscience Nursing, 25*(1), 22-29.

Santilli, N. (Ed.). (1996). *Managing seizure disorders: A handbook for health care professionals.* Philadelphia: J.B. Lippincott.

Self-Care Status—0313

Domain-Functional Health (I)

Class-Self-Care (D)

Scale(s)-Severely compromised to Not compromised (a)

Care Recipient:

Data Source:

Definition: Ability to perform basic personal care activities and instrumental activities of daily living

OUTCOME TARGET RATING: Maintain at_____   Increase to_____

Self-Care Status Overall Rating	Severely compromised 1	Substantially compromised 2	Moderately compromised 3	Mildly compromised 4	Not compromised 5	

INDICATORS:

031301	Bathes self	1	2	3	4	5	NA
031302	Dresses self	1	2	3	4	5	NA
031303	Prepares food and fluid for eating	1	2	3	4	5	NA
031304	Feeds self	1	2	3	4	5	NA
031305	Maintains personal cleanliness	1	2	3	4	5	NA
031306	Maintains oral hygiene	1	2	3	4	5	NA
031307	Toilets self independently	1	2	3	4	5	NA
031315	Manages own non-parenteral medication	1	2	3	4	5	NA
031309	Manages own parenteral medication	1	2	3	4	5	NA
031310	Performs household tasks	1	2	3	4	5	NA
031311	Manages household finances	1	2	3	4	5	NA
031312	Arranges for own transportation	1	2	3	4	5	NA
031313	Obtains required household items	1	2	3	4	5	NA
031314	Recognizes safety needs in the home	1	2	3	4	5	NA

3rd edition 2004; Revised 4th edition

Outcome Content References:

Armer, J. M., Conn, V. S., Decker, S. A., & Tripp-Reimer, T. (2001). Self-care deficit. In M. Maas, K. Buckwalter, M. Hardy, T. Tripp-Reimer, M. Titler, & J. Specht (Eds.), *Nursing care of older adults: Diagnoses, outcomes & interventions* (pp. 366-384). St. Louis: Mosby.

Head, B. J. (2001). Impaired home maintenance management. In M. Maas, K. Buckwalter, M. Hardy, T. Tripp-Reimer, M. Titler, & J. Specht (Eds.), *Nursing care of older adults: Diagnoses, outcomes & interventions* (pp. 64-74). St. Louis: Mosby.

Continued

Hickey, T. (1988). Self-care behavior of older adults. *Family and Community Health, 11*(3), 22-35.

Katz, S., & Akpom, C. A. (1976). A measure of primary sociobiological functions. *International Journal of Health Services, 6*(3), 493-507.

Katz, S., Ford, A. B., Moskowitz, R. W., Jackson, B. A., & Jaffe, M. W. (1963). Studies of illness in the aged. The Index of ADL: A standardized measure of biological and psychosocial function. *Journal of the American Medical Association, 185*(12), 914-919.

Klein, R. M., & Bell, B. (1982). Self-care skills: Behavioral measurement with Klein-Bell ADL Scale. *Archives of Physical Medicine and Rehabilitation, 63*(7), 335-338.

Leenerts, M. H., Teel, C. S., & Pendleton, M. K. (2002). Building a model of self-care for health promotion in aging. *Journal of Nursing Scholarship, 34*(4), 355-361.

Resnick, B. (2001). Motivating older adults to engage in self-care. *Patient Care for the Nurse Practitioner, 4*(9), 13-14, 16, 19.

S

Self-Care: Activities of Daily Living (ADL)—0300

Domain-Functional Health (I)

Class-Self-Care (D)

Scale(s)-Severely compromised to Not compromised (a)

Care Recipient:

Data Source:

Definition: Ability to perform the most basic physical tasks and personal care activities independently with or without assistive device

OUTCOME TARGET RATING: Maintain at_____   Increase to_____

Self-Care: Activities of Daily Living (ADL) Overall Rating	Severely compromised 1	Substantially compromised 2	Moderately compromised 3	Mildly compromised 4	Not compromised 5	
INDICATORS:						
030001 Eating	1	2	3	4	5	NA
030002 Dressing	1	2	3	4	5	NA
030003 Toileting	1	2	3	4	5	NA
030004 Bathing	1	2	3	4	5	NA
030005 Grooming	1	2	3	4	5	NA
030006 Hygiene	1	2	3	4	5	NA
030007 Oral hygiene	1	2	3	4	5	NA
030008 Walking	1	2	3	4	5	NA
030009 Wheelchair mobility	1	2	3	4	5	NA
030010 Transfer performance	1	2	3	4	5	NA
030012 Positions self	1	2	3	4	5	NA

1st edition 1997; Revised 3rd edition 2004

Outcome Content References:

Armer, J. M., Conn, V. S., Decker, S. A., & Tripp-Reimer, T. (2001). Self-care deficit. In M. Maas, K. Buckwalter, M. Hardy, T. Tripp-Reimer, M. Titler, & J. Specht (Eds.), *Nursing care of older adults: Diagnoses, outcomes & interventions* (pp. 366-384). St. Louis: Mosby.

Hickey, T. (1988). Self-care behavior of older adults. *Family and Community Health, 11*(3), 22-35.

Katz, S., & Akpom, C. A. (1976). A measure of primary sociobiological functions. *International Journal of Health Services, 6*(3), 493-507.

+Katz, S., Ford, A. B., Moskowitz, R. W., Jackson, B. A., & Jaffe, M. W. (1963). Studies of illness in the aged. The Index of ADL: A standardized measure of biological and psychosocial function. *Journal of the American Medical Association, 185*(12), 914-919.

Klein, R. M., & Bell, B. (1982). Self-care skills: Behavioral measurement with Klein-Bell ADL Scale. *Archives of Physical Medicine and Rehabilitation, 63*(7), 335-338.

Leenerts, M. H., Teel, C. S., & Pendleton, M. K. (2002). Building a model of self-care for health promotion in aging. *Journal of Nursing Scholarship, 34*(4), 355-361.

Resnick, B. (2001). Motivating older adults to engage in self-care. *Patient Care for the Nurse Practitioner, 4*(9), 13-14, 16, 19.

Weitzel, E. (2001). Unilateral neglect. In M. Maas, K. Buckwalter, M. Hardy, T. Tripp-Reimer, M. Titler, & J. Specht (Eds.), *Nursing care of older adults: Diagnoses, outcomes & interventions* (pp. 492-502). St. Louis: Mosby.

S

Self-Care: Bathing—0301

Domain-Functional Health (I)

Class-Self-Care (D)

Scale(s)-Severely compromised to Not compromised (a)

Care Recipient:

Data Source:

Definition: Ability to cleanse own body independently with or without assistive device

OUTCOME TARGET RATING: Maintain at_____   Increase to_____

Self-Care: Bathing Overall Rating	Severely compromised 1	Substantially compromised 2	Moderately compromised 3	Mildly compromised 4	Not compromised 5	
INDICATORS:						
030101 Gets in and out of bathroom	1	2	3	4	5	NA
030102 Gets bath supplies	1	2	3	4	5	NA
030103 Obtains bath water	1	2	3	4	5	NA
030104 Turns on water	1	2	3	4	5	NA
030105 Regulates water temperature	1	2	3	4	5	NA
030106 Regulates water flow	1	2	3	4	5	NA
030107 Bathes at sink	1	2	3	4	5	NA
030108 Bathes in tub	1	2	3	4	5	NA
030109 Bathes in shower	1	2	3	4	5	NA
030113 Washes face	1	2	3	4	5	NA
030114 Washes upper body	1	2	3	4	5	NA
030115 Washes lower body	1	2	3	4	5	NA
030116 Cleans perineal area	1	2	3	4	5	NA
030111 Dries body	1	2	3	4	5	NA

1st edition 1997; Revised 3rd edition 2004

S

Outcome Content References:

Armer, J. M., Conn, V. S., Decker, S. A., & Tripp-Reimer, T. (2001). Self-care deficit. In M. Maas, K. Buckwalter, M. Hardy, T. Tripp-Reimer, M. Titler, & J. Specht (Eds.), *Nursing care of older adults: Diagnoses, outcomes & interventions* (pp. 366-384). St. Louis: Mosby.

+*Guide for the Uniform Data Set for Medical Rehabilitation* (including the FIM™ instrument), (version 5.1) (1997). Buffalo, NY: University at Buffalo.

Gulick, E. E. (1990). The self-administered ADL scale for persons with multiple sclerosis. In C. F. Waltz & O. L. Strickland (Eds.), *Measurement of nursing outcomes* (pp. 128-147). New York: Springer.

Hickey, T. (1988). Self-care behavior of older adults. *Family and Community Health, 11*(3), 22-35.

Klein, R. M., & Bell, B. (1982). Self-care skills: Behavioral measurement with Klein-Bell ADL Scale. *Archives of Physical Medicine and Rehabilitation, 63*(7), 335-338.

Leenerts, M. H., Teel, C. S., & Pendleton, M. K. (2002). Building a model of self-care for health promotion in aging. *Journal of Nursing Scholarship, 34*(4), 355-361.

McKeighten, R. J., Mehmert, P. A., & Dickel, C. A. (1990). Bathing/hygiene self-care deficit: Defining characteristics and related factors across age groups and diagnosis-related groups in an acute care setting. *Nursing Diagnosis, 1*(4), 155-161.

Resnick, B. (2001). Motivating older adults to engage in self-care. *Patient Care for the Nurse Practitioner, 4*(9), 13-14, 16, 19.

Shillam, L. L., & Beeman, C., & Loshin, P. (1983). Effect of occupational therapy intervention on bathing independence of disabled persons. *The American Journal of Occupational Therapy, 37*(11), 744-748.

Self-Care: Dressing—0302

Domain-Functional Health (I)

Class-Self-Care (D)

Scale(s)-Severely compromised to Not compromised (a)

Care Recipient:

Data Source:

Definition: Ability to dress self independently with or without assistive device

OUTCOME TARGET RATING: Maintain at_____   Increase to_____

Self-Care: Dressing Overall Rating	Severely compromised 1	Substantially compromised 2	Moderately compromised 3	Mildly compromised 4	Not compromised 5	
INDICATORS:						
030201 Selects clothing	1	2	3	4	5	NA
030215 Gets clothing from drawer	1	2	3	4	5	NA
030216 Gets clothing from closet	1	2	3	4	5	NA
030203 Picks up clothing	1	2	3	4	5	NA
030204 Puts clothing on upper body	1	2	3	4	5	NA
030205 Puts clothing on lower body	1	2	3	4	5	NA
030206 Buttons clothing	1	2	3	4	5	NA
030207 Uses fasteners	1	2	3	4	5	NA
030208 Uses zippers	1	2	3	4	5	NA
030209 Puts on socks	1	2	3	4	5	NA
030210 Puts on shoes	1	2	3	4	5	NA
030213 Ties shoes	1	2	3	4	5	NA
030211 Removes clothes from upper body	1	2	3	4	5	NA
030214 Removes clothes from lower body	1	2	3	4	5	NA

1st edition 1997; Revised 3rd edition 2004; Revised 4th edition

S

Outcome Content References:

Armer, J. M., Conn, V. S., Decker, S. A., & Tripp-Reimer, T. (2001). Self-care deficit. In M. Maas, K. Buckwalter, M. Hardy, T. Tripp-Reimer, M. Titler, & J. Specht (Eds.), *Nursing care of older adults: Diagnoses, outcomes & interventions* (pp. 366-384). St. Louis: Mosby.

Beck, C. (1988). Measurement of dressing performance in persons with dementia. *American Journal of Alzheimer's Care and Related Disorders and Research, 3*(3), 21-25.

Cole, S. L. (1992). Dress for success: A nurse's knowledge of simple clothing adaptations and dressing aids may make the difference between rehabilitation success and failure. *Geriatric Nursing, 13*(4), 217-221.

Cook, E. A., Luschen, L., & Sikes, S. (1991). Dressing training for an elderly woman with cognitive and perceptual impairments. *The American Journal of Occupational Therapy, 45*(7), 652-654.

Dudgeon, B. J., DeLisa, J. A., & Miller, R. M. (1984). Optokinetic nystagmus and upper extremity dressing independence after stroke. *Archives of Physical Medicine & Rehabilitation, 66*(3), 164-167.

Ford, L. J. (1975). Teaching dressing skills to a severely retarded child. *The American Journal of Occupational Therapy, 2*(29), 87-92.

Continued

+*Guide for the Uniform Data Set for Medical Rehabilitation* (including the FIM™ instrument (version 5.1) (1997). Buffalo, NY: University at Buffalo.

Hickey, T. (1988). Self-care behavior of older adults. *Family and Community Health, 11*(3), 22-35.

Leenerts, M. H., Teel, C. S., & Pendleton, M. K. (2002). Building a model of self-care for health promotion in aging. *Journal of Nursing Scholarship, 34*(4), 355-361.

Panikoff, L. B. (1983). Recovery trends of functional skills in the head injured adult. *The American Journal of Occupational Therapy, 37*(11), 735-743.

Resnick, B. (2001). Motivating older adults to engage in self-care. *Patient Care for the Nurse Practitioner, 4*(9), 13-14, 16, 19.

Runge, M. (1967). Self-dressing techniques for patients with spinal cord injury. *The American Journal of Occupational Therapy, 21*(6), 367-375.

S

Self-Care: Eating—0303

Domain-Functional Health (I)

Class-Self-Care (D)

Scale(s)-Severely compromised to Not compromised (a)

Care Recipient:

Data Source:

Definition: Ability to prepare and ingest food and fluid independently with or without assistive device

OUTCOME TARGET RATING:　　Maintain at_____　　　Increase to_____

Self-Care: Eating Overall Rating	Severely compromised 1	Substantially compromised 2	Moderately compromised 3	Mildly compromised 4	Not compromised 5	
INDICATORS:						
030301　Prepares food for ingestion	1	2	3	4	5	NA
030302　Opens containers	1	2	3	4	5	NA
030316　Cuts up food	1	2	3	4	5	NA
030303　Uses utensils	1	2	3	4	5	NA
030304　Gets food onto the utensil	1	2	3	4	5	NA
030305　Picks up cup or glass	1	2	3	4	5	NA
030306　Brings food to mouth with fingers	1	2	3	4	5	NA
030307　Brings food to mouth with container	1	2	3	4	5	NA
030308　Brings food to mouth with utensil	1	2	3	4	5	NA
030309　Drinks from a cup or glass	1	2	3	4	5	NA
030310　Places food in mouth	1	2	3	4	5	NA
030311　Manipulates food in mouth	1	2	3	4	5	NA
030312　Chews food	1	2	3	4	5	NA
030313　Swallows food	1	2	3	4	5	NA
030317　Swallows fluid	1	2	3	4	5	NA
030314　Completes a meal	1	2	3	4	5	NA

1st edition 1997; Revised 3rd edition 2004

Outcome Content References:

Armer, J. M., Conn, V. S., Decker, S. A., & Tripp-Reimer, T. (2001). Self-care deficit. In M. Maas, K. Buckwalter, M. Hardy, T. Tripp-Reimer, M. Titler, & J. Specht (Eds.), *Nursing care of older adults: Diagnoses, outcomes & interventions* (pp. 366-384). St. Louis: Mosby.

Athlin, E., Norberg, A., Axelson, K., Moller, A., & Nordstrom, G. (1989). Aberrant eating behavior in elderly parkinsonian patients with and without dementia: Analysis of video-recorded meals. *Research in Nursing and Health, 12*(1), 41-51.

+*Guide for the Uniform Data Set for Medical Rehabilitation* (including the FIM™ instrument), (version 5.1). (1997). Buffalo, NY: University at Buffalo.

Hickey, T. (1988). Self-care behavior of older adults. *Family and Community Health, 11*(3), 22-35.

Continued

S

Leenerts, M. H., Teel, C. S., & Pendleton, M. K. (2002). Building a model of self-care for health promotion in aging. *Journal of Nursing Scholarship, 34*(4), 355-361.

Luiselli, J. K. (1993). Training self-feeding skills in children who are deaf and blind. *Behavior Modification, 17*(4), 457-473.

Piazza, C. C., Anderson, C., & Fisher, W. (1993). Teaching self-feeding skills to patients with Rett Syndrome. *Developmental Medicine and Child Neurology, 35*(11), 991-996.

Resnick, B. (2001). Motivating older adults to engage in self-care. *Patient Care for the Nurse Practitioner, 4*(9), 13-14, 16, 19.

Tandy, L., & Malan, S. (2001). Impaired swallowing. In M. Maas, K. Buckwalter, M. Hardy, T. Tripp-Reimer, M. Titler, & J. Specht (Eds.), *Nursing care of older adults: Diagnoses, outcomes & interventions* (pp. 158-171). St. Louis: Mosby.

S

Self-Care: Hygiene—0305

Domain-Functional Health (I)

Class-Self-Care (D)

Scale(s)-Severely compromised to Not compromised (a)

Care Recipient:

Data Source:

Definition: Ability to maintain own personal cleanliness and kempt appearance independently with or without assistive device

OUTCOME TARGET RATING: Maintain at_____   Increase to_____

Self-Care: Hygiene Overall Rating	Severely compromised 1	Substantially compromised 2	Moderately compromised 3	Mildly compromised 4	Not compromised 5	
INDICATORS:						
030501 Washes hands	1	2	3	4	5	NA
030503 Cleans perineal area	1	2	3	4	5	NA
030515 Wears protective pads	1	2	3	4	5	NA
030504 Cleans ears	1	2	3	4	5	NA
030505 Keeps nose blown and clean	1	2	3	4	5	NA
030506 Maintains oral hygiene	1	2	3	4	5	NA
030508 Shampoos hair	1	2	3	4	5	NA
030509 Combs or brushes hair	1	2	3	4	5	NA
030510 Shaves	1	2	3	4	5	NA
030511 Applies makeup	1	2	3	4	5	NA
030512 Cares for fingernails	1	2	3	4	5	NA
030516 Cares for toenails	1	2	3	4	5	NA
030513 Uses a mirror	1	2	3	4	5	NA
030514 Maintains neat appearance	1	2	3	4	5	NA
030517 Maintains body hygiene	1	2	3	4	5	NA

1st edition 1997; Revised 3rd edition 2004; Revised 4th edition

Outcome Content References:

Armer, J. M., Conn, V. S., Decker, S. A., & Tripp-Reimer, T. (2001). Self-care deficit. In M. Maas, K. Buckwalter, M. Hardy, T. Tripp-Reimer, M. Titler, & J. Specht (Eds.), *Nursing care of older adults: Diagnoses, outcomes & interventions* (pp. 366-384). St. Louis: Mosby.

Cole, G. (1991). Hygiene and care of the patient's environment. In G. Cole (Ed.), *Basic nursing skills and concepts* (pp. 261-290). St. Louis: Mosby.

Guide for the Uniform Data Set for Medical Rehabilitation (including the FIM™ instrument), (version 5.1). (1997). Buffalo, NY: University at Buffalo.

Hallstrom, R., & Beck, S. L. (1993). Implementation of the AORN skin shaving standard: Evaluation of a planned change. *AORN Journal, 58*(3), 498-506.

Hickey, T. (1988). Self-care behavior of older adults. *Family and Community Health, 11*(3), 22-35.

Leenerts, M. H., Teel, C. S., & Pendleton, M. K. (2002). Building a model of self-care for health promotion in aging. *Journal of Nursing Scholarship, 34*(4), 355-361.

McKeighten, R. J., Mehmert, P. A., & Dickel, C. A. (1990). Bathing/hygiene self-care deficit: Defining characteristics and related factors across age groups and diagnosis-related groups in an acute care setting. *Nursing Diagnosis, 1*(4), 155-161.

Ney, D. F. (1993). Cerumen impaction, ear hygiene practices, and hearing acuity. *Geriatric Nursing—American Journal of Care for the Aging, 14*(2), 70-73.

Resnick, B. (2001). Motivating older adults to engage in self-care. *Patient Care for the Nurse Practitioner, 4*(9), 13-14, 16, 19.

Wong, S. E., Flanagan, S. G., Kuehnel, T. G., Liberman, R. P., Hunnicut, R., & Adams-Badgett, J. (1988). Training chronic mental patients to independently practice personal grooming skills. *Hospital and Community Psychiatry, 39*(8), 874-879.

S

Self-Care: Instrumental Activities of Daily Living (IADL)—0306

Domain-Functional Health (I)   Care Recipient:

Class-Self-Care (D)   Data Source:

Scale(s)-Severely compromised to Not compromised (a)

Definition: Ability to perform activities needed to function in the home or community independently with or without assistive device

OUTCOME TARGET RATING: Maintain at_____   Increase to_____

Self-Care: Instrumental Activities of Daily Living (IADL) Overall Rating	Severely compromised 1	Substantially compromised 2	Moderately compromised 3	Mildly compromised 4	Not compromised 5	
INDICATORS:						
030601 Shops for groceries	1	2	3	4	5	NA
030602 Shops for clothing	1	2	3	4	5	NA
030603 Shops for household supplies	1	2	3	4	5	NA
030604 Prepares meals	1	2	3	4	5	NA
030605 Serves meals	1	2	3	4	5	NA
030606 Operates phone	1	2	3	4	5	NA
030607 Handles written communication	1	2	3	4	5	NA
030608 Opens containers	1	2	3	4	5	NA
030609 Performs housework	1	2	3	4	5	NA
030610 Performs household repairs	1	2	3	4	5	NA
030611 Performs yard work	1	2	3	4	5	NA
030612 Manages money	1	2	3	4	5	NA
030613 Manages business affairs	1	2	3	4	5	NA
030614 Travels on public transportation	1	2	3	4	5	NA
030615 Drives own car	1	2	3	4	5	NA
030616 Does own laundry	1	2	3	4	5	NA
030617 Manages own non-parenteral medication	1	2	3	4	5	NA
030619 Manages own parenteral medication	1	2	3	4	5	NA

1st edition 1997; Revised 3rd edition 2004; Revised 4th edition

Outcome Content References:

Armer, J. M., Conn, V. S., Decker, S. A., & Tripp-Reimer, T. (2001). Self-care deficit. In M. Maas, K. Buckwalter, M. Hardy, T. Tripp-Reimer, M. Titler, & J. Specht (Eds.), *Nursing care of older adults: Diagnoses, outcomes & interventions* (pp. 366-384). St. Louis: Mosby.

S

Fillenbaum, G. G., & Smyer, M. A. (1981). The development, validity, and reliability of the OARS Multidimensional Functional Assessment Questionnaire. *Journal of Gerontology, 36*(4), 428-434.

Head, B. J. (2001). Impaired home maintenance management. In M. Maas, K. Buckwalter, M. Hardy, T. Tripp-Reimer, M. Titler, & J. Specht (Eds.), *Nursing care of older adults: Diagnoses, outcomes & interventions* (pp. 64-74). St. Louis: Mosby.

Hickey, T. (1988). Self-care behavior of older adults. *Family and Community Health, 11*(3), 22-35.

Jette, A. M. (1980). Functional status index: Reliability of a chronic disease evaluation instrument. *Archives of Physical Medicine & Rehabilitation, 61*(9), 395-401.

+Katz, S., Ford, A. B., Moskowitz, R. W., Jackson, B. A., & Jaffe, M. W. (1963). Studies of illness in the aged. The Index of ADL: A standardized measure of biological and psychosocial function. *Journal of the American Medical Association, 185*(12), 914-919.

Lawton, M. P. (1983). Assessment of behaviors required to maintain residence in the community. In T. Crook, S. Ferris, & R. Bartus (Eds.), *Assessment in geriatric psychopharmacology* (pp. 119-135). New Canaan, CT: Mark Powley Associates.

Lawton, M. P., & Brody, E. M. (1969). Assessment of older people: Self-maintaining and instrumental activities of daily living. *Gerontologist, 9*(3), 179-186.

Leenerts, M. H., Teel, C. S., & Pendleton, M. K. (2002). Building a model of self-care for health promotion in aging. *Journal of Nursing Scholarship, 34*(4), 355-361.

Linn, M. W., & Linn, B. S. (1982). The Rapid Disability Rating Scale-2. *Journal of the American Geriatric Society, 30*(6), 378-382.

Meenan, R. F., Gertman, P. M., & Mason, J. H. (1980). Measuring health status in arthritis: The arthritis impact measurement scales. *Arthritis Rheumatism, 23*(2), 146-152.

Pearlman, R. (1987). Development of a functional assessment questionnaire for geriatric patients: The Comprehensive Older Persons' Evaluation (COPE). *Journal of Chronic Disease, 40*(56), 85S-94S.

Resnick, B. (2001). Motivating older adults to engage in self-care. *Patient Care for the Nurse Practitioner, 4*(9), 13-14, 16, 19.

Shanas, E., Townsend, P., Wedderburn, D., Friis, H., Milhoj, P., & Stehouwer, J. (1968). *Old people in three industrial societies.* New York: Atherton Press.

S

Self-Care: Non-Parenteral Medication—0307

Domain-Functional Health (I)

Class-Self-Care (D)

Scale(s)-Severely compromised to Not compromised (a)

Care Recipient:

Data Source:

Definition: Ability to administer oral and topical medications to meet therapeutic goals independently with or without assistive device

OUTCOME TARGET RATING: Maintain at_____   Increase to_____

Self-Care: Non-Parenteral Medication Overall Rating	Severely compromised 1	Substantially compromised 2	Moderately compromised 3	Mildly compromised 4	Not compromised 5	
INDICATORS:						
030701 Identifies medication	1	2	3	4	5	NA
030702 Administers correct dose	1	2	3	4	5	NA
030716 Monitors therapeutic effects	1	2	3	4	5	NA
030717 Adjusts medication to achieve therapeutic effects	1	2	3	4	5	NA
030705 Follows medication precautions	1	2	3	4	5	NA
030706 Monitors medication side effects	1	2	3	4	5	NA
030707 Uses memory aids	1	2	3	4	5	NA
030708 Performs self-monitoring activities	1	2	3	4	5	NA
030709 Uses monitoring equipment accurately	1	2	3	4	5	NA
030710 Maintains required supplies	1	2	3	4	5	NA
030718 Uses medication as prescribed	1	2	3	4	5	NA
030712 Stores medication properly	1	2	3	4	5	NA
030713 Disposes of medication properly	1	2	3	4	5	NA
030714 Obtains required laboratory tests	1	2	3	4	5	NA
030719 Understands implications of test results	1	2	3	4	5	NA

1st edition 1997; Revised 3rd edition 2004; Revised 4th edition

S

Outcome Content References:

Armer, J. M., Conn, V. S., Decker, S. A., & Tripp-Reimer, T. (2001). Self-care deficit. In M. Maas, K. Buckwalter, M. Hardy, T. Tripp-Reimer, M. Titler, & J. Specht (Eds.), *Nursing care of older adults: Diagnoses, outcomes & interventions* (pp. 366-384). St. Louis: Mosby.

Barry, K. (1993). Patient self-medication: An innovative approach to medication teaching. *Journal of Nursing Care Quality, 8*(1), 75-82.

Felsenthal, G., Glomski, N., & Jones, D. (1986). Medication education program in an inpatient geriatric rehabilitation unit. *Archives of Physical Medication and Rehabilitation, 67*(1), 27-29.

Hickey, T. (1988). Self-care behavior of older adults. *Family and Community Health, 11*(3), 22-35.

Leenerts, M. H., Teel, C. S., & Pendleton, M. K. (2002). Building a model of self-care for health promotion in aging. *Journal of Nursing Scholarship, 34*(4), 355-361.

Lorish, D. D., Richards, B., & Brown, S. (1990). Perspective of the patient with rheumatoid arthritis on issues related to missed medication. *Arthritis Care and Research, 3*(2), 78-84.

Resnick, B. (2001). Motivating older adults to engage in self-care. *Patient Care for the Nurse Practitioner, 4*(9), 13-14, 16, 19.

S

Self-Care: Oral Hygiene—0308

Domain-Functional Health (I)   Care Recipient:

Class-Self-Care (D)   Data Source:

Scale(s)-Severely compromised to Not compromised (a)

Definition: Ability to care for own mouth and teeth independently with or without assistive device

OUTCOME TARGET RATING: Maintain at_____   Increase to_____

Self-Care: Oral Hygiene Overall Rating	Severely compromised 1	Substantially compromised 2	Moderately compromised 3	Mildly compromised 4	Not compromised 5	
INDICATORS:						
030801 Brushes teeth	1	2	3	4	5	NA
030802 Flosses teeth	1	2	3	4	5	NA
030810 Uses mouthwash	1	2	3	4	5	NA
030803 Cleans mouth, gums, and tongue	1	2	3	4	5	NA
030804 Cleans dentures or dental appliances	1	2	3	4	5	NA
030806 Uses fluoridation	1	2	3	4	5	NA
030807 Obtains regular dental care	1	2	3	4	5	NA

1st edition 1997; Revised 3rd edition 2004

Outcome Content References:

Armer, J. M., Conn, V. S., Decker, S. A., & Tripp-Reimer, T. (2001). Self-care deficit. In M. Maas, K. Buckwalter, M. Hardy, T. Tripp-Reimer, M. Titler, & J. Specht (Eds.), *Nursing care of older adults: Diagnoses, outcomes & interventions* (pp. 366-384). St. Louis: Mosby.

Fischman, S. (1993). Self-care: Practical periodontal care in today's practice. *International Dental Journal, 43*(2 Suppl. 1), 179-183.

Hickey, T. (1988). Self-care behavior of older adults. *Family and Community Health, 11*(3), 22-35.

Horowitz, L. G. (1990). Dental patient education: Self-care to healthy human development. *Patient Education and Counseling, 15*(1), 65-71.

Leenerts, M. H., Teel, C. S., & Pendleton, M. K. (2002). Building a model of self-care for health promotion in aging. *Journal of Nursing Scholarship, 34*(4), 355-361.

+Niederman, R., & Sullivan, T. M. (1981). Oral hygiene skill achievement index I. *Journal of Periodontology, 52*(3), 143-149.

+Niederman, R., Sullivan, T. M., Weiss, D., Morhart, R., Robbins, W., & Maier, D. (1981). Oral hygiene skill achievement index II. *Journal of Periodontology, 52*(3), 150-154.

Rayant, G. A., & Sheiham, A. (1980). An analysis of factors affecting compliance with tooth-cleaning recommendations. *Journal of Clinical Periodontology, 7*(4), 289-299.

Resnick, B. (2001). Motivating older adults to engage in self-care. *Patient Care for the Nurse Practitioner, 4*(9), 13-14, 16, 19.

Richardson, A. (1987). A process standard for oral care. *Nursing Times, 83*(32), 38-40.

S

Self-Care: Parenteral Medication—0309

Domain-Functional Health (I)

Class-Self-Care (D)

Scale(s)-Severely compromised to Not compromised (a)

Care Recipient:

Data Source:

Definition: Ability to administer parenteral medications to meet therapeutic goals independently with or without assistive device

OUTCOME TARGET RATING: Maintain at_____   Increase to_____

Self-Care: Parenteral Medication Overall Rating	Severely compromised 1	Substantially compromised 2	Moderately compromised 3	Mildly compromised 4	Not compromised 5	
INDICATORS:						
030901 Identifies medication	1	2	3	4	5	NA
030902 Administers correct dose	1	2	3	4	5	NA
030918 Monitors therapeutic effects	1	2	3	4	5	NA
030919 Adjusts medication to achieve therapeutic effects	1	2	3	4	5	NA
030905 Follows medication precautions	1	2	3	4	5	NA
030906 Monitors medication side effects	1	2	3	4	5	NA
030907 Uses memory aids	1	2	3	4	5	NA
030908 Performs self-monitoring activities	1	2	3	4	5	NA
030909 Uses monitoring equipment accurately	1	2	3	4	5	NA
030910 Maintains required supplies	1	2	3	4	5	NA
030919 Uses medication as prescribed	1	2	3	4	5	NA
030912 Stores medication properly	1	2	3	4	5	NA
030913 Disposes of medication properly	1	2	3	4	5	NA
030920 Disposes of syringes and needles properly	1	2	3	4	5	NA
030914 Maintains asepsis	1	2	3	4	5	NA
030915 Monitors injection sites	1	2	3	4	5	NA
030916 Obtains required laboratory tests	1	2	3	4	5	NA

1st edition 1997; Revised 3rd edition 2004; Revised 4th edition

Continued

Outcome Content References:

Armer, J. M., Conn, V. S., Decker, S. A., & Tripp-Reimer, T. (2001). Self-care deficit. In M. Maas, K. Buckwalter, M. Hardy, T. Tripp-Reimer, M. Titler, & J. Specht (Eds.), *Nursing care of older adults: Diagnoses, outcomes & interventions* (pp. 366-384). St. Louis: Mosby.

Gilbert, D. N., Dworkin, R. J., Raber, S. R., & Leggett, J. E. (1997). Outpatient parenteral antimicrobial-drug therapy. *New England Journal of Medicine, 337*(12), 829-838.

Hickey, T. (1988). Self-care behavior of older adults. *Family and Community Health, 11*(3), 22-35.

Leenerts, M. H., Teel, C. S., & Pendleton, M. K. (2002). Building a model of self-care for health promotion in aging. *Journal of Nursing Scholarship, 34*(4), 355-361.

Resnick, B. (2001). Motivating older adults to engage in self-care. *Patient Care for the Nurse Practitioner, 4*(9), 13-14, 16, 19.

Robinson, J., Gould, M. A., Burrows-Hudson, S., Baltz, P., Currier, H., Piwkiewicz, D., & Smith, L. J. (1991). A care plan for self-administration of epoetin alpha. *ANNA Journal, 18*(6), 573-580.

Sarisley, C. (1987). Designing a teaching program for outpatient antibiotic therapy. *Journal of Nursing Staff Development, 3*(3), 128-135.

S

Self-Care: Toileting—0310

Domain-Functional Health (I)

Class-Self-Care (D)

Scale(s)-Severely compromised to Not compromised (a)

Care Recipient:

Data Source:

Definition: Ability to toilet self independently with or without assistive device

OUTCOME TARGET RATING: Maintain at_____   Increase to_____

Self-Care: Toileting Overall Rating	Severely compromised 1	Substantially compromised 2	Moderately compromised 3	Mildly compromised 4	Not compromised 5	
INDICATORS:						
031001 Responds to full bladder in timely manner	1	2	3	4	5	NA
031002 Responds to urge to have a bowel movement in timely manner	1	2	3	4	5	NA
031013 Gets in and out of bathroom	1	2	3	4	5	NA
031004 Removes clothing	1	2	3	4	5	NA
031005 Positions self on toilet or commode	1	2	3	4	5	NA
031014 Gets to toilet between urge and passage of urine	1	2	3	4	5	NA
031015 Gets to toilet between urge and evacuation of stool	1	2	3	4	5	NA
031006 Empties bladder	1	2	3	4	5	NA
031011 Empties bowel	1	2	3	4	5	NA
031007 Wipes self after urinating	1	2	3	4	5	NA
031012 Wipes self after bowel movement	1	2	3	4	5	NA
031008 Gets up from toilet or commode	1	2	3	4	5	NA
031009 Adjusts clothing after toileting	1	2	3	4	5	NA

1st edition 1997; Revised 3rd edition 2004; Revised 4th edition

Outcome Content References:

Armer, J. M., Conn, V. S., Decker, S. A., & Tripp-Reimer, T. (2001). Self-care deficit. In M. Maas, K. Buckwalter, M. Hardy, T. Tripp-Reimer, M. Titler, & J. Specht (Eds.), *Nursing care of older adults: Diagnoses, outcomes & interventions* (pp. 366-384). St. Louis: Mosby.

Burgio, K. L., Burgio, L. D., McCormick, K. A., & Engel, B. T. (1991). Assessing toileting skills and habits in an adult day care center. *Journal of Gerontological Nursing, 17*(12), 32-35.

+*Guide for the Uniform Data Set for Medical Rehabilitation* (including the FIM™ instrument), (version 5.1) (1997). Buffalo, NY: University at Buffalo.

Continued

Hickey, T. (1988). Self-care behavior of older adults. *Family and Community Health, 11*(3), 22-35.

+Katz, S., Ford, A. B., Moskowitz, R. W., Jackson, B. A., & Jaffe, M. W. (1963). Studies of illness in the aged. The Index of ADL: A standardized measure of biological and psychosocial function. *Journal of the American Medical Association, 185*(12), 914-919.

Leenerts, M. H., Teel, C. S., & Pendleton, M. K. (2002). Building a model of self-care for health promotion in aging. *Journal of Nursing Scholarship, 34*(4), 355-361.

Okamoto, G. A., Sousa, J., Telzrow, R. W., Holm, R. A., McCartin, R., & Shurtleff, D. B. (1984). Toileting skills in children with myelomeningocele: Rates of learning. *Archives of Physical Medicine and Rehabilitation, 65*(4), 182-185.

Resnick, B. (2001). Motivating older adults to engage in self-care. *Patient Care for the Nurse Practitioner, 4*(9), 13-14, 16, 19.

Seim, H. C. (1989). Toilet training in first children. *The Journal of Family Practice, 29*(6), 633-636.

S

Self-Direction of Care—1613

Domain-Health Knowledge & Behavior (IV)

Class-Health Behavior (Q)

Scale(s)-Never demonstrated to Consistently demonstrated (m)

Care Recipient:

Data Source:

Definition: Care recipient actions taken to direct others who assist with or perform physical tasks and personal health care

OUTCOME TARGET RATING: Maintain at_____   Increase to_____

Self-Direction of Care Overall Rating	Never demonstrated 1	Rarely demonstrated 2	Sometimes demonstrated 3	Often demonstrated 4	Consistently demonstrated 5	
INDICATORS:						
161301 Sets health care goals	1	2	3	4	5	NA
161302 Describes appropriate care	1	2	3	4	5	NA
161311 Obtains needed resources	1	2	3	4	5	NA
161304 Instructs others in appropriate care behaviors	1	2	3	4	5	NA
161305 Evaluates the care given by others	1	2	3	4	5	NA
161306 Determines that care is completed appropriately	1	2	3	4	5	NA
161307 Expresses confidence in problem solving	1	2	3	4	5	NA
161308 Takes corrective action when care is not appropriate	1	2	3	4	5	NA
161309 Instructs others in appropriate health maintenance activities	1	2	3	4	5	NA

2nd edition 2000; Revised 3rd edition 2004; Revised 4th edition

Outcome Content References:

Edwards, P. A. (Ed.). (2000). *The specialty practice of rehabilitation nursing: A core curriculum* (4th ed.). Glenview, IL: Association of Rehabilitation Nurses.

Orem, D. E. (1985). A concept of self-care for the rehabilitation client. *Rehabilitation Nursing, 10*(3), 33-36.

Rehabilitation Nursing Foundation. (1995). *Twenty-one rehabilitation nursing diagnoses: A guide to interventions and outcomes.* Glenview, IL: Author.

S

Self-Esteem—1205

Domain-Psychosocial Health (III)

Class-Psychological Well-Being (M)

Scale(s)-Never positive to Consistently positive (k)

Care Recipient:

Data Source:

Definition: Personal judgment of self-worth

OUTCOME TARGET RATING: Maintain at_____   Increase to_____

Self-Esteem Overall Rating	Never positive 1	Rarely positive 2	Sometimes positive 3	Often positive 4	Consistently positive 5	
INDICATORS:						
120501 Verbalizations of self-acceptance	1	2	3	4	5	NA
120502 Acceptance of self-limitations	1	2	3	4	5	NA
120503 Maintenance of erect posture	1	2	3	4	5	NA
120504 Maintenance of eye contact	1	2	3	4	5	NA
120505 Description of self	1	2	3	4	5	NA
120506 Regard for others	1	2	3	4	5	NA
120507 Open communication	1	2	3	4	5	NA
120508 Fulfillment of personally significant roles	1	2	3	4	5	NA
120509 Maintenance of grooming and hygiene	1	2	3	4	5	NA
120510 Balance of participation and listening in groups	1	2	3	4	5	NA
120511 Confidence level	1	2	3	4	5	NA
120512 Acceptance of compliments from others	1	2	3	4	5	NA
120513 Expected response from others	1	2	3	4	5	NA
120514 Acceptance of constructive criticism	1	2	3	4	5	NA
120515 Willingness to confront others	1	2	3	4	5	NA
120521 Description of success in work	1	2	3	4	5	NA
120522 Description of success in school	1	2	3	4	5	NA
120517 Description of success in social groups	1	2	3	4	5	NA
120518 Description of pride in self	1	2	3	4	5	NA
120519 Feelings about self-worth	1	2	3	4	5	NA

1st edition 1997; Revised 4th edition

Outcome Content References:

Bonham, P., & Cheney, A. (1982). Concept of self: A framework for nursing assessment. In P. L. Chinn (Ed.), *Advances in nursing theory development* (pp. 173-189). Rockville, MD: Aspen.

Coopersmith, S. (1967). *The antecedents of self-esteem.* San Francisco: W. H. Freeman.

Crandall, R. (1973). The measurement of self-esteem and related constructs. In J. P. Robinson & P. R. Shaver (Eds.), *Measures of social psychological attitudes.* Ann Arbor, MI: Institute for Social Research, University of Michigan.

Fitts, W. (1965). *Manual for the Tennessee Self-Concept Scale*. Nashville, TN: Counselor Recordings & Tests.

Groh, C. J., & Whall, A. L. (2001). Self-esteem disturbance. In M. Maas, K. Buckwalter, M. Hardy, T. Tripp-Reimer, M. Titler, & J. Specht (Eds.), *Nursing care of older adults: Diagnoses, outcomes & interventions* (pp. 593-600). St. Louis: Mosby.

Larson, J. (1989). Validation of the defining characteristics of disturbance in self-esteem in patients with anorexia nervosa. In R. Carroll-Johnson (Ed.) *Classification of nursing diagnoses: Proceedings of the eighth conference* (North American Nursing Diagnosis Association) (pp. 307-312). Philadelphia: J.B. Lippincott.

+Nugent, W. R., & Thomas, J. W. (1993). Validation of a clinical measure of self-esteem. *Research on Social Work Practice, 3*(2), 191-207.

Roid, G., & Fitts, W. (1988). *Tennessee Self-Concept Scale: Revised manual*. Los Angeles: Western Psychological Services.

Rosenberg, M. (1965). *Society & adolescent self image*. Princeton, NJ: Princeton University Press.

Stanwyck, D. (1983). Self-esteem through the life span. *Family and Community Health, 6*(2), 11-28.

S.

Self-Mutilation Restraint—1406

Domain-Psychosocial Health (III)

Class-Self-Control (O)

Scale(s)-Never demonstrated to Consistently demonstrated (m)

Care Recipient:

Data Source:

Definition: Personal actions to refrain from intentional self-inflicted injury (non-lethal)

OUTCOME TARGET RATING: Maintain at_____   Increase to_____

Self-Mutilation Restraint Overall Rating	Never demonstrated 1	Rarely demonstrated 2	Sometimes demonstrated 3	Often demonstrated 4	Consistently demonstrated 5	
INDICATORS:						
140601 Refrains from gathering means for self-injury	1	2	3	4	5	NA
140608 Obtains assistance as needed	1	2	3	4	5	NA
140604 Upholds contract to not harm self	1	2	3	4	5	NA
140605 Maintains self-control without supervision	1	2	3	4	5	NA
140606 Refrains from injuring self	1	2	3	4	5	NA
140609 Uses available support groups	1	2	3	4	5	NA
140610 Uses medication as prescribed	1	2	3	4	5	NA
140611 Participates in mental health promotion activities	1	2	3	4	5	NA
140612 Follows treatment regimen	1	2	3	4	5	NA
140613 Uses effective coping strategies	1	2	3	4	5	NA

1st edition 1997; Revised 3rd edition 2004; Revised 4th edition

Outcome Content References:

Burrow, S. (1994). Nursing management of self-mutilation. *British Journal of Nursing, 3*(8), 382-386.

Coler, M. S., & Vincent, K. G. (1995). Psychiatric mental health nursing. In K. V. Gettrust (Series Ed.), *Plans of care for specialty practice.* Albany, NY: Delmar.

Faye, P. (1995). Addictive characteristics of the behavior of self-mutilation. *Journal of Psychosocial Nursing and Mental Health Services, 33*(2), 19-22.

+Rojahn, J., Polster, L. M., Mulick, J. A., & Wisniewski, J. J. (1989). Reliability of the Behavior Problems Inventory. *Journal of the Multihandicapped Person, 2,* 283-293.

Stuart, G. W., & Laraia, M. T. (2001). *Principles and practice of psychiatric nursing* (7th ed.). St. Louis: Mosby.

Valente, S. M. (1991). Deliberate self-injury management in a psychiatric setting. *Journal of Psychosocial Nursing and Mental Health Services, 29*(12), 19-25.

Winchel, R. M. (1991). Self-injurious behavior. A review of the behavior and biology of self-mutilation. *American Journal of Psychiatry, 148*(3), 306-17.

S

Sensory Function—2405

Domain-Physiologic Health (II)

Class-Sensory (Y)

Scale(s)-Severe deviation from normal range to No deviation from normal range (b)

Care Recipient:

Data Source:

> **Definition:** Extent to which an individual correctly senses skin stimulation, sounds, proprioception, taste and smell, and visual images

OUTCOME TARGET RATING: Maintain at_____   Increase to_____

Sensory Function Overall Rating	Severe deviation from normal range 1	Substantial deviation from normal range 2	Moderate deviation from normal range 3	Mild deviation from normal range 4	No deviation from normal range 5	
INDICATORS:						
240501 Ability to sense skin stimulation	1	2	3	4	5	NA
240502 Ability to hear sounds	1	2	3	4	5	NA
240507 Ability to sense position changes of the head	1	2	3	4	5	NA
240508 Ability to sense position changes of the body	1	2	3	4	5	NA
240504 Ability to discriminate odors	1	2	3	4	5	NA
240505 Ability to discriminate taste	1	2	3	4	5	NA
240506 Ability to see	1	2	3	4	5	NA

3rd edition 2004; Revised 4th edition

Outcome Content References:

Cataract Management Guideline Panel. (1993). *Cataracts in adults: Management of functional impairment. Clinical practice guideline*, No. 4 (AHCPR Publication No. 93-0542). Rockville, MD: U.S. Department of Health and Human Services. Public Health Services, Agency for Health Care Policy and Research.

McCance, K. L., & Huether, S. E. (2002). *Pathophysiology: The biologic basis for disease in adults and children* (4th ed.). St. Louis: Mosby.

Phipps, W. J., Monahan, F. D., Sands, J. K., Marek, J., & Neighbors, M. (Eds.). (2003). *Medical-surgical nursing: Concepts and clinical practice* (7th ed) St. Louis: Mosby.

Swanson, E. A., & Drury, J. (2001). Sensory/perceptual alterations. In M. Maas, K. Buckwalter, M. Hardy, T. Tripp-Reimer, M. Titler, & J. Specht (Eds.), *Nursing care of older adults: Diagnoses, outcomes & interventions* (pp. 476-491). St. Louis: Mosby.

S

Sensory Function: Cutaneous—2400

Domain-Physiologic Health (II)

Class-Sensory (Y)

Scale(s)-Severe deviation from normal range to No deviation from normal range (b) and Severe to None (n)

Care Recipient:

Data Source:

Definition: Extent to which stimulation of the skin is correctly sensed

OUTCOME TARGET RATING: Maintain at_____   Increase to_____

Sensory Function: Cutaneous Overall Rating	Severe deviation from normal range 1	Substantial deviation from normal range 2	Moderate deviation from normal range 3	Mild deviation from normal range 4	No deviation from normal range 5	
INDICATORS:						
240001 Sharp versus dull discrimination	1	2	3	4	5	NA
240002 2-point discrimination	1	2	3	4	5	NA
240003 Vibration discrimination	1	2	3	4	5	NA
240004 Warmth discrimination	1	2	3	4	5	NA
240005 Cold discrimination	1	2	3	4	5	NA
240006 Tickle and itch discrimination	1	2	3	4	5	NA
240007 Noxious stimulus discrimination	1	2	3	4	5	NA
	Severe	**Substantial**	**Moderate**	**Mild**	**None**	
240008 Paresthesia	1	2	3	4	5	NA
240009 Hyperparesthesia	1	2	3	4	5	NA
240011 Tingling	1	2	3	4	5	NA
240012 Loss of sensation	1	2	3	4	5	NA

2nd edition 2000; Revised 3rd edition 2004

S

Outcome Content References:

Lewis, S. M., Collier, I. C., Heitkermper, M. M., & Dirksen, S. R. (2000). *Medical-surgical nursing: Assessment & management of clinical problems* (5th ed.). St. Louis: Mosby.

McCance, K. L., & Huether, S. E. (2002). *Pathophysiology: The biologic basis for disease in adults and children* (4th ed.). St. Louis: Mosby.

Swanson, E. A., & Drury, J. (2001). Sensory/perceptual alterations. In M. Maas, K. Buckwalter, M. Hardy, T. Tripp-Reimer, M. Titler, & J. Specht (Eds.), *Nursing care of older adults: Diagnoses, outcomes & interventions* (pp. 476-491). St. Louis: Mosby.

Sensory Function: Hearing—2401

Domain-Physiologic Health (II)

Class-Sensory (Y)

Scale(s)-Severe deviation from normal range to No deviation from normal range (b) and Severe to None (n)

Care Recipient:

Data Source:

Definition: Extent to which sounds are correctly sensed

OUTCOME TARGET RATING:　　Maintain at＿＿＿＿＿　　　Increase to＿＿＿＿＿

Sensory Function: Hearing Overall Rating	Severe deviation from normal range 1	Substantial deviation from normal range 2	Moderate deviation from normal range 3	Mild deviation from normal range 4	No deviation from normal range 5	
INDICATORS:						
240101　Auditory acuity (left)	1	2	3	4	5	NA
240102　Auditory acuity (right)	1	2	3	4	5	NA
240103　Air conduction of sound (left)	1	2	3	4	5	NA
240112　Air conduction of sound (right)	1	2	3	4	5	NA
240104　Bone conduction of sound (left)	1	2	3	4	5	NA
240113　Bone conduction of sound (right)	1	2	3	4	5	NA
240105　Ratio of air and bone conduction	1	2	3	4	5	NA
240107　Auditory discrimination of discrete sounds	1	2	3	4	5	NA
240108　Hears a whisper six inches from left ear (voice test)	1	2	3	4	5	NA
240114　Hears a whisper six inches from right ear (voice test)	1	2	3	4	5	NA
240109　Turns to sound	1	2	3	4	5	NA
240110　Shows interest in auditory stimuli	1	2	3	4	5	NA
240118　Recognizes source of sound	1	2	3	4	5	NA
	Severe	**Substantial**	**Moderate**	**Mild**	**None**	
240106　Tinnitus (left)	1	2	3	4	5	NA
240115　Tinnitus (right)	1	2	3	4	5	NA
240116　Loss of high pitch tones	1	2	3	4	5	NA

Continued

		Severe	Substantial	Moderate	Mild	None	
240117	Loss of ability to distinguish conversation from background environmental noise	1	2	3	4	5	NA

Assistive device YES / NO

2nd edition 2000; Revised 3rd edition 2004; Revised 4th edition

Outcome Content References:

Burrell, L. O. (Ed). (1992). *Adult nursing in hospital and community settings*. Norwalk, CT: Appleton & Lange.

May, J. J. (2000). Occupational hearing loss. *American Journal of Industrial Medicine, 37*(1), 112-120.

Phipps, W. J., Monahan, F. D., Sands, J. K., Marek, J., & Neighbors, M. (Eds.). (2003). *Medical-surgical nursing: Concepts and clinical practice* (7th ed). St. Louis: Mosby.

Sataloff, J., & Roberts, B. (1999). Differential diagnosis in occupation hearing loss compensation claims. *Journal of Occupation Hearing Loss, 2*(4), 183-189.

Smeltzer, S. C., & Bare, B. G. (Eds.). (2003). *Brunner and Suddarth's textbook of medical-surgical nursing* (10th ed.). Philadelphia: Lippincott, Williams & Wilkins.

Swanson, E. A., & Drury, J. (2001). Sensory/perceptual alterations. In M. Maas, K. Buckwalter, M. Hardy, T. Tripp-Reimer, M. Titler, & J. Specht (Eds.), *Nursing care of older adults: Diagnoses, outcomes & interventions* (pp. 476-491). St. Louis: Mosby.

S

Sensory Function: Proprioception—2402

Domain-Physiologic Health (II)

Class-Sensory (Y)

Care Recipient:

Data Source:

Scale(s)-Severe deviation from normal range to No deviation from normal range (b) and Severe to None (n)

Definition: Extent to which the position and movement of the head and body are correctly sensed

OUTCOME TARGET RATING: Maintain at_____   Increase to_____

Sensory Function: Proprioception Overall Rating	Severe deviation from normal range 1	Substantial deviation from normal range 2	Moderate deviation from normal range 3	Mild deviation from normal range 4	No deviation from normal range 5	

INDICATORS:

		Severe deviation from normal range 1	Substantial deviation from normal range 2	Moderate deviation from normal range 3	Mild deviation from normal range 4	No deviation from normal range 5	
240201	Head position discrimination	1	2	3	4	5	NA
240202	Head movement discrimination	1	2	3	4	5	NA
240203	Upper limb movement discrimination	1	2	3	4	5	NA
240210	Lower limb movement discrimination	1	2	3	4	5	NA
240204	Upper limb position discrimination	1	2	3	4	5	NA
240211	Lower limb position discrimination	1	2	3	4	5	NA
240212	Trunk movement discrimination	1	2	3	4	5	NA
240213	Trunk position discrimination	1	2	3	4	5	NA
240205	Sense of balance	1	2	3	4	5	NA
		Severe	**Substantial**	**Moderate**	**Mild**	**None**	
240206	Vertigo	1	2	3	4	5	NA
240207	Lightheadedness	1	2	3	4	5	NA
240208	Nystagmus	1	2	3	4	5	NA

2nd edition 2000; Revised 3rd edition 2004

Outcome Content References:

Lewis, S. M., Collier, I. C., Heitkermper, M. M., & Dirksen, S. R. (2000). *Medical-surgical nursing: Assessment & management of clinical problems* (5th ed.). St. Louis: Mosby.

McCance, K. L., & Huether, S. E. (2002). *Pathophysiology: The biologic basis for disease in adults and children* (4th ed.). St. Louis: Mosby.

Swanson, E. A., & Drury, J. (2001). Sensory/perceptual alterations. In M. Maas, K. Buckwalter, M. Hardy, T. Tripp-Reimer, M. Titler, & J. Specht (Eds.), *Nursing care of older adults: Diagnoses, outcomes & interventions* (pp. 476-491). St. Louis: Mosby.

S

Sensory Function: Taste & Smell—2403

Domain-Physiologic Health (II)

Class-Sensory (Y)

Care Recipient:

Data Source:

Scale(s)-Severe deviation from normal range to No deviation from normal range (b) and Severe to None (n)

Definition: Extent to which chemicals inhaled or dissolved in saliva are correctly sensed

OUTCOME TARGET RATING: Maintain at_____   Increase to_____

Sensory Function: Taste & Smell Overall Rating	Severe deviation from normal range 1	Substantial deviation from normal range 2	Moderate deviation from normal range 3	Mild deviation from normal range 4	No deviation from normal range 5	
INDICATORS:						
240301 Discriminates odors	1	2	3	4	5	NA
240304 Recognizes sweet flavor	1	2	3	4	5	NA
240305 Recognizes salty flavor	1	2	3	4	5	NA
240306 Recognizes bitter flavor	1	2	3	4	5	NA
240307 Recognizes sour flavor	1	2	3	4	5	NA
	Severe	Substantial	Moderate	Mild	None	
240302 Odor distortion	1	2	3	4	5	NA
240308 Taste distortion	1	2	3	4	5	NA
240310 Metallic taste	1	2	3	4	5	NA
240311 Hemianosmia	1	2	3	4	5	NA

2nd edition 2000; Revised 3rd edition 2004

Outcome Content References:

Burrell, L. O. (Ed). (1992). *Adult nursing in hospital and community settings.* Norwalk, CT: Appleton & Lange.

Phipps, W. J., Monahan, F. D., Sands, J. K., Marek, J., & Neighbors, M. (Eds.). (2003). *Medical-surgical nursing: Concepts and clinical practice* (7th ed). St. Louis: Mosby.

Smeltzer, S. C., & Bare, B. G. (Eds.). (2003). *Brunner and Suddarth's textbook of medical-surgical nursing* (10th ed.). Philadelphia: Lippincott, Williams & Wilkins.

Swanson, E. A., & Drury, J. (2001). Sensory/perceptual alterations. In M. Maas, K. Buckwalter, M. Hardy, T. Tripp-Reimer, M. Titler, & J. Specht (Eds.), *Nursing care of older adults: Diagnoses, outcomes & interventions* (pp. 476-491). St. Louis: Mosby.

S

Sensory Function: Vision—2404

Domain-Physiologic Health (II)

Class-Sensory (Y)

Scale(s)-Severe deviation from normal range to No deviation from normal range (b) and Severe to None (n)

Care Recipient:

Data Source:

Definition: Extent to which visual images are correctly sensed

OUTCOME TARGET RATING: Maintain at_____   Increase to_____

Sensory Function: Vision Overall Rating	Severe deviation from normal range 1	Substantial deviation from normal range 2	Moderate deviation from normal range 3	Mild deviation from normal range 4	No deviation from normal range 5	
INDICATORS:						
240401 Central visual acuity (left)	1	2	3	4	5	NA
240421 Central visual acuity (right)	1	2	3	4	5	NA
240402 Peripheral visual acuity (left)	1	2	3	4	5	NA
240422 Peripheral visual acuity (right)	1	2	3	4	5	NA
240403 Central visual fields (left)	1	2	3	4	5	NA
240423 Central visual fields (right)	1	2	3	4	5	NA
240404 Peripheral visual fields (left)	1	2	3	4	5	NA
240424 Peripheral visual fields (right)	1	2	3	4	5	NA
240416 Response to visual stimuli	1	2	3	4	5	NA

	Severe	Substantial	Moderate	Mild	None	
240405 Hemianopia	1	2	3	4	5	NA
240406 Floaters	1	2	3	4	5	NA
240407 Flashes of light	1	2	3	4	5	NA
240408 Halos around lights	1	2	3	4	5	NA
240409 Spiderwebs	1	2	3	4	5	NA
240410 Double vision	1	2	3	4	5	NA
240411 Blurred vision	1	2	3	4	5	NA
240412 Distorted vision	1	2	3	4	5	NA
240413 Color vision distortions	1	2	3	4	5	NA
240414 Night blindness	1	2	3	4	5	NA
240415 Day blindness	1	2	3	4	5	NA
240417 Headaches	1	2	3	4	5	NA

S

Continued

	Severe	Substantial	Moderate	Mild	None	
240418 Dizziness	1	2	3	4	5	NA
240419 Eye strain	1	2	3	4	5	NA

Assistive device YES / NO

2nd edition 2000; Revised 3rd edition 2004

Outcome Content References:

Burrell, L. O. (Ed). (1992). *Adult nursing in hospital and community settings*. Norwalk, CT: Appleton & Lange.

Phipps, W. J., Monahan, F. D., Sands, J. K., Marek, J., & Neighbors, M. (Eds.). (2003). *Medical-surgical nursing: Concepts and clinical practice* (7th ed). St. Louis: Mosby.

Smeltzer, S. C., & Bare, B. G. (Eds.). (2003). *Brunner and Suddarth's textbook of medical-surgical nursing* (10th ed.). Philadelphia: Lippincott, Williams & Wilkins.

Swanson, E. A., & Drury, J. (2001). Sensory/perceptual alterations. In M. Maas, K. Buckwalter, M. Hardy, T. Tripp-Reimer, M. Titler, & J. Specht (Eds.), *Nursing care of older adults: Diagnoses, outcomes & interventions* (pp. 476-491). St. Louis: Mosby.

S

Sexual Functioning—0119

Domain-Functional Health (I)

Class-Growth & Development (B)

Scale(s)-Never demonstrated to Consistently demonstrated (m)

Care Recipient:

Data Source:

Definition: Integration of physical, socioemotional, and intellectual aspects of sexual expression and performance

OUTCOME TARGET RATING: Maintain at_____   Increase to_____

Sexual Functioning Overall Rating	Never demonstrated 1	Rarely demonstrated 2	Sometimes demonstrated 3	Often demonstrated 4	Consistently demonstrated 5	
INDICATORS:						
011901 Attains sexual arousal	1	2	3	4	5	NA
011902 Sustains penile/clitoral erection through orgasm	1	2	3	4	5	NA
011903 Sustains arousal through orgasm	1	2	3	4	5	NA
011904 Uses assistive device as needed	1	2	3	4	5	NA
011905 Adapts sexual techniques as needed	1	2	3	4	5	NA
011906 Refrains from substance use that adversely affects sexual function	1	2	3	4	5	NA
011927 Uses hormone replacement therapy as needed	1	2	3	4	5	NA
011907 Expresses ability to perform sexually despite physical imperfections	1	2	3	4	5	NA
011908 Expresses comfort with sexual expression	1	2	3	4	5	NA
011909 Expresses self-esteem	1	2	3	4	5	NA
011910 Expresses comfort with body	1	2	3	4	5	NA
011911 Expresses sexual interest	1	2	3	4	5	NA
011912 Expresses ability to be intimate	1	2	3	4	5	NA
011913 Expresses willingness to be sexual	1	2	3	4	5	NA
011914 Reports available consenting partner	1	2	3	4	5	NA

S

Continued

		Never demonstrated	Rarely demonstrated	Sometimes demonstrated	Often demonstrated	Consistently demonstrated	
011915 NA	Expresses respect for partner	1	2	3	4	5	
011916	Expresses acceptance of partner	1	2	3	4	5	NA
011917	Expresses knowledge of partner's sexual capabilities	1	2	3	4	5	NA
011918	Expresses knowledge of personal sexual capabilities	1	2	3	4	5	NA
011919	Expresses knowledge of partner's sexual needs	1	2	3	4	5	NA
011920	Expresses knowledge of personal sexual needs	1	2	3	4	5	NA
011921	Communicates comfortably with partner	1	2	3	4	5	NA
011922	Communicates sexual needs with partner	1	2	3	4	5	NA
011923	Communicates sexual preferences with partner	1	2	3	4	5	NA
011924	Performs sexually if environment conducive	1	2	3	4	5	NA
011925	Performs sexually without coercion of partner	1	2	3	4	5	NA

2nd edition 2000; Revised 3rd edition 2004; Revised 4th edition

Outcome Content References:

Arcos, B. (2004). Female sexual function and response. *Journal of the American Osteopathic Association, 104*(1), 516-520.

Clark, J. C. (1993). Psychosocial responses of the patient: Altered sexual health. In S. I. Groenwald, M. H Frogge, M. Goodman, & C. H. Yarbro (Eds.), *Cancer nursing principles and practice* (3rd ed., pp. 449-467). Sudbury, MA: Jones and Bartlett.

Dobkin, P. L., & Bradley, I. (1991). Assessment of sexual dysfunction in oncology patients: Review, critique, and suggestions. *Journal of Psychosocial Oncology, 9*(1), 43-71.

Dunning, P. (1993). Sexuality and women with diabetes. *Patient Education and Counseling, 21*(1-2), 5-14.

Kralik, D., Koch, T., & Telford, K. (2001). Constructions of sexuality for midlife women living with chronic illness. *Journal of Advanced Nursing, 35*(2), 180-187.

Masters, W. H., & Johnson, V. E. (1970). *Human sexual inadequacy.* Boston: Little, Brown and Company.

Tuttle, B. (1984). Adult sexual response. In L. P. Higgins & J. W. Hawkins (Eds.), *Human sexuality across the life span: Implications for nursing practice* (pp. 39-76). Monterey, CA: Wadsworth Health Sciences Division.

S

Sexual Identity—1207

Domain-Psychosocial Health (III)

Class-Psychological Well-Being (M)

Scale(s)-Never demonstrated to Consistently demonstrated (m)

Care Recipient:

Data Source:

Definition: Acknowledgment and acceptance of own sexual identity

OUTCOME TARGET RATING: Maintain at_____   Increase to_____

Sexual Identity Overall Rating	Never demonstrated 1	Rarely demonstrated 2	Sometimes demonstrated 3	Often demonstrated 4	Consistently demonstrated 5	

INDICATORS:

		Never demonstrated 1	Rarely demonstrated 2	Sometimes demonstrated 3	Often demonstrated 4	Consistently demonstrated 5	
120701	Affirms self as a sexual being	1	2	3	4	5	NA
120702	Exhibits clear sense of sexual orientation	1	2	3	4	5	NA
120703	Exhibits comfort with sexual orientation	1	2	3	4	5	NA
120704	Integrates sexual orientation into life roles	1	2	3	4	5	NA
120706	Uses healthy coping behaviors to resolve sexual identity issues	1	2	3	4	5	NA
120707	Challenges negative images of sexual self	1	2	3	4	5	NA
120708	Seeks social support	1	2	3	4	5	NA
120709	Reports healthy intimate relationships	1	2	3	4	5	NA
120710	Reports healthy sexual functioning	1	2	3	4	5	NA
120711	Describes risks associated with sexual activity	1	2	3	4	5	NA
120712	Uses precautions to minimize risks associated with sexual activity	1	2	3	4	5	NA
120713	Describes personal sexual value system	1	2	3	4	5	NA
120714	Sets personal sexual boundaries	1	2	3	4	5	NA

2nd edition 2000; Revised 3rd edition 2004; Revised 4th edition

S

Continued

Outcome Content References:

Bohan, J. S. (1996). *Psychology and sexual orientation: Coming to terms*. New York: Routledge.

Cain, R. (1991). Stigma management and gay identity development. *Social Work, 36*(1), 67-73.

Cass, V. E. (1984). Homosexual identity formation: Testing a theoretical model. *The Journal of Sex Research, 20*(2), 143-167.

Eliason, M. J. (1996). *Who cares? Institutional barriers to health care for lesbian, gay, and bisexual persons*. New York: NLN Press.

Kinsey, A. C., Pomeroy, W. B., & Martin, C. E. (1948). *Sexual behavior in the human male*. Philadelphia: W.B. Saunders.

Nass, G., Libby, R., & Fischer, M. P. (1989). *Sexual choices: An introduction to human sexuality* (2nd ed.). Monterey, CA: Wadsworth Health Sciences.

Troiden, R. R. (1989). The formation of homosexual identities. *Journal of Homosexuality, 17*(1-2), 43-73.

Tuttle, B. (1984). Adult sexual response. In L. P. Higgins & J. W. Hawkins (Eds.), *Human sexuality across the life span: Implications for nursing practice* (pp. 39-76). Monterey, CA: Wadsworth Health Sciences Division.

S

Skeletal Function—0211

Domain-Functional Health (I)

Class-Mobility (C)

Scale(s)-Severely compromised to Not compromised (a)

Care Recipient:

Data Source:

Definition: Ability of the bones to support the body and facilitate movement

OUTCOME TARGET RATING: Maintain at_____   Increase to_____

Skeletal Function Overall Rating	Severely compromised 1	Substantially compromised 2	Moderately compromised 3	Mildly compromised 4	Not compromised 5	
INDICATORS:						
021101 Bone integrity	1	2	3	4	5	NA
021102 Bone density	1	2	3	4	5	NA
021103 Joint movement	1	2	3	4	5	NA
021104 Weight bearing	1	2	3	4	5	NA
021105 Skeletal alignment	1	2	3	4	5	NA
021106 Joint stability	1	2	3	4	5	NA

2nd edition 2000; Revised 3rd edition 2004

Outcome Content References:

Bouxsein, M. L., Myers, E. R., & Hayes, W. C. (1996). Biomechanics of age—related fractures. In R. Marcus, D. Feldman, & J. Kelsey (Eds.), *Osteoporosis*. San Diego: Academic Press.

Carter, D. R., Van Der Meulen, M. C. H., & Beaupre, G. S. (1996). Skeletal development: Mechanical consequences of growth, aging, and disease. In R. Marcus, D. Feldman, & J. Kelsey (Eds.), *Osteoporosis*. San Diego: Academic Press.

Krahl, H., Michaelis, U., Peiper, H., Quack, G., & Montag, M. (1994). Stimulation of bone growth through sports: A radiologic investigation of the upper extremities in professional tennis players. *The American Journal of Sports Medicine, 22*(6), 751-758.

Melton, L. J. (1997). Epidemiology of spinal osteoporosis. *Spine, 22*(Suppl. 24), 2S-11S.

Mourad, L. (1991). *Orthopedic disorders*. St. Louis: Mosby.

Sowers, M. (1997). Clinical epidemiology and osteoporosis: Measures and their interpretation. *Epidemiology and Clinical Decision Making, 26*(1), 219-231.

Vincente-Rodriguez, G. (2006). How does exercise affect bone development during growth? *Sports Medicine, 36*(7), 561-569.

S

Sleep—0004

Domain-Functional Health (I)   *Care Recipient:*

Class-Energy Maintenance (A)   *Data Source:*

Scale(s)-Severely compromised to Not compromised (a) and Severe to None (n)

Definition: Natural periodic suspension of consciousness during which the body is restored

OUTCOME TARGET RATING: Maintain at_____   Increase to_____

Sleep Overall Rating	Severely compromised 1	Substantially compromised 2	Moderately compromised 3	Mildly compromised 4	Not compromised 5	
INDICATORS:						
000401 Hours of sleep	1	2	3	4	5	NA
000402 Observed hours of sleep	1	2	3	4	5	NA
000403 Sleep pattern	1	2	3	4	5	NA
000404 Sleep quality	1	2	3	4	5	NA
000405 Sleep efficiency	1	2	3	4	5	NA
000407 Sleep routine	1	2	3	4	5	NA
000418 Sleeps through the night consistently	1	2	3	4	5	NA
000408 Feelings of rejuvenation after sleep	1	2	3	4	5	NA
000410 Wakeful at appropriate times	1	2	3	4	5	NA
000419 Comfortable bed	1	2	3	4	5	NA
000420 Comfortable temperature in room	1	2	3	4	5	NA
000411 Electroencephalogram findings	1	2	3	4	5	NA
000412 Electromyogram findings	1	2	3	4	5	NA
000413 Electrooculogram findings	1	2	3	4	5	NA

	Severe	Substantial	Moderate	Mild	None	
000421 Difficulty getting to sleep	1	2	3	4	5	NA
000406 Interrupted sleep	1	2	3	4	5	NA
000409 Inappropriate napping	1	2	3	4	5	NA
000416 Sleep apnea	1	2	3	4	5	NA
000417 Dependence on sleep aids	1	2	3	4	5	NA
000422 Nightmares	1	2	3	4	5	NA
000423 Nocturia	1	2	3	4	5	NA

S

		Severe	Substantial	Moderate	Mild	None	
000424	Snoring	1	2	3	4	5	NA
000425	Pain	1	2	3	4	5	NA

1st edition 1997; Revised 2nd edition 2000; Revised 3rd edition 2004; Revised 4th edition

Outcome Content References:

+Buysse, D. J., Reynolds, C. F, III, Monk, T. H., Berman, S. R., & Kupfer, D. J. (1989). The Pittsburgh Sleep Quality Index: A new instrument for psychiatric practice and research. *Psychiatry Research, 28*(2), 193-213.

Ellis, J. R., & Nowlis, E. A. (1994). *Providing nursing care within the nursing process* (5th ed.). Philadelphia: J.B. Lippincott.

Hoch, C. C., Reynolds, C. F., & Houck, P. (1988). Sleep patterns in Alzheimer, depressed, and healthy elderly. *Western Journal of Nursing Research, 10*(3), 239-256.

Mead-Bennet, E. (1989). The relationship of primigravid sleep experience and select moods on the first postpartum day. *Journal of Obstetric, Gynecologic, & Neonatal Nursing, 19*(2), 146-152.

Paulsen, V. M., & Shaver, J. L. (1991). Stress, support, psychological states and sleep. *Social Science and Medicine, 32*(11), 1237-1243.

Porth, C. M. (2002). *Pathophysiology: Concepts of altered health states* (6th ed.). Philadelphia: Lippincott Williams & Wilkins.

Potter, P. A., & Perry, A. G. (2001). *Fundamentals of nursing* (5th ed.). St. Louis: Mosby.

Redeker, N. S. (2000). Sleep in acute care settings: An integrative review. *Journal of Nursing Scholarship, 32*(1), 31-38.

Schoenfelder, D. P., & Culp, K. R. (2001). Sleep pattern disturbance. In M. Maas, K. Buckwalter, M. Hardy, T. Tripp-Reimer, M. Titler, & J. Specht (Eds.), *Nursing care of older adults: Diagnoses, outcomes & interventions* (pp. 401-413). St. Louis: Mosby.

Topf, M. (1992). Effects of personal control over hospital noise on sleep. *Research in Nursing and Health, 15*(1), 19-28.

Topf, M., & Davis, J. E. (1993). Critical care unit noise and rapid eye movement sleep. *Heart & Lung, 22*(3), 252-258.

Williams, P. D., White, M. A., Powell, G. M., Alexander, D. J., & Conlon, M. (1988). Activity level in hospitalized children during sleep onset latency. *Computers in Nursing, 6*(2), 70-76.

S

Smoking Cessation Behavior—1625

Domain-Health Knowledge & Behavior (IV)

Class-Health Behavior (Q)

Scale(s)-Never demonstrated to Consistently demonstrated (m)

Care Recipient:

Data Source:

Definition: Personal actions to eliminate tobacco use

OUTCOME TARGET RATING: Maintain at_____   Increase to_____

Smoking Cessation Behavior Overall Rating	Never demonstrated 1	Rarely demonstrated 2	Sometimes demonstrated 3	Often demonstrated 4	Consistently demonstrated 5	
INDICATORS:						
162501 Expresses willingness to stop smoking	1	2	3	4	5	NA
162502 Expresses belief in the ability to stop smoking	1	2	3	4	5	NA
162503 Identifies benefits of smoking cessation	1	2	3	4	5	NA
162504 Identifies negative consequences of tobacco use	1	2	3	4	5	NA
162505 Develops effective strategies to eliminate tobacco use	1	2	3	4	5	NA
162506 Identifies barriers to tobacco elimination	1	2	3	4	5	NA
162507 Adjusts tobacco elimination strategies as needed	1	2	3	4	5	NA
162508 Commits to tobacco elimination strategies	1	2	3	4	5	NA
162509 Follows selected tobacco elimination strategies	1	2	3	4	5	NA
162510 Participates in screening for associated health problems	1	2	3	4	5	NA
162511 Uses strategies to cope with withdrawal symptoms	1	2	3	4	5	NA
162512 Uses behavior modification strategies	1	2	3	4	5	NA

S

	Never demonstrated	Rarely demonstrated	Sometimes demonstrated	Often demonstrated	Consistently demonstrated	
162513 Uses effective coping strategies	1	2	3	4	5	NA
162514 Obtains assistance from health professional	1	2	3	4	5	NA
162515 Uses personal support system	1	2	3	4	5	NA
162516 Uses reputable sources of information	1	2	3	4	5	NA
162517 Uses nicotine replacement therapy	1	2	3	4	5	NA
162518 Uses alternative therapies	1	2	3	4	5	NA
162519 Identifies emotional states that affect tobacco use	1	2	3	4	5	NA
162520 Adjusts lifestyle to promote tobacco elimination	1	2	3	4	5	NA
162521 Uses prescribed medication as recommended	1	2	3	4	5	NA
162522 Uses non-prescription medication as recommended	1	2	3	4	5	NA
162523 Uses available support groups	1	2	3	4	5	NA
162524 Uses available community resources	1	2	3	4	5	NA
162525 Participates in counseling	1	2	3	4	5	NA
162526 Participates in telephone counseling	1	2	3	4	5	NA
162527 Monitors for signs of depression	1	2	3	4	5	NA
162528 Eliminates tobacco use	1	2	3	4	5	NA
162529 Commits to tobacco abstinence	1	2	3	4	5	NA

4th edition

Outcome Content References:

American Cancer Society. (2006). *Guide to quitting smoking*. Retrieved February 20, 2007, from http://www.cancer.org/docroot/PED/content/PED_10_13X_Guide_for_Quitting_Smoking.asp

Anderson, N. R. (2006). The role of the home healthcare nurse in smoking cessation: Guidelines for successful intervention. *Home Healthcare Nurse, 24*(7), 424-431.

Continued

S

Giarelli, E. (2006). Smoking cessation for women: Evidence of the effectiveness of nursing interventions. *Clinical Journal of Oncology Nursing, 10*(5), 667-671.

Higgins, S. T., Heil, S. H., Dumeer, A. M., Thomas, C. S., Solomon, L. J., & Bernstein, I. M. (2006). Smoking status in the initial weeks of quitting as a predictor of smoking-cessation outcomes in pregnant women. *Drug and Alcohol Dependence, 85*(2), 138-141.

Kassel, J. D., & Yates, M. (2002). Is there a role for assessment in smoking cessation treatment? *Behaviour Research and Therapy, 40*, 1457-1470.

McEwen, A., Hajek, P., McRobbie, H., & West, R. (2006). *Manual of smoking cessation: A guide for counselors and practitioners.* Malden, MA: Blackwell.

Molyneux, A., Lewis, S., Coleman, T., McNeill, A., Godfrey, C., Madeley, R., & Britton, J. (2006). Designing smoking cessation services for school-age smokers: A survey and qualitative study. *Nicotine & Tobacco Research, 8*(4), 539-546.

Price, J. H., Jordan, T. R., & Dake, J. A. (2006). Perceptions and use of smoking cessation in nurse-midwives practice. *Journal of Midwifery & Women's Health, 51*(3), 208-215.

Scheibmeir, M. S., & O'Connell, K. A. (2002). Promoting smoking cessation in adults. *Nursing Clinics of North America, 37*, 331-340.

Schofield, I. (2006). Supporting older people to quit smoking. *Nursing Older People, 18*(6), 29-33.

S

Social Interaction Skills—1502

Domain-Psychosocial Health (III)

Class-Social Interaction (P)

Scale(s)-Never demonstrated to Consistently demonstrated (m)

Care Recipient:

Data Source:

Definition: Personal behaviors that promote effective relationships

OUTCOME TARGET RATING: Maintain at_____   Increase to_____

Social Interaction Skills Overall Rating	Never demonstrated 1	Rarely demonstrated 2	Sometimes demonstrated 3	Often demonstrated 4	Consistently demonstrated 5	

INDICATORS:

150201	Uses disclosure as appropriate	1	2	3	4	5	NA
150202	Exhibits receptiveness	1	2	3	4	5	NA
150203	Cooperates with others	1	2	3	4	5	NA
150204	Exhibits sensitivity to others	1	2	3	4	5	NA
150205	Uses assertive behaviors as appropriate	1	2	3	4	5	NA
150206	Uses confrontation as appropriate	1	2	3	4	5	NA
150207	Exhibits consideration	1	2	3	4	5	NA
150208	Exhibits genuineness	1	2	3	4	5	NA
150209	Exhibits warmth	1	2	3	4	5	NA
150210	Exhibits poise	1	2	3	4	5	NA
150211	Appears relaxed	1	2	3	4	5	NA
150212	Engages others	1	2	3	4	5	NA
150213	Exhibits trust	1	2	3	4	5	NA
150214	Uses compromise as appropriate	1	2	3	4	5	NA
150216	Uses conflict resolution strategies	1	2	3	4	5	NA

1st edition 1997; Revised 3rd edition 2004

Outcome Content References:

Cutting, A. L., & Dunn, J. (2006). Conversations with siblings and with friends: Links between relationship quality and social understanding. *British Journal of Developmental Psychology, 24*(1), 73-87.

Erickson, D. H., Beiser, M., Iacono, W. G., Fleming, J. A. E., & Lin, T. (1989). The role of social relationships in the course of first-episode schizophrenia and affective psychosis. *American Journal of Psychiatry, 146*(11), 1456-1461.

Gotcher, J. M. (1992). Interpersonal communication and psychosocial adjustment. *Journal of Psychosocial Oncology, 10*(3), 21-39.

Heltsley, M. E., & Powers, R. C. (1975). Social interaction and perceived adequacy of interaction of the rural aged. *The Gerontologist, 15*(6), 533-536.

Levin, J., & Levin, W. C. (1981). Willingness to interact with an old person. *Research on Aging, 3*(2), 211-217.

Nussbaum, J. F. (1983). Relational closeness of elderly interaction: Implications for life satisfaction. *Western Journal of Speech Communication, 47*, 229-243.

Continued

S

Richter, G., & Richter, J. (1989). Social relationships reflected by depressive inpatients. *Acta Psychiatrica Scandinavica, 80*(6), 573-578.

+Ruehlman, L. S., & Karoly, P. (1991). With a little flak from my friends: Development and preliminary validation of the Test of Negative Social Exchange (TENSE). *Psychological Assessment: A Journal of Consulting and Clinical Psychology, 3*(1), 97-104.

Sheppard, M. (1993). Client satisfaction, extended intervention and interpersonal skills in community mental health. *Journal of Advanced Nursing, 18*(2), 246-259.

Waterman, J. D., Blegen, M., Clinton, P., & Specht, J. P. (2001). Social isolation. In M. Maas, K. Buckwalter, M. Hardy, T. Tripp-Reimer, M. Titler, & J. Specht (Eds.), *Nursing care of older adults: Diagnoses, outcomes & interventions* (pp. 651-663). St. Louis: Mosby.

Webb, L., Delaney, J. J., & Young, L. R. (1989). Age, interpersonal attraction, and social interaction. *Research on Aging, 11*(1), 107-123.

S

Social Involvement—1503

Domain-Psychosocial Health (III)

Class-Social Interaction (P)

Scale(s)-Never demonstrated to Consistently demonstrated (m)

Care Recipient:

Data Source:

Definition: Social interactions with persons, groups, or organizations

OUTCOME TARGET RATING: Maintain at_____   Increase to_____

Social Involvement Overall Rating	Never demonstrated 1	Rarely demonstrated 2	Sometimes demonstrated 3	Often demonstrated 4	Consistently demonstrated 5	
INDICATORS:						
150301 Interacts with close friends	1	2	3	4	5	NA
150302 Interacts with neighbors	1	2	3	4	5	NA
150303 Interacts with family members	1	2	3	4	5	NA
150304 Interacts with members of work group(s)	1	2	3	4	5	NA
150305 Participates as member of church	1	2	3	4	5	NA
150306 Participates in active church work	1	2	3	4	5	NA
150307 Participates in organized activity	1	2	3	4	5	NA
150308 Participates as officer in organization	1	2	3	4	5	NA
150309 Participates as a volunteer	1	2	3	4	5	NA
150311 Participates in leisure activities with others	1	2	3	4	5	NA
150313 Participates in team sports	1	2	3	4	5	NA

1st edition 1997; Revised 3rd edition 2004

Outcome Content References:

Cutting, A. L., & Dunn, J. (2006). Conversations with siblings and with friends: Links between relationship quality and social understanding. *British Journal of Developmental Psychology, 24*(1), 73-87.

Erickson, D. H., Beiser, M., Iacono, W. G., Fleming, J. A. E., & Lin, T. (1989). The role of social relationships in the course of first-episode schizophrenia and affective psychosis. *American Journal of Psychiatry, 146*(11), 1456-1461.

Gotcher, J. M. (1992). Interpersonal communication and psychosocial adjustment. *Journal of Psychosocial Oncology, 10*(3), 21-39.

Heltsley, M. E., & Powers, R. C. (1975). Social interaction and perceived adequacy of interaction of the rural aged. *The Gerontologist, 15*(6), 533-536.

Jylha, M., & Aro, S. (1989). Social ties and survival among the elderly in Tampere, Finland. *International Journal of Epidemiology, 18*(1), 158-164.

Levin, J., & Levin, W. C. (1981). Willingness to interact with an old person. *Research on Aging, 3*(2), 211-217.

Nussbaum, J. F. (1983). Relational closeness of elderly interaction: Implications for life satisfaction. *Western Journal of Speech Communication, 47*, 229-243.

S

Continued

Richter, G., & Richter, J. (1989). Social relationships reflected by depressive inpatients. *Acta Psychiatrica Scandinavica, 80*(6), 573-578.

Rohrer, J. E., Arif, A. A., Pierce, J. R., Jr., & Blackburn, C. (2004). Unsafe neighborhoods, social group activity, and self-rated health. *Journal of Public Health Management, 10*(2), 124-129.

Sheppard, M. (1993). Client satisfaction, extended intervention and interpersonal skills in community mental health. *Journal of Advanced Nursing, 18*(2), 246-259.

Waterman, J. D., Blegen, M., Clinton, P., & Specht, J. P. (2001). Social isolation. In M. Maas, K. Buckwalter, M. Hardy, T. Tripp-Reimer, M. Titler, & J. Specht (Eds.), *Nursing care of older adults: Diagnoses, outcomes & interventions* (pp. 651-663). St. Louis: Mosby.

Webb, L., Delaney, J. J., & Young, L. R. (1989). Age, interpersonal attraction, and social interaction. *Research on Aging, 11*(1), 107-123.

S

Social Support—1504

Domain-Psychosocial Health (III)

Class-Social Interaction (P)

Scale(s)-Not adequate to Totally adequate (f)

Care Recipient:

Data Source:

Definition: Reliable assistance from others

OUTCOME TARGET RATING: Maintain at_____   Increase to_____

Social Support Overall Rating	Not adequate 1	Slightly adequate 2	Moderately adequate 3	Substantially adequate 4	Totally adequate 5	
INDICATORS:						
150408 Willingness to call on others for assistance	1	2	3	4	5	NA
150401 Money available from others when needed	1	2	3	4	5	NA
150412 Assistance offered by others	1	2	3	4	5	NA
150402 Time provided by others	1	2	3	4	5	NA
150403 Labor provided by others	1	2	3	4	5	NA
150404 Information provided by others	1	2	3	4	5	NA
150405 Emotional assistance provided by others	1	2	3	4	5	NA
150406 Confidant relationship(s)	1	2	3	4	5	NA
150407 Persons who can help as needed	1	2	3	4	5	NA
150409 Assistive social network	1	2	3	4	5	NA
150410 Supportive social contacts	1	2	3	4	5	NA
150411 Stable social network	1	2	3	4	5	NA

1st edition 1997; Revised 3rd edition 2004; Revised 4th edition

Outcome Content References:

Akister, J., & Johnson, K. (2002). Parenting issues that may be addressed through a confidential helpline. *Health & Social Care in the Community, 10*(2), 106-111.

Bisconti, T. L., Bergeman, C. S., & Boker, S. M. (2006). Social support as a predictor of variability: An examination of the adjustment trajectories of recent widows. *Psychology and Aging, 21*(3), 590-599.

Dimond, M., & Jones, S. L. (1983). Social support: A review and theoretical integration. In P. L. Chinn (Ed.), *Advances in nursing theory development* (pp. 235-249). Rockville, MD: Aspen.

Gleeson-Kreig, J., Bernal, H., & Woolley, S. (2002). The role of social support in the self-management of diabetes mellitus among a Hispanic population. *Public Health Nursing, 19*(3), 215-222.

Hutchison, C. (1999). Social support: Factors to consider when designing studies that measure social support. *Journal of Advanced Nursing, 29*(6), 1520-1526.

Martire, L. M., Schulz, R., Mittelmark, M. B., & Newsom, J. T. (1999). Stability and change in older adults' social contact and social support: The cardiovascular health study. *Journals of Gerontology Series B—Psychological Sciences & Social Sciences, 54*(5), S302-311.

+Sarason, I. G., Sarason, B. R., Shearin, E. N., & Pierce, G. R. (1987). A brief measure of social support: Practical and theoretical implications. *Journal of Social and Personal Relationships, 4*, 497-510.

Tilden, V. P. (1985). Issues of conceptualization and measurement of social support in the construction of nursing theory. *Research in Nursing and Health, 8*(2), 199-206.

S

Continued

Travis, S., & Hunt, P. (2001). Supportive and palliative care networks: A new model for integrated care. *International Journal of Palliative Nursing, 7*(10), 501-504.

van Tilburg, T. (1998). Losing and gaining in old age: Changes in personal network size and social support in a four-year longitudinal study. *Journals of Gerontology Series B—Psychological Sciences & Social Sciences, 53*(6), S313-S323.

Warren, B. J. (1997). Depression, stressful life events, social support, and self-esteem in middle class African American women. *Archives of Psychiatric Nursing, 11*(3), 107-117.

Waterman, J. D., Blegen, M., Clinton, P., & Specht, J. P. (2001). Social isolation. In M. Maas, K. Buckwalter, M. Hardy, T. Tripp-Reimer, M. Titler, & J. Specht (Eds.), *Nursing care of older adults: Diagnoses, outcomes & interventions* (pp. 651-663). St. Louis: Mosby.

Wellisch, D., Kagawa-Singer, M., Reid, S. L., & Lin, Y., Nishikawa-Lee, S., & Wellisch, M. (1999). An exploratory study of social support: A cross-cultural comparison of Chinese, Japanese, and Anglo-American breast cancer patients. *Psycho-Oncology, 8*(3), 207-219.

S

Spiritual Health—2001

Domain-Perceived Health (V)

Class-Health & Life Quality (U)

Scale(s)-Severely compromised to Not compromised (a)

Care Recipient:

Data Source:

Definition: Connectedness with self, others, higher power, all life, nature, and the universe that transcends and empowers the self

OUTCOME TARGET RATING: Maintain at_____   Increase to_____

Spiritual Health Overall Rating	Severely compromised 1	Substantially compromised 2	Moderately compromised 3	Mildly compromised 4	Not compromised 5	
INDICATORS:						
200101 Quality of faith	1	2	3	4	5	NA
200102 Quality of hope	1	2	3	4	5	NA
200103 Meaning and purpose in life	1	2	3	4	5	NA
200104 Achievement of spiritual world view	1	2	3	4	5	NA
200105 Feelings of peacefulness	1	2	3	4	5	NA
200106 Ability to love	1	2	3	4	5	NA
200107 Ability to forgive	1	2	3	4	5	NA
200109 Ability to pray	1	2	3	4	5	NA
200110 Ability to worship	1	2	3	4	5	NA
200108 Spiritual experiences	1	2	3	4	5	NA
200122 Spiritual contentment	1	2	3	4	5	NA
200111 Participation in spiritual rites and passages	1	2	3	4	5	NA
200113 Participation in meditation	1	2	3	4	5	NA
200115 Participation in spiritual reading	1	2	3	4	5	NA
200112 Interaction with spiritual leaders	1	2	3	4	5	NA
200114 Expression through music	1	2	3	4	5	NA
200119 Expression through art	1	2	3	4	5	NA
200120 Expression through writing	1	2	3	4	5	NA
200116 Connectedness with inner-self	1	2	3	4	5	NA
200117 Connectedness with others	1	2	3	4	5	NA

S

Continued

		Severely compromised	Substantially compromised	Moderately compromised	Mildly compromised	Not compromised	
200121	Interaction with others to share thoughts, feelings, and beliefs	1	2	3	4	5	NA

1st edition 1997; Revised 3rd edition 2004

Outcome Content References:

Burkhardt, M. A. (1989). Spirituality: An analysis of the concept. *Holistic Nursing Practice, 3*(3), 69-77.

Burkhart, L., & Solari-Twadell, P. A. (2001). Spirituality and religiousness: Differentiating the diagnoses through a review of the nursing literature. *Nursing Diagnosis: The International Journal of Nursing Language and Classification, 12*(2), 45-54.

Emblen, J. D. (1992). Religion and spirituality defined according to current use in nursing literature. *Journal of Professional Nursing, 8*(1), 41-47.

Haase, J. E., Britt, T., Coward, D. D., Leidy, N. K., & Penn, P. E. (1992). Simultaneous concept analysis of spiritual perspective, hope, acceptance and self-transcendence. *Image—The Journal of Nursing Scholarship, 24*(2), 141-146.

Labun, E. (1988). Spiritual care: An element in nursing care planning. *Journal of Advanced Nursing, 13*(3), 314-320.

LeMone, P. (2001). Spiritual distress. In M. Maas, K. Buckwalter, M. Hardy, T. Tripp-Reimer, M. Titler, & J. Specht (Eds.), *Nursing care of older adults: Diagnoses, outcomes & interventions* (pp. 782-793). St. Louis: Mosby.

Pender, N., Murdaugh, C., & Parsons, M. A. (2001). *Health promotion in nursing practice* (4th ed.). Upper Saddle River, NJ: Prentice Hall.

Reed, P. G. (1992). An emerging paradigm for the investigation of spirituality in nursing. *Research in Nursing and Health, 15*(5), 349-357.

+Roberts, K. T., & Aspy, C. B. (1993). Development of the Serenity Scale. *Journal of Nursing Measurement, 1*(2), 145-164.

S

Stress Level—1212

Domain-Psychosocial Health (III)

Class-Psychological Well-Being (M)

Scale(s)-Severe to None (n)

Care Recipient:

Data Source:

Definition: Severity of manifested physical or mental tension resulting from factors that alter an existing equilibrium

OUTCOME TARGET RATING: Maintain at_____   Increase to_____

Stress Level Overall Rating	Severe 1	Substantial 2	Moderate 3	Mild 4	None 5	

INDICATORS:

		Severe 1	Substantial 2	Moderate 3	Mild 4	None 5	
121201	Increased blood pressure	1	2	3	4	5	NA
121202	Increased radial pulse rate	1	2	3	4	5	NA
121203	Increased respiratory rate	1	2	3	4	5	NA
121204	Dilated pupils	1	2	3	4	5	NA
121205	Increased muscle tension in neck, shoulders, and back	1	2	3	4	5	NA
121206	Tension headache	1	2	3	4	5	NA
121207	Sweaty palms	1	2	3	4	5	NA
121208	Dry mouth and throat	1	2	3	4	5	NA
121209	Diarrhea	1	2	3	4	5	NA
121210	Urinary frequency	1	2	3	4	5	NA
121211	Change in food intake	1	2	3	4	5	NA
121212	Upset stomach	1	2	3	4	5	NA
121213	Restlessness	1	2	3	4	5	NA
121214	Sleep disturbance	1	2	3	4	5	NA
121235	Interruption of thought process	1	2	3	4	5	NA
121215	Forgetfulness	1	2	3	4	5	NA
121216	Frequent cognitive mistakes	1	2	3	4	5	NA
121217	Diminished attention to detail	1	2	3	4	5	NA
121218	Inability to concentrate on tasks	1	2	3	4	5	NA
121219	Emotional outbursts	1	2	3	4	5	NA
121220	Irritability	1	2	3	4	5	NA
121221	Depression	1	2	3	4	5	NA
121222	Anxiety	1	2	3	4	5	NA
121223	Suspiciousness	1	2	3	4	5	NA
121224	Oppressive thoughts	1	2	3	4	5	NA

S

Continued

		Severe	Substantial	Moderate	Mild	None	
121225	Flashback episodes	1	2	3	4	5	NA
121226	Dissociation	1	2	3	4	5	NA
121227	Compulsive behavior	1	2	3	4	5	NA
121228	Increased alcohol use	1	2	3	4	5	NA
121229	Increased psychotropic medication use	1	2	3	4	5	NA
121230	Increased smoking	1	2	3	4	5	NA
121231	Absenteeism	1	2	3	4	5	NA
121232	Decreased productivity	1	2	3	4	5	NA
121233	Increased frequency of accidents	1	2	3	4	5	NA
121234	Change in libido	1	2	3	4	5	NA

3rd edition 2004; Revised 4th edition

Outcome Content References:

American Psychiatric Association. (2000). *Diagnostic and statistical manual of mental disorders* (4th ed., text revision). Washington DC: Author.

Campbell, R. J. (1989). *Psychiatric dictionary* (6th ed.). New York: Oxford University.

Curtis, R., Groarke, A.,. Coughlan, R., & Gsel, A. (2004). The influence of disease severity, perceived stress, social support and coping in patients with chronic illness: A 1 year follow up. *Psychology, Health & Medicine, 9*(4), 456-475.

Lazarus, R. S., & Folkman, S. (1984). *Stress, appraisal, and coping*. New York: Springer.

Richardson, C. G., & Ratner, P. A. (2005). Sense of coherence as a moderator of the effects of stressful life events of health. *Journal of Epidemiology & Community Health, 59*(11), 979-984.

Stanhope, M., & Lancaster, J. (1988). *Community health nursing: Process and practice for promoting health* (2nd ed.). St. Louis: Mosby.

Tasman, A., Kay, J., & Lieberman, J. A. (1997). *Psychiatry* (Vol. 2). Philadelphia: Saunders.

S

Student Health Status—2005

Domain-Perceived Health (V)
Class-Health & Life Quality (U)
Scale-Severely compromised to Not compromised (a) and Severe to None (n)

Care Recipient:
Data Source:

Definition: Physical, cognitive, emotional, and social status of a school-age child

OUTCOME TARGET RATING: Maintain at_____   Increase to_____

Student Health Status Overall Rating		Severely compromised 1	Substantially compromised 2	Moderately compromised 3	Mildly compromised 4	Not compromised 5	
200501	Physical health	1	2	3	4	5	NA
200502	Mental health	1	2	3	4	5	NA
200503	School attendance	1	2	3	4	5	NA
200504	Readiness to learn	1	2	3	4	5	NA
200505	Academic performance at grade level or higher	1	2	3	4	5	NA
200506	Standardized test performance at grade level or higher	1	2	3	4	5	NA
200507	Progression to graduation on expected schedule	1	2	3	4	5	NA
200508	Return to class after visit to health office	1	2	3	4	5	NA
200509	Physician office visits minimized	1	2	3	4	5	NA
200510	Emergency room visits minimized	1	2	3	4	5	NA
200511	Reports to the health office for medications at appropriate time	1	2	3	4	5	NA
200512	Participation in mandated screenings	1	2	3	4	5	NA
200513	Family follow-up of referrals	1	2	3	4	5	NA
200514	Participation in self-care activities	1	2	3	4	5	NA
200515	Students with chronic illness or special needs managed according to IHP*/IEP*	1	2	3	4	5	NA
200516	Financial resources for health care	1	2	3	4	5	NA

Continued

		Severely compromised	Substantially compromised	Moderately compromised	Mildly compromised	Not compromised	
200517	Participation in curricular school activities	1	2	3	4	5	NA
200518	Participation in extracurricular school activities	1	2	3	4	5	NA
200519	Participation in physical activities	1	2	3	4	5	NA
200520	Growth	1	2	3	4	5	NA
200521	Development	1	2	3	4	5	NA
200522	Optimum weight	1	2	3	4	5	NA
200523	Healthy dietary habits	1	2	3	4	5	NA
200524	Postponement of sexual activity	1	2	3	4	5	NA

		Severe	Substantial	Moderate	Mild	None	
200527	Alcohol use	1	2	3	4	5	NA
200528	Recreational drug use	1	2	3	4	5	NA
200533	Performance-enhancing drug use	1	2	3	4	5	NA
200529	Tobacco use	1	2	3	4	5	NA
200530	Occurrence of accidents	1	2	3	4	5	NA
200531	Disruptive behavior	1	2	3	4	5	NA
200534	Eating disorder	1	2	3	4	5	NA
200532	Occurrence of sexually transmitted disease	1	2	3	4	5	NA
200535	Risk for pregnancy	1	2	3	4	5	NA

*IHP = Individualized Healthcare Plan, IEP = Individualized Educational Plan

3rd edition 2004; Revised 4th edition

Outcome Content References:

Council of Chief State School Officers. (1998). *Incorporating health-related indicators in education accountability systems.* Washington, DC: Author.

Howard, M. (1991). *How to help your teenager postpone sexual involvement.* Lexington, NY: Continuum Publishing Co.

Marx, E., & Wooley, S. F. (Eds). (1998). *Health is academic: A guide to coordinated school health programs.* New York: Teachers College Columbia University.

Miller, B., Card, J., Paikoff, R. J., & Peterson, J. (1992). *Preventing adolescent pregnancy.* Newbury Park, CA: Sage.

Novello, A. C., DeGraw, C., & Kleinman, D. V. (1992). Healthy children ready to learn: An essential collaboration between health and education. *Public Health Reports, 107*(1), 3-10.

Tyson, H. (1999). A load off the teachers' backs: Coordinated school health programs. *Phi Delta Kappan, 80*(5), K1-K8.

Washington State Office of Superintendent of Public Instruction. (2001). *School nurse outcome measures.* Olympia, WA: Author.

Substance Addiction Consequences—1407

Domain-Perceived Health (v)

Class-Symptom Status (v)

Scale(s)-Severe to None (n)

Care Recipient:

Data Source:

Definition: Severity of change in health status and social functioning due to substance addiction

OUTCOME TARGET RATING: Maintain at_____ Increase to_____

Substance Addiction Consequences Overall Rating	Severe 1	Substantial 2	Moderate 3	Mild 4	None 5	

INDICATORS:

		Severe 1	Substantial 2	Moderate 3	Mild 4	None 5	
140701	Sustained decrease in physical activity	1	2	3	4	5	NA
140702	Chronic impaired motor function	1	2	3	4	5	NA
140703	Chronic decreased endurance	1	2	3	4	5	NA
140704	Chronic fatigue	1	2	3	4	5	NA
140705	Chronic impaired cognitive function	1	2	3	4	5	NA
140706	Chronic impaired breathing	1	2	3	4	5	NA
140707	Prolonged recovery from illnesses	1	2	3	4	5	NA
140718	Absenteeism from work	1	2	3	4	5	NA
140719	Absenteeism from school	1	2	3	4	5	NA
140720	Difficulty maintaining role performance	1	2	3	4	5	NA
140709	Difficulty maintaining employment	1	2	3	4	5	NA
140710	Difficulty maintaining adequate housing	1	2	3	4	5	NA
140711	Difficulty supporting self financially	1	2	3	4	5	NA
140721	Difficulty maintaining social interactions	1	2	3	4	5	NA
140722	Risk for infection from sharing needles	1	2	3	4	5	NA

S

Continued

		Severe (4+ occurrences)	Substantial (3 occurrences)	Moderate (2 occurrences)	Mild (1 occurrence)	None (no occurrence)	
140712	Traffic accidents within the last year	1	2	3	4	5	NA
140717	Traffic tickets within the last year	1	2	3	4	5	NA
140713	Arrests within the last year	1	2	3	4	5	NA
140714	Emergency room visits within the last year	1	2	3	4	5	NA
140715	Hospitalizations within the last year	1	2	3	4	5	NA

1st edition 1997; Revised 3rd edition 2004; Revised 4th edition

Outcome Content References:

Carruthers, S. (2003). The ins and outs of injection in Western Australia. *Journal of Substance Use, 8*, 11-18.

Leri, F., Bruneau, J., & Stewart, J. (2003). Understanding polydrug use: Review of heroin and cocaine co-use. *Addiction, 98*(1), 7-22.

McCuster, J., Stoddard, A. M., Zapka, J. G., & Lewis, B. F. (1993). Behavioral outcomes of AIDS educational interventions for drug users in short term treatment. *American Journal of Public Health, 83*(10), 1463-1466.

+McLellan, A. T., Luborsky, L., Woody, G. E., & O'Brien, C. P. (1980). An improved diagnostic evaluation instrument for substance abuse patients. *Journal of Nervous and Mental Disease, 168*(1), 26-33.

Millson, P. E., Challacombe, L., Villeneuve, P. J., Fischer, B., Strike, C. J., Myers, T., Shore, R., Hopkins, S., Raftis, S., & Pearson, M. (2004). Self-perceived health among Canadian opiate users: A comparison to the general population and to other chronic disease populations. *Canadian Journal of Public Health, 95*(2), 99-103.

Simons-Morton, D. G., Mullen, P. D., Mains, D. A., Tabak, E. R., & Green, L. W. (1992). Characteristics of controlled studies of patient education and counseling for preventive health behaviors. *Patient Education and Counseling, 19*(2), 174-204.

Talashek, M. L., Gerace, L. M., & Starr, K. L. (1994). The substance abuse pandemic: Determinants to guide interventions. *Public Health Nursing, 11*(2), 131-139.

S

Substance Withdrawal Severity—2108

Domain-Perceived Health (V)
Class-Symptom Status-(V)
Scale(s)-Severe to None (n)

Care Recipient:
Data Source:

Definition: Severity of physical and psychological signs or symptoms caused by withdrawal from addictive drugs, toxic chemicals, tobacco, or alcohol

OUTCOME TARGET RATING: Maintain at_____   Increase to_____

Substance Withdrawal Severity Overall Rating	Severe 1	Substantial 2	Moderate 3	Mild 4	None 5	
INDICATORS:						
210801 Substance-seeking behavior	1	2	3	4	5	NA
210802 Substance cravings	1	2	3	4	5	NA
210803 Irritability	1	2	3	4	5	NA
210804 Agitation	1	2	3	4	5	NA
210805 Emotional outbursts	1	2	3	4	5	NA
210806 Depression	1	2	3	4	5	NA
210807 Hyperreflexia	1	2	3	4	5	NA
210808 Myoclonus	1	2	3	4	5	NA
210809 Fasciculations	1	2	3	4	5	NA
210810 Muscle pain	1	2	3	4	5	NA
210811 Tremors	1	2	3	4	5	NA
210812 Change in vital signs	1	2	3	4	5	NA
210813 Dysrhythmia	1	2	3	4	5	NA
210814 Change in appetite	1	2	3	4	5	NA
210815 Nausea	1	2	3	4	5	NA
210816 Vomiting	1	2	3	4	5	NA
210817 Abdominal pain	1	2	3	4	5	NA
210818 Diarrhea	1	2	3	4	5	NA
210819 Rhinorrhea	1	2	3	4	5	NA
210820 Lacrimation	1	2	3	4	5	NA
210821 Pupil change	1	2	3	4	5	NA
210822 Goose bumps	1	2	3	4	5	NA
210823 Hot and cold flashes	1	2	3	4	5	NA
210824 Photophobia	1	2	3	4	5	NA
210825 Paresthesias	1	2	3	4	5	NA
210826 Abnormal sensitivity to sound	1	2	3	4	5	NA
210827 Headaches	1	2	3	4	5	NA
210828 Yawning	1	2	3	4	5	NA
210829 Impaired concentration	1	2	3	4	5	NA

S

Continued

		Severe	Substantial	Moderate	Mild	None	
210830	Disorientation	1	2	3	4	5	NA
210831	Sleeplessness	1	2	3	4	5	NA
210832	Hallucinations	1	2	3	4	5	NA
210833	Seizures	1	2	3	4	5	NA
210834	Fever	1	2	3	4	5	NA
210835	Chills	1	2	3	4	5	NA
210836	Flushing	1	2	3	4	5	NA
210837	Diaphoresis	1	2	3	4	5	NA
210838	Fatigue	1	2	3	4	5	NA
210839	Weakness	1	2	3	4	5	NA
210840	Alcohol level in blood	1	2	3	4	5	NA
210841	Substance level in blood	1	2	3	4	5	NA
210842	Substance level in urine	1	2	3	4	5	NA

Identify substance(s)_____

4th edition

Outcome Content References:

Boyd, M. A. (Ed.). (2005). *Psychiatric nursing contemporary practice* (3rd ed.). Philadelphia: Lippincott Williams & Wilkins.

Olmedo, R., & Hoffman, R. S. (2000). Withdrawal symptoms. *Emergency Medical Clinics of North America, 18*(2), 273-288.

S

Suffering Severity—2003

Domain-Perceived Health (V)

Class-Symptom Status (V)

Scale(s)-Severe to None (n)

Care Recipient:

Data Source:

Definition: Severity of anguish associated with a distressing symptom, injury, or loss that has potential long-term effects

OUTCOME TARGET RATING: Maintain at_____   Increase to_____

Suffering Severity Overall Rating	Severe 1	Substantial 2	Moderate 3	Mild 4	None 5	

INDICATORS:

200301	Self-absorption	1	2	3	4	5	NA
200302	Depression	1	2	3	4	5	NA
200303	Sadness	1	2	3	4	5	NA
200304	Powerlessness	1	2	3	4	5	NA
200305	Grief	1	2	3	4	5	NA
200306	Guilt	1	2	3	4	5	NA
200307	Hopelessness	1	2	3	4	5	NA
200308	Helplessness	1	2	3	4	5	NA
200309	Worthlessness	1	2	3	4	5	NA
200314	Vulnerability	1	2	3	4	5	NA
200315	Spiritual distress	1	2	3	4	5	NA
200316	Despair	1	2	3	4	5	NA
200319	Loneliness	1	2	3	4	5	NA
200310	Fear of reoccurrence	1	2	3	4	5	NA
200311	Fear of unbearable pain	1	2	3	4	5	NA
200312	Fear of unknown circumstances	1	2	3	4	5	NA
200313	Fear of being alone	1	2	3	4	5	NA
200317	Bitterness toward others	1	2	3	4	5	NA

2nd edition 2000; Revised 3rd edition 2004

Outcome Content References:

Ankri, J., Adrieu, S., Beaufils, B., Grand, A., & Henrard, J. C. (2005). Beyond the global score of the Zarit Burden Interview: useful dimensions for clinicians. *International Journal of Geriatric Psychiatry, 20*(3), 254-260.

Cherny, N. I., Coyle, N., & Foley, K. M. (1994). The treatment of suffering when patients request elective death. *Journal of Palliative Care, 10*(2), 71-79.

Copp, L. A. (1974). The spectrum of suffering. *American Journal of Nursing, 74*(3), 491-495.

Duffy, M. E. (1992). A theoretical and empirical review of the concept of suffering. In P. L. Starck & J. P. McGovern (Eds.), *The hidden dimension of illness: Human suffering* (Pub. No. 15-2451, pp. 291-303). New York: National League for Nursing Press.

Fochtman, D. (2006). The concept of suffering in children and adolescents with cancer. *Journal of Pediatric Oncology Nursing, 23*(2), 92-102.

Hall, P. (2006). Mothers' experiences of postnatal depression: An interpretative phenomenological analysis. *Community Practitioner, 79*(8), 256-260.

Jacob, S. R., & Scandrett-Hobdon, S. (1994). Mothers grieving the death of a child: Case reports of maternal grief. *The Nurse Practitioner, 19*(7), 60-65.

Continued

Mako, C., Galek, K., & Poppito, S. R. (2006). Spiritual pain among patients with advanced cancer in palliative care. *Journal of Palliative Medicine, 9*(5), 1106-1113.

Mount, B. M. (1984). Psychological and social aspects of cancer pain. In P. D. Wall & R. Melzack (Eds.), *Textbook of pain* (pp. 460-471). New York: Churchill Livingstone.

Price, D. D., & Harkins, S. W. (1992). Psychophysical approaches to pain measurement and assessment. In D. C. Turk & R. Melzack (Eds.), *Handbook of pain assessment* (pp. 111-134). New York: The Guilford Press.

Steeves, R. H., Kahn, D. L., & Benoliel, J. Q. (1990). Nurses' interpretation of the suffering of their patients. *Western Journal of Nursing Research, 12*(6), 714-731.

S

Suicide Self-Restraint—1408

Domain-Psychosocial Health (III)

Class-Self-Control (O)

Scale(s)-Never demonstrated to Consistently demonstrated (m)

Care Recipient:

Data Source:

Definition: Personal actions to refrain from gestures and attempts at killing self

OUTCOME TARGET RATING: Maintain at_____   Increase to_____

Suicide Self-Restraint Overall Rating		Never demonstrated 1	Rarely demonstrated 2	Sometimes demonstrated 3	Often demonstrated 4	Consistently demonstrated 5	
INDICATORS:							
140801	Expresses feelings	1	2	3	4	5	NA
140815	Expresses sense of hope	1	2	3	4	5	NA
140802	Maintains connectedness in relationships	1	2	3	4	5	NA
140823	Obtains assistance as needed	1	2	3	4	5	NA
140804	Verbalizes suicidal ideas	1	2	3	4	5	NA
140805	Control impulses	1	2	3	4	5	NA
140806	Refrains from gathering means for suicide	1	2	3	4	5	NA
140807	Refrains from giving away possessions	1	2	3	4	5	NA
140816	Refrains from inflicting serious injury	1	2	3	4	5	NA
140809	Refrains from using non-prescribed mood-altering substances	1	2	3	4	5	NA
140810	Discloses plan for suicide if present	1	2	3	4	5	NA
140811	Upholds suicide contract	1	2	3	4	5	NA
140812	Maintains self-control without supervision	1	2	3	4	5	NA
140813	Refrains from attempting suicide	1	2	3	4	5	NA
140824	Obtains treatment for depression	1	2	3	4	5	NA
140825	Obtains treatment for substance abuse	1	2	3	4	5	NA

S

Continued

		Never demonstrated	Rarely demonstrated	Sometimes demonstrated	Often demonstrated	Consistently demonstrated	
140819	Reports adequate pain control for chronic pain	1	2	3	4	5	NA
140826	Uses suicide prevention resources	1	2	3	4	5	NA
140827	Uses social support group	1	2	3	4	5	NA
140821	Uses available mental health care services	1	2	3	4	5	NA
140822	Plans for future	1	2	3	4	5	NA

1st edition 1997; Revised 2nd edition 2000; Revised 3rd edition 2004; Revised 4th edition

Outcome Content References:

Aubert, P., Daigle, M. S., & Dagile, J. (2004). Cultural traits and immigration: Hostility and suicidality in Chinese Canadian students. *Transcultural Psychiatry, 41*(4), 514-532.

Conwell, Y. (1997). Management of suicidal behavior in the elderly. *The Psychiatric Clinics of North America, 20*(3), 667-683.

Cugino, A., Markovich, E. I., Rosenblatt, S., Jarjoura, D., Blend, D., & Whittier, F. C. (1992). Searching for a pattern: Repeat suicide attempts. *Journal of Psychosocial Nursing, 30*(3), 23-25.

Forster, P. (1994). Accurate assessment of short-term suicide risk in a crisis. *Psychiatric Annals, 24*(11), 571-578.

Hirschfeld, R. M. A., & Russell, J. M. (1997). Assessment and treatment of suicidal patients. *The New England Journal of Medicine, 337*(13), 910-915.

Ingram, T. N. (2001). Risk for violence: Self-directed or directed at others. In M. Maas, K. Buckwalter, M. Hardy, T. Tripp-Reimer, M. Titler, & J. Specht (Eds.), *Nursing care of older adults: Diagnoses, outcomes & interventions* (pp. 696-705). St. Louis: Mosby.

+Ivanoff, A., Joon Jang, S., Smyth, N. J., & Linehan, M. M. (1994). Fewer reasons for staying alive when you are thinking of killing yourself: The Brief Reasons for Living Inventory. *Journal of Psychopathology and Behavioral Assessment, 16*(1), 1-13.

Josepho, S. A., & Plutchek, R. (1994). Stress, coping, and suicide risk in psychiatric inpatients. *Suicide and Life-Threatening Behavior, 24*(1), 48-57.

+Linehan, M. M., Goodstein, J. L., Nielsen, S. L., & Chiles, J. A. (1983). Reasons for staying alive when you are thinking of killing yourself: The Reasons for Living Inventory. *Journal of Consulting and Clinical Psychology, 51*(2), 276-286, 484-485.

Lipshitz, A. (1995). Suicide prevention in young adults (age 18-30). *Suicide and Life-Threatening Behavior, 25*(1), 155-169.

Mellick, E., Buckwalter, K. C., & Stolley, J. M. (1992). Suicide among elderly white men: Development of a profile. *Journal of Psychosocial Nursing, 30*(2), 29-34.

Robie, D., Edgemon-Hill, E. J., Phelps, B., Schmitz, C., & Laughlin, J. A. (1999). Suicide prevention protocol: One hospital's nursing protocol for identification and intervention. *American Journal of Nursing, 99*(12), 53, 55, 57.

Valente, S. M., & Trainor, D. (1998). Rational suicide among patients who are terminally ill. *Official Journal of the Association of Operating Room Nurses, 68*(2), 252-255, 257-258, 260-264.

S

Swallowing Status—1010

Domain-Physiologic Health (II)

Class-Digestion & Nutrition (K)

Scale(s)-Severely compromised to Not compromised (a) and Severe to None (n)

Care Recipient:

Data Source:

Definition: Safe passage of fluids and/or solids from the mouth to the stomach

OUTCOME TARGET RATING: Maintain at_____   Increase to_____

Swallowing Status Overall Rating	Severely compromised 1	Substantially compromised 2	Moderately compromised 3	Mildly compromised 4	Not compromised 5	
INDICATORS:						
101001	Maintains food in mouth	1	2	3	4	5	NA
101002	Handles oral secretions	1	2	3	4	5	NA
101003	Saliva production	1	2	3	4	5	NA
101004	Chewing ability	1	2	3	4	5	NA
101005	Delivery of bolus to hypopharynx is timed with swallow reflex	1	2	3	4	5	NA
101006	Ability to clear oral cavity	1	2	3	4	5	NA
101007	Timely bolus formation	1	2	3	4	5	NA
101008	Number of swallows appropriate for bolus size/texture	1	2	3	4	5	NA
101009	Meal duration with respect to amount consumed	1	2	3	4	5	NA
101010	Timely swallow reflex	1	2	3	4	5	NA
101015	Maintains neutral head and trunk position	1	2	3	4	5	NA
101016	Food acceptance	1	2	3	4	5	NA
101018	Swallow study findings	1	2	3	4	5	NA

		Severe	Substantial	Moderate	Mild	None	
101011	Changes in voice quality	1	2	3	4	5	NA
101012	Choking	1	2	3	4	5	NA
101020	Coughing	1	2	3	4	5	NA
101021	Gagging	1	2	3	4	5	NA
101013	Increased swallow effort	1	2	3	4	5	NA
101014	Gastric reflux	1	2	3	4	5	NA
101017	Discomfort with swallowing	1	2	3	4	5	NA

2nd edition 2000; Revised 3rd edition 2004

S

Outcome Content References:

Arvedson, J., & Brodsky, L. (Eds.). (2002). *Pediatric swallowing and feeding: Assessment and management* (2nd ed.). San Diego: Singular Publishing Group.

Bosch, J., Van Dyke, D., Smith, S., & Poulton, S. (1997). The role of medical condition in the exacerbation of self-injurious behavior: An exploratory study. *Mental Retardation, 35*(2), 124-130.

Christensen, J. R. (1989). Developmental approach to pediatric neurogenic dysphagia. *Dysphagia, 3*(3), 131-134.

Feinberg, M. (1997). The effects of medication on swallowing. In B. Sonies (Ed.), *Dysphagia: A Continuum of Care* (pp. 107-120). Gaithersburg, MD: Aspen.

Hendrix, T. R. (1993). Art and science of history taking in the patient with difficulty swallowing. *Dysphagia, 8*(2), 69-73.

The Joanna Briggs Institute for Evidence Based Nursing and Midwifery. (2000). Identification and nursing management of dysphagia in adults with neurological impairment. *Best Practice, 4*(2), Blackwell Science-Asia, Australia.

Kramer, S. S., & Eicher, P. M. (1993). The evaluation of pediatric feeding abnormalities. *Dysphagia, 8*(3), 215-24.

Langmore, S. (2000). *Endoscopic evaluation and treatment of swallowing disorders*. New York: Thieme Medical.

Lespargot, A., Langevin, M., Muller, S., & Guillemont, S. (1993). Swallowing disturbances associated with drooling in cerebral-palsied children. *Developmental Medicine and Child Neurology, 35*(4), 298-304.

Morris, S. E. (1989). Development of oral-motor skills in the neurologically impaired child receiving non-oral feedings. *Dysphagia, 3*(3), 135-154.

Ramsay, M., Gisel, E. G., & Boutry, M. (1993). Non-organic failure to thrive: Growth failure secondary to feeding skills disorder. *Developmental Medicine and Child Neurology, 35*(4), 285-297.

Tuchman, D., & Walter, R. (Eds.). (1994). *Disorders of feeding and swallowing in infants and children*. San Diego: Singular Publishing Group.

Wolf, L. S., & Glass, R. P. (1992). *Feeding and swallowing disorders in infancy*. Tucson: Therapy Skill Builders.

S

Swallowing Status: Esophageal Phase—1011

Domain-Physiologic Health (II)

Class-Digestion & Nutrition (K)

Scale(s)-Severely compromised to Not compromised (a) and Severe to None (n)

Care Recipient:

Data Source:

Definition: Safe passage of fluids and/or solids from the pharynx to the stomach

OUTCOME TARGET RATING: Maintain at_____   Increase to_____

Swallowing Status: Esophageal Phase Overall Rating	Severely compromised 1	Substantially compromised 2	Moderately compromised 3	Mildly compromised 4	Not compromised 5	
INDICATORS:						
101106 Maintains neutral head and neck position	1	2	3	4	5	NA
101114 Food acceptance	1	2	3	4	5	NA
101115 Volume acceptance	1	2	3	4	5	NA
101116 Swallow study findings: esophageal phase	1	2	3	4	5	NA

	Severe	Substantial	Moderate	Mild	None	
101101 Choking with swallowing	1	2	3	4	5	NA
101118 Coughing with swallowing	1	2	3	4	5	NA
101102 Gastric reflux	1	2	3	4	5	NA
101103 Epigastric pain	1	2	3	4	5	NA
101104 Discomfort with swallowing	1	2	3	4	5	NA
101108 Nighttime coughing	1	2	3	4	5	NA
101109 Nighttime vomiting	1	2	3	4	5	NA
101119 Nighttime choking	1	2	3	4	5	NA
101110 Repetitive swallowing	1	2	3	4	5	NA
101111 Hematemesis	1	2	3	4	5	NA
101112 Acidic breath odor	1	2	3	4	5	NA
101113 Bruxism	1	2	3	4	5	NA

2nd edition 2000; Revised 3rd edition 2004

Outcome Content References:

Arvedson, J., & Brodsky, L. (Eds.). (2002). *Pediatric swallowing and feeding: Assessment and management* (2nd ed.). San Diego: Singular Publishing Group.

Bosch, J., Van Dyke, D., Smith, S., & Poulton, S. (1997). The role of medical condition in the exacerbation of self injurious behavior: An exploratory study. *Mental Retardation, 35*(2), 124-130.

Christensen, J. R. (1989). Developmental approach to neurogenic pediatric dysphagia. *Dysphagia, 3*(3), 131-134.

Feinberg, M. (1997). The effects of medication on swallowing. In B. Sonies (Ed.), *Dysphagia: A continuum of care* (pp. 107-120). Gaithersburg, MD: Aspen.

Hendrix, T. R. (1993). Art and science of history taking in the patient with difficulty swallowing. *Dysphagia, 8*(2), 69-73.

Continued

S

Kramer, S., & Eicher, P. M. (1993). The evaluation of pediatric feeding abnormalities. *Dysphagia, 8*(3), 215-224.

Langmore, S. (2000). *Endoscopic evaluation and treatment of swallowing disorders*. New York: Thieme Medical Publishers.

Lespargot, A., Langevin, M., Muller, S., & Guillemont, S. (1993). Swallowing disturbances associated with drooling in cerebral-palsied children. *Developmental Medicine and Child Neurology, 35*(4), 298-304.

Morris, S. (1989). Development of oral-motor skills in the neurologically impaired child receiving non-oral feedings. *Dysphagia, 3*(3), 135-154.

Ramsay, M., Gisel, E. G., & Boutry, M. (1993). Non-organic failure to thrive: Growth failure secondary to feeding skills disorder. *Developmental Medicine and Child Neurology, 35*(4), 285-297.

Tuchman, D., & Walter, R. (Eds.). (1994). *Disorders of feeding and swallowing in infants and children*. San Diego: Singular Publishing.

Wolf, L. S., & Glass, R. P. (1992). *Feeding and swallowing disorders in infancy*. Tucson: Therapy Skill Builders.

S

Swallowing Status: Oral Phase—1012

Domain-Physiologic Health (II)   *Care Recipient:*

Class-Digestion & Nutrition (K)   *Data Source:*

Scale(s)-Severely compromised to Not compromised (a) and Severe to None (n)

Definition: Preparation, containment, and posterior movement of fluids and/or solids in the mouth

OUTCOME TARGET RATING: Maintain at_____   Increase to_____

Swallowing Status: Oral Phase Overall Rating	Severely compromised 1	Substantially compromised 2	Moderately compromised 3	Mildly compromised 4	Not compromised 5	
INDICATORS:						
101201 Maintains food in mouth	1	2	3	4	5	NA
101202 Handles oral secretions	1	2	3	4	5	NA
101203 Bolus formation	1	2	3	4	5	NA
101204 Timely bolus formation	1	2	3	4	5	NA
101205 Chewing ability	1	2	3	4	5	NA
101206 Delivery of bolus to hypopharynx timed with swallow reflex	1	2	3	4	5	NA
101207 Ability to clear oral cavity	1	2	3	4	5	NA
101209 Lip closure	1	2	3	4	5	NA
101210 Number of swallows appropriate for bolus size/ texture	1	2	3	4	5	NA
101211 Nippling efficiency	1	2	3	4	5	NA
101212 Rate of food consumption	1	2	3	4	5	NA
101214 Gag reflex						NA
101215 Swallow study findings: oral phase	1	2	3	4	5	NA

	Severe	Substantial	Moderate	Mild	None	
101208 Coughing before swallowing	1	2	3	4	5	NA
101217 Choking before swallowing	1	2	3	4	5	NA
101218 Gagging before swallowing	1	2	3	4	5	NA
101213 Nasal reflux	1	2	3	4	5	NA

2nd edition 2000; Revised 3rd edition 2004

S

Continued

Outcome Content References:

Arvedson, J., & Brodsky, L. (Eds.). (2002). *Pediatric swallowing and feeding: Assessment and management* (2nd ed.). San Diego: Singular Publishing Group.

Bosch, J., Van Dyke, D., Smith, S., & Poulton, S. (1997). The role of medical condition in the exacerbation of self injurious behavior: An exploratory study. *Mental Retardation, 35*(2), 124-130.

Christensen, J. R. (1989). Developmental approach to neurogenic pediatric dysphagia. *Dysphagia, 3*(3), 131-134.

Feinberg, M. (1997). The effects of medication on swallowing. In B. Sonies (Ed.), *Dysphagia: A continuum of care* (pp. 107-120). Gaithersburg, MD: Aspen.

Hendrix, T. R. (1993). Art and science of history taking in the patient with difficulty swallowing. *Dysphagia, 8*(2), 69-73.

Kramer, S., & Eicher, P. M. (1993). The evaluation of pediatric feeding abnormalities. *Dysphagia, 8*(3), 215-224.

Langmore, S. (2000). *Endoscopic evaluation and treatment of swallowing disorders.* New York: Thieme Medical Publishers.

Lespargot, A., Langevin, M., Muller, S., & Guillemont, S. (1993). Swallowing disturbances associated with drooling in cerebral-palsied children. *Developmental Medicine and Child Neurology, 35*(4), 298-304.

Morris, S. (1989). Development of oral-motor skills in the neurologically impaired child receiving non-oral feedings. *Dysphagia, 3*(3), 135-154.

Ramsay, M., Gisel, E. G., & Boutry, M. (1993). Non-organic failure to thrive: Growth failure secondary to feeding skills disorder. *Developmental Medicine and Child Neurology, 35*(4), 285-297.

Tuchman, D., & Walter, R. (Eds.). (1994). *Disorders of feeding and swallowing in infants and children.* San Diego: Singular Publishing Group.

Wolf, L. S., & Glass, R. P. (1992). *Feeding and swallowing disorders in infancy.* Tucson: Therapy Skill Builders.

S

Swallowing Status: Pharyngeal Phase—1013

Domain-Physiologic Health (II)   Care Recipient:

Class-Digestion & Nutrition (K)   Data Source:

Scale(s)-Severely compromised to Not compromised (a) and Severe to None (n)

Definition: Safe passage of fluids and/or solids from the mouth to the esophagus

OUTCOME TARGET RATING: Maintain at_____   Increase to_____

Swallowing Status: Pharyngeal Phase Overall Rating	Severely compromised 1	Substantially compromised 2	Moderately compromised 3	Mildly compromised 4	Not compromised 5	
INDICATORS:						
101301 Timely swallow reflex	1	2	3	4	5	NA
101304 Number of swallows appropriate for bolus size/ texture	1	2	3	4	5	NA
101305 Maintains neutral head and neck position	1	2	3	4	5	NA
101307 Laryngeal elevation	1	2	3	4	5	NA
101311 Food acceptance	1	2	3	4	5	NA
101312 Swallow study findings: pharyngeal phase	1	2	3	4	5	NA

	Severe	Substantial	Moderate	Mild	None	
101302 Changes in voice quality	1	2	3	4	5	NA
101303 Choking	1	2	3	4	5	NA
101314 Coughing	1	2	3	4	5	NA
101315 Gagging	1	2	3	4	5	NA
101306 Increased swallow effort	1	2	3	4	5	NA
101310 Nasal reflux	1	2	3	4	5	NA
101316 Aspirations	1	2	3	4	5	NA

2nd edition 2000; Revised 3rd edition 2004

S

Outcome Content References:

Arvedson, J., & Brodsky, L. (Eds.). (2002). *Pediatric swallowing and feeding: Assessment and management* (2nd ed.). San Diego: Singular Publishing Group.

Bosch, J., Van Dyke, D., Smith, S., & Poulton, S. (1997). The role of medical condition in the exacerbation of self injurious behavior: An exploratory study. *Mental Retardation, 35*(2), 124-130.

Christensen, J. R. (1989). Developmental approach to neurogenic pediatric dysphagia. *Dysphagia, 3*(3), 131-134.

Feinberg, M. (1997). The effects of medication on swallowing. In B. Sonies (Ed.), *Dysphagia: A continuum of care* (pp. 107-120). Gaithersburg, MD: Aspen.

Hendrix, T. R. (1993). Art and science of history taking in the patient with difficulty swallowing. *Dysphagia, 8*(2), 69-73.

Kramer, S., & Eicher, P. M. (1993). The evaluation of pediatric feeding abnormalities. *Dysphagia, 8*(3), 215-24.

Langmore, S. (2000). *Endoscopic evaluation and treatment of swallowing disorders.* New York: Thieme Medical Publishers.

Continued

Lespargot, A., Langevin, M., Muller, S., & Guillemont, S. (1993). Swallowing disturbances associated with drooling in cerebral-palsied children. *Developmental Medicine and Child Neurology, 35*(4), 298-304.

Morris, S. (1989). Development of oral-motor skills in the neurologically impaired child receiving non-oral feedings. *Dysphagia, 3*(3), 135-154.

Ramsay, M., Gisel, E. G., & Boutry, M. (1993). Non-organic failure to thrive: Growth failure secondary to feeding skills disorder. *Developmental Medicine and Child Neurology, 35*(4), 285-297.

Tuchman, D., & Walter, R. (Eds.). (1994). *Disorders of feeding and swallowing in infants and children.* San Diego: Singular Publishing Group.

Wolf, L. S., & Glass, R. P. (1992). *Feeding and swallowing disorders in infancy.* Tucson: Therapy Skill Builders.

S

Symptom Control—1608

Domain-Health Knowledge & Behavior (IV)

Class-Health Behavior (Q)

Scale(s)-Never demonstrated to Consistently demonstrated (m)

Care Recipient:

Data Source:

Definition: Personal actions to minimize perceived adverse changes in physical and emotional functioning

OUTCOME TARGET RATING: Maintain at_____   Increase to_____

Symptom Control Overall Rating	Never demonstrated 1	Rarely demonstrated 2	Sometimes demonstrated 3	Often demonstrated 4	Consistently demonstrated 5	
INDICATORS:						
160801 Monitors symptom onset	1	2	3	4	5	NA
160802 Monitors symptom persistence	1	2	3	4	5	NA
160803 Monitors symptom severity	1	2	3	4	5	NA
160804 Monitors symptom frequency	1	2	3	4	5	NA
160805 Monitors symptom variation	1	2	3	4	5	NA
160806 Uses preventive measures	1	2	3	4	5	NA
160807 Uses symptom relief measures	1	2	3	4	5	NA
160813 Obtains health care when warning signs occur	1	2	3	4	5	NA
160809 Uses available resources	1	2	3	4	5	NA
160810 Uses diary to monitor symptoms over time	1	2	3	4	5	NA
160811 Reports symptoms controlled	1	2	3	4	5	NA

1st edition 1997; Revised 2nd edition 2000; Revised 3rd edition 2004; Revised 4th edition

Outcome Content References:

Coleman, C. L., Holzemer, W. L., Eller, L. S., Corless, I., Reynolds, N., Nokes, K. M., Kemppainen, J. K., Dole, P., Kirksey, K., Seficik, L. Nicholas, P., & Hamilton, M. J. (2006). Gender differences in use of prayer as a self-care strategy for managing symptoms in African Americans living with HIV/AIDS. *Journal of the Association of Nurses in AIDS Care, 17*(4), 16-23.

Hegyvary, S. T. (1993). Patient care outcomes related to management of symptoms. In J. J. Fitzpatrick & J. S. Stevenson (Eds.), *Annual review of nursing research,* (Vol. 11, pp. 145-168). New York: Springer.

Kercsmar, C. M., Dearborn, D. G., Schluchter, M., Xue, L., Kirchner, H. L., Sobolewski, J., Greenberg, S. J., Vesper, S. J., & Allan, T. (2006). Reduction in asthma morbidity in children as a result of home remediation aimed at moisture sources. *Environmental Health Perspectives, 114*(10), 1574-1580.

Kim, S. H., Oh, E. G., & Lee, W. H. (2006). Symptom experience, psychological distress, and quality of life in Korean patients with liver cirrhosis: A cross-sectional survey. *International Journal of Nursing Studies, 43*(8), 1047-1056.

+McCorkle, R., & Benoliel, J. Q. (1983). Symptom distress, current concerns, and mood disturbances after diagnosis of life-threatening disease. *Social Science Medicine, 17*(7), 431-438.

Continued

S

+McCorkle, R., & Young, K. (1978). Development of a symptom distress scale. *Cancer Nursing, 1*(5), 373-378.

Segrin, T., Dorros, S. M., Meek, P., & Lopez, A. M. (2007). Depression and anxiety in women with breast cancer and their partners. *Nursing Research, 56*(1), 44-53.

Sherbourne, C. D., Allen, H. M., Kamberg, C. J., & Wells, K. B. (1992). Physical/psychophysiological symptoms measure. In A. L. Stewart & J. E. Ware, Jr. (Eds.), *Measuring functioning and well-being* (pp. 261-272). Durham, NC: Duke University Press.

Strauss, A. L., Corbin, J., Fagerhaugh, S., Glaser, B. G., Maines, D., Suczek, B., & Wiener, C. L. (1984). Symptom control. In *Chronic illness and the quality of life* (2nd ed., pp. 49-59). St. Louis: Mosby.

White, M. A., & Grilo, C. M. (2007). Symptom severity in obese women with binge eating disorder as a function of smoking history. *International Journal of Eating Disorders, 40*(1), 77-81.

Williams, P. D., Piamjariyakul, U., Ducey, K., Badura, J., Boltz, K. D., Olberding, K., Wingate, A., & Williams, A. R. (2006). Cancer treatment, symptom monitoring, and self-care in adults: Pilot study. *Cancer Nursing, 29*(5), 347-355.

S

Symptom Severity—2103

Domain-Perceived Health (V)

Class-Symptom Status (V)

Scale(s)-Severe to None (n)

Care Recipient:

Data Source:

Definition: Severity of perceived adverse changes in physical, emotional, and social functioning

OUTCOME TARGET RATING: Maintain at_____   Increase to_____

Symptom Severity Overall Rating	Severe 1	Substantial 2	Moderate 3	Mild 4	None 5	
INDICATORS:						
210301 Symptom intensity	1	2	3	4	5	NA
210302 Symptom frequency	1	2	3	4	5	NA
210303 Symptom persistence	1	2	3	4	5	NA
210304 Associated discomfort	1	2	3	4	5	NA
210305 Associated restlessness	1	2	3	4	5	NA
210306 Associated fear	1	2	3	4	5	NA
210307 Associated anxiety	1	2	3	4	5	NA
210308 Impaired physical mobility	1	2	3	4	5	NA
210309 Impaired role performance	1	2	3	4	5	NA
210310 Impaired interpersonal relationships	1	2	3	4	5	NA
210311 Impaired mood	1	2	3	4	5	NA
210312 Impaired life enjoyment	1	2	3	4	5	NA
210313 Inadequate sleep	1	2	3	4	5	NA
210316 Sleep deficit	1	2	3	4	5	NA
210314 Loss of appetite	1	2	3	4	5	NA

1st edition 1997; Revised 3rd edition 2004

Outcome Content References:

Banes, S., Gott, M., Payne, S., Parker, C., Seamark, D., Gariballa, S., & Small, N. (2006). Prevalence of symptoms in a community based sample of heart failure patients. *Journal of Pain & Symptom Management, 32*(3), 208-216.

Docherty, S. L., Sandelowski, M., & Preisser, J. S. (2006). Three months in the symptom life of a teenage girl undergoing treatment for cancer. *Research in Nursing & Health, 29*(4), 294-310.

Hartford, M., Karlson, B. W., Sjolin, M., Holmberg, S., & Herlitz, J. (1993). Symptoms, thoughts, and environmental factors in suspected acute myocardial infarction. *Heart & Lung, 22*(1), 64-70.

Hegyvary, S. T. (1993). Patient care outcomes related to management of symptoms. In J. J. Fitzpatrick & J. S. Stevenson (Eds.), *Annual review of nursing research* (Vol. 11, pp. 145-168). New York: Springer.

+McCorkle, R., & Benoliel, J. Q. (1983). Symptom distress, current concerns, and mood disturbances after diagnosis of life-threatening disease. *Social Science Medicine, 17*(7), 431-438.

+McCorkle, R., & Young, K. (1978). Development of a symptom distress scale. *Cancer Nursing, 1*(5), 373-378.

Payne, J. K., Piper, B. F., Rabinowitz, I., & Zimmerman, M. B. (2006). Biomarkers, fatigue, sleep, and depressive symptoms in women with breast cancer: A pilot study. *Oncology Nursing Forum, 33*(4), 775-783.

Sherbourne, C. D., Allen, H. M., Kamberg, C. J., & Wells, K. B. (1992). Physical/psychophysiologic symptoms measure. In A. L. Stewart & J. E. Ware, Jr. (Eds.), *Measure functioning and well-being* (pp. 261-272). Durham, NC: Duke University Press.

Strauss, A. L., Corbin, J., Fagerhaugh, S., Glaser, B. G., Maines, D., Suczek, B., & Wiener, C. L. (1984). Symptom control. In *Chronic illness and the quality of life* (2nd ed., pp. 49-59). St. Louis: Mosby.

S

Symptom Severity: Perimenopause—2104

Domain-Perceived Health (V)

Class-Symptom Status (V)

Scale(s)-Severe to None (n)

Care Recipient:

Data Source:

Definition: Severity of symptoms caused by declining hormonal levels

OUTCOME TARGET RATING: Maintain at_____   Increase to_____

Symptom Severity: Perimenopause Overall Rating	Severe 1	Substantial 2	Moderate 3	Mild 4	None 5	

INDICATORS:

210401	Menstrual irregularity	1	2	3	4	5	NA
210402	Abdominal cramps	1	2	3	4	5	NA
210403	Hot flashes	1	2	3	4	5	NA
210404	Night sweats	1	2	3	4	5	NA
210405	Vaginal dryness	1	2	3	4	5	NA
210406	Mood swings	1	2	3	4	5	NA
210407	Menstrual flow	1	2	3	4	5	NA
210408	Insomnia	1	2	3	4	5	NA
210409	Fatigue	1	2	3	4	5	NA
210410	Musculoskeletal pain	1	2	3	4	5	NA
210411	Weight gain	1	2	3	4	5	NA
210412	Decreased libido	1	2	3	4	5	NA
210413	Heart palpitations	1	2	3	4	5	NA
210414	Vertigo	1	2	3	4	5	NA
210415	Memory changes	1	2	3	4	5	NA

2nd edition 2000; Revised 3rd edition 2004

Outcome Content References:

Alexander, L. L., & LaRosa, J. (1994). *New dimensions in women's health.* Sudbury, MA: Jones and Bartlett.

Andrews, G. *Women's sexual health* (2nd ed.). London: Bailliere Tindall.

Clark, A. J., Flowers, J., Boots, L., & Shettar, S. (1995). Sleep disturbance in mid-life women. *Journal of Advanced Nursing, 22*(3), 562-568.

Dannels, A., & Charlifue, S. (2004). The perimenopause experience for women with spinal cord injuries. *SCI Nursing, 21*(1), 9-113.

Fogel, C. I., & Woods, N. F. (Eds.). (1995). *Women's health care: A comprehensive handbook.* Thousand Oaks: Sage.

Heger, M., Ventskovskey, B. M., Borzenko, I., Kneis, K. C., Rettengberger, R., Kaszkin-Bettag, M., & Heger, P. W. (2006). Efficacy and safety of a special extract of Rheum rhaponticum (ERr 731) in perimenopausal women with climacteric complaints: A 12-week randomized, double-blind, placebo-controlled trial. *Menopause, 13*(5), 744-759.

Logothetis, M. L. (1991). Women's decisions about estrogen replacement therapy. *Western Journal of Nursing Research, 13*(4), 458-474.

Lyndaker, C., & Hulton, L. (2004). The influence of age on symptoms of perimenopause. *Journal of Obstetric, Gynecologic, & Neonatal Nursing, 33*(3), 340-347.

Richards, M., Rubinow, D. R., Daly, R. C., & Schmidt, P. J. (2006). Premenstrual symptoms and perimenopausal depression. *American Journal of Psychiatry, 163*(1), 133-137.

Woods, N. F., & Mitchell, E. S. (1996). Patterns of depressed mood in midlife women: Observations from the Seattle Midlife Women's Health Study. *Research in Nursing and Health, 19*(2), 111-123.

S

Symptom Severity: Premenstrual Syndrome (PMS)—2105

Domain-Perceived Health (V)

Class-Symptom Status (V)

Scale(s)-Severe to None (n)

Care Recipient:

Data Source:

Definition: Severity of symptoms caused by cyclic hormonal fluctuations

OUTCOME TARGET RATING: Maintain at_____   Increase to_____

Symptom Severity: Premenstrual Syndrome (PMS) Overall Rating	Severe 1	Substantial 2	Moderate 3	Mild 4	None 5	
INDICATORS:						
210501 Abdominal bloating	1	2	3	4	5	NA
210502 Abdominal cramps	1	2	3	4	5	NA
210503 Disrupted bowel patterns	1	2	3	4	5	NA
210504 Decreased urine output	1	2	3	4	5	NA
210505 Acne	1	2	3	4	5	NA
210506 Anxiety	1	2	3	4	5	NA
210507 Backache	1	2	3	4	5	NA
210508 Breast tenderness	1	2	3	4	5	NA
210509 Decreased energy	1	2	3	4	5	NA
210510 Depression	1	2	3	4	5	NA
210511 Fluid retention	1	2	3	4	5	NA
210512 Food cravings	1	2	3	4	5	NA
210513 Headaches	1	2	3	4	5	NA
210514 Insomnia	1	2	3	4	5	NA
210515 Irritability	1	2	3	4	5	NA
210516 Mood swings	1	2	3	4	5	NA
210517 Nausea	1	2	3	4	5	NA
210518 Vertigo	1	2	3	4	5	NA
210519 Vomiting	1	2	3	4	5	NA

2nd edition 2000; Revised 3rd edition 2004

Outcome Content References:

Alexander, L. L., & LaRosa, J. (1994). *New dimensions in women's health*. Sudbury, MA: Jones and Bartlett.

Carter, J., & Verhoef, M. J. (1994). Efficacy of self-help and alternative treatments of premenstrual syndrome. *Women's Health Issues, 4*(3), 130-137.

Fogel, C. I., & Woods, N. F. (Eds.). (1995). *Women's health care: A comprehensive handbook*. Thousand Oaks: Sage.

Freeman, E. W., Kroll, R., Rapkin, A., Pearlstein, T., Brown, C., Parsey, K., Zhang, P., Patel, H., & Foegh, M. (2001). Evaluation of a unique oral contraceptive in the treatment of premenstrual dysphoric disorder. *Journal of Women's Health & Gender-Based Medicine, 10*(6), 561-569.

Lewis, L. L. (1995). One year in the life of a woman with premenstrual syndrome: A case study. *Nursing Research, 44*(2), 111-116.

Mitchell, E. S., Woods, N. F., & Lentz, M. J. (1994). Differentiation of women with three premenstrual symptom patterns. *Nursing Research, 43*(1), 25-30.

Richards, M., Rubinow, D. R., Daly, R. C., & Schmidt, P. J. (2006). Premenstrual symptoms and perimenopausal depression. *American Journal of Psychiatry, 163*(1), 133-137.

S

Continued

Taylor, D. L. (1994). Evaluating therapeutic change in symptom severity at the level of the individual woman experiencing severe PMS. *Image—The Journal of Nursing Scholarship, 26*(1), 25-33.

Woods, N. F., Lentz, M., Mitchell, E., Taylor, D., & Lee, K. (1986). *The daily health diary. The prevalence of PMS: Final report* (NV01054). Washington, DC: Division of Nursing U.S. Public Health Services, U.S. Department of Health and Human Services.

Woods, N. F., Mitchell, E. S., & Lentz, M. F. (1995). Social pathways to premenstrual symptoms. *Research in Nursing & Health, 18*(3), 225-237.

S

Systemic Toxin Clearance: Dialysis—2302

Domain-Physiologic Health (II)

Class-Therapeutic Response (a)

Scale(s)-Severe deviation from normal range to No deviation from normal range (b) and Severe to None (n)

Care Recipient:

Data Source:

Definition: Clearance of toxins from the body with peritoneal dialysis or hemodialysis

OUTCOME TARGET RATING: Maintain at_____   Increase to_____

Systemic Toxin Clearance: Dialysis Overall Rating	Severe deviation from normal range 1	Substantial deviation from normal range 2	Moderate deviation from normal range 3	Mild deviation from normal range 4	No deviation from normal range 5	
INDICATORS:						
230212 Urea reduction ratio (URR) ≥ 65%	1	2	3	4	5	NA
230216 Blood pressure	1	2	3	4	5	NA
230214 Serum potassium	1	2	3	4	5	NA
230217 Serum sodium	1	2	3	4	5	NA
230220 Serum creatinine	1	2	3	4	5	NA
230221 Serum calcium	1	2	3	4	5	NA
230222 Serum bicarbonate	1	2	3	4	5	NA
230223 Serum magnesium	1	2	3	4	5	NA
230224 Serum phosphorus	1	2	3	4	5	NA
230225 Creatinine clearance	1	2	3	4	5	NA
230226 Blood urea nitrogen to creatinine ratio	1	2	3	4	5	NA

	Severe	Substantial	Moderate	Mild	None	
230203 Nausea	1	2	3	4	5	NA
230204 Vomiting	1	2	3	4	5	NA
230205 Weakness	1	2	3	4	5	NA
230206 Malaise	1	2	3	4	5	NA
230207 Anorexia	1	2	3	4	5	NA
230208 Insomnia	1	2	3	4	5	NA
230209 Edema	1	2	3	4	5	NA
230210 Dizziness	1	2	3	4	5	NA
230211 Pruritus	1	2	3	4	5	NA
230218 Ascites	1	2	3	4	5	NA
230219 Muscle cramps	1	2	3	4	5	NA
230227 Anemia	1	2	3	4	5	NA
230228 Weight gain	1	2	3	4	5	NA
230229 Impaired concentration	1	2	3	4	5	NA

2nd edition 2000; Revised 3rd edition 2004; Revised 4th edition

S

Continued

Outcome Content References:

Broscious, S. K., & Castagnola, J. (2006). Chronic kidney disease: Acute manifestations and role of critical care nurses. *Critical Care Nurse, 26*(4), 17-28.

Brundage, D. J. (1992). *Renal disorders*. St. Louis: Mosby.

Gutch, C. F., Stoner, M. H., & Corea, A. L. (1999). *Review of hemodialysis for nurses and dialysis personnel* (6th ed). St. Louis: Mosby.

Guzman, N. J., & Peterson, J. C. (1993). In C. C. Tisher & C. S. Wilcox (Eds.), *House officers series: Nephrology* (2nd ed., pp. 60-87). Baltimore: Williams & Wilkins.

Lancaster, L. E. (Ed.). (1995). *ANNA's core curriculum for nephrology nurses* (3rd ed.) (Section X.). Pitman, NJ: Anthony J. Janetti.

Smeltzer, S. C., & Bare, B. G. (2004). *Brunner & Suddarth's textbook of medical surgical nursing* (10th ed.). Philadelphia: Lippincott Williams & Wilkins.

S

Thermoregulation—0800

Domain-Physiologic Health (II)

Class-Metabolic Regulation (I)

Scale(s)-Severely compromised to Not compromised (a) and Severe to None (n)

Care Recipient:

Data Source:

Definition: Balance among heat production, heat gain, and heat loss

OUTCOME TARGET RATING: Maintain at_____   Increase to_____

Thermoregulation Overall Rating	Severely compromised 1	Substantially compromised 2	Moderately compromised 3	Mildly compromised 4	Not compromised 5	
INDICATORS:						
080009 Presence of goose bumps when cold	1	2	3	4	5	NA
080010 Sweating when hot	1	2	3	4	5	NA
080011 Shivering when cold	1	2	3	4	5	NA
080017 Apical heart rate	1	2	3	4	5	NA
080012 Radial pulse rate	1	2	3	4	5	NA
080013 Respiratory rate	1	2	3	4	5	NA
080015 Reported thermal comfort	1	2	3	4	5	NA
	Severe	Substantial	Moderate	Mild	None	
080001 Increased skin temperature	1	2	3	4	5	NA
080018 Decreased skin temperature	1	2	3	4	5	NA
080019 Hyperthermia	1	2	3	4	5	NA
080020 Hypothermia	1	2	3	4	5	NA
080003 Headache	1	2	3	4	5	NA
080004 Muscle aches	1	2	3	4	5	NA
080005 Irritability	1	2	3	4	5	NA
080006 Drowsiness	1	2	3	4	5	NA
080007 Skin color changes	1	2	3	4	5	NA
080008 Muscle twitching	1	2	3	4	5	NA
080014 Dehydration	1	2	3	4	5	NA
080021 Heat cramps	1	2	3	4	5	NA
080022 Heat stroke	1	2	3	4	5	NA
080023 Frostbite	1	2	3	4	5	NA

1st edition 1997; Revised 3rd edition 2004; Revised 4th edition

T

Continued

Outcome Content References:

Ainslie, P. N., Campbell, I. T., Lambert, J. P., MacLaren, D. P. M., & Reilly, R. (2005). Physiological and metabolic aspects of very prolonged exercise with particular reference to hill walking. *Sports Medicine, 35*(7), 619-647.

Ballester, J. M., & Harchelroad, F. P. (1999). Hyperthermia: How to recognize and prevent heat-related illnesses. *Geriatrics, 54*(7), 20-24.

Caruso, C., Hadley, B., Shuklou, R., & Frame, P. (1992). Cooling effects and comfort of four cooling blanket temperatures in humans with fever. *Nursing Research, 41*(2), 68-72.

Charkoudian, N. (2003). Skin blood flow in adult human thermoregulation: How it works, when it does not, and why. *Mayo Clinic Proceedings, 78*(5), 603-612.

Elliott, F. (2005). Do the prep work. *Occupational Health & Safety, 74*(11), 68, 70.

Erickson, R., & Kerklin, S. (1992). Comparison of methods for core temperature measurement. *Heart & Lung, 21*(3), 297.

Finke, C. (1991). Measurement of the thermoregulatory response: A review. *Focus on Critical Care, 18*(5), 408-412.

Franceschl, V. (1991). Accuracy and feasibility of measuring oral temperature in critically ill adults. *Focus on Critical Care, 18*(3), 221-228.

Holtzclaw, B. J. (2001). Risk for altered body temperature. In M. Maas, K. Buckwalter, M. Hardy, T. Tripp-Reimer, M. Titler, & J. Specht (Eds.), *Nursing care of older adults: Diagnoses, outcomes & interventions* (pp. 201-216). St. Louis: Mosby.

Murphy, K. (1992). Acetaminophen and ibuprofen: Finer control and overdose. *Pediatric Nursing, 18*(4), 428-431.

Parker, R. J., & Davidson, A. C. (2005). Hypothyroidism—An unexpected diagnosis following emergency treatment for heatstroke. *International Journal of Clinical Practice, 59*(Suppl. 147), 31-33.

Segatore, M. (1992). Fever after traumatic brain injury. *American Association of Neuroscience Nurse, 24*(2), 104-109.

Stewart, G., & Webster, D. (1992). Re-evaluation of the tympanic thermometer in the emergency department. *Annals of Emergency Medicine, 21*(2), 158-161.

Summers, S., Dudgeon, N., Byram, K., & Zingsheim, K. (1990). The effects of two warming methods on core and surface temperatures, hemoglobin oxygen saturation, blood pressure, and perceived comfort of hypothermic postanesthesia patients. *Journal of Post Anesthesia Nursing, 5*(5), 354-364.

Watson, G., Casa, D. J., Fiala, K. A., Hile, A., Roti, M. W., Healey, J. C., Armstrong, L. E., & Maresh, C. M. (2006). Creatine use and exercise heat tolerance in dehydrated men. *Journal of Athletic Training, 41*(1), 18-29.

T

Thermoregulation: Newborn—0801

Domain-Physiologic Health (II)   *Care Recipient:*

Class-Metabolic Regulation (I)   *Data Source:*

Scale(s)-Severely compromised to Not compromised (a) and Severe to None (n)

Definition: Balance among heat production, heat gain, and heat loss during the first 28 days of life

OUTCOME TARGET RATING: Maintain at_____   Increase to_____

Thermoregulation: Newborn Overall Rating	Severely compromised 1	Substantially compromised 2	Moderately compromised 3	Mildly compromised 4	Not compromised 5	
INDICATORS:						
080106 Weight gain	1	2	3	4	5	NA
080107 Non-shivering thermogenesis	1	2	3	4	5	NA
080108 Assumes heat retention posture with hypothermia	1	2	3	4	5	NA
080109 Assumes heat dissipation posture with hyperthermia	1	2	3	4	5	NA
080110 Weaning from Isolette to crib	1	2	3	4	5	NA
080113 Acid/base balance	1	2	3	4	5	NA
	Severe	**Substantial**	**Moderate**	**Mild**	**None**	
080116 Temperature instability	1	2	3	4	5	NA
080117 Hyperthermia	1	2	3	4	5	NA
080118 Hypothermia	1	2	3	4	5	NA
080119 Irregular respirations	1	2	3	4	5	NA
080120 Tachypnea	1	2	3	4	5	NA
080103 Restlessness	1	2	3	4	5	NA
080104 Lethargy	1	2	3	4	5	NA
080105 Skin color changes	1	2	3	4	5	NA
080111 Dehydration	1	2	3	4	5	NA
080112 Blood glucose instability	1	2	3	4	5	NA
080114 Hyperbilirubinemia	1	2	3	4	5	NA

1st edition 1997; Revised 3rd edition 2004

Outcome Content References:

Bliss-Holtz, J. (1992). Temperature relationships in cold-stressed infants. *Neonatal Network, 11*(2), 72.

Bohnhorst, B., Heyne, T., Peter, C. S., & Poets, C. F. (2001). Skin-to-skin (kangaroo) care, respiratory control, and thermoregulation. *Journal of Pediatrics, 138*(2), 193-197.

Deacon, J., & O'Neill, P. (Eds.). (1999). *Core curriculum for neonatal intensive care nursing* (2nd ed.). Philadelphia: W.B. Saunders.

Continued

Greer, P. (1988). Head coverings for newborns under radiant warmers. *Journal of Obstetric, Gynecologic, and Neonatal Nursing, 17*(4), 265-270.

Keeling, E. B. (1992). Thermoregulation and axillary temperature measurements in neonates: A review of the literature. *Maternal-Child Nursing Journal, 20*(3-4), 124-140.

Konrad, C. (1980). *Nursing interventions to assess and control fever in infants and small children.* Unpublished master's thesis, The University of Iowa, Iowa City.

Mattson, S., & Smith, J. E. (Eds.). (2000). *Core curriculum for maternal-newborn nursing* (2nd ed.). Philadelphia: W.B. Saunders.

Truman, P. (2006). Jaundice in the preterm infant. *Paediatric Nursing, 18*(5), 20-22.

T

Tissue Integrity: Skin & Mucous Membranes—1101

Domain-Physiologic Health (II)

Class-Tissue Integrity (L)

Scale(s)-Severely compromised to Not compromised (a) and Severe to None (n)

Care Recipient:

Data Source:

Definition: Structural intactness and normal physiological function of skin and mucous membranes

OUTCOME TARGET RATING: Maintain at_____   Increase to_____

Tissue Integrity: Skin & Mucous Membranes Overall Rating	Severely compromised 1	Substantially compromised 2	Moderately compromised 3	Mildly compromised 4	Not compromised 5	
INDICATORS:						
110101 Skin temperature	1	2	3	4	5	NA
110102 Sensation	1	2	3	4	5	NA
110103 Elasticity	1	2	3	4	5	NA
110104 Hydration	1	2	3	4	5	NA
110106 Perspiration	1	2	3	4	5	NA
110108 Texture	1	2	3	4	5	NA
110109 Thickness	1	2	3	4	5	NA
110111 Tissue perfusion	1	2	3	4	5	NA
110112 Hair growth on skin	1	2	3	4	5	NA
110113 Skin integrity	1	2	3	4	5	NA
	Severe	Substantial	Moderate	Mild	None	
110105 Abnormal pigmentation	1	2	3	4	5	NA
110115 Skin lesions	1	2	3	4	5	NA
110116 Mucous membrane lesions	1	2	3	4	5	NA
110117 Scar tissue	1	2	3	4	5	NA
110118 Skin cancers	1	2	3	4	5	NA
110119 Skin flaking	1	2	3	4	5	NA
110120 Skin scaling	1	2	3	4	5	NA
110121 Erythema	1	2	3	4	5	NA
110122 Blanching	1	2	3	4	5	NA
110123 Necrosis	1	2	3	4	5	NA
110124 Induration	1	2	3	4	5	NA

1st edition 1997; Revised 3rd edition 2004

Outcome Content References:

+Bergstrom, N., Braden, B. J., Laguzza, A., & Holman, V. (1987). The Braden Scale for predicting pressure sore risk. *Nursing Research, 36*(4), 205-210.

Cohen, I. K., Diegelmann, R. F., & Lindblad, W. L. (1992). *Wound healing: Biochemical and clinical aspects*. Philadelphia: W.B. Saunders.

Continued

T

Hardy, M. D. (2001). Impaired skin integrity: Dry skin. In M. Maas, K. Buckwalter, M. Hardy, T. Tripp-Reimer, M. Titler, & J. Specht (Eds.), *Nursing care of older adults: Diagnoses, outcomes & interventions* (pp. 137-144). St. Louis: Mosby.

Lazarus, G. S., Cooper, D. M., Knighton, D. R., Margohs, D. J., Pecoraro, R. E., Rodeheaver, G., & Robson, M. C. (1994). Definitions and guidelines for assessment of wounds and evaluation of healing. *Archives of Dermatology, 130*(4), 489-493.

Maklebust, J., & Sieggreen, M., (1996). *Pressure ulcers: Guidelines for prevention and nursing management* (2nd ed.). Springhouse, PA: Springhouse.

Potter, P. A., & Perry, A. G. (2001). *Fundamentals of nursing* (5th ed.). St. Louis: Mosby.

U.S. Department of Health and Human Services. (1992). *Pressure ulcers in adults: Prediction and prevention* (AHCPR Publication No. 92-0047). Rockville, MD: Public Health Service Agency for Health Care Policy and Research.

U.S. Department of Health and Human Services. (1994). *Treatment of pressure ulcers* (AHCPR Publication No. 95-0652). Rockville, MD: Public Health Service Agency for Health Care Policy and Research.

Van Rijswijk, L. (1993). Full-thickness leg ulcers: Patient demographics and predictors of healing. *The Journal of Family Practice, 36*(6), 625-632.

T

Tissue Perfusion: Abdominal Organs—0404

Domain-Physiologic Health (II)   *Care Recipient:*

Class-Cardiopulmonary (E)   *Data Source:*

Scale(s)-Severe deviation from normal range to No deviation from normal range (b) and Severe to None (n)

Definition: Adequacy of blood flow through the small vessels of the abdominal viscera to maintain organ function

OUTCOME TARGET RATING: Maintain at_____   Increase to_____

Tissue Perfusion: Abdominal Organs Overall Rating	Severe deviation from normal range 1	Substantial deviation from normal range 2	Moderate deviation from normal range 3	Mild deviation from normal range 4	No deviation from normal range 5	
INDICATORS:						
040424 Diastolic blood pressure	1	2	3	4	5	NA
040425 Systolic blood pressure	1	2	3	4	5	NA
040426 Mean blood pressure	1	2	3	4	5	NA
040402 Urine output	1	2	3	4	5	NA
040403 Electrolyte and acid/ base balance	1	2	3	4	5	NA
040405 Bowel sounds	1	2	3	4	5	NA
040418 Urine specific gravity	1	2	3	4	5	NA
040419 Blood urea nitrogen	1	2	3	4	5	NA
040420 Plasma creatinine	1	2	3	4	5	NA
040421 Liver function test findings	1	2	3	4	5	NA
040422 Pancreatic enzymes	1	2	3	4	5	NA
	Severe	Substantial	Moderate	Mild	None	
040407 Abnormal thirst	1	2	3	4	5	NA
040408 Abdominal pain	1	2	3	4	5	NA
040409 Nausea	1	2	3	4	5	NA
040410 Vomiting	1	2	3	4	5	NA
040411 Malabsorption deficiencies	1	2	3	4	5	NA
040412 Chronic gastritis	1	2	3	4	5	NA
040413 Abdominal distention	1	2	3	4	5	NA
040414 Ascites	1	2	3	4	5	NA
040415 Gastrointestinal varices	1	2	3	4	5	NA
040416 Constipation	1	2	3	4	5	NA
040417 Diarrhea	1	2	3	4	5	NA
040427 Altered fluid balance	1	2	3	4	5	NA
040428 Loss of appetite	1	2	3	4	5	NA

T

Continued

1st edition 1997; Revised 3rd edition 2004; Revised 4th edition

Outcome Content References:

Lewis, S. M., Collier, I. C., Heitkermper, M. M., & Dirksen, S. R. (2000). *Medical-surgical nursing: Assessment & management of clinical problems* (5th ed.). St. Louis: Mosby.

McCance, K. L., & Huether, S. E. (2002). *Pathophysiology: The biologic basis for disease in adults and children* (4th ed.). St. Louis: Mosby.

Smeltzer, S. C., & Bare, B. G. (2004). *Brunner & Suddarth's textbook of medical surgical nursing* (10th ed.). Philadelphia: Lippincott Williams & Wilkins.

T

Tissue Perfusion: Cardiac—0405

Domain-Physiologic Health (II)

Class-Cardiopulmonary (E)

Scale(s)-Severe deviation from normal range to No deviation from normal range (b) and Severe to None (n)

Care Recipient:

Data Source:

Definition: Adequacy of blood flow through the coronary vasculature to maintain heart function

OUTCOME TARGET RATING: Maintain at_____   Increase to_____

Tissue Perfusion: Cardiac Overall Rating	Severe deviation from normal range 1	Substantial deviation from normal range 2	Moderate deviation from normal range 3	Mild deviation from normal range 4	No deviation from normal range 5	
INDICATORS:						
040515 Apical heart rate	1	2	3	4	5	NA
040516 Radial pulse rate	1	2	3	4	5	NA
040517 Systolic blood pressure	1	2	3	4	5	NA
040518 Diastolic blood pressure	1	2	3	4	5	NA
040519 Mean blood pressure	1	2	3	4	5	NA
040501 Ejection fraction	1	2	3	4	5	NA
040502 Pulmonary wedge pressure	1	2	3	4	5	NA
040503 Cardiac index	1	2	3	4	5	NA
040509 Electrocardiogram findings	1	2	3	4	5	NA
040510 Cardiac enzymes	1	2	3	4	5	NA
040511 Coronary angiogram findings	1	2	3	4	5	NA
040512 Exercise stress test findings	1	2	3	4	5	NA
040513 Thallium scan findings	1	2	3	4	5	NA
	Severe	**Substantial**	**Moderate**	**Mild**	**None**	
040504 Angina	1	2	3	4	5	NA
040520 Arrhythmia	1	2	3	4	5	NA
040521 Tachycardia	1	2	3	4	5	NA
040522 Bradycardia	1	2	3	4	5	NA
040505 Profuse diaphoresis	1	2	3	4	5	NA
040506 Nausea	1	2	3	4	5	NA
040507 Vomiting	1	2	3	4	5	NA

1st edition 1997; Revised 2nd edition 2000; Revised 3rd edition 2004; Revised 4th edition

Outcome Content References:

Lewis, S. M., Collier, I. C., Heitkermper, M. M., & Dirksen, S. R. (2000). *Medical-surgical nursing: Assessment & management of clinical problems* (5th ed.). St. Louis: Mosby.

Continued

T

McCance, K. L., & Huether, S. E. (2002). *Pathophysiology: The biologic basis for disease in adults and children* (4th ed.). St. Louis: Mosby.

Smeltzer, S. C., & Bare, B. G. (2004). *Brunner & Suddarth's textbook of medical surgical nursing* (10th ed.). Philadelphia: Lippincott Williams & Wilkins.

Wenger, N. K., Froelicher, E. S., Smith, L. K., et al. (1995). *Cardiac rehabilitation as secondary prevention, Clinical practice guideline, No. 17*. (AHCPR Publication No. 96-0673). Rockville, MD: U.S. Department of Health and Human Services. Public Health Services, Agency for Health Care Policy and Research and the National Heart, Lung, and Blood Institute.

T

Tissue Perfusion: Cellular—0416

Domain-Physiologic Health (II)

Class-Cardiopulmonary (E)

Scale(s)-Severe deviation from normal range to No deviation from normal range (b) and Severe to None (n)

Care Recipient:

Data Source:

Definition: Adequacy of blood flow through the vasculature to maintain function at the cellular level

OUTCOME TARGET RATING: Maintain at_____   Increase to_____

Tissue Perfusion: Cellular Overall Rating	Severe deviation from normal range 1	Substantial deviation from normal range 2	Moderate deviation from normal range 3	Mild deviation from normal range 4	No deviation from normal range 5	
INDICATORS:						
041601 Systolic blood pressure	1	2	3	4	5	NA
041602 Diastolic blood pressure	1	2	3	4	5	NA
041603 Mean arterial blood gases	1	2	3	4	5	NA
041604 Oxygen saturation	1	2	3	4	5	NA
041605 Fluid balance	1	2	3	4	5	NA
041606 Apical heart rate	1	2	3	4	5	NA
041607 Heart rhythm	1	2	3	4	5	NA
041608 Electrolyte and acid / base balance	1	2	3	4	5	NA
041609 Capillary refill	1	2	3	4	5	NA
041610 Urine output	1	2	3	4	5	NA
041611 Creatinine clearance	1	2	3	4	5	NA

	Severe	Substantial	Moderate	Mild	None	
041612 Agitation	1	2	3	4	5	NA
041613 Necrosis	1	2	3	4	5	NA
041614 Nausea	1	2	3	4	5	NA
041615 Vomiting	1	2	3	4	5	NA
041616 Pain	1	2	3	4	5	NA
041617 Decreased level of consciousness	1	2	3	4	5	NA
041618 Pale, cool skin	1	2	3	4	5	NA
041619 Skin breakdown	1	2	3	4	5	NA

4th edition

T

Outcome Content References:

Bridges, E. J., & Dukes, M. S. (2005). Cardiovascular aspects of septic shock: Pathophysiology, monitoring, and treatment. *Critical Care Nursing, 25*, 14-36.

Goodrich, D. (2006). Continuous central venous oximetry monitoring. *Critical Care Nursing Clinics, 18*(2), 203-209.

O'Donnell, J. M., & Nacul, F. (Eds.). (2001). *Surgical intensive care medicine* (pp. 411-425). Boston: Kluwer Academic Publishers.

Swearingen, P. L., & Keen, J. H. (Eds.). (2001). *Manual of critical care nursing: Nursing interventions and collaborative management* (4th ed., pp. 593-604). St. Louis: Mosby.

Tissue Perfusion: Cerebral—0406

Domain-Physiologic Health (II)

Class-Cardiopulmonary (E)

Scale(s)-Severe deviation from normal range to No deviation from normal range (b) and Severe to None (n)

Care Recipient:

Data Source:

Definition: Adequacy of blood flow through the cerebral vasculature to maintain brain function

OUTCOME TARGET RATING: Maintain at_____   Increase to_____

Tissue Perfusion: Cerebral Overall Rating	Severe deviation from normal range 1	Substantial deviation from normal range 2	Moderate deviation from normal range 3	Mild deviation from normal range 4	No deviation from normal range 5	
INDICATORS:						
040602 Intracranial pressure	1	2	3	4	5	NA
040613 Systolic blood pressure	1	2	3	4	5	NA
040614 Diastolic blood pressure	1	2	3	4	5	NA
040617 Mean blood pressure	1	2	3	4	5	NA
040615 Cerebral angiogram findings	1	2	3	4	5	NA
	Severe	Substantial	Moderate	Mild	None	
040603 Headache	1	2	3	4	5	NA
040604 Carotid bruit	1	2	3	4	5	NA
040605 Restlessness	1	2	3	4	5	NA
040606 Listlessness	1	2	3	4	5	NA
040607 Unexplained anxiety	1	2	3	4	5	NA
040608 Agitation	1	2	3	4	5	NA
040609 Vomiting	1	2	3	4	5	NA
040610 Hiccoughs	1	2	3	4	5	NA
040611 Syncope	1	2	3	4	5	NA
040616 Fever	1	2	3	4	5	NA
040618 Impaired cognition	1	2	3	4	5	NA
040619 Decreased level of consciousness	1	2	3	4	5	NA
040620 Impaired neurological reflexes	1	2	3	4	5	NA

1st edition 1997; Revised 3rd edition 2004; Revised 4th edition

Outcome Content References:

Lewis, S. M., Collier, I. C., Heitkermper, M. M., & Dirksen, S. R. (2000). *Medical-surgical nursing: Assessment & management of clinical problems* (5th ed.). St. Louis: Mosby.

McCance, K. L., & Huether, S. E. (2002). *Pathophysiology: The biologic basis for disease in adults and children* (4th ed.). St. Louis: Mosby.

Smeltzer, S. C., & Bare, B. G. (2004). *Brunner & Suddarth's textbook of medical surgical nursing* (10th ed.). Philadelphia: Lippincott Williams & Wilkins.

T

Tissue Perfusion: Peripheral—0407

Domain-Physiologic Health (II)

Class-Cardiopulmonary (E)

Scale(s)-Severe deviation from normal range to No deviation from normal range (b) and Severe to None (n)

Care Recipient:

Data Source:

> **Definition:** Adequacy of blood flow through the small vessels of the extremities to maintain tissue function

OUTCOME TARGET RATING: Maintain at_____   Increase to_____

Tissue Perfusion: Peripheral Overall Rating	Severe deviation from normal range 1	Substantial deviation from normal range 2	Moderate deviation from normal range 3	Mild deviation from normal range 4	No deviation from normal range 5	

INDICATORS:

040715	Capillary refill fingers	1	2	3	4	5	NA
040716	Capillary refill toes	1	2	3	4	5	NA
040710	Extremity skin temperature	1	2	3	4	5	NA
040730	Carotid pulse strength (right)	1	2	3	4	5	NA
040731	Carotid pulse strength (left)	1	2	3	4	5	NA
040732	Brachial pulse strength (right)	1	2	3	4	5	NA
040733	Brachial pulse strength (left)	1	2	3	4	5	NA
040734	Radial pulse strength (right)	1	2	3	4	5	NA
040735	Radial pulse strength (left)	1	2	3	4	5	NA
040736	Femoral pulse strength (right)	1	2	3	4	5	NA
040737	Femoral pulse strength (left)	1	2	3	4	5	NA
040738	Pedal pulse strength (right)	1	2	3	4	5	NA
040739	Pedal pulse strength (left)	1	2	3	4	5	NA
040727	Systolic blood pressure	1	2	3	4	5	NA
040728	Diastolic blood pressure	1	2	3	4	5	NA
040740	Mean blood pressure	1	2	3	4	5	NA

T

Continued

		Severe	Substantial	Moderate	Mild	None	
040711	Extremity bruits	1	2	3	4	5	NA
040712	Peripheral edema	1	2	3	4	5	NA
040713	Localized extremity pain	1	2	3	4	5	NA
040729	Necrosis	1	2	3	4	5	NA
040741	Numbness	1	2	3	4	5	NA
040742	Tingling	1	2	3	4	5	NA
040743	Pallor	1	2	3	4	5	NA
040744	Muscle weakness	1	2	3	4	5	NA
040745	Muscle cramps	1	2	3	4	5	NA
040746	Skin breakdown	1	2	3	4	5	NA
040747	Rubor	1	2	3	4	5	NA
040748	Paresthesia	1	2	3	4	5	NA

1st edition 1997; Revised 3rd edition 2004; Revised 4th edition

Outcome Content References:

Cohen, I. K., Diegelmann, R. F., & Lindblad, W. L. (1992). *Wound healing: Biochemical and clinical aspects*. Philadelphia: W.B. Saunders.

Lazarus, G. S., Cooper, D. M., Knighton, D. R., Margohs, D. J., Pecoraro, R. E., Rodeheaver, G., & Robson, M. C. (1994). Definitions and guidelines for assessment of wounds and evaluation of healing. *Archives of Dermatology, 130*(4), 489-493.

Maklebust, J., & Sieggreen, M. (1996). *Pressure ulcers: Guidelines for prevention and nursing management* (2nd ed.). Springhouse, PA: Springhouse.

Potter, P. A., & Perry, A. G. (2001). *Fundamentals of nursing* (5th ed.). St. Louis: Mosby.

Smeltzer, S. C., & Bare, B. G. (2004). *Brunner & Suddarth's textbook of medical surgical nursing* (10th ed.). Philadelphia: Lippincott Williams & Wilkins.

Van Rijswijk, L. (1993). Full-thickness leg ulcers: Patient demographics and predictors of healing. *The Journal of Family Practice, 36*(6), 625-632.

T

Tissue Perfusion: Pulmonary—0408

Domain-Physiologic Health (II) Care Recipient:

Class-Cardiopulmonary (E) Data Source:

Scale(s)-Severe deviation from normal range to No deviation from normal range (b) and Severe to None (n)

Definition: Adequacy of blood flow through pulmonary vasculature to perfuse alveoli/capillary unit

OUTCOME TARGET RATING: Maintain at_____   Increase to_____

Tissue Perfusion: Pulmonary Overall Rating	Severe deviation from normal range 1	Substantial deviation from normal range 2	Moderate deviation from normal range 3	Mild deviation from normal range 4	No deviation from normal range 5	
INDICATORS:						
040810 Ventilation-perfusion scan	1	2	3	4	5	NA
040811 Pulmonary artery pressure (PAP)	1	2	3	4	5	NA
040814 Respiratory rhythm	1	2	3	4	5	NA
040815 Respiratory rate	1	2	3	4	5	NA
040816 Systolic blood pressure	1	2	3	4	5	NA
040817 Diastolic blood pressure	1	2	3	4	5	NA
040822 Mean blood pressure	1	2	3	4	5	NA
040818 Partial pressure of oxygen in arterial blood (PaO_2)	1	2	3	4	5	NA
040819 Partial pressure of carbon dioxide in arterial blood ($PaCO_2$)	1	2	3	4	5	NA
040820 Arterial pH	1	2	3	4	5	NA
040821 Oxygen saturation	1	2	3	4	5	NA
	Severe	Substantial	Moderate	Mild	None	
040805 Chest pain	1	2	3	4	5	NA
040806 Pleural friction rub	1	2	3	4	5	NA
040807 Hemoptysis	1	2	3	4	5	NA
040808 Unexplained anxiety	1	2	3	4	5	NA
040823 Shortness of breath	1	2	3	4	5	NA
040824 Impaired gas exchange	1	2	3	4	5	NA

1st edition 1997; Revised 3rd edition 2004; Revised 4th edition

Outcome Content References:

Lewis, S. M., Collier, I. C., Heitkermper, M. M., & Dirksen, S. R. (2000). *Medical-surgical nursing: Assessment & management of clinical problems* (5th ed.). St. Louis: Mosby.

McCance, K. L., & Huether, S. E. (2002). *Pathophysiology: The biologic basis for disease in adults and children* (4th ed.). St. Louis: Mosby.

Smeltzer, S. C., & Bare, B. G. (2004). *Brunner & Suddarth's textbook of medical surgical nursing* (10th ed.). Philadelphia: Lippincott Williams & Wilkins.

Transfer Performance—0210

Domain-Functional Health (I)

Class-Mobility (C)

Scale(s)-Severely compromised to Not compromised (a)

Care Recipient:

Data Source:

Definition: Ability to change body location independently with or without assistive device

OUTCOME TARGET RATING: Maintain at_____   Increase to_____

Transfer Performance Overall Rating	Severely compromised 1	Substantially compromised 2	Moderately compromised 3	Mildly compromised 4	Not compromised 5	
INDICATORS:						
021009 Transfers from one surface to another while lying	1	2	3	4	5	NA
021001 Transfers from bed to chair	1	2	3	4	5	NA
021002 Transfers from chair to bed	1	2	3	4	5	NA
021003 Transfers from chair to chair	1	2	3	4	5	NA
021004 Transfers from wheelchair to vehicle	1	2	3	4	5	NA
021005 Transfers from vehicle to wheelchair	1	2	3	4	5	NA
021007 Transfers from wheelchair to toilet	1	2	3	4	5	NA
021008 Transfers from toilet to wheelchair	1	2	3	4	5	NA

1st edition 1997; Revised 3rd edition 2004; Revised 4th edition

Outcome Content References:

+*Guide for the Uniform Data Set for Medical Rehabilitation* (including the FIM™ instrument), (version 5.1) (1997). Buffalo, NY: University at Buffalo.

Kane, R. L., & Kane, R. A. (2000). *Assessing older persons: Measures, meaning, and practical applications*. New York: Oxford University Press.

Mikulic, M. A., Griffith, E. R., & Jebsen, R. H. (1976). Clinical application of a standardized mobility test. *Archives of Physical Medicine and Rehabilitation, 57*(3), 143-146.

T

Treatment Behavior: Illness or Injury—1609

Domain-Health Knowledge & Behavior (IV)

Class-Health Behavior (Q)

Scale-Never demonstrated to Consistently demonstrated (m)

Care Recipient:

Data Source:

Definition: Personal actions to palliate or eliminate pathology

OUTCOME TARGET RATING: Maintain at_____   Increase to_____

Treatment Behavior: Illness or Injury Overall Rating	Never demonstrated 1	Rarely demonstrated 2	Sometimes demonstrated 3	Often demonstrated 4	Consistently demonstrated 5	
INDICATORS:						
160901 Follows recommended precautions	1	2	3	4	5	NA
160902 Follows recommended treatment regimen	1	2	3	4	5	NA
160918 Performs prescribed procedure	1	2	3	4	5	NA
160904 Follows prescribed activity level	1	2	3	4	5	NA
160905 Follows medication regimen	1	2	3	4	5	NA
160919 Follows prescribed diet	1	2	3	4	5	NA
160906 Avoids behaviors that potentiate pathology	1	2	3	4	5	NA
160907 Performs self-care consistent with ability	1	2	3	4	5	NA
160908 Monitors treatment therapeutic effects	1	2	3	4	5	NA
160909 Monitors treatment side effects	1	2	3	4	5	NA
160910 Monitors disease side effects	1	2	3	4	5	NA
160911 Monitors changes in disease status	1	2	3	4	5	NA
160912 Uses treatment devices correctly	1	2	3	4	5	NA
160913 Alters role activities to meet treatment requirements	1	2	3	4	5	NA
160920 Balances activity and rest	1	2	3	4	5	NA
160921 Obtains advice from professional as needed	1	2	3	4	5	NA

Continued

		Never demonstrated	Rarely demonstrated	Sometimes demonstrated	Often demonstrated	Consistently demonstrated	
160916	Makes appointments with health professional as needed	1	2	3	4	5	NA

1st edition 1997; Revised 3rd edition 2004; Revised 4th edition

Outcome Content References:

Conn, V., Taylor, S., & Casey, B. (1992). Cardiac rehabilitation program participation and outcomes after myocardial infarction. *Rehabilitation Nursing, 17*(2), 58-62.

Gorski, J. A., Slifer, K. J., Townsend, V., Kelly-Suttka, J., & Amari, A. (2005). Behavioural treatment of non-compliance in adolescents with newly acquired spinal cord injuries. *Pediatric Rehabilitation, 8*(3), 187-198.

Hensold, T. C., Guercio, J. M., Grubbs, E. E., Upton, J. C., & Faw, G. (2006). A personal intervention substance abuse treatment approach: Substance abuse treatment in a least restrictive residential model. *Brain Injury, 20*(4), 369-381.

See, J., & Murray, J. A. (2006). Gluten-free diet: The medical and nutrition management of celiac disease. *Nutrition in Clinical Practice, 21*(1), 1-15.

Shaw, S. E., Morris, D. M., Uswatte, G., McKay, S., Meythaler, J. M., & Taub, E. (2005). Constraint-induced movement therapy for recovery of upper-limb function following traumatic brain injury. *Journal of Rehabilitation Research & Development, 42*(6), 769-778.

Wenger, N. K., Froelicher, E. S., Smith, L. K., et al. (1995). *Cardiac rehabilitation as secondary prevention, Clinical practice guideline*, No. 17. (AHCPR Publication No. 96-0673). Rockville, MD: U.S. Department of Health and Human Services. Public Health Services, Agency for Health Care Policy and Research and the National Heart, Lung, and Blood Institute.

Woods, N. (1989). Conceptualizations of self-care: Toward health-oriented models. *Advances in Nursing Science, 12*(1), 1-13.

T

Urinary Continence—0502

Domain-Physiologic Health (II)

Class-Elimination (F)

Care Recipient:

Data Source:

Scale(s)-Never demonstrated to Consistently Demonstrated (m) and Consistently demonstrated to Never demonstrated (t)

Definition: Control of elimination of urine from the bladder

OUTCOME TARGET RATING: Maintain at_____   Increase to_____

Urinary Continence Overall Rating	Never demonstrated 1	Rarely demonstrated 2	Sometimes demonstrated 3	Often demonstrated 4	Consistently demonstrated 5	
INDICATORS:						
050201 Recognizes urge to void	1	2	3	4	5	NA
050202 Maintains predictable pattern of voiding	1	2	3	4	5	NA
050203 Responds to urge in timely manner	1	2	3	4	5	NA
050204 Voids in appropriate receptacle	1	2	3	4	5	NA
050205 Gets to toilet between urge and passage of urine	1	2	3	4	5	NA
050218 Maintains barrier-free environment for independent toileting	1	2	3	4	5	NA
050206 Voids >150 cc each time	1	2	3	4	5	NA
050208 Starts and stops stream	1	2	3	4	5	NA
050209 Empties bladder completely	1	2	3	4	5	NA
050215 Ingests adequate amount of fluid	1	2	3	4	5	NA
050216 Manages clothing independently	1	2	3	4	5	NA
050217 Toilets independently	1	2	3	4	5	NA
050219 Identifies medication that interferes with urinary control	1	2	3	4	5	NA

	Consistently demonstrated	Often demonstrated	Sometimes demonstrated	Rarely demonstrated	Never demonstrated	
050207 Urine leakage between voidings	1	2	3	4	5	NA
050210 Post void residual >100-200 cc	1	2	3	4	5	NA

U

Continued

		Consistently demonstrated	Often demonstrated	Sometimes demonstrated	Rarely demonstrated	Never demonstrated	
050211	Urine leakage with increased abdominal pressure (e.g., sneezing, laughing, lifting)	1	2	3	4	5	NA
050212	Wets clothing during day	1	2	3	4	5	NA
050213	Wets clothing or bedding during night	1	2	3	4	5	NA
050214	Urinary tract infection	1	2	3	4	5	NA

1st edition 1997; Revised 3rd edition 2004

Outcome Content References:

Lewthwaite, B., & Girouard, L. (2006). Urinary drainage following continence surgery: Development of Canadian best practice guidelines. *Urologic Nursing, 26*(1), 33-39.

+Morris, J. N., Hawes, C., Fries, B. E., Phillips, C. D., Mor, V., Katz, S., Murphy, K., Drugovich, M. L., & Friedlob, A. S. (1990). Designing the national resident assessment instrument for nursing homes. *Gerontologist 30*(3), 293-307.

+O'Donnell, P. D., & Calandro, V. J. (1991). Incontinence Management Scale for elderly inpatient men. *Urology, 37*(3), 220-223.

Palmer, M. H., McCormick, K. A., Langford, A., Langlais, J., & Alvaran, M. (1992). Continence outcomes: Documentation on medical records in the nursing home environment. *Journal of Nursing Care Quality, 6*(3), 36-43.

Specht, J. P., & Maas, M. L. (2001). Urinary incontinence: Functional, iatrogenic, overflow, reflex, stress, total, and urge. In M. Maas, K. Buckwalter, M. Hardy, T. Tripp-Reimer, M. Titler, & J. Specht (Eds.), *Nursing care of older adults: Diagnoses, outcomes & interventions* (pp. 252-278). St. Louis: Mosby.

Viktrup, L., Summers, K. H., & Dennett, S. L. (2004). Clinical practice guidelines for the initial management of urinary incontinence in women: A European-focused review. *BJU International Journal, 94*(Suppl. 1), 14-22.

U

Urinary Elimination—0503

Domain-Physiologic Health (II)

Class-Elimination (F)

Scale(s)-Severely compromised to Not compromised (a) and Severe to None (n)

Care Recipient:

Data Source:

Definition: Collection and discharge of urine

OUTCOME TARGET RATING: Maintain at_____   Increase to_____

Urinary Elimination Overall Rating	Severely compromised 1	Substantially compromised 2	Moderately compromised 3	Mildly compromised 4	Not compromised 5	
INDICATORS:						
050301 Elimination pattern	1	2	3	4	5	NA
050302 Urine odor	1	2	3	4	5	NA
050303 Urine amount	1	2	3	4	5	NA
050304 Urine color	1	2	3	4	5	NA
050306 Urine clarity	1	2	3	4	5	NA
050307 Fluid intake	1	2	3	4	5	NA
050313 Empties bladder completely	1	2	3	4	5	NA
050314 Recognition of urge	1	2	3	4	5	NA
	Severe	Substantial	Moderate	Mild	None	
050305 Visible urine particles	1	2	3	4	5	NA
050329 Visible blood in urine	1	2	3	4	5	NA
050309 Pain with urination	1	2	3	4	5	NA
050330 Burning with urination						
050310 Hesitancy with urination	1	2	3	4	5	NA
050331 Urinary frequency	1	2	3	4	5	NA
050311 Urgency with urination	1	2	3	4	5	NA
050332 Urinary retention	1	2	3	4	5	NA
050333 Nocturia	1	2	3	4	5	NA
050312 Urinary incontinence	1	2	3	4	5	NA
050334 Stress incontinence	1	2	3	4	5	NA
050335 Urge incontinence	1	2	3	4	5	NA
050336 Functional incontinence	1	2	3	4	5	NA

1st edition 1997; Revised 3rd edition 2004

Outcome Content References:

Anonymous. (2006). In brief. Kegels hold up as urinary continence treatment. *Harvard Women's Health Watch, 13*(9), 7.

Anonymous. (2006). Promoting urinary continence in older people. *Nursing Older People, 18*(3), 35-36.

Borello-France, D. F., Zyczynski, H. M., Downey, P. A., Rause, C. R., & Wister, J. A. (2006). Effect of pelvic-floor muscle exercise position on continence and quality-of-life outcomes in women with stress urinary incontinence. *Physical Therapy, 86*(7), 974-986.

U

Continued

Brundage, D. J., & Linton, A. D. (1997). Age related changes in the genitourinary system. In M. A. Matteson, E. S. McConnell, & A. D. Linton (Eds.), *Gerontological nursing: Concepts in practice* (2nd ed.). Philadelphia, W.B. Saunders.

Burns, P. A. (2006). A nurse led continence service reduced symptoms of incontinence, frequency, urgency, and nocturia. *Evidence-Based Nursing, 9*(3), 85.

Morton, P. G. (1989). *Health assessment in nursing.* Springhouse, PA: Springhouse.

Palmer, M. H., McCormick, K. A., Langford, A., Langlais, J., & Alvaran, M. (1992). Continence outcomes: Documentation on medical records in the nursing home environment. *Journal of Nursing Care Quality, 6*(3), 36-43.

Potter, P. A., & Perry, A. G. (2001). *Fundamentals of nursing* (5th ed.). St. Louis: Mosby.

U

Vision Compensation Behavior—1611

Domain-Health & Knowledge Behavior (IV)

Class-Health Behavior (Q)

Scale(s)-Never demonstrated to Consistently demonstrated (m)

Care Recipient:

Data Source:

Definition: Personal actions to compensate for visual impairment

OUTCOME TARGET RATING: Maintain at_____   Increase to_____

Vision Compensation Behavior Overall Rating	Never demonstrated 1	Rarely demonstrated 2	Sometimes demonstrated 3	Often demonstrated 4	Consistently demonstrated 5	
INDICATORS:						
161101 Monitors symptoms of vision deterioration	1	2	3	4	5	NA
161102 Positions self to advantage vision	1	2	3	4	5	NA
161103 Reminds others to use techniques that advantage vision	1	2	3	4	5	NA
161104 Uses adequate lighting for activity being performed	1	2	3	4	5	NA
161105 Wears eyeglasses correctly	1	2	3	4	5	NA
161106 Wears contact lens correctly	1	2	3	4	5	NA
161107 Cares for eyewear correctly	1	2	3	4	5	NA
161108 Uses vision assistive devices	1	2	3	4	5	NA
161109 Uses computer assistive devices	1	2	3	4	5	NA
161113 Uses animal assistance	1	2	3	4	5	NA
161110 Uses support services for low-vision	1	2	3	4	5	NA
161111 Uses Braille	1	2	3	4	5	NA

2nd edition 2000; Revised 3rd edition 2004

Outcome Content References:

Burrell, L. O. (Ed). (1992). *Adult nursing in hospital and community settings.* Norwalk, CT: Appleton & Lange.

Phipps, W. J., Monahan, F. D., Sands J. K., Marek, J., & Neighbors, M. (Eds.). (2003). *Medical-surgical nursing: Concepts and clinical practice* (7th ed). St. Louis: Mosby.

Smeltzer, S. C., & Bare, B. G. (Eds.). (2003). *Brunner and Suddarth's textbook of medical-surgical nursing* (10th ed.). Philadelphia: Lippincott Williams & Wilkins.

V

Vital Signs—0802

Domain-Physiologic Health (II)

Class-Metabolic Regulation (I)

Scale(s)-Severe deviation from normal range to No deviation from normal range (b)

Care Recipient:

Data Source:

> **Definition:** Extent to which temperature, pulse, respiration, and blood pressure are within normal range

OUTCOME TARGET RATING: Maintain at_____   Increase to_____

Vital Signs Overall Rating	Severe deviation from normal range 1	Substantial deviation from normal range 2	Moderate deviation from normal range 3	Mild deviation from normal range 4	No deviation from normal range 5	
INDICATORS:						
080201 Body temperature	1	2	3	4	5	NA
080202 Apical heart rate	1	2	3	4	5	NA
080208 Apical heart rhythm	1	2	3	4	5	NA
080203 Radial pulse rate	1	2	3	4	5	NA
080204 Respiratory rate	1	2	3	4	5	NA
080210 Respiratory rhythm	1	2	3	4	5	NA
080205 Systolic blood pressure	1	2	3	4	5	NA
080206 Diastolic blood pressure	1	2	3	4	5	NA
080209 Pulse pressure	1	2	3	4	5	NA
080211 Depth of inspiration	1	2	3	4	5	NA

1st edition 1997; Revised 3rd edition 2004; Revised 4th edition

Outcome Content References:

Caruso, C., Hadley, B., Shukla, R., & Frame, P. (1992). Cooling effects and comfort of four cooling blanket temperatures in humans with fever. *Nursing Research, 41*(2), 68-72.

Finke, C. (1991). Measurement of the thermoregulatory response: A review. *Focus on Critical Care, 18*(5), 408-412.

Summers, S., Dudgeon, N., Byram, K., & Zingsheim, K. (1990). The effects of two warming methods on core and surface temperatures, hemoglobin oxygen saturation, blood pressure, and perceived comfort of hypothermic postanesthesia patients. *Journal of Post Anesthesia Nursing, 5*(5), 354-364.

Thomas, S. A., Liehr, P., DeKeyser, F., Frazier, L., & Friedmann, E. (2002). A review of nursing research on blood pressure. *Journal of Nursing Scholarship, 34*(4), 313-321.

V

Weight: Body Mass—1006

Domain-Physiologic Health (II)

Class-Metabolic Regulation (I)

Scale(s)-Severe deviation from normal range to No deviation from normal range (b)

Care Recipient:

Data Source:

Definition: Extent to which body weight, muscle, and fat are congruent to height, frame, gender, and age

OUTCOME TARGET RATING: Maintain at_____   Increase to_____

Weight: Body Mass Overall Rating	Severe deviation from normal range 1	Substantial deviation from normal range 2	Moderate deviation from normal range 3	Mild deviation from normal range 4	No deviation from normal range 5	
INDICATORS:						
100601 Weight	1	2	3	4	5	NA
100602 Triceps skinfold thickness	1	2	3	4	5	NA
100603 Subscapular skinfold thickness	1	2	3	4	5	NA
100604 Waist/hip circumference ratio (women)	1	2	3	4	5	NA
100605 Neck/waist circumference ratio (men)	1	2	3	4	5	NA
100606 Body fat percentage	1	2	3	4	5	NA
100607 Head circumference percentile (child)	1	2	3	4	5	NA
100608 Height percentile (child)	1	2	3	4	5	NA
100609 Weight percentile (child)	1	2	3	4	5	NA

1st edition 1997; Revised 3rd edition 2004

Outcome Content References:

Collinsworth, R., & Boyle, K. (1989). Nutritional assessment of the elderly. *Journal of Gerontological Nursing, 15*(12), 17-21.

Curtas, S., Chapman, G., & Meguid, M. (1989). Evaluation of nutritional status. *Nursing Clinics of North America, 24*(2), 301-313.

Flegal, K. M., Tabak, C. J., & Ogden, C. L. (2006). Overweight in children: Definitions and interpretation. *Health Education Research, 21*(6), 755-760.

Folsom, A. R., Kaye, S. A., Sellers, T. A., Hang, C. P., Cerhan, J. R., Potter, J. D., & Prineas, R. J. (1993). Body fat distribution and five year risk of death in older women. *Journal of the American Medical Association, 269*(4), 483-487.

Gianino, S., & St. John, R. E. (1993). Nutritional assessment of the patient in the intensive care unit. *Critical Care Nursing Clinics of North America, 5*(1), 1-16.

Koo, W. W., & Hockman, E. M. (2006). Posthospital discharge feeding for preterm infants: Effects of standard compared with enriched milk formula on growth, bone mass, and body composition. *American Journal of Clinical Nutrition, 84*(6), 1357-1364.

Moscicki, A., Ellenberg, J. H., Murphy, D. A., & Jiahong, X. (2006). Associations among body composition, androgen levels, and human immunodeficiency virus status in adolescents. *Journal of Adolescent Health, 39*(2), 164-173.

Yang, F., Lv, J. H., Lei, S. F., Chen, X. D., Liu, M. Y., Jian, W. X., Xu, H., Tan, L. J., Deng, F. Y., Yang, Y. J., Wang, Y. B., Sun, X., Xiao, S. M., Jiang, C., Guo, Y. F., Guo, J. J., Li, Y. N., Zhu, X. Z., Papasian, C. J., & Deng, H. W. (2006). Receiver-operating characteristic analysis of body mass index, waist circumference and waist-to-hip ratio for obesity: Screening in young adults in central south of China. *Clinical Nutrition, 25*(6), 1030-1039.

W

Weight Gain Behavior—1626

Domain-Health Knowledge & Behavior (IV)

Class-Health Behavior (Q)

Scale(s)-Never demonstrated to Consistently demonstrated (m)

Care Recipient:

Data Source:

Definition: Personal actions to gain weight following voluntary or involuntary significant weight loss				

OUTCOME TARGET RATING: Maintain at_____   Increase to_____

Weight Gain Behavior Overall Rating	Never demonstrated 1	Rarely demonstrated 2	Sometimes demonstrated 3	Often demonstrated 4	Consistently demonstrated 5	
INDICATORS:						
162601 Obtains assistance for weight from health professional	1	2	3	4	5	NA
162602 Identifies cause of weight loss	1	2	3	4	5	NA
162603 Receives proper dental care	1	2	3	4	5	NA
162604 Sets achievable weight gain goals	1	2	3	4	5	NA
162605 Selects a healthy target weight	1	2	3	4	5	NA
162606 Commits to a healthy eating plan	1	2	3	4	5	NA
162607 Identifies caloric intake requirements	1	2	3	4	5	NA
162608 Maintains an adequate supply of nutritious food and fluid	1	2	3	4	5	NA
162609 Obtains financial assistance for purchasing food	1	2	3	4	5	NA
162610 Prepares food to enhance swallowing	1	2	3	4	5	NA
162611 Uses flavor enhancers	1	2	3	4	5	NA
162612 Obtains assistance with food preparation	1	2	3	4	5	NA
162613 Identifies food and fluid preferences and dislikes	1	2	3	4	5	NA
162614 Identifies food allergies	1	2	3	4	5	NA

W

		Never demonstrated	Rarely demonstrated	Sometimes demonstrated	Often demonstrated	Consistently demonstrated	
162615	Uses vitamin/mineral supplements	1	2	3	4	5	NA
162616	Drinks eight glasses of water daily	1	2	3	4	5	NA
162617	Recognizes signs and symptoms of electrolyte imbalance	1	2	3	4	5	NA
162618	Obtains treatment for electrolyte imbalance	1	2	3	4	5	NA
162619	Monitors appetite level	1	2	3	4	5	NA
162620	Uses prescribed medication to increase appetite	1	2	3	4	5	NA
162621	Uses prescribed medication to enhance weight gain	1	2	3	4	5	NA
162622	Uses nutrient supplements	1	2	3	4	5	NA
162623	Selects high-protein, high-caloric food and fluid	1	2	3	4	5	NA
162624	Eats nutritious food and fluid between meals	1	2	3	4	5	NA
162625	Maintains fluid balance	1	2	3	4	5	NA
162626	Maintains adequate sleep	1	2	3	4	5	NA
162627	Uses diary to monitor food and fluid intake	1	2	3	4	5	NA
162628	Administers enteral tube feedings as recommended	1	2	3	4	5	NA
162629	Administers parenteral nutrition as recommended	1	2	3	4	5	NA
162630	Monitors exercise for caloric requirements	1	2	3	4	5	NA
162631	Uses personal support system to enhance weight gain	1	2	3	4	5	NA

W

Continued

		Never demonstrated	Rarely demonstrated	Sometimes demonstrated	Often demonstrated	Consistently demonstrated	
162632	Participates in support groups	1	2	3	4	5	NA
162633	Participates in nutritional monitoring	1	2	3	4	5	NA
162634	Monitors body mass index	1	2	3	4	5	NA
162635	Monitors body weight	1	2	3	4	5	NA

Target weight _____ kg/lb

4th edition

Outcome Content References:

Ferguson, M., Cook, A., Bender, S., Rimmasch, H., & Voss, A. (2001). Diagnosing and treating involuntary weight loss. *MEDSURG Nursing, 10*(4), 165-177.

Huffman, G. B. (2002). Evaluating and treating unintentional weight loss in the elderly. *American Family Physician, 65*(4), 640-650.

Martin, H., & Ammerman, S. D. (2002). Adolescents with eating disorders: Primary care screening, identification, and early intervention. *Nursing Clinics of North America, 37*(3), 537-551.

NIH Technology Assessment Conference Panel. Methods for voluntary weight loss and control. *Annals of Internal Medicine, 119*(7), 764-770.

National Institute for Health and Clinical Excellence. (2006). *Nutrition support in adults: Oral nutrition support, enteral tube feeding and parenteral nutrition.* London: Author.

Orphanidou, C. I., McCargar, L. J., Birmingham, C. L., & Belzberg, A. S. (1997). Changes in body composition and fat distribution after short-term weight gain in patients with anorexia nervosa. *American Journal of Clinical Nutrition, 65,* 1034-1041.

Wolfe, B. E., & Gimby, L. B. (2003). Caring for the hospitalized patient with an eating disorder. *Nursing Clinics of North America, 38*(1), 75-99.

Yaari, S., & Goldbourt, U. (1998). Voluntary and involuntary weight loss: Associations with long term mortality in 9,228 middle-aged and elderly men. *American Journal of Epidemiology, 148*(6), 546-555.

Yeh, S., DeGuzman, B., & Kramer, T. (2002). Reversal of COPD-associated weight loss using the anabolic agent oxandrolone. *Chest, 122*(2), 421-428.

W

Weight Loss Behavior—1627

Domain-Health Knowledge & Behavior (IV)

Class-Health Behavior (Q)

Scale(s)-Never demonstrated to Consistently demonstrated (m)

Care Recipient:

Data Source:

Definition: Personal actions to lose weight through diet, exercise, and behavior modification

OUTCOME TARGET RATING: Maintain at_____   Increase to_____

Weight Loss Behavior Overall Rating	Never demonstrated 1	Rarely demonstrated 2	Sometimes demonstrated 3	Often demonstrated 4	Consistently demonstrated 5	

INDICATORS:

162701	Obtains information on weight loss strategies from health professional	1	2	3	4	5	NA
162702	Selects a healthy target weight	1	2	3	4	5	NA
162703	Commits to a healthy eating plan	1	2	3	4	5	NA
162704	Selects nutritious food and fluid	1	2	3	4	5	NA
162705	Controls food portion	1	2	3	4	5	NA
162706	Establishes an exercise routine	1	2	3	4	5	NA
162707	Caloric expenditure exceeds caloric intake	1	2	3	4	5	NA
162708	Controls preoccupation with food	1	2	3	4	5	NA
162709	Identifies emotional states that affect food and fluid intake	1	2	3	4	5	NA
162710	Identifies social situations that affect food and fluid intake	1	2	3	4	5	NA
162711	Plans for situations that affect food and fluid intake	1	2	3	4	5	NA
162712	Uses behavior modification strategies	1	2	3	4	5	NA
162713	Uses self-talk motivation	1	2	3	4	5	NA

W

Continued

		Never demonstrated	Rarely demonstrated	Sometimes demonstrated	Often demonstrated	Consistently demonstrated	
162714	Avoids high caloric food and fluid	1	2	3	4	5	NA
162715	Drinks eight glasses of water daily	1	2	3	4	5	NA
162716	Includes vitamins in weight loss plan	1	2	3	4	5	NA
162717	Uses appetite suppressants as prescribed	1	2	3	4	5	NA
162718	Uses weight loss medication as prescribed	1	2	3	4	5	NA
162719	Uses personal support system to enhance weight loss	1	2	3	4	5	NA
162720	Participates in weight loss support group	1	2	3	4	5	NA
162721	Manages setbacks by resuming weight loss efforts	1	2	3	4	5	NA
162722	Monitors body weight	1	2	3	4	5	NA
162723	Monitors body mass index	1	2	3	4	5	NA
162724	Uses diary to monitor food and fluid intake	1	2	3	4	5	NA
162725	Uses diary to monitor exercise over time	1	2	3	4	5	NA
162726	Maintains progress toward target weight	1	2	3	4	5	NA
162727	Uses commercial diet products safely	1	2	3	4	5	NA

Target weight _____ kg/lb

4th edition

Outcome Content References:

Budd, G. M., & Volpe, S. L. (2006). School-based obesity prevention: Research, challenges, and recommendations. *Journal of School Health, 76*(10), 485-495.

Dennis, K. E. (2004). Weight management in women. *Nursing Clinics of North America, 39*(1), 231-241.

Fabricatore, A. N. (2007). Behavior therapy and cognitive-behavioral therapy of obesity: Is there a difference? *Journal of the American Dietetic Association, 107*(1), 92-99.

W

National Institutes of Health. (2000). *The practical guide: Identification, evaluation, and treatment of overweight and obesity in adults.* Bethesda, MD: U.S. Department of Health and Human Services.

Patel, S. R., Malhotra, A., White, D. P., Gottlieb, D. J., & Hu, F. B. (2006). Association between reduced sleep and weight gain in women. *American Journal of Epidemiology, 164*(10), 947-954.

Tyler, D. O., Allan, J. D., & Alcozer, F. R. (1997). Weight loss methods used by African American and Euro-American women. *Research in Nursing & Health, 20,* 413-423.

W

Weight Maintenance Behavior—1628

Domain-Health Knowledge & Behavior (IV)

Class-Health Behavior (Q)

Scale(s)-Never demonstrated to Consistently demonstrated (m)

Care Recipient:

Data Source:

Definition: Personal actions to maintain optimum body weight					

OUTCOME TARGET RATING: Maintain at_____   Increase to_____

Weight Maintenance Behavior Overall Rating	Never demonstrated 1	Rarely demonstrated 2	Sometimes demonstrated 3	Often demonstrated 4	Consistently demonstrated 5	
INDICATORS:						
162801 Monitors body weight	1	2	3	4	5	NA
162802 Maintains optimal daily caloric intake	1	2	3	4	5	NA
162803 Balances exercise with caloric intake	1	2	3	4	5	NA
162804 Selects nutritious meals	1	2	3	4	5	NA
162805 Selects nutritious snacks	1	2	3	4	5	NA
162806 Drinks eight glasses of water daily	1	2	3	4	5	NA
162807 Uses nutrient supplements as needed	1	2	3	4	5	NA
162808 Eats in response to hunger	1	2	3	4	5	NA
162809 Maintains recommended eating pattern	1	2	3	4	5	NA
162810 Retains ingested foods	1	2	3	4	5	NA
162811 Maintains fluid balance	1	2	3	4	5	NA
162812 Obtains assistance from health professional	1	2	3	4	5	NA
162813 Uses personal support systems	1	2	3	4	5	NA
162814 Identifies social situations that affect food and fluid intake	1	2	3	4	5	NA
162815 Identifies emotional states that affect food and fluid intake	1	2	3	4	5	NA

W

		Never demonstrated	Rarely demonstrated	Sometimes demonstrated	Often demonstrated	Consistently demonstrated	
162816	Plans for situations that affect food and fluid intake	1	2	3	4	5	NA
162817	Controls preoccupation with food	1	2	3	4	5	NA
162818	Controls preoccupation with weight	1	2	3	4	5	NA
162819	Expresses realistic body image	1	2	3	4	5	NA
162820	Maintains adequate sleep	1	2	3	4	5	NA
162821	Maintains optimum weight	1	2	3	4	5	NA

Target weight _____ kg/lb

4th edition

Outcome Content References:

American Psychiatric Association. (1993). Practice guideline for eating disorders. *American Journal of Psychiatry, 150*(2), 212-223.

Bruce, B., & Wilfley, D. (1996). Binge eating among the overweight population: A serious and prevalent problem. *Journal of the American Dietetic Association, 96*(1), 58-62.

Chang, B. L., Uman, G. C., Linn, L. S., Ware, J. E., & Kane, R. L. (1985). Adherence to healthcare regimens among elderly women. *Nursing Research, 34*(1) 27-31.

Curtas, S., Chapman, G., & Meguid, M. (1989). Evaluation of nutritional status. *Nursing Clinics of North America, 24*(2), 301-313.

Farrow, J. (1992). The adolescent male with an eating disorder. *Pediatric Annals, 21*(11), 769-774.

Fisher, M., Golden, N. H., Katzman, D. K., Kreipe, R. E., Rees, J., Schebendach, J., Sigman, G., Ammerman, S., & Hobeman, H. M. (1995). Eating disorders in adolescents: A background paper. *Journal of Adolescent Health, 16*(6), 420-437.

Halmi, K. (1994). A multimodal model for understanding and treating eating disorders. *Journal of Women's Health, 3*(6), 487-493.

Hawks, S. R., & Richins, P. (1994). Toward a new paradigm for the management of obesity. *Journal of Health Education, 25*(3), 147-153.

National Heart, Lung and Blood Institute. (2005). *Aim for a healthy weight* (NIH Publication No. 05-5213). Bethesda, MD: U.S. Department of Health and Human Services.

Wilson, P., Herman, J., & Chubon, S. J. (1991). Eating strategies used by persons with head and neck cancer during and after radiotherapy. *Cancer Nursing, 14*(2), 98-104.

Yates, A. (1992). Biologic considerations in the etiology of eating disorders. *Pediatric Annuals, 21*(11), 739-744.

W

Will to Live—1206

Domain-Psychosocial Health (III)   Care Recipient:

Class-Psychological Well-Being (M)   Data Source:

Scale(s)-Severely compromised to Not compromised (a) and Severe to None (n)

Definition: Desire, determination, and effort to survive

OUTCOME TARGET RATING: Maintain at_____   Increase to_____

Will to Live Overall Rating	Severely compromised 1	Substantially compromised 2	Moderately compromised 3	Mildly compromised 4	Not compromised 5	
INDICATORS:						
120601 Expression of determination to live	1	2	3	4	5	NA
120602 Expression of hope	1	2	3	4	5	NA
120603 Expression of optimism	1	2	3	4	5	NA
120604 Expression of sense of control	1	2	3	4	5	NA
120605 Expression of feelings	1	2	3	4	5	NA
120617 Interest in one's illness	1	2	3	4	5	NA
120618 Interest in one's treatment	1	2	3	4	5	NA
120608 Use of strategies to compensate for problems associated with disease	1	2	3	4	5	NA
120613 Use of treatments to lengthen life	1	2	3	4	5	NA
120609 Use of strategies to enhance health	1	2	3	4	5	NA
120610 Use of strategies to lengthen life	1	2	3	4	5	NA
	Severe	Substantial	Moderate	Mild	None	
120614 Depression	1	2	3	4	5	NA
120615 Suicidal thoughts	1	2	3	4	5	NA
120616 Pessimistic thoughts	1	2	3	4	5	NA

1st edition 1997; Revised 3rd edition 2004; Revised 4th edition

Outcome Content References:

Chochinov, H. M., Hack, T., Hassard, T., Kristjanson, L. J., McClement, S., & Harlos, M. (2005). Dignity therapy: A novel psychotherapeutic intervention for patients near the end of life. *Journal of Clinical Oncology, 23*(24), 5520-5525.

Dickerson, S. S., Boehmke, M., Ogle, C., & Brown, J. K. (2006). Seeking and managing hope: Patients' experiences using the Internet for cancer care. *Oncology Nursing Forum, 33*(1), E8-E17.

Gaskins, S., & Brown, K. (1992). Psychosocial responses among individuals with human immunodeficiency virus infection. *Applied Nursing Research, 5*(3), 111-121.

W

Greer, S., Morris, T., & Pettingale, K. (1979). Psychological response to breast cancer: Effect on outcome. *The Lancet, 2*(8146), 785-787.

Hagopian, G. (1993). Cognitive strategies used in adapting to a cancer diagnosis. *Oncology Nursing Forum, 20*(5), 759-763.

+Ivanoff, A., Joon Jang, S., Smyth, N. J., & Linehan, M. M. (1994). Fewer reasons for staying alive when you are thinking of killing yourself: The Brief Reasons for Living Inventory. *Journal of Psychopathology and Behavioral Assessment, 16*(1), 1-13.

Katz, R., & Lowe, L. (1989). The "will to live" as perceived by nurses and physicians. *Issues in Mental Health Nursing, 10*(1), 15-22.

+Linehan, M. M., Goodstein, J. L., Nielsen, S. L., & Chiles, J. A. (1983). Reasons for staying alive when you are thinking of killing yourself: The Reasons for Living Inventory. *Journal of Consulting and Clinical Psychology, 51*(2), 276-286, 484-485.

Lipman, M. M. (2005). Office visit: Creating a will to live by. *Consumer Reports on Health, 17*(6), 11.

Richardson, A. (2004). Creating a culture of compassion: Developing supportive care for people with cancer. *European Journal of Oncology Nursing, 8*(4), 293-305.

Weisman, A. (1972). *On death and denying: A psychiatric study of terminality*. New York: Behavioral Publications.

W

Wound Healing: Primary Intention—1102

Domain-Physiologic Health (II)

Class-Tissue Integrity (L)

Scale(s)-None to Extensive (i) and Extensive to None (h)

Care Recipient:

Data Source:

Definition: Extent of regeneration of cells and tissues following intentional closure

OUTCOME TARGET RATING: Maintain at_____   Increase to_____

Wound Healing: Primary Intention Overall Rating	None 1	Limited 2	Moderate 3	Substantial 4	Extensive 5	

INDICATORS:

		None 1	Limited 2	Moderate 3	Substantial 4	Extensive 5	
110201	Skin approximation	1	2	3	4	5	NA
110213	Wound edge approximation	1	2	3	4	5	NA
110214	Scar formation	1	2	3	4	5	NA

		Extensive	Substantial	Moderate	Limited	None	
110202	Purulent drainage	1	2	3	4	5	NA
110203	Serous drainage	1	2	3	4	5	NA
110204	Sanguineous drainage	1	2	3	4	5	NA
110205	Serosanguineous drainage	1	2	3	4	5	NA
110206	Sanguineous drainage from drain	1	2	3	4	5	NA
110207	Serosanguineous drainage from drain	1	2	3	4	5	NA
110208	Surrounding skin erythema	1	2	3	4	5	NA
110215	Surrounding skin bruising	1	2	3	4	5	NA
110209	Periwound edema	1	2	3	4	5	NA
110210	Increased skin temperature	1	2	3	4	5	NA
110211	Foul wound odor	1	2	3	4	5	NA

Location of wound (# from picture): _____

1st edition 1997; Revised 3rd edition 2004

1. Front of head
2. Right ear
3. Left ear
4. Front of neck
5. Right chest
6. Left chest
7. Sternum
8. Right upper quadrant
9. Left upper quadrant
10. Right lower quadrant
11. Left lower quadrant
12. Abdominal midline
13. Navel
14. Pubic and perineal area
15. Right trochanter (hip)
16. Left trochanter (hip)
17. Right anterior thigh
18. Right knee
19. Right lower anterior leg
20. Right ankle (inner/outer)
21. Right foot
22. Right toes
23. Left anterior thigh
24. Left knee
25. Left lower anterior leg
26. Left ankle (inner/outer)
27. Left foot
28. Left toes
29. Right upper interior arm
30. Right interior forearm
31. Right wrist
32. Right palm
33. Right fingers _____(specify)

W

34. Left upper interior arm
35. Left interior forearm
36. Left wrist
37. Left palm
38. Left fingers _____ (specify)
39. Back of head
40. Back of neck
41. Left scapula
42. Right scapula
43. Spine
44. Left back
45. Right back
46. Left buttock
47. Right buttock
48. Sacrum
49. Left posterior thigh

50. Left lower posterior leg
51. Left heel
52. Left bottom foot
53. Right posterior thigh
54. Right lower posterior leg
55. Right heel
56. Right bottom foot
57. Left upper posterior arm
58. Left elbow
59. Left posterior forearm
60. Left dorsal hand
61. Right upper posterior arm
62. Right elbow
63. Right posterior forearm
64. Right dorsal hand

Outcome Content References:

Cohen, I. K., Diegelmann, R. F., & Lindblad, W. L. (1992). *Wound healing: Biochemical and clinical aspects*. Philadelphia: W.B. Saunders.

+Holden-Lund, C. (1988). Effects of relaxation with guided imagery on surgical stress and wound healing. *Research in Nursing & Health, 11*(4), 235-244.

Lazarus, G. S., Cooper, D. M., Knighton, D. R., Margohs, D. J., Pecoraro, R. E., Rodeheaver, G., & Robson, M. C. (1994). Definitions and guidelines for assessment of wounds and evaluation of healing. *Archives of Dermatology, 130*(4), 489-493.

Potter, P. A., & Perry, A. G. (2001). *Fundamentals of nursing* (5th ed.). St. Louis: Mosby.

W

Wound Healing: Secondary Intention—1103

Domain-Physiologic Health (II)

Class-Tissue Integrity (L)

Scale(s)-None to Extensive (i) and Extensive to None (h)

Care Recipient:

Data Source:

Definition: Extent of regeneration of cells and tissues in an open wound

OUTCOME TARGET RATING: Maintain at_____   Increase to_____

Wound Healing: Secondary Intention Overall Rating	None 1	Limited 2	Moderate 3	Substantial 4	Extensive 5	

INDICATORS:

		None 1	Limited 2	Moderate 3	Substantial 4	Extensive 5	
110301	Granulation	1	2	3	4	5	
110320	Scar formation	1	2	3	4	5	
110321	Decreased wound size	1	2	3	4	5	

		Extensive	Substantial	Moderate	Limited	None	
110303	Purulent drainage	1	2	3	4	5	NA
110304	Serous drainage	1	2	3	4	5	NA
110305	Sanguineous drainage	1	2	3	4	5	NA
110306	Serosanguineous drainage	1	2	3	4	5	NA
110307	Surrounding skin erythema	1	2	3	4	5	NA
110322	Wound inflammation	1	2	3	4	5	NA
110308	Periwound edema	1	2	3	4	5	NA
110310	Blistered skin	1	2	3	4	5	NA
110311	Macerated skin	1	2	3	4	5	NA
110312	Necrosis	1	2	3	4	5	NA
110313	Sloughing	1	2	3	4	5	NA
110314	Tunneling	1	2	3	4	5	NA
110315	Undermining	1	2	3	4	5	NA
110316	Sinus tract formation	1	2	3	4	5	NA
110317	Foul wound odor	1	2	3	4	5	NA

Location of wound (# from picture) _____

1st edition 1997; Revised 3rd edition 2004

1. Front of head

2. Right ear

3. Left ear

4. Front of neck

5. Right chest

6. Left chest

7. Sternum

8. Right upper quadrant

9. Left upper quadrant

10. Right lower quadrant

11. Left lower quadrant

12. Abdominal midline

13. Navel

14. Pubic and perineal area

15. Right trochanter (hip)

16. Left trochanter (hip)

17. Right anterior thigh

18. Right knee

19. Right lower anterior leg

20. Right ankle (inner/outer)

21. Right foot

22. Right toes

23. Left anterior thigh

24. Left knee

25. Left lower anterior leg

26. Left ankle (inner/outer)

27. Left foot

28. Left toes

29. Right upper interior arm

30. Right interior forearm

31. Right wrist

32. Right palm

33. Right fingers _____(specify)

34. Left upper interior arm

35. Left interior forearm

36. Left wrist

37. Left palm

38. Left fingers _____(specify)

39. Back of head

40. Back of neck

41. Left scapula

42. Right scapula

43. Spine

44. Left back

45. Right back

46. Left buttock

47. Right buttock

48. Sacrum

49. Left posterior thigh

50. Left lower posterior leg

51. Left heel

52. Left bottom foot

53. Right posterior thigh

54. Right lower posterior leg

55. Right heel

56. Right bottom foot

57. Left upper posterior arm

58. Left elbow

59. Left posterior forearm

60. Left dorsal hand

61. Right upper posterior arm

62. Right elbow

63. Right posterior forearm

64. Right dorsal hand

Outcome Content References:

Bergstrom, N., Bennett, M. A., Carlson, C. E., et al. (1994). *Treatment of pressure ulcers. Clinical practice guideline*, No. 15 (AHCPR Publication No. 95-0652). Rockville, MD: U.S. Department of Health and Human Services, Agency for Health Care Policy and Research.

Cohen, I. K., Diegelmann, R. F., & Lindblad, W. L. (1992). *Wound healing: Biochemical and clinical aspects*. Philadelphia: W.B. Saunders.

Flanagan, M. (1994). Assessment criteria. *Nursing Times, 90*(35), 76-88.

Frantz, R. A. (2001). Impaired skin integrity: Pressure ulcer. In M. Maas, K. Buckwalter, M. Hardy, T. Tripp-Reimer, M. Titler, & J. Specht (Eds.), *Nursing care of older adults: Diagnoses, outcomes & interventions* (pp. 121-136). St. Louis: Mosby.

Frantz, R. A., & Gardner, S. (1994). Elderly skin care: Principles of chronic wound care. *Journal of Gerontological Nursing, 20*(9), 35-44.

Lazarus, G. S., Cooper, D. M., Knighton, D. R., Margohs, D. J., Pecoraro, R. E., Rodeheaver, G., & Robson, M. C. (1994). Definitions and guidelines for assessment of wounds and evaluation of healing. *Archives of Dermatology, 130*(4), 489-493.

Maklebust, J., & Sieggreen, M. (1996). *Pressure ulcers: Guidelines for prevention and nursing management* (2nd ed.). Springhouse, PA: Springhouse.

Potter, P. A., & Perry, A. G. (2001). *Fundamentals of nursing* (5th ed.). St. Louis: Mosby.

+Thomas, D. R., Rodeheaver, G. T., Bartolucci, A. A., Frantz, R. A., Sussman, C., Ferrell, B. A., Cuddigan, J., Stotts, N. A., & Macklebust, J. (1997). Pressure ulcer scale for healing: Derivation and validation of the PUSH tool. *Advances in Wound Care, 10*(5), 96-101.

Van Rijswijk, L. (1993). Full-thickness leg ulcers: Patient demographics and predictors of healing. *The Journal of Family Practice, 36*(6), 625-632.

W

PART FOUR

NOC Linkages
Health Patterns
NANDA—International
International
Classification
Functioning

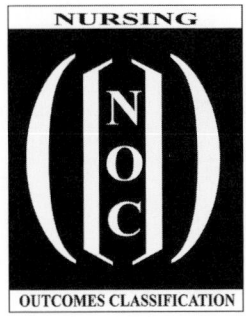

NOC Linkages—Health Patterns

This section provides updated linkages among the Health Patterns identified by Gordon[1] and the NOC outcomes developed to date at three levels of abstraction: the individual, family, and community. These linkages were first published in the second edition of NOC. Early work by Gordon suggests the importance of the nurse assessing 11 health concepts utilizing patterns of behavior over time rather than isolated patient events. This approach examines the *sequence of behavior* over time incorporating a broad view of behavior as physiological, psychological, or sociological in nature. The patterns were proposed by Gordon to serve as a means of identifying nursing diagnoses during the early development of patient problem statements that were standardized for use in clinical practice. The patterns areas provide a structured framework for the assessment of a client. The nurse uses an interview approach and perfroms a physical examination for each patient receiving nursing care to assess each of the 11 health patterns.

Due to the popularity and long history of use of these health patterns in nursing, linkages among the NOC outcomes and the 11 health patterns were developed to assist nurses who routinely use the health patterns as an assessment structure in practice. In addition, many educational institutions use the patterns as an assessment tool to teach the assessment phase of the nursing process to nursing students. The linkages provide one way of identifying relevant outcomes for nurses using the NOC in education, practice, and research. Each outcome is placed under a specific pattern based on the pattern name and definition developed by Gordon. Outcomes that describe the actual health status of a more general nature were placed in the Health-Perception-Health-Management Pattern when they did not fit into a more specific pattern. Many of these outcomes would be assessed primarily by physical examination rather than by interviewing the client about his or her perceptions of health.

Several specific outcomes could not be easily placed in this structure and appear as a list at the end of the linkages. Linkages of the NOC to the 11 health patterns are important for: (1) assisting individuals to learn and use the NOC; (2) improving diagnostic reasoning skills in nursing; (3) identifying new outcomes for development of the NOC, especially as the family and community level outcomes are further developed; and (4) emphasizing the effectiveness of nursing interventions with the current emphasis in health care on outcomes. Current use of this pattern focus by nurses is predominant in the United States, as well as in many countries worldwide.

Reference

1. Gordon, M. (1994). *Nursing diagnosis: Process and application,* (3rd ed.). New York: McGraw-Hill.

Nursing Outcomes Classification (NOC) Organized by the Eleven Health Patterns (Gordon, 1994)

HEALTH-PERCEPTION-HEALTH MANAGEMENT PATTERN: This pattern describes the client's perceived pattern of health and well-being and how health is managed across time. It includes general perceptions about health, general health management, prevention practices, potential or actual noncompliance, motivation for health promotion, and unrealistic health or illness perceptions. At the family level general perceptions of the family's health status are the focus of this pattern. Assessment of this pattern may reveal the influential member of the family for health-related decisions. At the community level general concerns about community health problems and services available are assessed. For example, this may include objective data from mortality and morbidity statistics, accident rates, and violence statistics.

INDIVIDUAL LEVEL:

Acceptance: Health Status
Adherence Behavior
Adherence Behavior: Healthy Diet
Aspiration Prevention
Asthma Self-Management
Burn Recovery
Cardiac Disease Self-Management
Cardiopulmonary Status
Caregiver Emotional Health
Caregiver Home Care Readiness
Caregiver Performance: Direct Care
Caregiver Performance: Indirect Care
Caregiver Physical Health
Caregiver Well-Being
Child Development: 1 Month
Child Development: 2 Months
Child Development: 4 Months
Child Development: 6 Months
Child Development: 12 Months
Child Development: 2 Years
Child Development: 3 Years
Child Development: 4 Years
Child Development: 5 Years
Child Development: Middle Childhood
Child Development: Adolescence
Compliance Behavior
Compliance Behavior: Prescribed Diet
Compliance Behavior: Prescribed Medication
Development: Late Adulthood
Development: Middle Adulthood
Development: Young Adulthood
Diabetes Self-Management
Discharge Readiness: Independent Living
Discharge Readiness: Supported Living
Fall Prevention Behavior

Falls Occurrence
Fetal Status: Antepartum
Fetal Status: Intrapartum
Health Promoting Behavior
Health Seeking Behavior
Immune Hypersensitivity Response
Immune Status
Immunization Behavior
Infection Severity
Infection Severity: Newborn
Maternal Status: Antepartum
Maternal Status: Intrapartum
Maternal Status: Postpartum
Medication Response
Motivation
Multiple Sclerosis Self-Management
Participation in Health Care Decisions
Personal Health Status
Personal Resiliency
Personal Safety Behavior
Personal Well-Being
Physical Aging
Physical Injury Severity
Postpartum Maternal Health Behavior
Post-Procedure Recovery
Prenatal Health Behavior
Pre-Procedure Readiness
Preterm Infant Organization
Quality of Life
Respiratory Status
Risk Control
Risk Control: Alcohol Use
Risk Control: Cancer
Risk Control: Cardiovascular Health
Risk Control: Drug Use

INDIVIDUAL LEVEL: CONT'D

Risk Control: Hearing Impairment
Risk Control: Hyperthermia
Risk Control: Hypothermia
Risk Control: Infectious Process
Risk Control: Sexually Transmitted Diseases
Risk Control: Sun Exposure
Risk Control: Tobacco Use
Risk Control: Unintended Pregnancy
Risk Control: Visual Impairment
Risk Detection
Safe Home Environment
Seizure Control
Self-Care: Non-Parenteral Medication

Self-Care: Parenteral Medication
Self-Direction of Care
Student Health Status
Substance Withdrawal Severity
Symptom Control
Tissue Perfusion: Abdominal Organs
Tissue Perfusion: Cardiac
Tissue Perfusion: Cellular
Tissue Perfusion: Peripheral
Tissue Perfusion: Pulmonary
Treatment Behavior: Illness or Injury
Vital Signs
Will to Live

FAMILY LEVEL:

Family Health Status
Family Participation in Professional Care

COMMUNITY LEVEL:

Community Disaster Readiness
Community Disaster Response
Community Health Status
Community Health Status: Immunity
Community Risk Control: Chronic Disease

Community Risk Control: Communicable
   Disease
Community Risk Control: Lead Exposure
Community Risk Control: Violence

NUTRITION-METABOLIC PATTERN: This pattern describes the pattern of food and fluid consumption relative to metabolic need. Physical examination for this pattern focuses on the skin, bony prominences, hair, oral mucous membranes, teeth, height and weight for life stage, and body temperature. At the family level assessment focuses on patterns of food consumption and identifies who makes decisions about the nutritional intake of family members, while the community assessment focuses of these patterns in geographic neighborhoods.

INDIVIDUAL LEVEL:

Appetite
Blood Glucose Level
Breastfeeding Establishment: Infant
Breastfeeding Establishment: Maternal
Breastfeeding Maintenance
Breastfeeding Weaning
Burn Healing
Electrolyte & Acid/Base Balance
Fluid Balance
Fluid Overload Severity
Gastrointestinal Function
Growth
Hydration
Nausea & Vomiting Control
Nausea & Vomiting: Disruptive Effects
Nausea & Vomiting Severity
Nutritional Status
Nutritional Status: Biochemical Measures

Nutritional Status: Energy
Nutritional Status: Food & Fluid Intake
Nutritional Status: Nutrient Intake
Oral Hygiene
Swallowing Status
Swallowing Status: Esophageal Phase
Swallowing Status: Oral Phase
Swallowing Status: Pharyngeal Phase
Thermoregulation
Thermoregulation: Newborn
Tissue Integrity: Skin & Mucous
   Membranes
Weight: Body Mass
Weight Gain Behavior
Weight Loss Behavior
Weight Maintenance Behavior
Wound Healing: Primary Intention
Wound Healing: Secondary Intention

NOC currently has no outcomes focused on the nutrition-metabolic pattern at the family or community level.

ELIMINATION PATTERN: Describes patterns of excretory function (bowel, bladder, and skin) at the individual level. Physical examination includes gross screening of specimens and prostheses such as ostomy bags. The nurse identifies patterns of urinary or bowel incontinence, difficulty with urination, and constipation. At the family and community level the focus is on waste disposal and related hygiene practices.

INDIVIDUAL LEVEL:

Bowel Continence
Bowel Elimination
Kidney Function
Ostomy Self-Care

Systemic Toxin Clearance:
    Dialysis
Urinary Continence
Urinary Elimination

NOC currently has no outcomes focused on the elimination pattern at the family or community level.

ACTIVITY-EXERCISE PATTERN: This pattern focuses on exercise, activity, leisure, and recreation and includes perceived capabilities for movement, self-care, and home management. Physical examination includes gait, posture, muscle tone, absence of body part, and the use of assistive devices. At the family and community level patterns of activity are assessed. This includes recreational and cultural activities at the community level and public transportation.

INDIVIDUAL LEVEL:

Activity Tolerance
Ambulation
Ambulation: Wheelchair
Balance
Body Mechanics Performance
Body Positioning: Self-Initiated
Bone Healing
Cardiac Pump Effectiveness
Circulation Status
Coordinated Movement
Elopement Occurrence
Elopement Propensity Risk
Endurance
Energy Conservation
Fatigue Level
Hyperactivity Level
Immobility Consequences: Physiological
Immobility Consequences: Psycho-Cognitive
Joint Movement
Joint Movement: Ankle
Joint Movement: Elbow
Joint Movement: Fingers
Joint Movement: Hip
Joint Movement: Knee
Joint Movement: Neck

Joint Movement: Passive
Joint Movement: Shoulder
Joint Movement: Spine
Joint Movement: Wrist
Leisure Participation
Mobility
Physical Fitness
Play Participation
Psychomotor Energy
Respiratory Status: Airway Patency
Respiratory Status: Gas Exchange
Respiratory Status: Ventilation
Safe Wandering
Self-Care Status
Self-Care: Activities of Daily Living (ADL)
Self-Care: Bathing
Self-Care: Dressing
Self-Care: Eating
Self-Care: Hygiene
Self-Care: Instrumental Activities of Daily
    Living (IADL)
Self-Care: Oral Hygiene
Self-Care: Toileting
Skeletal Function
Transfer Performance

NOC currently has no outcomes focused on the activity-exercise pattern at the family or community level.

COGNITIVE-PERCEPTUAL PATTERN: This pattern describes sensory, perceptual, and cognitive function. The areas of concern are the adequacy of language skills, memory, problem solving, and decision-making skills and the sensory functions of vision, hearing, touch, taste, and smell. In addition, pain perception and compensation for sensory loss are included. The focus of the family and community pattern is on how decisions are made.

INDIVIDUAL LEVEL:

Acute Confusion Level
Cognition
Cognitive Orientation
Concentration
Decision-Making
Distorted Thought Self-Control
Hearing Compensation Behavior
Heedfulness of Affected Side
Information Processing
Knowledge: Arthritis Management
Knowledge: Asthma Management
Knowledge: Body Mechanics
Knowledge: Breastfeeding
Knowledge: Cancer Management
Knowledge: Cancer Threat Reduction
Knowledge: Cardiac Disease Management
Knowledge: Child Physical Safety
Knowledge: Conception Prevention
Knowledge: Congestive Heart Failure
   Management
Knowledge: Depression Management
Knowledge: Diabetes Management
Knowledge: Diet
Knowledge: Disease Process
Knowledge: Energy Conservation
Knowledge: Fall Prevention
Knowledge: Fertility Promotion
Knowledge: Health Behavior
Knowledge: Health Promotion
Knowledge: Health Resources
Knowledge: Hypertension Management
Knowledge: Illness Care
Knowledge: Infant Care
Knowledge: Infection Management
Knowledge: Labor & Delivery
Knowledge: Medication

Knowledge: Multiple Sclerosis Management
Knowledge: Ostomy Care
Knowledge: Pain Management
Knowledge: Parenting
Knowledge: Personal Safety
Knowledge: Postpartum Maternal Health
Knowledge: Preconception Maternal Health
Knowledge: Pregnancy
Knowledge: Pregnancy and Postpartum
   Sexual Functioning
Knowledge: Prescribed Activity
Knowledge: Preterm Infant Care
Knowledge: Sexual Functioning
Knowledge: Substance Use Control
Knowledge: Treatment Procedure
Knowledge: Treatment Regimen
Knowledge: Weight Management
Memory
Neurological Status
Neurological Status: Autonomic
Neurological Status: Central Motor Control
Neurological Status: Consciousness
Neurological Status: Cranial Sensory/Motor
   Function
Neurological Status: Peripheral
Neurological Status: Spinal Sensory/Motor
   Function
Pain: Disruptive EffectsSensory Function
Sensory Function: Cutaneous
Sensory Function: Hearing
Sensory Function: Proprioception
Sensory Function: Taste & Smell
Sensory Function: Vision
Tissue Perfusion: Cerebral
Vision Compensation Behavior

COMMUNITY LEVEL:

Community Competence

NOC currently has no outcomes focused on the cognitive-perceptual pattern at the family level.

SLEEP-REST PATTERN: Describes pattern of sleep, rest, and relaxation at the individual, family, and community level. The family and community level focuses on disturbances such as noise, family schedules, and patterns of relaxation focused on group activities

INDIVIDUAL LEVEL:

Rest
Sleep

NOC currently has no outcomes focused on the sleep-rest pattern at the family or community level.

Self-Perception-Self-Concept Pattern: Describes self-concept pattern and perceptions of self such as body image, social self, self-competency, and subjective mood states. Negative evaluations of self include discomfort, change, loss, and threat. At the family and community level the focus is on status in the community, competency, and image.

Individual Level:

Body Image
Comfort Status
Comfort Status: Environment
Comfort Status: Physical
Comfort Status: Psychospiritual
Comfort Status: Sociocultural
Discomfort Level
Hope

Identity
Mood Equilibrium
Pain: Adverse Psychological Response
Pain Level
Personal Autonomy
Self-Esteem
Suffering Severity
Symptom Severity

Family Level:

Family Functioning

Community Level:

Community Competence

Role-Relationship Pattern: Describes pattern of role-engagements and relationships. This pattern includes family roles, work or student roles, and social roles. Loss, change, and threat are some of the major challenges included in this pattern. At the family level the dynamics of the family are the focus and center on supportive and close relationships or on the negative relationships such as abuse and violence.

Individual Level:

Abuse Cessation
Abuse Protection
Abusive Behavior Self-Restraint
Caregiver-Patient Relationship
Communication
Communication: Expressive
Communication: Receptive
Loneliness Severity
Neglect Cessation
Neglect Recovery
Parent-Infant Attachment

Parenting Performance
Parenting: Psychosocial Safety
Parenting: Adolescent Physical Safety
Parenting: Early/Middle Childhood Physical
  Safety
Parenting: Infant/Toddler Physical
  Safety
Role Performance
Social Interaction Skills
Social Involvement
Social Support

Family Level:

Family Integrity
Family Social Climate
Family Support During Treatment

Community Level:

Community Violence Level

Sexuality-Reproductive Pattern: Describes client's patterns of satisfaction and dissatisfaction with sexuality and reproductive patterns. At the family level the focus is on the couple, while the community level focuses on attitudes toward sexuality.

INDIVIDUAL LEVEL:

Abuse Recovery: Sexual
Physical Maturation: Female
Physical Maturation: Male
Sexual Functioning

Sexual Identity
Symptom Severity: Perimenopause
Symptom Severity: Premenstrual
   Syndrome (PMS)

NOC currently has no outcomes focused on the sexuality-reproductive pattern at the family or community level.

COPING-STRESS-TOLERANCE PATTERN: Describes general coping pattern and effectiveness of the pattern in terms of stress tolerance. At the family level similar patterns are the focus. The community level focuses on such problem areas as unemployment, racial or ethnic tensions, drug problems, or accident rates.

INDIVIDUAL LEVEL:

Abuse Recovery
Abuse Recovery: Emotional
Abuse Recovery: Financial
Abuse Recovery: Physical
Adaptation to Physical Disability
Aggression Self-Control
Agitation Level
Alcohol Abuse Cessation Behavior
Anxiety Level
Anxiety Self-Control
Caregiver Adaptation to Patient
   Institutionalization
Caregiver Lifestyle Disruption
Caregiver Role Endurance
Caregiver Stressors
Child Adaptation to Hospitalization
Comfortable Death
Coping

Depression Level
Depression Self-Control
Dignified Life Closure
Drug Abuse Cessation Behavior
Fear Level
Fear Level: Child
Fear Self-Control
Grief Resolution
Impulse Self-Control
Newborn Adaptation
Pain Control
Psychosocial Adjustment:
   Life Change
Self-Mutilation Restraint
Smoking Cessation Behavior
Stress Level
Substance Addiction Consequences
Suicide Self-Restraint

FAMILY LEVEL:

Family Coping
Family Normalization
Family Resiliency

NOC currently has no outcomes focused on the coping-stress-tolerance pattern at the community level.

VALUE-BELIEF PATTERN: Describes patterns of values, beliefs (including spiritual), or goals that guide choices and decisions. This pattern provides guidelines for ways of behaving at the individual, family, and community levels.

INDIVIDUAL LEVEL:

Health Beliefs
Health Beliefs: Perceived Ability
   to Perform
Health Beliefs: Perceived Control

Health Beliefs: Perceived Resources
Health Beliefs: Perceived Threat
Health Orientation
Spiritual Health

NOC currently has no outcomes focused on the value-belief pattern at the family or community level.

OUTCOMES NOT PLACED WITHIN A PATTERN:

Allergic Response: Localized
Allergic Response: Systemic
Blood Coagulation
Blood Loss Severity
Blood Transfusion Reaction
Client Satisfaction
Client Satisfaction: Access to Care Resources
Client Satisfaction: Caring
Client Satisfaction: Case Management
Client Satisfaction: Communication
Client Satisfaction: Continuity of Care
Client Satisfaction: Cultural Needs Fulfillment
Client Satisfaction: Functional Assistance
Client Satisfaction: Pain Management
Client Satisfaction: Physical Care
Client Satisfaction: Physical Environment
Client Satisfaction: Protection of Rights
Client Satisfaction: Psychological Care
Client Satisfaction: Safety
Client Satisfaction: Symptom Control
Client Satisfaction: Teaching
Client Satisfaction: Technical Aspects of Care
Hemodialysis Access
Mechanical Ventilation Response: Adult
Mechanical Ventilation Weaning Response: Adult

NOC Linkages–NANDA-I

This section of the book contains suggested linkages between the NANDA-I classification[1] published in 2007 and the current edition of NOC. The 385 NOC outcomes in this edition are linked to 188 nursing diagnoses. In some cases the diagnosis was divided into more specific type of diagnosis listed, so this provides linkages to 196 diagnoses. A linkage is an association or relationship that exists between a patient problem (nursing diagnosis) and a desired outcome (resolution or improvement of the problem). The change in outcome is usually a result of an intervention by a nurse or other health care provider. Treatments for a diagnosis will vary depending on the outcome selected. Linkages among NANDA, NOC, and NIC are available in a separate publication.[2] Linkages assist the nurse to select an outcome for a specific patient problem, thus facilitating clinical decision-making and diagnostic reasoning. The linkages also assist in the development of standardized care plans for specific populations and efforts to computerize nursing data in electronic health records. The linkage work supports the continuing refinement of the classification by helping to identify missing outcomes for future development.

The linkages identified in this section are options from which the nurse can select. Other outcomes may also be appropriate for a specific clinical problem. The linkages are based on expert judgement and clinical data from our test sites. This section is organized by key terms, and each problem has the NANDA definition included. Two categories of outcomes are available for each diagnosis. Outcomes considered to be the closest match to the diagnosis are listed under the category Suggested Outcomes; Outcomes closely associated to the diagnosis are listed under the category Additional Associated Outcomes. For the Risk Diagnoses only suggested outcomes are included.

References

1. NANDA-I. (2007). *NANDA nursing diagnoses: Definition and classification 2007-2008.* Philadelphia: Author.

2. Johnson, M., Bulechek, G., Butcher, H., Dochterman, J. Maas, M., Moorhead, S. & Swanson, E. (2006). *NANDA, NOC and NIC Linkages: Nursing diagnoses, outcomes and interventions* (2nd ed.). St. Louis: Mosby.

Activity Intolerance

DEFINITION: Insufficient physiological or psychological energy to endure or complete required or desired daily activities

SUGGESTED OUTCOMES:

Activity Tolerance
Discomfort Level
Endurance
Fatigue Level
Psychomotor Energy

Self-Care Status
Self-Care: Activities of Daily Living (ADL)
Self-Care: Instrumental Activities of Daily
   Living (IADL)
Vital Signs

ADDITIONAL ASSOCIATED OUTCOMES

Ambulation
Ambulation: Wheelchair
Asthma Self-Management
Cardiac Disease Self-Management
Cardiac Pump Effectiveness
Cardiopulmonary Status
Circulation Status
Client Satisfaction: Functional Assistance
Client Satisfaction: Symptom Control
Coordinated Movement
Discharge Readiness: Independent Living
Energy Conservation

Health Beliefs: Perceived Ability to Perform
Immobility Consequences: Physiological
Mobility
Mood Equilibrium
Multiple Sclerosis Self-Management
Nutritional Status: Energy
Pain: Disruptive Effects
Physical Fitness
Respiratory Status
Respiratory Status: Gas Exchange
Respiratory Status: Ventilation
Symptom Severity

Activity Intolerance, Risk for

DEFINITION: At risk for experiencing insufficient physiological or psychological energy to endure or complete required or desired daily activities

SUGGESTED OUTCOMES:

Activity Tolerance
Asthma Self-Management
Cardiac Disease Self-Management
Cardiac Pump Effectiveness
Cardiopulmonary Status
Circulation Status
Coordinated Movement
Depression Level
Discomfort Level
Endurance
Energy Conservation
Fatigue Level
Health Beliefs: Perceived Control
Knowledge: Disease Process
Knowledge: Prescribed Activity

Mood Equilibrium
Multiple Sclerosis Self-Management
Nutritional Status: Energy
Pain: Disruptive Effects
Pain Level
Physical Fitness
Respiratory Status
Respiratory Status: Gas Exchange
Respiratory Status: Ventilation
Risk Control
Risk Detection
Symptom Control
Symptom Severity
Weight Gain Behavior
Weight Loss Behavior

Airway Clearance, Ineffective

DEFINITION: Inability to clear secretions or obstructions from the respiratory tract to maintain a clear airway

SUGGESTED OUTCOMES:
Aspiration Prevention
Mechanical Ventilation Response: Adult
Respiratory Status: Airway Patency
Respiratory Status: Ventilation

ADDITIONAL ASSOCIATED OUTCOMES:
Allergic Response: Systemic
Anxiety Level
Asthma Self-Management
Cognition
Endurance
Fatigue Level
Immune Hypersensitivity Response
Infection Severity
Mechanical Ventilation Weaning Response: Adult
Neurological Status

Pain Level
Post-Procedure Recovery
Respiratory Status
Respiratory Status: Gas Exchange
Risk Control: Infectious Process
Risk Control: Tobacco Use
Smoking Cessation Behavior
Symptom Control
Treatment Behavior: Illness or Injury
Vital Signs

Anxiety

DEFINITION: Vague uneasy feeling of discomfort or dread accompanied by an autonomic response (the source often nonspecific or unknown to the individual); a feeling of apprehension caused by anticipation of danger. It is an alerting signal that warns of impending danger and enables the individual to take measures to deal with threat.

SUGGESTED OUTCOMES:
Anxiety Level
Anxiety Self-Control
Concentration

Coping
Hyperactivity Level

ADDITIONAL ASSOCIATED OUTCOMES:
Acceptance: Health Status
Aggression Self-Control
Agitation Level
Child Adaptation to Hospitalization
Client Satisfaction: Caring
Client Satisfaction: Psychological Care
Elopement Propensity Risk
Fatigue Level
Grief Resolution
Impulse Self-Control
Information Processing
Nausea & Vomiting Control

Nausea & Vomiting Severity
Neurological Status: Autonomic
Parent-Infant Attachment
Psychosocial Adjustment: Life Change
Safe Wandering
Self-Mutilation Restraint
Sleep
Social Interaction Skills
Stress Level
Substance Withdrawal Severity
Symptom Control
Vital Signs

Aspiration, Risk for

DEFINITION: At risk for entry of gastrointestinal secretions, oropharyngeal secretions, solids, or fluids into tracheobronchial passages

SUGGESTED OUTCOMES: CONT'D

Aspiration Prevention
Body Positioning: Self-Initiated
Cognition
Cognitive Orientation
Gastrointestinal Function
Immobility Consequences: Physiological
Knowledge: Treatment Procedure
Mechanical Ventilation Response: Adult
Nausea & Vomiting Control
Nausea & Vomiting Severity

Neurological Status
Post-Procedure Recovery
Pre-Procedure Readiness
Respiratory Status
Respiratory Status: Ventilation
Risk Control
Risk Detection
Seizure Control
Self-Care: Non-Parenteral Medication
Swallowing Status

Autonomic Dysreflexia

DEFINITION: Life-threatening, uninhibited sympathetic response of the nervous system to a noxious stimulus after a spinal cord injury at T7 or above

SUGGESTED OUTCOMES:

Neurological Status: Autonomic
Sensory Function: Cutaneous
Vital Signs

ADDITIONAL ASSOCIATED OUTCOMES:

Circulation Status
Knowledge: Disease Process
Neurological Status
Neurological Status: Peripheral
Sensory Function

Sensory Function: Vision
Symptom Severity
Tissue Integrity: Skin & Mucous
    Membranes
Treatment Behaviors: Illness or Injury

Autonomic Dysreflexia, Risk for

DEFINITION: At risk for life-threatening, uninhibited response of the sympathetic nervous system, post spinal shock, in an individual with a spinal cord injury or lesion at T6 or above (has been demonstrated in patients with injuries at T7 and T8)

SUGGESTED OUTCOMES:

Bowel Elimination
Caregiver Home Care Readiness
Discomfort Level
Gastrointestinal Function
Infection Severity

Knowledge: Disease Process
Knowledge: Medication
Medication Response
Neurological Status: Autonomic
Pain Level

Suggested Outcomes: Cont'd

Risk Control

Risk Control: Hyperthermia

Risk Control: Infectious Process

Risk Detection

Substance Withdrawal Severity

Symptom Severity

Thermoregulation

Tissue Integrity: Skin & Mucous
   Membranes

Treatment Behavior: Illness or Injury

Urinary Elimination

Vital Signs

Blood Glucose, Risk for Unstable

Definition: Risk for variation of blood glucose/sugar levels from the normal range

Suggested Outcomes:

Acceptance: Health Status

Adherence Behavior: Healthy Diet

Blood Glucose Level

Caregiver Stressors

Compliance Behavior: Prescribed Healthy Diet

Compliance Behavior: Prescribed Medication

Coping

Diabetes Self-Management

Health Promoting Behavior

Health Seeking Behavior

Knowledge: Diabetes Management

Knowledge: Diet

Knowledge: Medication

Knowledge: Weight Management

Nutritional Status

Personal Health Status

Physical Fitness

Prenatal Health Behavior

Risk Control

Risk Detection

Sleep

Stress Level

Weight Gain Behavior

Weight Loss Behavior

Body Image, Disturbed

Definition: Confusion in mental picture of one's physical self

Suggested Outcomes:

Adaptation to Physical Disability

Body Image

Child Development: Adolescence

Self-Esteem

Additional Associated Outcomes:

Acceptance: Health Status

Burn Recovery

Child Development: 2 Years

Child Development: 3 Years

Child Development: 4 Years

Child Development: 5 Years

Child Development: Middle
   Childhood

Coping

Development: Late Adulthood

Development: Middle Adulthood

Development: Young Adulthood

Distorted Thought Self-Control

Heedfulness of Affected Side

Identity

Sexual Functioning

Sexual Identity

Weight: Body Mass

Weight Gain Behavior

Weight Loss Behavior

Body Temperature, Risk for Imbalanced

DEFINITION: At risk for failure to maintain body temperature within normal range

SUGGESTED OUTCOMES:

Burn Healing
Hydration
Immune Status
Infection Severity
Infection Severity: Newborn
Medication Response
Neglect Recovery
Neurological Status: Autonomic
Post-Procedure Recovery

Risk Control
Risk Control: Hyperthermia
Risk Control: Hypothermia
Risk Control: Infectious Process
Risk Control: Sun Exposure
Risk Detection
Substance Withdrawal Severity
Thermoregulation
Thermoregulation: Newborn

Bowel Incontinence

DEFINITION: Change in normal bowel habits characterized by involuntary passage of stool

SUGGESTED OUTCOMES:

Bowel Continence
Bowel Elimination
Tissue Integrity: Skin & Mucous Membranes

ADDITIONAL ASSOCIATED OUTCOMES:

Acute Confusion Level
Cognition
Fluid Overload Severity
Gastrointestinal Function
Knowledge: Ostomy Care
Neurological Status: Spinal Sensory/Motor
    Function

Nutritional Status: Food & Fluid Intake
Ostomy Self-Care
Self-Care: Hygiene
Self-Care: Toileting

Breastfeeding, Effective

DEFINITION: Mother-infant dyad/family exhibits adequate proficiency and satisfaction with breastfeeding process

SUGGESTED OUTCOMES:

Breastfeeding Establishment: Infant
Breastfeeding Establishment: Maternal

Breastfeeding Maintenance
Breastfeeding Weaning

ADDITIONAL ASSOCIATED OUTCOMES:

Anxiety Self-Control
Child Development: 1 Month
Child Development: 2 Months
Cognition
Fluid Balance
Growth

Hydration
Knowledge: Breastfeeding
Nutritional Status: Food &
    Fluid Intake
Parent-Infant Attachment
Postpartum Maternal Health Behavior

ADDITIONAL ASSOCIATED OUTCOMES: CONT'D

Social Support

Swallowing Status

Urinary Elimination

Weight: Body Mass

Breastfeeding, Ineffective

DEFINITION: Dissatisfaction or difficulty a mother, infant, or child experiences with the breastfeeding process

SUGGESTED OUTCOMES:

Breastfeeding Establishment: Infant

Breastfeeding Establishment: Maternal

Breastfeeding Maintenance

Breastfeeding Weaning

Knowledge: Breastfeeding

ADDITIONAL ASSOCIATED OUTCOMES:

Anxiety Self-Control

Child Development: 1 Month

Child Development: 2 Months

Cognition

Fatigue Level

Fluid Balance

Growth

Hydration

Knowledge: Infant Care

Nutritional Status: Food & Fluid Intake

Pain Level

Parent-Infant Attachment

Personal Health Status

Postpartum Maternal Health Behavior

Social Support

Swallowing Status

Urinary Elimination

Weight: Body Mass

Breastfeeding, Interrupted

DEFINITION: Break in the continuity of the breastfeeding process as a result of inability or inadvisability to put baby to breast for feeding

SUGGESTED OUTCOMES:

Breastfeeding Maintenance

Breastfeeding Weaning

Knowledge: Breastfeeding

Parent-Infant Attachment

ADDITIONAL ASSOCIATED OUTCOMES:

Fatigue Level

Infection Severity

Medication Response

Motivation

Parenting Performance

Personal Health Status

Postpartum Maternal Health Behavior

Risk Control: Alcohol Use

Risk Control: Drug Use

Role Performance

Stress Level

Breathing Pattern, Ineffective

DEFINITION: Inspiration and/or expiration that does not provide adequate ventilation

SUGGESTED OUTCOMES:

Allergic Response: Systemic

Mechanical Ventilation Response: Adult

Respiratory Status: Airway Patency

Respiratory Status: Gas Exchange

Respiratory Status: Ventilation

Vital Signs

ADDITIONAL ASSOCIATED OUTCOMES: CONT'D

Anxiety Level
Asthma Self-Management
Cardiopulmonary Status
Cognition
Discomfort Level
Electrolyte & Acid/Base Balance
Energy Conservation
Fatigue Level
Fluid Overload Severity
Infection Severity

Neurological Status: Autonomic
Neurological Status: Central Motor Control
Pain Level
Pre-Procedure Readiness
Respiratory Status
Risk Control: Infectious Process
Smoking Cessation Behavior
Weight: Body Mass
Weight Loss Behavior
Weight Maintenance Behavior

Cardiac Output, Decreased

DEFINITION: Inadequate blood pumped by the heart to meet metabolic demands of the body

SUGGESTED OUTCOMES:

Anxiety Level
Cardiac Pump Effectiveness
Cardiopulmonary Status
Circulation Status
Fluid Overload Severity
Tissue Perfusion: Abdominal Organs

Tissue Perfusion: Cardiac
Tissue Perfusion: Cellular
Tissue Perfusion: Cerebral
Tissue Perfusion: Peripheral
Vital Signs

ADDITIONAL ASSOCIATED OUTCOMES:

Acute Confusion Level
Agitation Level
Blood Coagulation
Blood Loss Severity
Cardiac Disease Self-Management
Cognition
Electrolyte & Acid/Base Balance
Endurance
Energy Conservation
Fatigue Level

Fluid Balance
Fluid Overload Severity
Hydration
Neurological Status: Autonomic
Respiratory Status
Respiratory Status: Gas Exchange
Respiratory Status: Ventilation
Tissue Perfusion: Pulmonary
Urinary Elimination

Caregiver Role Strain

DEFINITION: Difficulty in performing family caregiver role

SUGGESTED OUTCOMES:

Caregiver Emotional Health
Caregiver Lifestyle Disruption
Caregiver-Patient Relationship
Caregiver Performance: Direct Care
Caregiver Performance: Indirect Care
Caregiver Physical Health
Caregiver Role Endurance

Caregiver Stressors
Caregiver Well-Being
Family Support During Treatment
Parenting Performance
Personal Resiliency
Postpartum Maternal Health Behavior
Role Performance

ADDITIONAL ASSOCIATED OUTCOMES:

Caregiver Home Care Readiness
Depression Level
Depression Self-Control
Family Coping
Family Functioning
Family Resiliency

Fatigue Level
Knowledge: Health Resources
Leisure Participation
Social Involvement
Social Support
Stress Level

Caregiver Role Strain, Risk for

DEFINITION: Caregiver is vulnerable for felt difficulty in performing the family caregiver role

SUGGESTED OUTCOMES:

Caregiver Emotional Health
Caregiver Home Care Readiness
Caregiver Lifestyle Disruption
Caregiver-Patient Relationship
Caregiver Performance: Direct Care
Caregiver Performance: Indirect Care
Caregiver Physical Health
Caregiver Role Endurance
Caregiver Stressors
Coping
Depression Level
Discharge Readiness: Supported Living
Family Coping
Family Functioning
Family Resiliency

Family Support During Treatment
Fatigue Level
Knowledge: Energy Conservation
Knowledge: Health Behavior
Knowledge: Health Resources
Leisure Participation
Parenting Performance
Personal Resiliency
Rest
Risk Control
Risk Detection
Role Performance
Sleep
Stress Level
Substance Withdrawal Severity

Comfort, Readiness for Enhanced

DEFINITION: A pattern of ease, relief, and transcendence in physical, psychospiritual, environmental, and/or social dimensions that can be strengthened

SUGGESTED OUTCOMES:

Comfort Status
Comfort Status: Environment
Comfort Status: Physical
Comfort Status: Psychospiritual
Comfort Status: Sociocultural
Comfortable Death
Dignified Life Closure
Grief Resolution

Hope
Leisure Participation
Personal Autonomy
Personal Resiliency
Personal Well-Being
Quality of Life
Spiritual Health

ADDITIONAL ASSOCIATED OUTCOMES:

Abuse Recovery
Anxiety Level
Coping

Depression Level
Discomfort Level
Fatigue Level

ADDITIONAL ASSOCIATED OUTCOMES: CONT'D

Fear Level
Health-Seeking Behavior
Loneliness Severity
Mood Equilibrium
Neglect Recovery
Pain Level
Personal Health Status
Psychosocial Adjustment: Life Change
Rest
Risk Control

Risk Detection
Sleep
Social Interaction Skills
Social Involvement
Social Support
Stress Level
Suffering Severity
Suicide Self-Restraint
Will to Live

Communication, Impaired Verbal

DEFINITION: Decreased, delayed, or absent ability to receive, process, transmit, and/or use a system of symbols

SUGGESTED OUTCOMES:

Communication
Communication: Expressive
Communication: Receptive

ADDITIONAL ASSOCIATED OUTCOMES:

Acute Confusion Level
Agitation Level
Child Development: 3 Years
Child Development: 4 Years
Child Development: 5 Years
Child Development: Middle Childhood
Child Development: Adolescent
Client Satisfaction: Communication
Cognition
Cognitive Orientation
Development: Late Adulthood
Development: Middle Adulthood
Development: Young Adulthood

Distorted Thought Self-Control
Information Processing
Neurological Status
Neurological Status: Cranial Sensory/Motor
  Function
Respiratory Status
Self-Esteem
Sensory Function
Sensory Function: Hearing
Sensory Function: Vision
Stress Level
Tissue Perfusion: Cerebral

Communication, Readiness for Enhanced

DEFINITION: A pattern of exchanging information and ideas with others that is sufficient for meeting one's needs and life's goals, and can be strengthened

SUGGESTED OUTCOMES:

Communication
Communication: Expressive
Communication: Receptive

ADDITIONAL ASSOCIATED OUTCOMES:

Child Development: Adolescence
Client Satisfaction: Communication
Development: Late Adulthood
Development: Middle Adulthood
Development: Young Adulthood

Health-Seeking Behavior
Hearing Compensation Behavior
Motivation
Social Interaction Skills

Community Coping, Ineffective

DEFINITION: Pattern of community activities for adaptation and problem solving that is unsatisfactory for meeting the demands or needs of the community

SUGGESTED OUTCOMES:

Community Competence
Community Disaster Readiness
Community Risk Control: Chronic Disease
Community Risk Control: Communicable
   Disease

Community Risk Control: Lead Exposure
Community Risk Control: Violence
Community Violence Level

ADDITIONAL ASSOCIATED OUTCOMES:

Community Disaster Response
Community Health Status

Community Health Status: Immunity

Community Coping, Readiness for Enhanced

DEFINITION: Pattern of community activities for adaptation and problem solving that is satisfactory for meeting the demands or needs of the community but can be improved for management of current and future problems/stressors

SUGGESTED OUTCOMES:
Community Competence
Community Disaster Readiness
Community Disaster Response

ADDITIONAL ASSOCIATED OUTCOMES:
Community Risk Control: Chronic Disease
Community Risk Control: Communicable Disease
Community Risk Control: Lead Exposure
Community Risk Control: Violence

Community Therapeutic Regimen Management, Ineffective

DEFINITION: Pattern of regulating and integrating into community processes programs for treatment of illness and the sequelae of illness that are unsatisfactory for meeting health-related goals

SUGGESTED OUTCOMES:
Community Risk Control: Chronic Disease
Community Risk Control: Communicable Disease
Community Risk Control: Lead Exposure

ADDITIONAL ASSOCIATED OUTCOMES:
Community Disaster Readiness
Community Disaster Response
Community Health Status
Community Health Status: Immunity

Confusion, Acute

DEFINITION: Abrupt onset of reversible disturbances of consciousness, attention, cognition, and perception that develop over a short period of time

SUGGESTED OUTCOMES:
Acute Confusion Level
Agitation Level
Cognitive Orientation
Information Processing
Neurological Status: Consciousness

ADDITIONAL ASSOCIATED OUTCOMES:

Alcohol Abuse Cessation Behavior
Anxiety Level
Blood Glucose Level
Cardiopulmonary Status
Cognition
Concentration
Development: Late Adulthood
Distorted Thought Self-Control
Drug Abuse Cessation Behavior
Electrolyte & Acid/Base Balance
Elopement Propensity Risk
Fatigue Level

Fluid Balance
Infection Severity
Memory
Personal Resiliency
Respiratory Status
Respiratory Status: Gas Exchange
Safe Home Environment
Safe Wandering
Sleep
Substance Withdrawal Severity
Thermoregulation
Tisssue Perfusion: Cerebral

Confusion, Chronic

DEFINITION: Irreversible, long-standing, and/or progressive deterioration of intellect and personality characterized by decreased ability to interpret environmental stimuli; decreased capacity for intellectual thought processes; and manifested by disturbances of memory, orientation, and behavior

SUGGESTED OUTCOMES:
Cognition
Cognitive Orientation
Concentration
Decision-Making

Distorted Thought Self-Control
Identity
Information Processing
Memory

ADDITIONAL ASSOCIATED OUTCOMES:

Agitation Level

Client Satisfaction

Client Satisfaction: Access to Care Resources

Client Satisfaction: Case Management

Client Satisfaction: Continuity of Care

Client Satisfaction: Pain Management

Client Satisfaction: Protection of Rights

Client Satisfaction: Safety

Communication

Elopement Occurrence

Elopement Propensity Risk

Fatigue Level

Personal Autonomy

Risk Control: Alcohol Use

Risk Control: Drug Use

Safe Home Environment

Safe Wandering

Social Interaction Skills

Confusion, Risk for Acute

DEFINITION: At risk for reversible disturbances of consciousness, attention, cognition, and perception that develop over a short period of time

SUGGESTED OUTCOMES:

Acute Confusion Level

Cognition

Cognitive Orientation

Concentration

Development: Late Adulthood

Electrolyte & Acid/Base Balance

Elopement Occurrence

Elopement Propensity Risk

Fatigue Level

Fluid Balance

Gastrointestinal Function

Hydration

Infection Severity

Information Processing

Kidney Function

Medication Response

Memory

Mobility

Neurological Status: Consciousness

Pain Level

Personal Resiliency

Physical Aging

Respiratory Status

Risk Control

Risk Control: Alcohol Use

Risk Control: Drug Use

Risk Control: Infectious Process

Risk Detection

Sleep

Urinary Elimination

Constipation

DEFINITION: Decrease in normal frequency of defecation accompanied by difficult or incomplete passage of stool and/or passage of excessively hard, dry stool

SUGGESTED OUTCOMES:

Bowel Elimination

Gastrointestinal Function

Hydration

Nausea & Vomiting Severity

Symptom Control

ADDITIONAL ASSOCIATED OUTCOMES:

Adherence Behavior: Healthy Diet

Appetite

Compliance Behavior: Prescribed Diet

Discomfort Level

Medication Response

Mobility

Nutritional Status: Food & Fluid Intake

Self-Care: Non-Parenteral Medication

Self-Care: Toileting

Constipation, Perceived

DEFINITION: Self-diagnosis of constipation and abuse of laxatives, enemas, and suppositories to ensure a daily bowel movement

SUGGESTED OUTCOMES:
Bowel Elimination
Gastrointestinal Function
Health Beliefs
Knowledge: Health Behavior

ADDITIONAL ASSOCIATED OUTCOMES:

Adherence Behavior
Adherence Behavior: Healthy Diet
Compliance Behavior: Prescribed Diet
Health Beliefs: Perceived Threat
Hydration

Knowledge: Ostomy Care
Medication Response
Mobility
Nutritional Status: Food & Fluid Intake
Treatment Behavior: Illness or Injury

Constipation, Risk for

DEFINITION: At risk for a decrease in normal frequency of defecation accompanied by difficult or incomplete passage of stool and/or passage of excessively hard, dry stool

SUGGESTED OUTCOMES:

Adherence Behavior: Healthy Diet
Appetite
Bowel Elimination
Compliance Behavior: Prescribed Diet
Gastrointestinal Function
Hydration
Immobility Consequences: Physiological
Knowledge: Medication
Medication Response

Mobility
Nutritional Status: Food & Fluid Intake
Risk Control
Risk Detection
Self-Care: Non-Parenteral Medication
Self-Care: Toileting
Symptom Control
Treatment Behavior: Illness or Injury

Contamination

DEFINITION: Exposure to environmental contaminants in doses sufficient to cause adverse health effects

SUGGESTED OUTCOMES:

Allergic Response: Localized
Community Disaster Response
Gastrointestinal Function
Immune Status

Kidney Function
Neurological Status
Respiratory Status

ADDITIONAL ASSOCIATED OUTCOMES:

Allergic Response: Systemic
Circulation Status
Community Competence
Community Disaster Readiness
Community Health Status
Community Health Status: Immunity
Community Risk Control: Chronic Disease
Community Risk Control: Communicable
    Disease
Community Risk Control: Lead Exposure
Immune Hypersensitivity Response

Knowledge: Cancer Reduction Threat
Nutritional Status
Personal Safety Behavior
Risk Control: Cancer
Risk Control: Infectious Process
Risk Control: Sun Exposure
Risk Control: Tobacco Use
Safe Home Environment
Substance Addiction Consequences
Tissue Integrity: Skin & Mucous Membranes

Contamination, Risk for

DEFINITION: Accentuated risk of exposure to environmental contaminants in doses sufficient to cause adverse health effects

SUGGESTED OUTCOMES:

Community Risk Control: Communicable
    Disease
Community Risk Control: Lead Exposure
Immune Status
Nutritional Status: Nutrient Intake
Personal Safety Behavior
Personal Resiliency
Risk Control

Risk Control: Cancer
Risk Control: Infectious Process
Risk Control: Tobacco Use
Risk Detection
Safe Home Environment
Self-Care: Bathing
Self-Care: Hygiene

Coping, Defensive

DEFINITION: Repeated projection of falsely positive self-evaluation based on a self-protective pattern that defends against underlying perceived threats to positive self-regard

SUGGESTED OUTCOMES:

Acceptance: Health Status
Adaptation to Physical Disability
Child Development: Adolescence
Coping

Personal Resiliency
Self-Esteem
Social Interaction Skills

ADDITIONAL ASSOCIATED OUTCOMES:

Grief Resolution
Impulse Self-Control
Psychosocial Adjustment: Life Change
Risk Control: Alcohol Use
Risk Control: Drug Use

Risk Control: Tobacco Use
Smoking Cessation Behavior
Social Involvement
Social Support
Substance Withdrawal Severity

Coping, Ineffective

DEFINITION: Inability to form a valid appraisal of the stressors, inadequate choices of practiced responses, and/or inability to use available resources

SUGGESTED OUTCOMES:

Acceptance: Health Status
Adaptation to Physical Disability
Child Adaptation to Hospitalization
Coping
Decision-Making
Impulse Self-Control

Knowledge: Health Resources
Personal Resiliency
Psychosocial Adjustment:
    Life Change
Role Performance
Stress Level

ADDITIONAL ASSOCIATED OUTCOMES:

Abusive Behavior Self-Restraint
Aggression Self-Control
Alcohol Abuse Cessation Behavior
Anxiety Self-Control
Caregiver Stressors
Concentration
Depression Self-Control
Drug Abuse Cessation Behavior
Fatigue Level
Grief Resolution
Information Processing
Personal Well-Being

Quality of Life
Risk Control: Alcohol Use
Risk Control: Drug Use
Risk Control: Tobacco Use
Self-Esteem
Self-Mutilation Restraint
Sleep
Smoking Cessation Behavior
Social Interaction Skills
Social Support
Substance Withdrawal Severity
Suicide Self-Restraint

Coping, Readiness for Enhanced

DEFINITION: A pattern of cognitive and behavioral efforts to manage demands that is sufficient for well-being and can be strengthened

SUGGESTED OUTCOMES:

Acceptance: Health Status
Adaptation to Physical Disability
Coping
Personal Resiliency

Personal Well-Being
Role Performance
Stress Level

ADDITIONAL ASSOCIATED OUTCOMES:

Caregiver Emotional Health
Caregiver Stressors
Child Adaptation to Hospitalization
Decision-Making
Health-Seeking Behavior

Motivation
Psychological Adjustment Life Change
Quality of Life
Self-Esteem
Social Interaction Skills

Death Anxiety

DEFINITION: Vague uneasy feeling of discomfort or dread generated by perceptions of a real or imagined threat to one's existence

SUGGESTED OUTCOMES:

Acceptance: Health Status
Anxiety Level
Comfortable Death
Dignified Life Closure

Fear Level
Psychosocial Adjustment: Life Change
Spiritual Health

ADDITIONAL ASSOCIATED OUTCOMES:

Coping
Anxiety Self-control
Depression Level
Depression Self-Control
Development: Late Adulthood
Discomfort Level
Fatigue Level
Fear Self-Control
Grief Resolution

Health Beliefs: Perceived Threat
Hope
Pain Control
Participation in Health Care Decisions
Personal Autonomy
Personal Resiliency
Social Support
Stress Level

Decision Making, Readiness for Enhanced

DEFINITION: A pattern of choosing courses of action that is sufficient for meeting short- and long-term health-related goals and can be strengthened

SUGGESTED OUTCOMES:

Adherence Behavior: Healthy Diet
Alcohol Abuse Cessation Behavior
Client Satisfaction: Protection of Rights
Compliance Behavior: Prescribed Diet
Compliance Behavior: Prescribed Medication
Decision-Making
Drug Abuse Cessation Behavior

Personal Autonomy
Postpartum Maternal Health Behavior
Risk Control
Risk Detection
Smoking Cessation Behavior
Weight Gain Behavior
Weight Loss Behavior

ADDITIONAL ASSOCIATED OUTCOMES:

Adaptation to Physical Disability
Family Participation in Professional Care
Health Beliefs: Perceived Ability to Perform
Health Beliefs: Perceived Control

Health-Seeking Behavior
Motivation
Participation in Health Care Decisions

Decisional Conflict

DEFINITION: Uncertainty about course of action to be taken when choice among competing actions involves risk, loss, or challenge to values and beliefs

SUGGESTED OUTCOMES:

Decision-Making
Information Processing
Participation in Health Care Decisions

Personal Autonomy
Stress Level

ADDITIONAL ASSOCIATED OUTCOMES:

Coping
Family Coping
Family Functioning
Family Social Climate
Health Beliefs

Health Orientation
Knowledge: Disease Process
Knowledge: Treatment Regimen
Psychosocial Adjustment: Life Change
Social Support

Denial, Ineffective

DEFINITION: Conscious or unconscious attempt to disavow the knowledge or meaning of an event to reduce anxiety/fear, but leading to the detriment of health

SUGGESTED OUTCOMES:

Acceptance: Health Status
Anxiety Self-Control
Fear Self-Control

Health Beliefs: Perceived Threat
Personal Resiliency
Symptom Severity

ADDITIONAL ASSOCIATED OUTCOMES:

Anxiety Level
Coping
Fear Level
Fear Level: Child
Health Beliefs
Health Seeking Behavior

Mood Equilibrium
Psychosocial Adjustment: Life Change
Social Support
Stress Level
Symptom Control

Dentition, Impaired

DEFINITION: Disruption in tooth development/eruption patterns or structural integrity of individual teeth

SUGGESTED OUTCOMES:

Oral Hygiene
Self-Care: Oral Hygiene

ADDITIONAL ASSOCIATED OUTCOMES:

Alcohol Abuse Cessation Behavior
Health Beliefs: Perceived Resources
Infection Severity
Knowledge: Health Behavior
Knowledge: Health Resources
Medication Response
Nausea & Vomiting Severity

Nutritional Status: Nutrient Intake
Pain Level
Risk Control: Drug Use
Risk Control: Infectious Process
Risk Control: Tobacco Use
Smoking Cessation Behavior
Weight Gain Behavior

Development, Risk for Delayed

DEFINITION: At risk for delay of 25% or more in one or more of the areas of social or self-regulatory behavior, or in cognitive, language, gross or fine motor skills

SUGGESTED OUTCOMES:

Abuse Recovery
Abuse Recovery: Physical
Abusive Behavior Self-Restraint
Caregiver Emotional Health
Caregiver Physical Health
Child Development: 1 Month
Child Development: 2 Months
Child Development: 4 Months
Child Development: 6 Months
Child Development: 12 Months
Child Development: 2 Years
Child Development: 3 Years
Child Development: 4 Years
Child Development: 5 Years
Child Development: Middle Childhood
Child Development: Adolescence
Development: Late Adulthood
Development: Middle Adulthood
Development: Young Adulthood
Family Functioning
Family Integrity
Family Social Climate
Fetal Status: Antepartum
Fetal Status: Intrapartum
Growth
Knowledge: Infant Care

Knowledge: Parenting
Maternal Status: Antepartum
Maternal Status: Intrapartum
Neglect Recovery
Newborn Adaptation
Parent-Infant Attachment
Parenting: Adolescent Physical Safety
Parenting: Early/Middle Childhood
   Physical Safety
Parenting: Infant/Toddler
   Physical Safety
Parenting Performance
Parenting: Psychosocial Safety
Personal Autonomy
Personal Health Status
Play Participation
Postpartum Maternal Health Behavior
Prenatal Health Behavior
Preterm Infant Organization
Risk Control
Risk Control: Alcohol Use
Risk Control: Drug Use
Risk Detection
Social Interaction Skills
Student Health Status
Substance Addiction Consequences

Diarrhea

DEFINITION: Passage of loose, unformed stools

SUGGESTED OUTCOMES:

Bowel Continence
Bowel Elimination
Electrolyte & Acid/Base Balance
Fluid Balance

Gastrointestinal Function
Hydration
Ostomy Self-Care
Symptom Severity

ADDITIONAL ASSOCIATED OUTCOMES:

Adherence Behavior: Healthy Diet
Anxiety Level
Anxiety Self-Control
Compliance Behavior: Prescribed Diet
Infection Severity
Medication Response
Nutritional Status: Biochemical Measures
Nutritional Status: Food & Fluid Intake

Risk Control: Alcohol Use
Risk Control: Drug Use
Risk Control: Infectious Process
Self-Care: Non-Parenteral Medication
Stress Level
Symptom Control
Treatment Behavior: Illness or Injury

Disuse Syndrome, Risk for

DEFINITION: At risk for deterioration of body systems as the result of prescribed or unavoidable musculoskeletal inactivity

SUGGESTED OUTCOMES:

Burn Recovery
Coordinated Movement
Discomfort Level
Endurance
Heedfulness of Affected Side
Immobility Consequences: Physiological
Immobility Consequences: Psycho-Cognitive
Joint Movement
Joint Movement: Ankle
Joint Movement: Elbow
Joint Movement: Fingers
Joint Movement: Hip
Joint Movement: Knee

Joint Movement: Neck
Joint Movement: Passive
Joint Movement: Shoulder
Joint Movement: Spine
Joint Movement: Wrist
Mobility
Neurological Status: Consciousness
Pain Level
Risk Control
Risk Detection
Skeletal Function
Transfer Performance

Diversional Activity, Deficient

DEFINITION: Decreased stimulation from (or interest or engagement in) recreational or leisure activities

SUGGESTED OUTCOMES:

Leisure Participation
Motivation

Play Participation
Social Involvement

ADDITIONAL ASSOCIATED OUTCOMES:

Child Development: 2 Years

Child Development: 3 Years

Child Development: 4 Years

Child Development: 5 Years

Child Development: Middle
  Childhood

Child Development: Adolescence

Development: Late Adulthood

Development: Middle Adulthood

Development: Young Adulthood

Health Promoting Behavior

Loneliness Severity

Personal Well-Being

Social Interaction Skills

Energy Field, Disturbed

DEFINITION: Disruption of the flow of energy surrounding a person's being results in disharmony of the body, mind, and/or spirit

SUGGESTED OUTCOMES:

Personal Health Status

Personal Well-Being

Spiritual Health

ADDITIONAL ASSOCIATED OUTCOMES:

Discomfort Level

Health Beliefs

Health Orientation

Pain Level

Personal Resiliency

Self-Esteem

Suffering Severity

Environmental Interpretation Syndrome, Impaired

DEFINITION: Consistent lack of orientation to person, place, time, or circumstances over more than 3 to 6 months necessitating a protective environment

SUGGESTED OUTCOMES:

Cognitive Orientation

Concentration

Memory

Neurological Status: Consciousness

Safe Home Environment

ADDITIONAL ASSOCIATED OUTCOMES:

Acute Confusion Level

Anxiety Level

Cognition

Communication

Decision-Making

Depression Level

Depression Self-Control

Elopement Occurrence

Elopement Propensity Risk

Family Resiliency

Information Processing

Loneliness Severity

Personal Resiliency

Safe Wandering

Failure to Thrive, Adult

DEFINITION: Progressive functional deterioration of a physical and cognitive nature. The individual's ability to live with multisystem diseases, cope with ensuing problems, and manage his/her care is remarkably diminished.

SUGGESTED OUTCOMES:

Appetite
Cardiopulmonary Status
Cognition
Endurance
Gastrointestinal Function
Nutritional Status

Nutritional Status: Food & Fluid Intake
Personal Resiliency
Physical Aging
Weight: Body Mass
Will to Live

ADDITIONAL ASSOCIATED OUTCOMES:

Acceptance: Health Status
Acute Confusion Level
Bowel Continence
Communication
Decision-Making
Depression Level
Depression Self-Control
Development: Late Adulthood
Development: Middle Adulthood
Discharge Readiness: Independent Living
Hydration
Infection Severity
Information Processing
Leisure Participation
Mood Equilibrium

Nausea & Vomiting Severity
Neglect Cessation
Neglect Recovery
Nutritional Status: Nutrient Intake
Personal Health Status
Psychosocial Adjustment: Life Change
Risk Control: Infectious Process
Self-Care: Activities of Daily
    Living (ADL)
Social Involvement
Suffering Severity
Treatment Behavior: Illness or Injury
Urinary Continence
Weight Gain Behavior
Weight Maintenance Behavior

Falls, Risk for

DEFINITION: Increased susceptibility to falling that may cause physical harm

SUGGESTED OUTCOMES:

Acute Confusion Level
Agitation Level
Ambulation
Balance
Blood Glucose Level
Cognition
Coordinated Movement
Elopement Occurrence
Endurance
Fall Prevention Behavior
Falls Occurrence
Fatigue Level
Heedfulness of Affected Side
Knowledge: Child Physical Safety

Knowledge: Fall Prevention
Medication Response
Mobility
Neurological Status: Central Motor Control
Nutritional Status
Pain Level
Parenting: Early/Middle Childhood Physical
    Safety
Parenting: Infant/Toddler Physical Safety
Physical Injury Severity
Post-Procedure Recovery
Risk Control
Risk Detection
Safe Home Environment

SUGGESTED OUTCOMES: CONT'D

Safe Wandering
Seizure Control
Self-Care: Toileting
Sensory Function
Sensory Function: Hearing

Sensory Function: Vision
Skeletal Function
Transfer Performance
Vision Compensation Behavior

Family Coping, Compromised

DEFINITION: Usually supportive primary person (family member or close friend) provides insufficient, ineffective, or compromised support, comfort, assistance, or encouragement that may be needed by the client to manage or master adaptive tasks related to his/her health challenge

SUGGESTED OUTCOMES:

Caregiver Emotional Health
Caregiver-Patient Relationship
Caregiver Performance:
   Direct Care

Caregiver Performance: Indirect Care
Caregiving Role Endurance
Family Coping
Family Normalization

ADDITIONAL ASSOCIATED OUTCOMES:

Caregiver Stressors
Family Participation in
   Professional Care
Family Resiliency

Family Support During Treatment
Neglect Cessation
Parent-Infant Attachment
Parenting Performance

Family Coping, Disabled

DEFINITION: Behavior of significant person (family member or other primary person) that disables his/her capacities and the client's capacities to effectively address tasks essential to either person's adaptation to the health challenge

SUGGESTED OUTCOMES:

Caregiver-Patient Relationship
Caregiver Performance: Direct Care
Caregiver Performance: Indirect Care
Caregiver Role Endurance

Caregiver Well-Being
Family Coping
Family Normalization
Neglect Recovery

ADDITIONAL ASSOCIATED OUTCOMES:

Adaptation to Physical Disability
Adherence Behavior: Healthy Diet
Agitation Level
Caregiver Emotional Health
Caregiver Stressors
Compliance Behavior: Prescribed Diet
Coping
Depression Level
Depression Self-Control
Development: Late Adulthood

Development: Middle Adulthood
Development: Young Adulthood
Family Health Status
Family Resiliency
Family Social Climate
Family Support During Treatment
Fatigue Level
Personal Resiliency
Psychosocial Adjustment: Life Change

Family Coping, Readiness for Enhanced

DEFINITION: Effective management of adaptive tasks by family member involved with the client's health challenge, who now exhibits desire and readiness for enhanced health and growth in regard to self and in relation to the client

SUGGESTED OUTCOMES:

Caregiver-Patient Relationship
Caregiver Well-Being
Family Coping
Family Normalization

Health Promoting Behavior
Health Seeking Behavior
Participation in Health Care Decisions

ADDITIONAL ASSOCIATED OUTCOMES:

Caregiver Emotional Health
Caregiver Lifestyle Disruption
Caregiver Performance: Indirect Care
Family Functioning
Family Health Status
Family Participation in Professional Care

Family Resiliency
Family Support During Treatment
Parent-Infant Attachment
Parenting Performance
Personal Resiliency

Family Processes, Dysfunctional: Alcoholism

DEFINITION: Psychosocial, spiritual, and physiological functions of the family unit are chronically disorganized, which leads to conflict, denial of problems, resistance to change, ineffective problem solving, and a series of self-perpetuating crises

SUGGESTED OUTCOMES:

Alcohol Abuse Cessation Behavior
Family Coping
Family Functioning
Family Resiliency
Family Social Climate

Parenting Performance
Role Performance
Substance Addiction Consequences
Substance Withdrawal Severity

ADDITIONAL ASSOCIATED OUTCOMES:

Agitation Level
Aggression Self-Control
Compliance Behavior
Decision-Making
Depression Level
Depression Self-Control
Family Health Status
Family Integrity

Family Normalization
Family Support During Treatment
Knowledge: Substance Use Control
Personal Resiliency
Social Interaction Skills
Social Involvement
Stress Level
Treatment Behavior: Illness or Injury

Family Processes, Interrupted

DEFINITION: Change in family relationships and/or functioning

SUGGESTED OUTCOMES:

Adaptation to Physical Disability
Family Coping
Family Functioning
Family Normalization

Family Resiliency
Family Social Climate
Parenting Performance

ADDITIONAL ASSOCIATED OUTCOMES:

Abuse Protection
Coping
Decision-Making
Family Health Status
Family Participation in Professional Care
Grief Resolution
Loneliness Severity
Parent-Infant Attachment

Personal Resiliency
Psychosocial Adjustment: Life Change
Role Performance
Social Interaction Skills
Social Involvement
Social Support
Stress Level

Family Processes, Readiness for Enhanced

DEFINITION: A pattern of family functioning that is sufficient to support the well-being of family members and can be strengthened

SUGGESTED OUTCOMES:

Family Coping
Family Functioning

Family Resiliency
Family Social Climate

ADDITIONAL ASSOCIATED OUTCOMES:

Family Health Status
Family Integrity
Family Normalization

Family Participation in Professional Care
Family Support During Treatment

Family Therapeutic Regimen Management, Ineffective

DEFINITION: Pattern of regulating and integrating into family processes a program for treatment of illness and the sequelae of illness that is unsatisfactory for meeting specific health goals

SUGGESTED OUTCOMES:

Caregiver Performance: Direct Care
Caregiver Performance: Indirect Care
Family Coping
Family Functioning

Family Normalization
Family Participation in Professional Care
Family Resiliency
Knowledge: Treatment Regimen

ADDITIONAL ASSOCIATED OUTCOMES:

Adherence Behavior
Adherence Behavior: Healthy Diet
Alcohol Abuse Cessation Behavior
Compliance Behavior
Compliance Behavior: Prescribed Diet
Drug Abuse Cessation Behavior
Elopement Occurrence

Elopement Propensity Risk
Family Health Status
Family Integrity
Family Social Climate
Family Support During Treatment
Smoking Cessation Behavior

Fatigue

DEFINITION: An overwhelming sustained sense of exhaustion and decreased capacity for physical and mental work at usual level

SUGGESTED OUTCOMES:

Activity Tolerance
Concentration
Endurance
Energy Conservation

Fatigue Level
Nutritional Status: Energy
Psychomotor Energy

ADDITIONAL ASSOCIATED OUTCOMES:

Anxiety Level
Blood Glucose Level
Depression Level
Mobility
Mood Equilibrium
Pain Level
Personal Health Status
Personal Well-Being

Quality of Life
Rest
Self-Care Status
Self-Care: Activities of Daily Living (ADL)
Self-Care: Instrumental Activities of Daily Living (IADL)
Sleep
Stress Level

Fear

DEFINITION: Response to perceived threat that is consciously recognized as a danger

SUGGESTED OUTCOMES:

Fatigue Level
Fear Level
Fear Level: Child
Fear Self-Control

Nausea & Vomiting Control
Nausea & Vomiting Severity
Self-Esteem
Vital Signs

ADDITIONAL ASSOCIATED OUTCOMES:

Acute Confusion Level
Anxiety Self-Control
Comfortable Death
Coping
Discomfort Level

Health Beliefs: Perceived Threat
Pain Level
Personal Resiliency
Social Support
Stress Level

Fluid Balance, Readiness for Enhanced

DEFINITION: A pattern of equilibrium between fluid volume and chemical composition of body fluids that is sufficient for meeting physical needs and can be strengthened

SUGGESTED OUTCOMES:
Fluid Balance
Hydration
Kidney Function
Nutritional Status: Food & Fluid Intake

ADDITIONAL ASSOCIATED OUTCOMES:
Appetite
Cardiac Pump Effectiveness
Cardiopulmonary Status
Compliance Behavior: Prescribed Diet
Gastrointestinal Function
Health-Seeking Behavior

Nausea & Vomiting Severity
Thermoregulation
Thermoregulation: Newborn
Vital Signs
Weight: Body Mass

Fluid Volume, Deficient

DEFINITION: Decreased intravascular, interstitial, and/or intracellular fluid. This refers to dehydration, water loss alone without change in sodium.

SUGGESTED OUTCOMES:
Acute Confusion Level
Fluid Balance
Hydration
Kidney Function

Thermoregulation
Thermoregulation: Newborn
Vital Signs

ADDITIONAL ASSOCIATED OUTCOMES:
Agitation Level
Appetite
Blood Loss Severity
Bowel Elimination
Breastfeeding Establishment: Infant
Breastfeeding Maintenance
Burn Healing
Burn Recovery

Cognition
Gastrointestinal Function
Knowledge: Medication
Nausea & Vomiting Severity
Nutritional Status: Food & Fluid Intake
Tissue Integrity: Skin & Mucous Membranes
Urinary Elimination

Fluid Volume, Excess

DEFINITION: Increased isotonic fluid retention

SUGGESTED OUTCOMES:

Cardiopulmonary Status
Fluid Balance
Fluid Overload Severity
Kidney Function

Respiratory Status
Vital Signs
Weight: Body Mass

ADDITIONAL ASSOCIATED OUTCOMES:

Cardiac Pump Effectiveness
Compliance Behavior: Prescribed Diet
Electrolyte & Acid/Base Balance
Knowledge: Congestive Heart Failure
    Management
Knowledge: Disease Process

Knowledge: Hypertension Management
Knowledge: Treatment Regimen
Nutritional Status: Food & Fluid Intake
Respiratory Status: Gas Exchange
Self-Care: Parenteral Medication
Urinary Elimination

Fluid Volume, Risk for Deficient

DEFINITION: At risk for experiencing vascular, cellular, or intracellular dehydration

SUGGESTED OUTCOMES:

Acute Confusion Level
Agitation Level
Appetite
Blood Loss Severity
Bowel Elimination
Breastfeeding Maintenance
Burn Healing
Burn Recovery
Compliance Behavior: Prescribed Diet
Electrolyte & Acid/Base Balance
Fluid Balance
Gastrointestinal Function
Hydration
Knowledge: Disease Process
Knowledge: Health Behavior

Knowledge: Medication
Knowledge: Treatment Regimen
Medication Response
Nausea & Vomiting Severity
Nutritional Status: Food & Fluid Intake
Risk Control
Risk Control: Hyperthermia
Risk Control: Sun Exposure
Risk Detection
Self-Care Status
Swallowing Status
Thermoregulation
Thermoregulation: Newborn
Urinary Elimination

Fluid Volume, Risk for Imbalanced

DEFINITION: At risk for a decrease, increase, or rapid shift from one to the other of intravascular, interstitial, and/or intracellular fluid. This refers to body fluid loss, gain, or both.

SUGGESTED OUTCOMES:

Appetite
Blood Loss Severity

Bowel Elimination
Breastfeeding Establishment: Infant

Suggested Outcomes: Cont'd

Breastfeeding Maintenance
Burn Healing
Burn Recovery
Cardiac Pump Effectiveness
Cardiopulmonary Status
Electrolyte & Acid/Base Balance
Fluid Balance
Fluid Overload Severity
Gastrointestinal Function
Hydration
Kidney Function
Knowledge: Congestive Heart Failure
  Management
Knowledge: Disease Process
Knowledge: Health Behavior
Knowledge: Hypertension Management
Knowledge: Medication
Knowledge: Treatment Regimen
Nausea & Vomiting Severity
Nutritional Status: Food & Fluid Intake
Physical Aging
Post-Procedure Recovery
Risk Control
Risk Control: Hyperthermia
Risk Detection
Self-Care Status
Thermoregulation
Thermoregulation: Newborn
Urinary Elimination
Vital Signs
Wound Healing: Secondary Intention

Gas Exchange, Impaired

DEFINITION: Excess or deficit in oxygenation and/or carbon dioxide elimination at the alveolar-capillary membrane

Suggested Outcomes:

Acute Confusion Level
Allergic Response: Systemic
Mechanical Ventilation Response: Adult
Respiratory Status
Respiratory Status: Gas Exchange
Respiratory Status: Ventilation
Tissue Perfusion: Pulmonary
Vital Signs

Additional Associated Outcomes:

Asthma Self-Management
Cardiopulmonary Status
Cognition
Cognitive Orientation
Tissue Perfusion: Abdominal Organs
Tissue Perfusion: Cardiac
Tissue Perfusion: Cellular
Tissue Perfusion: Peripheral

Grieving

DEFINITION: A normal complex process that includes emotional, physical, spiritual, social, and intellectual responses and behaviors by which individuals, families, and communities incorporate an actual, anticipated, or perceived loss into their daily lives

Suggested Outcomes:

Adaptation to Physical Disability
Coping
Family Coping
Grief Resolution
Psychosocial Adjustment: Life Change

ADDITIONAL ASSOCIATED OUTCOMES:

Aggression Self-Control
Appetite
Burn Recovery
Caregiver Adaptation to Patient
    Institutionalization
Caregiver Emotional Health
Comfort Status: Psychospiritual
Communication
Depression Level
Depression Self-Control

Dignified Life Closure
Family Social Climate
Family Resiliency
Fatigue Level
Hope
Knowledge: Depression Management
Personal Resiliency
Role Performance
Sleep
Spiritual Health

Grieving, Complicated

DEFINITION: A disorder that occurs after the death of a significant other, in which the experience of distress accompanying bereavement fails to follow normative expectations and manifests in functional impairment

SUGGESTED OUTCOMES:

Comfort Status: Psychospiritual
Coping
Family Coping
Family Resiliency
Fatigue Level

Grief Resolution
Personal Resiliency
Personal Well-Being
Psychosocial Adjustment: Life Change
Role Performance

ADDITIONAL ASSOCIATED OUTCOMES:

Aggression Self-Control
Anxiety Level
Appetite
Communication
Depression Level
Depression Self-Control

Mood Equilibrium
Motivation
Personal Health Status
Self-Esteem
Sleep

Grieving, Complicated, Risk for

DEFINITION: At risk for a disorder that occurs after the death of a significant other, in which the experience of distress accompanying bereavement fails to follow normative expectations and manifests in functional impairment

SUGGESTED OUTCOMES:

Anxiety Level
Caregiver Emotional Health
Caregiver Role Endurance
Comfort Status: Psychospiritual
Coping
Depression Level
Family Coping
Family Normalization
Family Resiliency

Grief Resolution
Loneliness Severity
Personal Resiliency
Risk Control
Risk Detection
Self-Esteem
Social Support
Stress Level

Growth and Development, Delayed

DEFINITION: Deviations from age-group norms

SUGGESTED OUTCOMES:

Child Development: 1 Month
Child Development: 2 Months
Child Development: 4 Months
Child Development: 6 Months
Child Development: 12 Months
Child Development: 2 Years
Child Development: 3 Years
Child Development: 4 Years
Child Development: 5 Years

Child Development: Middle Childhood
Child Development: Adolescence
Development: Late Adulthood
Development: Middle Adulthood
Development: Young Adulthood
Growth
Physical Aging
Physical Maturation: Female
Physical Maturation: Male

ADDITIONAL ASSOCIATED OUTCOMES:

Abuse Recovery
Abuse Recovery: Emotional
Abuse Recovery: Physical
Community Risk Control: Lead Exposure
Knowledge: Parenting
Neglect Recovery

Parenting Performance
Personal Autonomy
Personal Resiliency
Psychosocial Adjustment: Life Change
Weight: Body Mass

Growth, Risk for Disproportionate

DEFINITION: At risk for growth above the 97th percentile or below the 3rd percentile for age, crossing two percentile channels

SUGGESTED OUTCOMES:

Appetite
Body Image
Child Development: 1 Month
Child Development: 2 Months
Child Development: 4 Months
Child Development: 6 Months
Child Development: 12 Months
Child Development: 2 Years
Child Development: 3 Years
Child Development: 4 Years
Child Development: 5 Years
Child Development: Middle Childhood
Child Development: Adolescence
Community Risk Control: Lead Exposure

Growth
Infection Severity: Newborn
Knowledge: Infant Care
Knowledge: Preconception
   Maternal Health
Knowledge: Pregnancy
Knowledge: Preterm Infant Care
Parenting Performance
Physical Maturation: Female
Physical Maturation: Male
Prenatal Health Behavior
Risk Control
Risk Detection
Weight: Body Mass

Health Maintenance, Ineffective

DEFINITION: Inability to identify, manage, and/or seek out help to maintain health

SUGGESTED OUTCOMES:

Health Beliefs: Perceived Resources
Health Promoting Behavior
Health Seeking Behavior
Knowledge: Arthritis Management
Knowledge: Asthma Management
Knowledge: Cancer Management
Knowledge: Cancer Threat Reduction
Knowledge: Cardiac Disease Management
Knowledge: Congestive Heart Failure
   Management
Knowledge: Depression Management
Knowledge: Health Behavior
Knowledge: Health Promotion

Knowledge: Health Resources
Knowledge: Hypertension Management
Knowledge: Infection Management
Knowledge: Multiple Sclerosis Management
Knowledge: Pain Management
Knowledge: Pregnancy & Postpartum Sexual
   Functioning
Knowledge: Preterm Infant Care
Knowledge: Treatment Regimen
Knowledge: Weight Management
Participation in Health Care Decisions
Personal Health Status
Risk Detection

ADDITIONAL ASSOCIATED OUTCOMES:

Adaptation to Physical Disability
Adherence Behavior: Healthy Diet
Anxiety Self-Control
Cognition
Communication
Community Risk Control: Chronic Disease
Coping
Decision-Making
Family Coping
Grief Resolution

Information Processing
Motivation
Postpartum Maternal Health Behavior
Psychosocial Adjustment: Life Change
Risk Control
Self-Direction of Care
Social Support
Spiritual Health
Symptom Control
Treatment Behavior: Illness or Injury

Health Behavior, Risk-Prone

DEFINITION: Inability to modify lifestyle/behaviors in a manner consistent with a change in health status

SUGGESTED OUTCOMES:

Acceptance: Health Status
Adaptation to Physical Disability
Compliance Behavior
Coping

Health Seeking Behavior
Motivation
Psychosocial Adjustment: Life Change
Treatment Behavior: Illness or Injury

ADDITIONAL ASSOCIATED OUTCOMES:

Adherence Behavior
Adherence Behavior: Healthy Diet
Asthma Self-Management
Cardiac Disease Self-Management
Child Adaptation to Hospitalization
Cognition

Compliance Behavior: Prescribed Diet
Compliance Behavior: Prescribed Medication
Diabetes Self-Management
Discharge Readiness: Independent Living
Family Resiliency
Grief Resolution

ADDITIONAL ASSOCIATED OUTCOMES: CONT'D

Health Belief: Perceived Ability to Perform

Health Belief: Perceived Control

Impulse Self-Control

Mood Equilibrium

Multiple Sclerosis Self-Management

Participation in Health Care Decisions

Personal Resiliency

Postpartum Maternal Health Behavior

Self-Esteem

Smoking Cessation Behavior

Social Support

Stress Level

Substance Withdrawal Severity

Weight Gain Behavior

Weight Loss Behavior

Health-Seeking Behaviors (Specify)

DEFINITION: Active seeking (by a person in stable health) of ways to alter personal health habits and/or the environment in order to move toward a higher level of health

SUGGESTED OUTCOMES:

Adherence Behavior

Adherence Behavior: Healthy Diet

Alcohol Abuse Cessation Behavior

Cardiac Disease Self-Management

Compliance Behavior: Prescribed Diet

Diabetes Self-Management

Drug Abuse Cessation Behavior

Health Beliefs

Health Orientation

Health Promoting Behavior

Health Seeking Behavior

Knowledge: Arthritis Management

Knowledge: Asthma Management

Knowledge: Cancer Management

Knowledge: Cancer Threat Reduction

Knowledge: Cardiac Disease Management

Knowledge: Congestive Heart Failure
   Management

Knowledge: Depression Management

Knowledge: Diabetes Management

Knowledge: Hypertension Management

Knowledge: Health Promotion

Knowledge: Health Resources

Knowledge: Infection Management

Knowledge: Multiple Sclerosis Management

Knowledge: Pain Management

Knowledge: Weight Management

Multiple Sclerosis Self-Management

Personal Health Status

Personal Well-Being

Postpartum Maternal Health Behavior

Risk Detection

Smoking Cessation Behavior

Weight Gain Behavior

Weight Loss Behavior

ADDITIONAL ASSOCIATED OUTCOMES:

Adaptation to Physical Disability

Body Mechanics Performance

Energy Conservation

Motivation

Participation in Health Care Decisions

Personal Safety Behavior

Psychosocial Adjustment: Life Change

Quality of Life

Risk Control: Alcohol Use

Risk Control: Cancer

Risk Control: Cardiovascular Health

Risk Control: Drug Use

Risk Control: Hyperthermia

Risk Control: Hypothermia

Risk Control: Hearing Impairment

Risk Control: Infectious Process

Risk Control: Sexually Transmitted
   Diseases (STD)

Risk Control: Sun Exposure

Risk Control: Tobacco Use

Risk Control: Unintended Pregnancy

Risk Control: Visual Impairment

Safe Home Environment

Home Maintenance, Impaired

DEFINITION: Inability to independently maintain a safe, growth-promoting immediate environment

SUGGESTED OUTCOMES:

Family Functioning
Parenting Performance
Parenting: Psychosocial Safety
Role Performance

Safe Home Environment
Self-Care: Instrumental Activities of Daily
    Living (IADL)

ADDITIONAL ASSOCIATED OUTCOMES:

Caregiver Emotional Health
Caregiver Physical Health
Client Satisfaction: Physical Environment
Cognition

Discharge Readiness:
    Independent Living
Fatigue Level
Mobility

Hope, Readiness for Enhanced

DEFINITION: A pattern of expectations and desires that is sufficient for mobilizing energy on one's own behalf and can be strengthened

SUGGESTED OUTCOMES:

Hope
Personal Well-Being

Personal Resiliency
Spiritual Health

ADDITIONAL ASSOCIATED OUTCOMES:

Comfortable Death
Comfort Status: Psychospiritual
Coping
Decision-Making
Family Coping
Family Resiliency
Family Social Climate
Grief Resolution
Health-Seeking Behavior
Loneliness Severity

Pain Control
Personal Autonomy
Psychomotor Energy
Psychosocial Adjustment
    Life Change
Quality of Life
Self-Esteem
Suicide Self-Restraint
Will to Live

Hopelessness

DEFINITION: Subjective state in which an individual sees limited or no alternatives or personal choices available and is unable to mobilize energy on own behalf

SUGGESTED OUTCOMES:

Appetite
Comfort Status: Psychospiritual
Depression Self-Control
Hope
Mood Equilibrium

Personal Resiliency
Psychomotor Energy
Quality of Life
Sleep
Will to Live

ADDITIONAL ASSOCIATED OUTCOMES:

Acceptance: Health Status
Adaptation to Physical Disability
Coping
Decision-Making
Depression Level
Fatigue Level
Fear Self-Control
Grief Resolution
Immobility Consequences:
   Psycho-Cognitive

Knowledge: Depression Management
Motivation
Pain: Adverse Psychological Response
Pain Control
Pain: Disruptive Effects
Rest
Spiritual Health
Stress Level
Suffering Severity
Symptom Severity

Human Dignity, Risk for Compromised

DEFINITION: At risk for perceived loss of respect and honor

SUGGESTED OUTCOMES:

Abuse Recovery
Acceptance: Health Status
Adaptation to Physical Disability
Body Image
Bowel Continence
Client Satisfaction: Caring
Client Satisfaction: Cultural Needs Fulfillment
Client Satisfaction: Protection of Rights
Client Satisfaction: Psychological Care
Comfortable Death
Comfort Status: Sociocultural
Coping
Decision-Making
Depression Level
Dignified Life Closure
Family Coping

Family Functioning
Family Social Climate
Hope
Information Processing
Neglect Recovery
Pain Control
Participation in Health Care Decisions
Personal Autonomy
Personal Resiliency
Personal Well-Being
Risk Control
Risk Detection
Self-Esteem
Sexual Identity
Social Support
Urinary Continence

Hyperthermia

DEFINITION: Body temperature elevated above normal range

SUGGESTED OUTCOMES:

Thermoregulation
Thermoregulation: Newborn
Vital Signs

ADDITIONAL ASSOCIATED OUTCOMES:

Blood Transfusion Reaction
Comfort Status: Physical
Discomfort Level
Hydration

Immune Status
Infection Severity
Neurological Status: Autonomic
Risk Control: Hyperthermia

Hypothermia

DEFINITION: Body temperature below normal range

SUGGESTED OUTCOMES:
Thermoregulation
Thermoregulation: Newborn
Vital Signs

ADDITIONAL ASSOCIATED OUTCOMES:
Comfort Status: Physical
Neurological Status: Autonomic
Risk Control: Hypothermia

Immunization Status, Readiness for Enhanced

DEFINITION: A pattern of conforming to local, national, and/or international standards of immunization to prevent infectious disease(s) that is sufficient to protect a person, family, or community and can be strengthened

SUGGESTED OUTCOMES:
Community Health Status: Immunity
Community Risk Control: Communicable
    Disease
Compliance Behavior

Compliance Behavior: Prescribed Medication
Immune Status
Immunization Behavior
Risk Control: Infectious Process

ADDITIONAL ASSOCIATED OUTCOMES:
Community Disaster Readiness
Community Disaster Response
Health-Seeking Behavior

Knowledge: Disease Process
Knowledge: Infection Management

Infant Behavior, Disorganized

DEFINITION: Disintegrated physiological and neurobehavioral responses of infant to the environment

SUGGESTED OUTCOMES:
Coordinated Movement
Neurological Status
Preterm Infant Organization

Sleep
Thermoregulation: Newborn
Vital Signs

ADDITIONAL ASSOCIATED OUTCOMES:
Breastfeeding Establishment: Infant
Child Development: 1 Month
Child Development: 2 Months
Discomfort Level

Knowledge: Infant Care
Knowledge: Preterm Infant Care
Nutritional Status: Food & Fluid Intake

Infant Behavior, Risk for Disorganized

DEFINITION: Risk for alteration in integrating and modulation of the physiological and behavioral systems of functioning (i.e., autonomic, motor, state, organizational, self-regulatory, and attentional-interactional systems)

SUGGESTED OUTCOMES:

Child Development: 1 Month
Child Development: 2 Months
Coordinated Movement
Discomfort Level
Knowledge: Infant Care
Knowledge: Parenting
Knowledge: Preterm Infant Care

Neurological Status
Pain Level
Preterm Infant Organization
Risk Control
Risk Detection
Sleep
Thermoregulation: Newborn

Infant Behavior, Organized, Readiness for Enhanced

DEFINITION: A pattern of modulation of the physiologic and behavioral systems of functioning (i.e., autonomic, motor, state-organizational, self-regulatory, and attentional-interactional systems) in an infant that is satisfactory but that can be improved

SUGGESTED OUTCOMES:

Child Development: 1 Month
Child Development: 2 Months
Coordinated Movement
Neurological Status
Sensory Function: Hearing

Sensory Function: Vision
Sleep
Thermoregulation: Newborn
Vital Signs

ADDITIONAL ASSOCIATED OUTCOMES:

Discomfort Level
Knowledge: Infant Care
Knowledge: Parenting

Knowledge: Preterm Infant Care
Pain Level
Parent-Infant Attachment

Infant Feeding Pattern, Ineffective

DEFINITION: Impaired ability of an infant to suck or coordinate the suck/swallow response resulting in inadequate oral nutrition for metabolic needs

SUGGESTED OUTCOMES:

Aspiration Prevention
Breastfeeding Establishment: Infant
Breastfeeding Maintenance

Hydration
Nutritional Status: Food & Fluid Intake
Swallowing Status

ADDITIONAL ASSOCIATED OUTCOMES:

Bowel Elimination
Breastfeeding Establishment: Maternal
Gastrointestinal Function
Growth
Knowledge: Breastfeeding
Knowledge: Preterm Infant Care
Neurological Status

Nutritional Status: Biochemical Measures
Respiratory Status
Swallowing Status: Esophageal Phase
Swallowing Status: Oral Phase
Swallowing Status: Pharyngeal Phase
Urinary Elimination
Weight: Body Mass

Infection, Risk for

DEFINITION: At increased risk for being invaded by pathogenic organisms

SUGGESTED OUTCOMES:

Aspiration Prevention
Burn Healing
Burn Recovery
Community Risk Control: Communicable
 Disease
Health Beliefs
Hemodialysis Access
Immobility Consequences: Physiological
Immune Status
Immunization Behavior
Infection Severity
Infection Severity: Newborn
Knowledge: Infection Management

Knowledge: Treatment Procedure
Nutritional Status
Pre-Procedure Readiness
Risk Control
Risk Control: Infectious Process
Risk Control: Sexually Transmitted
 Diseases (STD)
Risk Detection
Self-Care: Hygiene
Tissue Integrity: Skin & Mucous Membranes
Treatment Behavior: Illness or Injury
Wound Healing: Primary Intention
Wound Healing: Secondary Intention

Injury, Risk for

DEFINITION: At risk of injury as a result of environmental conditions interacting with the individual's adaptive and defensive resources

SUGGESTED OUTCOMES:

Abuse Protection
Allergic Response: Systemic
Aspiration Prevention
Balance
Blood Glucose Level
Blood Loss Severity
Body Positioning: Self-Initiated
Coordinated Movement
Elopement Propensity Risk
Fall Prevention Behavior
Falls Occurrence
Fatigue Level
Knowledge: Body Mechanics
Knowledge: Child Physical Safety
Knowledge: Fall Prevention

Knowledge: Personal Safety
Maternal Status: Postpartum
Mobility
Nutritional Status
Parenting: Adolescent Physical Safety
Parenting: Early/Middle Childhood Physical
 Safety
Parenting: Infant/Toddler Physical Safety
Parenting: Psychosocial Safety
Personal Safety Behavior
Risk Control
Risk Control: Hearing Impairment
Risk Control: Visual Impairment
Risk Detection
Safe Home Environment

SUGGESTED OUTCOMES: CONT'D

Safe Wandering
Seizure Control
Self-Care Status

Sensory Function
Tissue Integrity: Skin & Mucous Membranes
Transfer Performance

Insomnia

DEFINITION: A disruption in amount and quality of sleep that impairs functioning

SUGGESTED OUTCOMES:

Concentration
Endurance
Fatigue Level
Mood Equilibrium
Personal Health Status

Personal Well-Being
Quality of Life
Rest
Sleep

ADDITIONAL ASSOCIATED OUTCOMES:

Anxiety Level
Bowel Elimination
Comfort Status
Depression Level
Discomfort Level
Fear Level
Fear Level: Child

Leisure Participation
Medication Response
Pain Level
Respiratory Status: Ventilation
Stress Level
Urinary Continence
Urinary Elimination

Intracranial Adaptive Capacity, Decreased

DEFINITION: Intracranial fluid dynamic mechanisms that normally compensate for increases in intracranial volumes are compromised, resulting in repeated disproportionate increases in intracranial pressure (ICP) in response to a variety of noxious and nonnoxious stimuli

SUGGESTED OUTCOMES:

Neurological Status
Neurological Status: Consciousness

Seizure Control
Tissue Perfusion: Cerebral

ADDITIONAL ASSOCIATED OUTCOMES:

Cognition
Cognitive Orientation
Communication
Electrolyte & Acid/Base Balance
Fluid Balance
Neurological Status: Autonomic

Neurological Status: Central Motor Control
Neurological Status: Cranial Sensory/Motor
    Function
Neurological Status: Spinal Sensory/Motor
    Function
Vital Signs

Knowledge, Deficient (Specify)

DEFINITION: Absence or deficiency of cognitive information related to a specific topic

SUGGESTED OUTCOMES:

Knowledge: Arthritis Management
Knowledge: Asthma Management
Knowledge: Body Mechanics
Knowledge: Breastfeeding
Knowledge: Cancer Management
Knowledge: Cancer Threat Reduction
Knowledge: Cardiac Disease Management
Knowledge: Child Physical Safety
Knowledge: Conception Prevention
Knowledge: Congestive Heart Failure
   Management
Knowledge: Depression Management
Knowledge: Diabetes Management
Knowledge: Diet
Knowledge: Disease Process
Knowledge: Energy Conservation
Knowledge: Fall Prevention
Knowledge: Fertility Promotion
Knowledge: Health Behavior
Knowledge: Health Promotion
Knowledge: Health Resources
Knowledge: Hypertension Management

Knowledge: Illness Care
Knowledge: Infant Care
Knowledge: Infection Management
Knowledge: Labor & Delivery
Knowledge: Medication
Knowledge: Multiple Sclerosis Management
Knowledge: Ostomy Care
Knowledge: Pain Management
Knowledge: Parenting
Knowledge: Personal Safety
Knowledge: Postpartum Maternal Health
Knowledge: Preconception Maternal Health
Knowledge: Pregnancy
Knowledge: Pregnancy & Postpartum Sexual
   Functioning
Knowledge: Prescribed Activity
Knowledge: Preterm Infant Care
Knowledge: Sexual Functioning
Knowledge: Substance Use Control
Knowledge: Treatment Procedure
Knowledge: Treatment Regimen
Knowledge: Weight Management

ADDITIONAL ASSOCIATED OUTCOMES:

Client Satisfaction: Teaching
Cognition
Communication: Receptive
Concentration
Information Processing

Memory
Motivation
Pre-Procedure Readiness
Stress Level

Knowledge, Readiness for Enhanced

DEFINITION: The presence or acquisition of cognitive information related to a specific topic is sufficient for meeting health-related goals and can be strengthened

SUGGESTED OUTCOMES:

Knowledge: Arthritis Management
Knowledge: Asthma Management
Knowledge: Body Mechanics
Knowledge: Breastfeeding
Knowledge: Cancer Management
Knowledge: Cancer Threat Reduction
Knowledge: Cardiac Disease Management

Knowledge: Child Physical Safety
Knowledge: Conception Prevention
Knowledge: Congestive Heart Failure
   Management
Knowledge: Depression Management
Knowledge: Diabetes Management
Knowledge: Diet

SUGGESTED OUTCOMES: CONT'D

Knowledge: Disease Process
Knowledge: Energy Conservation
Knowledge: Fall Prevention
Knowledge: Fertility Promotion
Knowledge: Health Behavior
Knowledge: Health Promotion
Knowledge: Health Resources
Knowledge: Hypertension Management
Knowledge: Illness Care
Knowledge: Infant Care
Knowledge: Infection Management
Knowledge: Labor & Delivery
Knowledge: Medication
Knowledge: Multiple Sclerosis
  Management
Knowledge: Ostomy Care

Knowledge: Pain Management
Knowledge: Parenting
Knowledge: Personal Safety
Knowledge: Postpartum Maternal Health
Knowledge: Preconception Maternal Health
Knowledge: Pregnancy
Knowledge: Pregnancy & Postpartum
  Sexual Functioning
Knowledge: Prescribed Activity
Knowledge: Preterm Infant Care
Knowledge: Sexual Functioning
Knowledge: Substance Use Control
Knowledge: Treatment Procedure
Knowledge: Treatment Regimen
Knowledge: Weight Management

ADDITIONAL ASSOCIATED OUTCOMES:

Client Satisfaction: Teaching
Cognition
Communication: Receptive
Concentration
Health-Seeking Behavior

Information Processing
Memory
Motivation
Pre-Procedure Readiness
Stress Level

Latex Allergy Response

DEFINITION: A hypersensitive reaction to natural latex rubber products

SUGGESTED OUTCOMES:

Allergic Response: Localized
Allergic Response: Systemic
Cardiopulmonary Status
Discomfort Level

Immune Hypersensitivity Response
Respiratory Status
Tissue Integrity: Skin & Mucous Membranes

ADDITIONAL ASSOCIATED OUTCOMES:

Knowledge: Treatment Regimen
Nausea & Vomiting Severity
Symptom Severity

Latex Allergy Response, Risk for

DEFINITION: Risk of hypersensitivity to natural latex rubber products

SUGGESTED OUTCOMES:

Allergic Response: Localized
Immune Hypersensitivity Response
Knowledge: Health Behavior
Pre-Procedure Readiness

Risk Control
Risk Detection
Tissue Integrity: Skin & Mucous Membranes

Lifestyle, Sedentary

DEFINITION: Reports a habit of life that is characterized by a low physical activity level

SUGGESTED OUTCOMES:

Activity Tolerance
Compliance Behavior
Endurance

Fatigue Level
Personal Health Status
Physical Fitness

ADDITIONAL ASSOCIATED OUTCOMES:

Adherence Behavior
Health Promoting Behavior
Knowledge: Health Behavior
Knowledge: Health Promotion

Leisure Participation
Motivation
Weight Loss Behavior

Liver Function, Risk for Impaired

DEFINITION: At risk for liver dysfunction

SUGGESTED OUTCOMES:

Alcohol Abuse Cessation Behavior
Blood Coagulation
Drug Abuse Cessation Behavior
Electrolyte & Acid/Base Balance
Knowledge: Medication
Medication Response
Risk Control
Risk Control: Alcohol Use

Risk Control: Drug Use
Risk Control: Infectious Process
Risk Control: Sexually Transmitted
    Diseases (STD)
Risk Detection
Substance Withdrawal Severity
Tissue Perfusion: Cellular

Loneliness, Risk for

DEFINITION: At risk for experiencing discomfort associated with a desire or need for more contact with others

SUGGESTED OUTCOMES:

Adaptation to Physical Disability
Communication
Development: Late Adulthood
Family Functioning
Family Integrity
Family Social Climate
Grief Resolution
Immobility Consequences: Psycho-Cognitive
Leisure Participation

Loneliness Severity
Neglect Cessation
Personal Resiliency
Psychosocial Adjustment: Life Change
Risk Control
Risk Detection
Social Interaction Skills
Social Involvement
Social Support

Memory, Impaired

DEFINITION: Inability to remember or recall bits of information or behavioral skills

SUGGESTED OUTCOMES:

Acute Confusion Level
Cognition
Cognitive Orientation
Concentration

Memory
Neurological Status
Neurological Status: Consciousness

ADDITIONAL ASSOCIATED OUTCOMES:

Agitation Level
Anxiety Level
Cardiac Pump Effectiveness
Cardiopulmonary Status
Circulation Status
Depression Level
Development: Late Adulthood
Discharge Readiness: Supported Living
Electrolyte & Acid/Base Balance
Fatigue Level

Hydration
Medication Response
Physical Aging
Respiratory Status
Respiratory Status: Gas Exchange
Respiratory Status: Ventilation
Safe wandering
Stress Level
Tissue Perfusion: Cerebral

Mobility: Bed, Impaired

DEFINITION: Limitation of independent movement from one bed position to another

SUGGESTED OUTCOMES:

Body Mechanics Performance
Body Positioning: Self-Initiated
Coordinated Movement

Immobility Consequences: Physiological
Mobility

ADDITIONAL ASSOCIATED OUTCOMES:

Cardiopulmonary Status
Cognition
Discomfort Level
Endurance
Fatigue Level
Immobility Consequences: Psycho-Cognitive
Joint Movement
Joint Movement: Ankle
Joint Movement: Elbow
Joint Movement: Fingers
Joint Movement: Hip
Joint Movement: Knee
Joint Movement: Neck

Joint Movement: Passive
Joint Movement: Shoulder
Joint Movement: Spine
Joint Movement: Wrist
Knowledge: Body Mechanics
Neurological Status
Neurological Status: Central Motor Control
Neurological Status: Spinal Sensory/Motor
   Function
Pain Level
Respiratory Status
Rest
Skeletal Function

Mobility: Physical, Impaired

DEFINITION: Limitation in independent, purposeful physical movement of the body or of one or more extremities

SUGGESTED OUTCOMES:

Ambulation
Ambulation: Wheelchair
Balance
Body Mechanics Performance

Body Positioning: Self-Initiated
Coordinated Movement
Mobility
Transfer Performance

ADDITIONAL ASSOCIATED OUTCOMES:

Activity Tolerance
Anxiety Level
Cardiopulmonary Status
Cognition
Depression Level
Discomfort Level
Endurance
Energy Conservation
Fall Prevention Behavior
Fatigue Level
Health Beliefs: Perceived Ability to Perform
Health Orientation
Immobility Consequences: Physiological
Immobility Consequences: Psycho-Cognitive
Joint Movement
Joint Movement: Ankle
Joint Movement: Elbow
Joint Movement: Hip
Joint Movement: Knee

Joint Movement: Shoulder
Joint Movement: Spine
Knowledge: Prescribed Activity
Motivation
Neurological Status: Spinal Sensory/Motor Function
Nutritional Status: Energy
Pain Level
Psychomotor Energy
Risk Control: Cardiovascular Health
Respiratory Status
Self-Care: Activities of Daily Living (ADL)
Sensory Function
Sensory Function: Cutaneous
Sensory Function: Proprioception
Sensory Function: Vision
Skeletal Function
Weight: Body Mass

Mobility: Wheelchair, Impaired

DEFINITION: Limitation of independent operation of wheelchair within environment

SUGGESTED OUTCOMES:

Adaptation to Physical Disability
Ambulation: Wheelchair
Balance

Coordinated Movement
Mobility
Transfer Performance

ADDITIONAL ASSOCIATED OUTCOMES:

Body Mechanics Performance
Cardiopulmonary Status
Cognition
Depression Level
Endurance
Fall Prevention Behavior

Fatigue Level
Immobility Consequences: Physiological
Immobility Consequences: Psycho-Cognitive
Joint Movement
Joint Movement: Elbow
Joint Movement: Fingers

ADDITIONAL ASSOCIATED OUTCOMES: CONT'D

Joint Movement: Shoulder
Joint Movement: Wrist
Knowledge: Body Mechanics
Neurological Status
Pain Level

Physical Fitness
Respiratory Status
Sensory Function: Vision
Skeletal Function

Moral Distress

DEFINITION: Response to the inability to carry out one's chosen ethical/moral decision/action

SUGGESTED OUTCOMES:

Anxiety Level
Client Satisfaction: Protection of Rights
Comfortable Death
Decision-Making
Dignified Life Closure

Family Integrity
Family Participation in Professional Care
Fear Level
Participation in Health Care Decisions

ADDITIONAL ASSOCIATED OUTCOMES:

Anxiety Self-Control
Client Satisfaction: Cultural Needs
    Fulfillment
Comfort Status: Psychospiritual
Coping
Family Coping
Family Functioning
Family Resiliency
Family Social Climate

Family Support During Treatment
Fear Self-Control
Information Processing
Knowledge: Treatment Regimen
Personal Autonomy
Personal Resiliency
Self-Esteem
Stress Level

Nausea

DEFINITION: A subjective unpleasant, wavelike sensation in the back of the throat, epigastrium, or abdomen that may lead to the urge or need to vomit

SUGGESTED OUTCOMES:

Appetite
Discomfort Level
Hydration
Nausea & Vomiting Control

Nausea & Vomiting: Disruptive Effects
Nausea & Vomiting Severity
Nutritional Status: Food & Fluid Intake

ADDITIONAL ASSOCIATED OUTCOMES:

Anxiety Level
Client Satisfaction: Symptom Control
Comfort Status: Physical
Electrolyte & Acid/Base Balance
Fear Level
Fluid Balance
Gastrointestinal Function
Infection Severity

Kidney Function
Maternal Status: Antepartum
Medication Response
Pain Level
Suffering Severity
Symptom Control
Symptom Severity

Noncompliance

DEFINITION: Behavior of person and/or caregiver that fails to coincide with a health-promoting or therapeutic plan agreed on by the person (and/or family and/or community) and health-care professional. In the presence of an agreed-on, health-promoting, or therapeutic plan, person's or caregiver's behavior is fully or partially nonadherent and may lead to clinically ineffective or partially ineffective outcomes.

SUGGESTED OUTCOMES:

Caregiver Performance: Direct Care
Caregiver Performance: Indirect Care
Compliance Behavior
Compliance Behavior: Prescribed Diet

Symptom Control
Compliance Behavior: Prescribed Medication
Treatment Behavior: Illness or Injury

ADDITIONAL ASSOCIATED OUTCOMES:

Acceptance: Health Status
Adaptation to Physical Disability
Alcohol Abuse Cessation Behavior
Caregiver Stressors
Caregiver-Patient Relationship
Client Satisfaction
Client Satisfaction: Case Management
Client Satisfaction: Communication
Drug Abuse Cessation Behavior
Family Coping
Family Participation in Professional Care
Family Resiliency
Health Beliefs
Health Beliefs: Perceived Ability to Perform
Health Beliefs: Perceived Control

Health Beliefs: Perceived Resources
Health Beliefs: Perceived Threat
Health Orientation
Knowledge: Disease Process
Knowledge: Treatment Regimen
Motivation
Participation in Health Care Decisions
Self-Care: Non-Parenteral Medication
Self-Care: Parenteral Medication
Smoking Cessation Behavior
Social Support
Weight Gain Behavior
Weight Loss Behavior
Will to Live

Nutrition: Imbalanced, Less Than Body Requirements

DEFINITION: Intake of nutrients insufficient to meet metabolic needs

SUGGESTED OUTCOMES:

Appetite
Breastfeeding Establishment: Infant
Gastrointestinal Function
Nutritional Status

Nutritional Status: Food & Fluid Intake
Nutritional Status: Nutrient Intake
Self-Care: Eating
Weight: Body Mass

ADDITIONAL ASSOCIATED OUTCOMES:

Adherence Behavior
Adherence Behavior: Healthy Diet
Body Image
Bowel Elimination

Compliance Behavior
Compliance Behavior: Prescribed Diet
Depression Level
Endurance

ADDITIONAL ASSOCIATED OUTCOMES: CONT'D

Fatigue Level

Health Beliefs

Hydration

Knowledge: Diet

Knowledge: Weight Management

Nausea & Vomiting Severity

Nutritional Status: Biochemical Measures

Nutritional Status: Energy

Prenatal Health Behavior

Sensory Function: Taste & Smell

Symptom Control

Symptom Severity

Weight Gain Behavior

Weight Maintenance Behavior

Nutrition: Imbalanced, More Than Body Requirements

DEFINITION: Intake of nutrients that exceeds metabolic needs

SUGGESTED OUTCOMES:

Nutritional Status

Nutritional Status: Food & Fluid Intake

Nutritional Status: Nutrient Intake

Weight: Body Mass

Weight Loss Behavior

ADDITIONAL ASSOCIATED OUTCOMES:

Adherence Behavior

Adherence Behavior: Healthy Diet

Body Image

Compliance Behavior

Compliance Behavior: Prescribed Diet

Depression Level

Health Beliefs

Health Beliefs: Perceived Ability
  to Perform

Knowledge: Diet

Knowledge: Weight Management

Motivation

Stress Level

Weight Maintenance Behavior

Nutrition: Imbalanced, Risk for More Than Body Requirements

DEFINITION: At risk for an intake of nutrients that exceeds metabolic needs

SUGGESTED OUTCOMES:

Adherence Behavior: Healthy Diet

Compliance Behavior: Prescribed Diet

Knowledge: Diet

Knowledge: Weight Management

Nutritional Status

Nutritional Status: Food & Fluid Intake

Nutritional Status: Nutrient Intake

Risk Control

Risk Detection

Stress Level

Weight: Body Mass

Weight Maintenance Behavior

Nutrition, Readiness for Enhanced

DEFINITION: A pattern of nutrient intake that is sufficient for meeting metabolic needs and can be strengthened

SUGGESTED OUTCOMES:

Adherence Behavior: Healthy Diet
Knowledge: Diet
Knowledge: Weight Management
Nutritional Status

Nutritional Status: Food & Fluid Intake
Nutritional Status: Nutrient Intake
Risk Control: Alcohol Use

ADDITIONAL ASSOCIATED OUTCOMES:

Appetite
Breastfeeding Establishment: Infant
Compliance Behavior: Prescribed Diet
Gastrointestinal Function
Health-Seeking Behavior

Sensory Function: Taste & Smell
Stress Level
Symptom Control
Symptom Severity
Weight Maintenance Behavior

Oral Mucous Membrane, Impaired

DEFINITION: Disruption of the lips and/or soft tissue of the oral cavity

SUGGESTED OUTCOMES:

Oral Hygiene
Tissue Integrity: Skin & Mucous Membranes

ADDITIONAL ASSOCIATED OUTCOMES:

Allergic Response: Localized
Hydration
Immune Status
Infection Severity
Infection Severity: Newborn
Nausea & Vomiting Severity
Nutritional Status

Nutritional Status: Food & Fluid Intake
Pain Level
Risk Control: Infectious Process
Risk Control: Tobacco Use
Self-Care: Oral Hygiene
Swallowing Status
Swallowing Status: Oral Phase

Pain, Acute

DEFINITION: Unpleasant sensory and emotional experience arising from actual or potential tissue damage or described in terms of such damage (International Association for the Study of Pain); sudden or slow onset of any intensity from mild to severe with an anticipated or predictable end and a duration of less than 6 months

SUGGESTED OUTCOMES:

Comfort Status: Physical
Discomfort Level
Pain Control

Pain Level
Stress Level
Vital Signs

ADDITIONAL ASSOCIATED OUTCOMES:

Anxiety Level
Appetite
Burn Recovery
Client Satisfaction: Pain Management
Client Satisfaction: Symptom Control
Comfort Status
Fear Level
Fear Level: Child
Knowledge: Pain Management

Nausea & Vomiting Severity
Personal Well-Being
Rest
Sleep
Symptom Control
Symptom Severity
Symptom Severity: Perimenopause
Symptom Severity: Premenstrual
   Syndrome (PMS)

Pain, Chronic

DEFINITION: Unpleasant sensory and emotional experience arising from actual or potential tissue damage or described in terms of such damage (International Association for the Study of Pain); sudden or slow onset of any intensity from mild to severe, constant, or recurring without an anticipated or predictable end and a duration of greater than 6 months

SUGGESTED OUTCOMES:

Depression Level
Discomfort Level
Pain Control

Pain Level
Pain: Adverse Psychological Response
Pain: Disruptive Effects

ADDITIONAL ASSOCIATED OUTCOMES:

Client Satisfaction: Pain Management
Client Satisfaction: Symptom Control
Depression Self-Control
Fatigue Level
Knowledge: Pain Management
Personal Well-Being
Quality of Life

Rest
Sleep
Stress Level
Suffering Severity
Symptom Control
Symptom Severity
Will to Live

Parent/Child Attachment, Risk for Impaired

DEFINITION: Disruption of the interactive process between parent/significant other and child/infant that fosters the development of a protective and nurturing reciprocal relationship

SUGGESTED OUTCOMES:

Caregiver Adaptation to Patient
   Institutionalization
Caregiver Performance: Direct Care
Child Development: 1 Month
Child Development: 2 Months
Child Development: 4 Months
Child Development: 6 Months
Child Development: 12 Months
Cognition

Coping
Depression Self-Control
Family Functioning
Family Social Climate
Knowledge: Parenting
Knowledge: Preterm Infant Care
Parent-Infant Attachment
Parenting Performance

SUGGESTED OUTCOMES: CONT'D

Risk Control

Risk Detection

Role Performance

Social Interaction Skills

Stress Level

Substance Addiction Consequences

Parental Role Conflict

DEFINITION: Parent experience of role confusion and conflict in response to crisis

SUGGESTED OUTCOMES:

Anxiety Level

Caregiver Adaptation to Patient
   Institutionalization

Caregiver Home Care Readiness

Caregiver Lifestyle Disruption

Coping

Family Functioning

Family Participation in Professional Care

Family Social Climate

Fear Level

Parenting Performance

Personal Resiliency

Psychosocial Adjustment: Life Change

Role Performance

ADDITIONAL ASSOCIATED OUTCOMES:

Anxiety Self-Control

Caregiver Performance: Direct Care

Caregiver Performance: Indirect Care

Caregiver Physical Health

Caregiver Stressors

Family Coping

Family Health Status

Family Normalization

Family Resiliency

Knowledge: Infant Care

Knowledge: Preterm Infant Care

Parent-Infant Attachment

Parenting, Impaired

DEFINITION: Inability of the primary caretaker to create, maintain, or regain an environment that promotes the optimum growth and development of the child

SUGGESTED OUTCOMES:

Child Development: 1 Month

Child Development: 2 Months

Child Development: 4 Months

Child Development: 6 Months

Child Development: 12 Months

Child Development: 2 Years

Child Development: 3 Years

Child Development: 4 Years

Child Development: 5 Years

Child Development: Middle Childhood

Child Development: Adolescence

Family Coping

Family Functioning

Family Social Climate

Parent-Infant Attachment

Parenting Performance

Parenting: Psychosocial Safety

Role Performance

ADDITIONAL ASSOCIATED OUTCOMES:

Abuse Cessation

Abuse Protection

Abuse Recovery

Abusive Behavior Self-Restraint

Anxiety Level

Anxiety Self-Control

ADDITIONAL ASSOCIATED OUTCOMES: CONT'D

Caregiver Performance: Direct Care
Caregiver Performance: Indirect Care
Cognition
Coping
Depression Level
Depression Self-Control
Fatigue Level
Knowledge: Child Physical Safety
Knowledge: Infant Care
Knowledge: Parenting
Knowledge: Preterm Infant Care
Motivation

Neglect Recovery
Parenting: Adolescent Physical Safety
Parenting: Early/Middle Childhood Physical Safety
Parenting: Infant/Toddler Physical Safety
Personal Resiliency
Psychosocial Adjustment: Life Change
Social Interaction Skills
Social Support
Stress Level
Substance Withdrawal Severity

Parenting, Readiness for Enhanced

DEFINITION: A pattern of providing an environment for children or other dependent person(s) that is sufficient to nurture growth and development and can be strengthened

SUGGESTED OUTCOMES:

Family Functioning
Knowledge: Child Physical Safety
Knowledge: Infant Care
Knowledge: Parenting

Knowledge: Preterm Infant Care
Parenting Performance
Parenting: Psychosocial Safety

ADDITIONAL ASSOCIATED OUTCOMES:

Child Development: 1 Month
Child Development: 2 Months
Child Development: 4 Months
Child Development: 6 Months
Child Development: 12 Months
Child Development: 2 Years
Child Development: 3 Years
Child Development: 4 Years
Child Development: 5 Years

Child Development: Middle Childhood
Child Development: Adolescence
Family Coping
Family Normalization
Family Social Climate
Parenting: Adolescent Physical Safety
Parenting: Early/Middle Childhood Physical Safety
Parenting: Infant/Toddler Physical Safety

Parenting, Risk for Impaired

DEFINITION: Risk for inability of the primary caretaker to create, maintain, or regain an environment that promotes the optimum growth and development of the child

SUGGESTED OUTCOMES:

Abusive Behavior Self-Restraint
Aggression Self-Control

Caregiver Emotional Health
Caregiver Physical Health

SUGGESTED OUTCOMES: CONT'D

Caregiver Role Endurance
Caregiver Stressors
Caregiver Well-Being
Cognition
Coping
Decision-Making
Depression Self-Control
Distorted Thought Self-Control
Family Coping
Family Health Status
Family Normalization
Family Resiliency
Family Social Climate
Fatigue Level
Knowledge: Health Resources
Knowledge: Infant Care
Knowledge: Parenting
Knowledge: Preterm Infant Care

Parent-Infant Attachment
Parenting Performance
Personal Health Status
Personal Resiliency
Risk Control
Risk Control: Alcohol Use
Risk Control: Drug Use
Risk Control: Tobacco Use
Risk Detection
Role Performance
Safe Home Environment
Self-Esteem
Sensory Function
Sleep
Social Interaction Skills
Social Support
Stress Level
Substance Withdrawal Severity

Perioperative Positioning Injury, Risk for

DEFINITION: At risk for inadvertent anatomical and physical changes as a result of posture or equipment used during an invasive/surgical procedure

SUGGESTED OUTCOMES:

Acute Confusion Level
Aspiration Prevention
Blood Coagulation
Blood Loss Severity
Circulation Status
Cognition
Cognitive Orientation
Fluid Overload Severity
Neurological Status: Spinal Sensory/Motor
   Function

Pre-Procedure Readiness
Respiratory Status: Gas Exchange
Respiratory Status: Ventilation
Risk Control
Risk Detection
Thermoregulation
Tissue Integrity: Skin & Mucous Membranes
Tissue Perfusion: Cellular
Tissue Perfusion: Peripheral

Peripheral Neurovascular Dysfunction, Risk for

DEFINITION: At risk for disruption in circulation, sensation, or motion of an extremity

SUGGESTED OUTCOMES:

Blood Coagulation
Body Positioning: Self-Initiated

Bone Healing
Burn Healing

SUGGESTED OUTCOMES: CONT'D

Burn Recovery
Cardiopulmonary Status
Circulation Status
Coordinated Movement
Heedfulness of Affected Side
Joint Movement: Ankle
Joint Movement: Elbow
Joint Movement: Hip
Joint Movement: Knee
Mobility
Neurological Status
Neurological Status: Cranial Sensory/Motor
   Function

Neurological Status: Peripheral
Neurological Status: Spinal Sensory/Motor
   Function
Physical Injury Severity
Respiratory Status
Risk Control
Risk Detection
Sensory Function: Cutaneous
Tissue Perfusion: Cellular
Tissue Perfusion: Peripheral

Personal Identity, Disturbed

DEFINITION: Inability to distinguish between self and nonself

SUGGESTED OUTCOMES:
Distorted Thought Self-Control
Identity
Self-Mutilation Restraint

ADDITIONAL ASSOCIATED OUTCOMES:

Acute Confusion Level
Anxiety Level
Anxiety Self-Control

Comfort Status: Psychospiritual
Depression Level
Sexual Identity

Poisoning, Risk for

DEFINITION: Accentuated risk of accidental exposure to, or ingestion of, drugs or dangerous products in doses sufficient to cause poisoning

SUGGESTED OUTCOMES:

Acute Confusion Level
Caregiver Performance: Direct Care
Cognition
Community Risk Control: Lead Exposure
Knowledge: Medication
Parenting: Adolescent Physical Safety
Parenting: Early/Middle Childhood
   Physical Safety
Parenting: Infant/Toddler Physical Safety

Personal Safety Behavior
Risk Control
Risk Control: Alcohol Use
Risk Control: Drug Use
Risk Detection
Safe Home Environment
Self-Care: Non-Parenteral Medication
Self-Care: Parental Medication
Vision Compensation Behavior

Post-Trauma Syndrome

DEFINITION: Sustained maladaptive response to a traumatic, overwhelming event

SUGGESTED OUTCOMES:

Abuse Recovery: Emotional
Abuse Recovery: Financial
Abuse Recovery: Physical
Abuse Recovery: Sexual
Aggression Self-Control
Anxiety Level
Comfort Status: Psychospiritual
Coping
Depression Level

Fear Level
Fear Level: Child
Hope
Impulse Self-Control
Mood Equilibrium
Personal Resiliency
Self-Mutilation Restraint
Stress Level
Suicide Self-Restraint

ADDITIONAL ASSOCIATED OUTCOMES:

Abuse Cessation
Abuse Protection
Abuse Recovery
Adaptation to Physical Disability
Agitation Level
Anxiety Self-Control
Body Image
Cognition
Community Disaster Response
Concentration
Depression Self-Control
Distorted Thought Self-Control

Fear Self-Control
Grief Resolution
Information Processing
Personal Safety Behavior
Psychosocial Adjustment: Life Change
Quality of Life
Risk Detection
Self-Esteem
Sleep
Social Support
Will to Live

Post-Trauma Syndrome, Risk for

DEFINITION: At risk for sustained maladaptive response to a traumatic, overwhelming event

SUGGESTED OUTCOMES:

Abuse Cessation
Abuse Protection
Abuse Recovery
Abuse Recovery: Emotional
Abuse Recovery: Sexual
Adaptation to Physical Disability
Aggression Self-Control
Anxiety Level
Anxiety Self-Control
Body Image
Comfort Status: Psychospiritual
Cognition
Coping

Depression Level
Depression Self-Control
Distorted Thought Self-Control
Grief Resolution
Impulse Self-Control
Information Processing
Mood Equilibrium
Personal Resiliency
Psychosocial Adjustment: Life Change
Quality of Life
Risk Control
Risk Control: Alcohol Use

SUGGESTED OUTCOMES: CONT'D

Risk Control: Drug Use

Risk Detection

Self-Esteem

Self-Mutilation Restraint

Sleep

Social Support

Spiritual Health

Stress Level

Suicide Self-Restraint

Power, Readiness for Enhanced

DEFINITION: A pattern of participating knowingly in change that is sufficient for well-being and can be strengthened

SUGGESTED OUTCOMES:

Adaptation to Physical Disability

Caregiver Adaptation to Patient
    Institutionalization

Health-Seeking Behavior

Personal Autonomy

Personal Resiliency

Personal Well-Being

Psychosocial Adjustment: Life Change

ADDITIONAL ASSOCIATED OUTCOMES:

Decision-Making

Family Resiliency

Health Beliefs

Health Beliefs: Perceived Ability to Perform

Health Beliefs: Perceived Control

Health-Promoting Behavior

Information Processing

Participation in Health Care Decisions

Self-Direction of Care

Powerlessness

DEFINITION: Perception that one's own action will not significantly affect an outcome; a perceived lack of control over a current situation or immediate happening

SUGGESTED OUTCOMES:

Acceptance: Health Status

Health Beliefs

Health Beliefs: Perceived Ability to Perform

Health Beliefs: Perceived Control

Health Beliefs: Perceived Resources

Hope

Participation in Health Care Decisions

Personal Autonomy

Personal Resiliency

Role Performance

Self-Esteem

ADDITIONAL ASSOCIATED OUTCOMES:

Abuse Recovery

Anxiety Level

Anxiety Self-Control

Client Satisfaction

Client Satisfaction: Access to Care Resources

Client Satisfaction: Case Management

Client Satisfaction: Pain Management

Client Satisfaction: Protection of Rights

Decision-Making

Depression Level

Depression Self-Control

Family Resiliency

ADDITIONAL ASSOCIATED OUTCOMES: CONT'D

Fatigue Level

Health Orientation

Information Processing

Knowledge: Disease Process

Self-Direction of Care

Social Interaction Skills

Social Involvement

Social Support

Stress Level

Powerlessness, Risk for

DEFINITION: At risk for perceived lack of control over a situation and/or one's ability to significantly affect an outcome

SUGGESTED OUTCOMES:

Abuse Recovery

Adaptation to Physical Disability

Anxiety Level

Anxiety Self-Control

Body Image

Coping

Decision-Making

Depression Level

Depression Self-Control

Dignified Life Closure

Endurance

Fatigue Level

Fear Level

Fear Self-Control

Health Beliefs

Health Beliefs: Perceived Ability to Perform

Health Beliefs: Perceived Control

Health Beliefs: Perceived Resources

Immobility Consequences: Psycho-Cognitive

Information Processing

Knowledge: Disease Process

Participation in Health Care Decisions

Personal Autonomy

Personal Resiliency

Risk Control

Risk Detection

Role Performance

Self-Direction of Care

Self-Esteem

Social Interaction Skills

Social Involvement

Social Support

Stress Level

Protection, Ineffective

DEFINITION: Decrease in the ability to guard self from internal or external threats such as illness or injury

SUGGESTED OUTCOMES:

Abuse Protection

Health Beliefs: Perceived Ability to Perform

Health Promoting Behavior

Immune Status

Immunization Behavior

Knowledge: Personal Safety

Personal Autonomy

Personal Resiliency

ADDITIONAL ASSOCIATED OUTCOMES:

Acute Confusion Level

Alcohol Abuse Cessation Behavior

Blood Coagulation

Cardiopulmonary Status

Client Satisfaction: Safety

Cognition

Cognitive Orientation

Community Health Status: Immunity

ADDITIONAL ASSOCIATED OUTCOMES: CONT'D

Community Risk Control: Violence
Coping
Development: Late Adulthood
Drug Abuse Cessation Behavior
Endurance
Fatigue Level
Infection Severity
Infection Severity: Newborn
Information Processing
Knowledge: Body Mechanics
Knowledge: Cancer Threat Reduction
Knowledge: Health Promotion
Knowledge: Health Resources
Knowledge: Infection Management
Knowledge: Pain Management
Neurological Status: Consciousness

Nutritional Status
Participation in Health Care Decisions
Respiratory Status
Respiratory Status: Ventilation
Risk Control
Risk Control: Infectious Process
Risk Detection
Self-Direction of Care
Sleep
Smoking Cessation Behavior
Stress Level
Substance Withdrawal Severity
Symptom Severity
Tissue Integrity: Skin & Mucous Membranes
Wound Healing: Primary Intention
Wound Healing: Secondary Intention

Rape-Trauma Syndrome

DEFINITION: Sustained maladaptive response to a forced, violent sexual penetration against the victim's will and consent

SUGGESTED OUTCOMES:

Abuse Protection
Abuse Recovery: Emotional
Abuse Recovery: Sexual
Comfort Status: Psychospiritual

Coping
Personal Resiliency
Sexual Functioning
Stress Level

ADDITIONAL ASSOCIATED OUTCOMES:

Abuse Cessation
Abuse Recovery
Agitation Level
Anxiety Level
Anxiety Self-Control
Body Image
Cognition
Decision Making
Depression Level
Depression Self-Control
Distorted Thought Self-Control
Fear Level
Fear Self-Control

Grief Resolution
Impulse Self-Control
Mood Equilibrium
Personal Autonomy
Personal Well-Being
Quality of Life
Self-Esteem
Self-Mutilation Restraint
Sleep
Social Involvement
Suicide Self-Restraint
Will to Live

Rape-Trauma Syndrome: Compound Reaction

DEFINITION: Forced violent sexual penetration against the victim's will and consent. The trauma syndrome that develops from this attack or attempted attack includes an acute phase of disorganization, of the victim's lifestyle and a long-term process of reorganization of lifestyle.

SUGGESTED OUTCOMES:

Abuse Recovery: Emotional
Abuse Recovery: Sexual
Comfort Status: Psychospiritual
Personal Autonomy
Personal Resiliency

Psychosocial Adjustment: Life Change
Self-Esteem
Sexual Functioning
Stress Level

ADDITIONAL ASSOCIATED OUTCOMES:

Abuse Cessation
Abuse Protection
Abuse Recovery
Agitation Level
Anxiety Level
Anxiety Self-Control
Decision-Making
Depression Level
Depression Self-Control
Family Coping
Family Normalization

Fear Level
Fear Self-Control
Mood Equilibrium
Personal Well-Being
Quality of Life
Risk Control: Alcohol Use
Risk Control: Drug Use
Sleep
Social Interaction Skills
Social Involvement
Will to Live

Rape-Trauma Syndrome: Silent Reaction

DEFINITION: Forced, violent sexual penetration against the victim's will and consent. The trauma syndrome that develops from this attack or attempted attack includes an acute phase of disorganization of the victim's lifestyle and a long-term process of reorganization of lifestyle.

SUGGESTED OUTCOMES:

Abuse Protection
Abuse Recovery: Emotional
Abuse Recovery: Sexual
Anxiety Level

Anxiety Self-Control
Comfort Status: Psychospiritual
Personal Resiliency
Sexual Functioning

ADDITIONAL ASSOCIATED OUTCOMES:

Abuse Cessation
Abuse Recovery
Agitation Level
Depression Level
Depression Self-Control
Fear Level
Fear Self-Control

Mood Equilibrium
Personal Autonomy
Personal Well-Being
Self-Esteem
Social Interaction Skills
Social Involvement
Stress Level

Religiosity, Impaired

DEFINITION: Impaired ability to exercise reliance on beliefs and/or participate in rituals of a particular faith tradition

SUGGESTED OUTCOMES:

Comfort Status: Psychospiritual
Dignified Life Closure
Hope

Psychosocial Adjustment: Life Change
Spiritual Health

ADDITIONAL ASSOCIATED OUTCOMES:

Acceptance: Health Status
Anxiety Level
Client Satisfaction: Cultural Needs
  Fulfillment
Comfortable Death
Coping
Development: Late Adulthood
Development: Middle Adulthood
Development: Young Adulthood

Fear Level
Personal Health Status
Personal Resiliency
Personal Well-Being
Quality of Life
Social Involvement
Social Support
Stress Level
Suffering Severity

Religiosity, Readiness for Enhanced

DEFINITION: Ability to increase reliance on religious beliefs and/or participate in rituals of a particular faith tradition

SUGGESTED OUTCOMES:

Hope
Personal Well-Being
Spiritual Health

ADDITIONAL ASSOCIATED OUTCOMES:

Client Satisfaction: Cultural Needs Fulfillment
Coping
Decision-Making
Dignified Life Closure

Grief Resolution
Personal Resiliency
Psychosocial Adjustment: Life Change
Quality of Life

Religiosity, Risk for Impaired

DEFINITION: At risk for impaired ability to exercise reliance on religious beliefs and/or participate in rituals of a particular faith tradition

SUGGESTED OUTCOMES:

Anxiety Level
Client Satisfaction: Cultural Needs Fulfillment
Coping
Depression Level
Development: Late Adulthood
Grief Resolution
Hope
Loneliness Severity
Mobility
Mood Equilibrium

Pain: Disruptive Effects
Personal Resiliency
Risk Control
Risk Detection
Self-Care: Instrumental Activities of Daily
    Living (IADL)
Social Involvement
Social Support
Spiritual Health
Suffering Severity

Relocation Stress Syndrome

DEFINITION: Physiological and/or psychosocial disturbance following transfer from one environment to another

SUGGESTED OUTCOMES:

Acute Confusion Level
Anxiety Level
Child Adaptation to Hospitalization
Coping
Depression Level
Fear Level
Loneliness Severity

Personal Autonomy
Personal Resiliency
Psychosocial Adjustment: Life Change
Self-Esteem
Sleep
Symptom Severity

ADDITIONAL ASSOCIATED OUTCOMES:

Agitation Level
Anxiety Self-Control
Caregiver Adaptation to Patient
    Institutionalization
Caregiver Home Care Readiness
Cognition
Depression Self-Control
Discharge Readiness: Independent Living
Discharge Readiness: Supported Living
Elopement Propensity Risk
Family Participation in Professional Care
Fatigue Level

Grief Resolution
Information Processing
Memory
Mood Equilibrium
Participation in Health Care Decisions
Quality of Life
Safe Wandering
Self-Care: Activities of Daily Living (ADL)
Self-Direction of Care
Social Involvement
Social Support
Stress Level

Relocation Stress Syndrome, Risk for

DEFINITION: At risk for physiological and/or psychosocial disturbance following transfer from one environment to another

SUGGESTED OUTCOMES:

Acceptance: Health Status
Acute Confusion Level
Agitation Level
Anxiety Level
Anxiety Self-Control
Child Adaptation to Hospitalization
Cognition
Coping
Discharge Readiness: Supported Living
Elopement Propensity Risk
Family Participation in Professional Care
Fatigue Level
Information Processing
Knowledge: Health Resources
Memory
Participation in Health Care Decisions
Personal Autonomy
Personal Health Status
Role Performance
Self-Care: Activities of Daily Living (ADL)
Self-Care: Instrumental Activities of Daily Living (IADL)
Self-Direction of Care
Social Interaction Skills
Social Involvement
Social Support
Stress Level

Role Performance, Ineffective

DEFINITION: Patterns of behavior and self-expression that do not match the environmental context, norms, and expectations

SUGGESTED OUTCOMES:

Anxiety Level
Caregiver Lifestyle Disruption
Cognition
Coping
Depression Level
Motivation
Parenting Performance
Personal Resiliency
Psychosocial Adjustment: Life Change
Role Performance

ADDITIONAL ASSOCIATED OUTCOMES:

Adaptation to Physical Disability
Agitation Level
Anxiety Self-Control
Body Image
Caregiver Adaptation to Patient Institutionalization
Caregiver Home Care Readiness
Caregiver Performance: Direct Care
Caregiver Performance: Indirect Care
Depression Self-Control
Elopement Propensity Risk
Family Functioning
Fatigue Level
Information Processing
Knowledge: Parenting
Memory
Pain Level
Parent-Infant Attachment
Parenting: Adolescent Physical Safety
Parenting: Early/Middle Childhood Physical Safety
Parenting: Infant/Toddler Physical Safety
Psychomotor Energy
Self-Esteem
Social Support
Stress Level
Substance Addiction Consequences

Self-Care Deficit: Bathing/Hygiene

DEFINITION: Impaired ability to perform or complete bathing/hygiene activities for oneself

SUGGESTED OUTCOMES:

Ostomy Self-Care
Self-Care: Activities of Daily Living (ADL)
Self-Care: Bathing
Self-Care: Hygiene

ADDITIONAL ASSOCIATED OUTCOMES:

Acute Confusion Level
Adaptation to Physical Disability
Agitation Level
Anxiety Self-Control
Body Mechanics Performance
Cardiopulmonary Status
Client Satisfaction: Functional Assistance
Client Satisfaction: Physical Care
Cognition
Coordinated Movement
Discomfort Level
Endurance
Energy Conservation
Fatigue Level
Heedfulness of Affected Side
Knowledge: Body Mechanics
Knowledge: Ostomy Care
Mobility
Motivation
Neurological Status
Neurological Status: Peripheral
Oral Hygiene
Pain Level
Psychomotor Energy
Respiratory Status
Self-Care: Oral Hygiene
Skeletal Function
Vision Compensation Behavior

Self-Care Deficit: Dressing/Grooming

DEFINITION: Impaired ability to perform or complete dressing and grooming activities for self

SUGGESTED OUTCOMES:

Self-Care: Activities of Daily Living (ADL)
Self-Care: Dressing
Self-Care: Hygiene

ADDITIONAL ASSOCIATED OUTCOMES:

Acute Confusion Level
Adaptation to Physical Disability
Agitation Level
Anxiety Level
Anxiety Self-Control
Balance
Body Mechanics Performance
Cardiopulmonary Status
Client Satisfaction: Functional Assistance
Client Satisfaction: Physical Care
Cognition
Coordinated Movement
Discomfort Level
Endurance
Energy Conservation
Fatigue Level
Heedfulness of Affected Side
Joint Movement: Fingers
Knowledge: Body Mechanics
Mobility
Motivation
Neurological Status
Neurological Status: Peripheral
Pain Level
Psychomotor Energy
Respiratory Status
Skeletal Function
Vision Compensation Behavior

Self-Care Deficit: Feeding

DEFINITION: Impaired ability to perform or complete feeding activities

SUGGESTED OUTCOMES:

Nutritional Status: Food & Fluid Intake
Self-Care: Activities of Daily Living (ADL)
Self-Care: Eating
Swallowing Status

ADDITIONAL ASSOCIATED OUTCOMES:

Acute Confusion Level
Adaptation to Physical Disability
Agitation Level
Anxiety Self-Control
Appetite
Aspiration Prevention
Client Satisfaction: Functional Assistance
Client Satisfaction: Physical Care
Cognition
Discomfort Level
Endurance
Fatigue Level
Joint Movement: Elbow
Joint Movement: Fingers
Joint Movement: Shoulder
Joint Movement: Wrist
Motivation
Nausea & Vomiting Control
Neurological Status: Central Motor Control
Neurological Status: Peripheral
Nutritional Status
Pain Control
Pain Level
Psychomotor Energy
Respiratory Status
Vision Compensation Behavior

Self-Care Deficit: Toileting

DEFINITION: Impaired ability to perform or complete own toileting activities

SUGGESTED OUTCOMES:

Knowledge: Ostomy Care
Ostomy Self-Care
Self-Care: Activities of Daily Living (ADL)
Self-Care: Hygiene
Self-Care: Toileting

ADDITIONAL ASSOCIATED OUTCOMES:

Acute Confusion Level
Agitation Level
Ambulation
Anxiety Level
Anxiety Self-Control
Balance
Cardiopulmonary Status
Client Satisfaction: Functional Assistance
Client Satisfaction: Physical Care
Cognition
Coordinated Movement
Discomfort Level
Endurance
Energy Conservation
Fatigue Level
Joint Movement
Mobility
Neurological Status
Neurological Status: Central Motor Control
Neurological Status: Spinal Sensory/Motor Function
Pain Level
Respiratory Status
Skeletal Function
Transfer Performance
Vision Compensation Behavior

Self-Care, Readiness for Enhanced

DEFINITION: A pattern of performing activities for oneself that helps to meet health-related goals and can be strengthened

SUGGESTED OUTCOMES:

Adherence Behavior
Compliance Behavior: Prescribed Diet
Compliance Behavior: Prescribed Medication
Personal Autonomy
Postpartum Maternal Health Behavior
Risk Control: Infectious Process
Risk Control: Sun Exposure
Self-Care Status
Self-Care: Activities of Daily Living (ADL)
Self-Care: Bathing
Self-Care: Dressing

Self-Care: Eating
Self-Care: Hygiene
Self-Care: Instrumental Activities of Daily
    Living (IADL)
Self-Care: Non-Parenteral Medication
Self-Care: Oral Hygiene
Self-Care: Parenteral Medication
Self-Care: Toileting
Smoking Cessation Behavior
Weight Gain Behavior
Weight Loss Behavior

ADDITIONAL ASSOCIATED OUTCOMES:

Adherence Behavior: Healthy Diet
Asthma Self-Management
Cardiac Disease Self-Management
Diabetes Self-Management

Health-Seeking Behavior
Multiple Sclerosis Self-Management
Personal Well-Being
Self-Direction of Care

Self-Concept, Readiness for Enhanced

DEFINITION: A pattern of perceptions or ideas about the self that is sufficient for well-being and can be strengthened

SUGGESTED OUTCOMES:

Abuse Recovery
Body Image
Identity
Personal Autonomy

Personal Resiliency
Role Performance
Self-Esteem

ADDITIONAL ASSOCIATED OUTCOMES:

Abuse Recovery: Emotional
Abuse Recovery: Financial
Abuse Recovery: Physical
Abuse Recovery: Sexual
Adaptation to Physical Disability
Child Development: Adolescence
Comfort Status: Psychospiritual

Depression Self-Control
Development: Late Adulthood
Development: Middle Adulthood
Development: Young Adulthood
Neglect Recovery
Personal Well-Being
Psychosocial Adjustment: Life Change

Self-Esteem: Chronic Low

DEFINITION: Long-standing negative self-evaluation/feelings about self or self-capabilities

SUGGESTED OUTCOMES:

Depression Level   Personal Resiliency
Personal Autonomy   Self-Esteem

ADDITIONAL ASSOCIATED OUTCOMES:

Body Image   Motivation
Comfort Status: Psychospiritual   Quality of Life
Depression Self-Control   Role Performance
Hope   Social Interaction Skills
Mood Equilibrium   Stress Level

Self-Esteem: Situational Low

DEFINITION: Development of a negative perception of self-worth in response to a current situation (specify)

SUGGESTED OUTCOMES:

Adaptation to Physical Disability   Psychosocial Adjustment: Life Change
Grief Resolution   Self-Esteem
Personal Resiliency

ADDITIONAL ASSOCIATED OUTCOMES:

Abuse Recovery   Development: Middle Adulthood
Abuse Recovery: Emotional   Development: Young Adulthood
Abuse Recovery: Physical   Fear Level
Abuse Recovery: Sexual   Fear Level: Child
Anxiety Level   Neglect Recovery
Body Image   Personal Autonomy
Burn Recovery   Role Performance
Coping   Stress Level
Development: Late Adulthood

Self-Esteem: Situational Low, Risk for

DEFINITION: At risk for developing negative perception of self-worth in response to a current situation (specify)

SUGGESTED OUTCOMES:

Abuse Recovery   Abuse Recovery: Sexual
Abuse Recovery: Emotional   Adaptation to Physical Disability
Abuse Recovery: Financial   Body Image
Abuse Recovery: Physical   Burn Recovery

SUGGESTED OUTCOMES: CONT'D

Child Development: Adolescence
Coping
Development: Late Adulthood
Development: Middle Adulthood
Development: Young Adulthood
Grief Resolution
Neglect Recovery
Personal Autonomy

Personal Resiliency
Psychosocial Adjustment: Life Change
Risk Control
Risk Detection
Role Performance
Self-Esteem
Weight Loss Behavior

Self-Mutilation

DEFINITION: Deliberate self-injurious behavior causing tissue damage with the intent of causing nonfatal injury to attain relief of tension

SUGGESTED OUTCOMES:

Impulse Self-Control
Self-Mutilation Restraint

ADDITIONAL ASSOCIATED OUTCOMES:

Abuse Recovery
Abuse Recovery: Emotional
Abuse Recovery: Physical
Abuse Recovery: Sexual
Alcohol Abuse Cessation Behavior
Anxiety Level
Body Image
Coping
Distorted Thought Self-Control

Drug Abuse Cessation Behavior
Identity
Loneliness Severity
Personal Resiliency
Self-Esteem
Sexual Identity
Social Support
Stress Level

Self-Mutilation, Risk for

DEFINITION: At risk for deliberate self-injurious behavior causing tissue damage with the intent of causing nonfatal injury to attain relief of tension

SUGGESTED OUTCOMES:

Abuse Recovery
Abuse Recovery: Emotional
Abuse Recovery: Physical
Abuse Recovery: Sexual
Anxiety Level
Body Image
Distorted Thought Self-Control
Impulse Self-Control
Mood Equilibrium
Personal Resiliency

Risk Control
Risk Control: Alcohol Use
Risk Control: Drug Use
Risk Detection
Self-Esteem
Self-Mutilation Restraint
Sexual Identity
Stress Level
Substance Addiction Consequences

Sensory Perception: Auditory, Disturbed

DEFINITION: Change in the amount or patterning of incoming stimuli accompanied by a diminished, exaggerated, distorted, or impaired response to such stimuli

SUGGESTED OUTCOMES:

Communication: Receptive
Concentration

Hearing Compensation Behavior
Sensory Function: Hearing

ADDITIONAL ASSOCIATED OUTCOMES:

Acute Confusion Level
Agitation Level
Cognitive Orientation
Distorted Thought Self-Control

Neurological Status: Cranial Sensory / Motor
    Function
Risk Control: Hearing Impairment

Sensory Perception: Gustatory, Disturbed

DEFINITION: Change in the amount or patterning of incoming stimuli accompanied by a diminished, exaggerated, distorted, or impaired response to such stimuli

SUGGESTED OUTCOMES:

Appetite
Nutritional Status: Food & Fluid Intake
Sensory Function: Taste & Smell

ADDITIONAL ASSOCIATED OUTCOMES:

Cognitive Orientation
Distorted Thought Self-Control
Nausea & Vomiting Severity

Neurological Status: Cranial Sensory / Motor
    Function
Stress Level

Sensory Perception: Kinesthetic, Disturbed

DEFINITION: Change in the amount or patterning of incoming stimuli accompanied by a diminished, exaggerated, distorted, or impaired response to such stimuli

SUGGESTED OUTCOMES:

Balance
Body Positioning: Self-Initiated

Coordinated Movement
Sensory Function: Proprioception

ADDITIONAL ASSOCIATED OUTCOMES:

Ambulation
Body Mechanics Performance
Cognitive Orientation
Distorted Thought Self-Control

Heedfulness of Affected Side
Multiple Sclerosis Self-Management
Neurological Status: Central Motor Control

Sensory Perception: Olfactory, Disturbed

DEFINITION: Change in the amount or patterning of incoming stimuli accompanied by a diminished, exaggerated, distorted, or impaired response to such stimuli

SUGGESTED OUTCOMES:
Appetite
Nutritional Status: Food & Fluid Intake
Sensory Function: Taste & Smell

ADDITIONAL ASSOCIATED OUTCOMES:
Cognitive Orientation
Distorted Thought Self-Control
Nausea & Vomiting Severity

Neurological Status: Cranial Sensory/Motor
   Function

Sensory Perception: Tactile, Disturbed

DEFINITION: Change in the amount or patterning of incoming stimuli accompanied by a diminished, exaggerated, distorted, or impaired response to such stimuli

SUGGESTED OUTCOMES:
Sensory Function: Cutaneous

ADDITIONAL ASSOCIATED OUTCOMES:
Cognitive Orientation
Distorted Thought Self-Control
Heedfulness to Affected Side
Neurological Status: Spinal Sensory/Motor
   Function

Pain Level
Tissue Integrity: Skin & Mucous Membranes

Sensory Perception: Visual, Disturbed

DEFINITION: Change in the amount or patterning of incoming stimuli accompanied by a diminished, exaggerated, distorted, or impaired response to such stimuli

SUGGESTED OUTCOMES:
Sensory Function: Vision
Vision Compensation Behavior

ADDITIONAL ASSOCIATED OUTCOMES:
Cognitive Orientation
Distorted Thought Self-Control
Neurological Status: Cranial Sensory/Motor Function
Risk Control: Visual Impairment

Sexual Dysfunction

DEFINITION: The state in which an individual experiences a change in sexual function during the sexual response phases of desire, excitation, and/or orgasm, which is viewed as unsatisfying, unrewarding or inadequate

SUGGESTED OUTCOMES:
Abuse Recovery: Sexual
Sexual Functioning
Sexual Identity

ADDITIONAL ASSOCIATED OUTCOMES:
Abuse Cessation
Abuse Recovery
Abuse Recovery: Emotional
Abuse Recovery: Physical
Adaptation to Physical Disability
Anxiety Level
Body Image
Fatigue Level
Fear Level
Knowledge: Cardiac Disease Management
Knowledge: Pregnancy & Postpartum
   Sexual Functioning

Personal Resiliency
Physical Aging
Physical Maturation: Female
Physical Maturation: Male
Risk Control: Sexually Transmitted
   Diseases (STD)
Role Performance
Self-Esteem
Social Interaction Skills
Stress Level

Sexuality Pattern, Ineffective

DEFINITION: Expressions of concern regarding own sexuality

SUGGESTED OUTCOMES:
Abuse Recovery: Sexual
Body Image
Personal Resiliency
Physical Maturation: Female

Physical Maturation: Male
Role Performance
Self-Esteem
Sexual Identity

ADDITIONAL ASSOCIATED OUTCOMES:
Abuse Cessation
Abuse Recovery
Anxiety Level
Anxiety Self-Control
Child Development: Adolescence
Development: Late Adulthood
Development: Middle Adulthood
Development: Young Adulthood

Fatigue Level
Personal Well-Being
Physical Aging
Psychosocial Adjustment: Life Change
Risk Control: Sexually Transmitted
   Diseases (STD)
Risk Control: Unintended Pregnancy
Stress Level

Skin Integrity, Impaired

DEFINITION: Altered epidermis and/or dermis

SUGGESTED OUTCOMES:

Allergic Response: Localized
Burn Healing
Tissue Integrity: Skin & Mucous Membranes

Wound Healing: Primary Intention
Wound Healing: Secondary Intention

ADDITIONAL ASSOCIATED OUTCOMES:

Burn Recovery
Circulation Status
Fluid Balance
Fluid Overload Severity
Hemodialysis Access
Immobility Consequences: Physiological
Infection Severity
Infection Severity: Newborn
Knowledge: Infection Management
Medication Response
Neurological Status: Peripheral
Nutritional Status
Ostomy Self-Care

Risk Control: Hyperthermia
Risk Control: Hypothermia
Risk Control: Infectious Process
Risk Control: Sun Exposure
Self-Care: Bathing
Self-Care: Hygiene
Sensory Function: Cutaneous
Thermoregulation
Thermoregulation: Newborn
Tissue Perfusion: Cellular
Tissue Perfusion: Peripheral
Treatment Behavior: Illness or Injury

Skin Integrity, Risk for Impaired

DEFINITION: At risk for skin being adversely altered

SUGGESTED OUTCOMES:

Allergic Response: Localized
Body Positioning: Self-Initiated
Burn Healing
Burn Recovery
Child Development: Adolescence
Fluid Overload Severity
Hemodialysis Access
Immobility Consequences: Physiological
Infection Severity
Infection Severity: Newborn
Neurological Status: Peripheral
Nutritional Status
Nutritional Status: Biochemical Measures
Ostomy Self-Care

Physical Aging
Risk Control
Risk Control: Hyperthermia
Risk Control: Hypothermia
Risk Control: Infectious Process
Risk Control: Sun Exposure
Risk Detection
Self-Mutilation Restraint
Tissue Integrity: Skin & Mucous Membrane
Tissue Perfusion: Cellular
Tissue Perfusion: Peripheral
Wound Healing: Primary Intention
Wound Healing: Secondary Intention

Sleep Deprivation

DEFINITION: Prolonged periods of time without sleep (sustained natural, periodic suspension of relative consciousness)

SUGGESTED OUTCOMES:

Acute Confusion Level
Agitation Level
Anxiety Level
Concentration
Discomfort Level
Fatigue Level

Mood Equilibrium
Pain: Disruptive Effects
Pain Level
Psychomotor Energy
Rest
Sleep

ADDITIONAL ASSOCIATED OUTCOMES:

Anxiety Self-Control
Cognition
Comfort Status: Environment
Depression Level
Distorted Thought Self-Control
Endurance
Energy Conservation

Information Processing
Medication Response
Memory
Pain Control
Postpartum Maternal Health Behavior
Stress Level
Symptom Severity

Sleep, Readiness for Enhanced

DEFINITION: A pattern of natural, periodic suspension of consciousness that provides adequate rest, sustains a desired lifestyle, and can be strengthened

SUGGESTED OUTCOMES:

Motivation
Rest
Sleep

ADDITIONAL ASSOCIATED OUTCOMES:

Comfort Status: Environment
Concentration
Discomfort Level
Energy Conservation

Health-Seeking Behavior
Mood Equilibrium
Personal Well-Being
Stress Level

Social Interaction, Impaired

DEFINITION: Insufficient or excessive quantity or ineffective quality of social exchange

SUGGESTED OUTCOMES:

Child Development: Middle Childhood
Child Development: Adolescence
Development: Late Adulthood
Development: Middle Adulthood
Development: Young Adulthood

Family Social Climate
Leisure Participation
Play Participation
Social Interaction Skills
Social Involvement

ADDITIONAL ASSOCIATED OUTCOMES:

Adaptation to Physical Disability

Body Image

Comfort Status: Sociocultural

Communication

Distorted Thought Self-Control

Family Functioning

Family Integrity

Fatigue Level

Fear Level

Fear Level: Child

Hyperactivity Level

Immobility Consequences: Psycho-Cognitive

Loneliness Severity

Mobility

Psychomotor Energy

Role Performance

Self-Esteem

Stress Level

Student Health Status

Social Isolation

DEFINITION: Aloneness experienced by the individual and perceived as imposed by others and as a negative or threatening state

SUGGESTED OUTCOMES:

Family Social Climate

Leisure Participation

Loneliness Severity

Social Interaction Skills

Social Involvement

Social Support

ADDITIONAL ASSOCIATED OUTCOMES:

Adaptation to Physical Disability

Aggression Self-Control

Body Image

Client Satisfaction: Communication

Communication

Depression Level

Fatigue Level

Fear Level

Fear Level: Child

Hearing Compensation Behavior

Mobility

Mood Equilibrium

Personal Well-Being

Play Participation

Self-Esteem

Vision Compensation Behavior

Sorrow: Chronic

DEFINITION: Cyclical, recurring, and potentially progressive pattern of pervasive sadness experienced (by a parent, caregiver, individual with chronic illness or disability) in response to continual loss, throughout the trajectory of an illness or disability

SUGGESTED OUTCOMES:

Acceptance: Health Status

Depression Level

Depression Self-Control

Grief Resolution

Hope

Loneliness Severity

Mood Equilibrium

Personal Well-Being

Psychosocial Adjustment: Life Change

Self-Esteem

Suffering Severity

ADDITIONAL ASSOCIATED OUTCOMES:

Adaptation to Physical Disability

Coping

Fear Level

Personal Resiliency

Physical Aging

Quality of Life

Social Involvement

Spiritual Health

Spiritual Distress

DEFINITION: Impaired ability to experience and integrate meaning and purpose in life through a connectedness with self, others, art, music, literature, nature, and/or a power greater than oneself

SUGGESTED OUTCOMES:

Comfort Status: Psychospiritual

Coping

Hope

Spiritual Health

Social Involvement

ADDITIONAL ASSOCIATED OUTCOMES:

Anxiety Level

Client Satisfaction: Cultural Needs Fulfillment

Comfortable Death

Dignified Life Closure

Fatigue Level

Grief Resolution

Loneliness Severity

Pain Control

Pain: Disruptive Effects

Pain Level

Personal Autonomy

Personal Resiliency

Personal Well-Being

Psychosocial Adjustment: Life Change

Quality of Life

Social Interaction Skills

Stress Level

Suicide Self-Restraint

Will to Live

Spiritual Distress, Risk for

DEFINITION: At risk for an impaired ability to experience and integrate meaning and purpose in life though connectedness with self, others, art, music, literature, nature, and/or a power greater than oneself

SUGGESTED OUTCOMES:

Anxiety Level

Client Satisfaction: Cultural Needs Fulfillment

Comfortable Death

Coping

Depression Level

Dignified Life Closure

Fatigue Level

Grief Resolution

Hope

Loneliness Severity

Mood Equilibrium

Pain: Disruptive Effects

Personal Autonomy

SUGGESTED OUTCOMES: CONT'D

Personal Resiliency
Personal Well-Being
Psychosocial Adjustment: Life Change
Quality of Life
Risk Control
Risk Detection

Self-Esteem
Social Interaction Skills
Social Involvement
Spiritual Health
Stress Level

Spiritual Well-Being, Readiness for Enhanced

DEFINITION: Ability to experience and integrate meaning and purpose in life through connectedness with self, others, art, music, literature, nature, and/or a power greater than oneself

SUGGESTED OUTCOMES:

Coping
Hope
Personal Well-Being

Quality of Life
Spiritual Health

ADDITIONAL ASSOCIATED OUTCOMES:

Client Satisfaction: Cultural Needs Fulfillment
Comfort Status: Sociocultural
Dignified Life Closure
Grief Resolution

Personal Health Status
Personal Resiliency
Psychosocial Adjustment: Life Change
Social Involvement

Stress Overload

DEFINITION: Excessive amounts and types of demands that require action

SUGGESTED OUTCOMES:

Abusive Behavior Self-Restraint
Acceptance: Health Status
Adaptation to Physical Disability
Aggression Self-Control
Anxiety Self-Control
Caregiver Adaptation to Institutionalization
Comfort Status: Psychospiritual
Coping

Decision-Making
Dignified Life Closure
Discomfort Level
Family Coping
Psychosocial Adjustment: Life Change
Self-Mutilation Restraint
Stress Level
Suicide Self-Restraint

ADDITIONAL ASSOCIATED OUTCOMES:

Abuse Protection
Community Risk Control: Violence
Coping
Depression Self-Control
Fall Prevention Behavior
Fear Self-Control

Personal Resiliency
Smoking Cessation Behavior
Symptom Control
Symptom Severity
Treatment Behavior: Illness or Injury

Sudden Infant Death Syndrome, Risk for

DEFINITION: Presence of risk factors for sudden death of an infant under 1 year of age

SUGGESTED OUTCOMES:

Knowledge: Infant Care
Knowledge: Parenting
Knowledge: Preterm Infant Care
Parenting Performance
Parenting: Infant/Toddler Physical Safety
Prenatal Health Behavior
Preterm Infant Organization

Risk Control
Risk Control: Hyperthermia
Risk Control: Hypothermia
Risk Control: Infectious Process
Risk Control: Tobacco Use
Risk Detection
Thermoregulation: Newborn

Suffocation, Risk for

DEFINITION: Accentuated risk of accidental suffocation (inadequate air available for inhalation)

SUGGESTED OUTCOMES:

Aspiration Prevention
Asthma Self-Management
Body Positioning: Self-Initiated
Knowledge: Child Physical Safety
Knowledge: Infant Care
Knowledge: Personal Safety
Knowledge: Preterm Infant Care
Neurological Status: Consciousness
Parenting: Infant/Toddler Physical Safety
Personal Safety Behavior

Post-Procedure Recovery
Respiratory Status
Respiratory Status: Airway Patency
Respiratory Status: Ventilation
Risk Control
Risk Detection
Safe Home Environment
Substance Addiction Consequences
Swallowing Status

Suicide, Risk for

DEFINITION: At risk for self-inflicted, life-threatening injury

SUGGESTED OUTCOMES:

Abuse Recovery
Abuse Recovery: Emotional
Abuse Recovery: Financial

Abuse Recovery: Physical
Abuse Recovery: Sexual
Adaptation to Physical Disability

SUGGESTED OUTCOMES: CONT'D

Depression Level
Fatigue Level
Grief Resolution
Hope
Impulse Self-Control
Loneliness Severity
Mood Equilibrium
Pain: Adverse Psychological Response
Pain Control
Personal Autonomy
Personal Resiliency
Personal Well-Being
Psychomotor Energy
Risk Control
Risk Control: Alcohol Use

Risk Control: Drug Use
Risk Detection
Self-Esteem
Sexual Identity
Social Interaction Skills
Social Involvement
Social Support
Stress Level
Substance Addiction Consequences
Substance Withdrawal Severity
Suffering Severity
Suicide Self-Restraint
Symptom Control
Will to Live

Surgical Recovery, Delayed

DEFINITION: Extension of the number of postoperative days required to initiate and perform activities that maintain life, health, and well-being

SUGGESTED OUTCOMES:

Acute Confusion Level
Ambulation
Appetite
Blood Loss Severity
Discomfort Level
Endurance
Fatigue Level
Fluid Overload Severity
Hydration

Immobility Consequences: Physiological
Infection Severity
Mobility
Nausea & Vomiting Severity
Pain Level
Post-Procedure Recovery Status
Self-Care: Activities of Daily Living (ADL)
Wound Healing: Primary Intention

ADDITIONAL ASSOCIATED OUTCOMES:

Allergic Response: Systemic
Cardiopulmonary Status
Client Satisfaction: Physical Care
Client Satisfaction: Safety
Client Satisfaction: Technical Aspects of Care
Discharge Readiness: Independent Living
Discharge Readiness: Supported Living
Gastrointestinal Function
Health Beliefs
Immobility Consequences: Psycho-Cognitive
Infection Severity: Newborn
Kidney Function
Knowledge: Infection Management

Knowledge: Treatment Regimen
Maternal Status: Postpartum
Mechanical Ventilation Weaning Response:
   Adult
Medication Response
Nutritional Status: Energy
Nutritional Status: Food & Fluid Intake
Nutritional Status: Nutrient Intake
Pain Control
Pain: Disruptive Effects
Respiratory Status
Role Performance
Self-Care Status

ADDITIONAL ASSOCIATED OUTCOMES: CONT'D

Self-Care: Bathing
Self-Care: Dressing
Self-Care: Eating
Self-Care: Hygiene

Self-Care: Instrumental Activities
   of Daily Living (IADL)
Transfer Performance

Swallowing, Impaired

DEFINITION: Abnormal functioning of the swallowing mechanism associated with deficits in oral, pharyngeal, or esophageal structure or function

SUGGESTED OUTCOMES:

Aspiration Prevention
Swallowing Status
Swallowing Status: Esophageal Phase

Swallowing Status: Oral Phase
Swallowing Status: Pharyngeal Phase

ADDITIONAL ASSOCIATED OUTCOMES:

Appetite
Cognition
Neurological Status: Consciousness
Neurological Status: Cranial Sensory/
   Motor Function

Nutritional Status: Food & Fluid Intake
Respiratory Status: Airway Patency
Self-Care: Eating

Therapeutic Regimen Management, Effective

DEFINITION: Pattern of regulating and integrating into daily living a program for treatment of illness and its sequelae that is satisfactory for meeting specific health goals

SUGGESTED OUTCOMES:

Adherence Behavior
Compliance Behavior
Family Participation in Professional Care
Knowledge: Treatment Regimen

Participation in Health Care Decisions
Risk Control
Symptom Control
Treatment Behavior: Illness or Injury

ADDITIONAL ASSOCIATED OUTCOMES:

Adherence: Healthy Diet
Alcohol Abuse Cessation Behavior
Asthma Self-Management
Body Mechanics Performance
Cardiac Disease Self-Management
Client Satisfaction
Client Satisfaction: Case Management
Client Satisfaction: Pain Management
Client Satisfaction: Teaching
Compliance Behavior: Prescribed Diet

Compliance Behavior: Prescribed Medication
Diabetes Self-Management
Drug Abuse Cessation Behavior
Energy Conservation
Health Beliefs: Perceived Ability to Perform
Health Promoting Behavior
Knowledge: Arthritis Management
Knowledge: Asthma Management
Knowledge: Cancer Management
Knowledge: Cardiac Disease Management

ADDITIONAL ASSOCIATED OUTCOMES: CONT'D

Knowledge: Congestive Heart Failure
  Management
Knowledge: Depression Management
Knowledge: Diabetes Management
Knowledge: Diet
Knowledge: Disease Process
Knowledge: Energy Conservation
Knowledge: Hypertension Management
Knowledge: Illness Care
Knowledge: Infection Management
Knowledge: Medication
Knowledge: Multiple Sclerosis Management
Knowledge: Pain Management
Knowledge: Prescribed Activity

Knowledge: Treatment Procedure
Knowledge: Weight Management
Multiple Sclerosis Self-Management
Ostomy Self-Care
Pain Control
Seizure Control
Self-Care: Non-Parenteral Medication
Self-Care: Parenteral Medication
Self-Direction of Care
Smoking Cessation Behavior
Weight Gain Behavior
Weight Loss Behavior
Weight Maintenance Behavior

Therapeutic Regimen Management, Ineffective

DEFINITION: Pattern of regulating and integrating into daily living a program for treatment of illness and the sequelae of illness that is unsatisfactory for meeting specific health goals

SUGGESTED OUTCOMES:

Compliance Behavior
Knowledge: Diet
Knowledge: Treatment Regimen

Participation in Health Care Decisions
Symptom Control
Treatment Behavior: Illness or Injury

ADDITIONAL ASSOCIATED OUTCOMES:

Adherence Behavior
Adherence Behavior: Healthy Diet
Asthma Self-Management
Cardiac Disease Self-Management
Client Satisfaction
Client Satisfaction: Case Management
Client Satisfaction: Pain Management
Compliance Behavior: Prescribed Diet
Compliance Behavior: Prescribed Medication
Diabetes Self-Management
Discharge Readiness: Independent Living
Family Support During Treatment
Health Beliefs
Health Beliefs: Perceived Ability to Perform
Health Beliefs: Perceived Control
Health Beliefs: Perceived Resources
Health Beliefs: Perceived Threat
Health Orientation
Knowledge: Arthritis Management
Knowledge: Asthma Management
Knowledge: Cancer Management
Knowledge: Cancer Threat Reduction

Knowledge: Cardiac Disease Management
Knowledge: Congestive Heart Failure
  Management
Knowledge: Depression Management
Knowledge: Diabetes Management
Knowledge: Disease Process
Knowledge: Hypertension Management
Knowledge: Illness Care
Knowledge: Infection Management
Knowledge: Multiple Sclerosis Management
Knowledge: Pain Management
Knowledge: Treatment Procedure
Knowledge: Weight Management
Motivation
Multiple Sclerosis Self-Management
Ostomy Self-Care
Risk Control: Infectious Process
Self-Care: Non-Parenteral Medication
Self-Care: Parenteral Medication
Self-Direction of Care
Weight Gain Behavior
Weight Loss Behavior

Therapeutic Regimen Management, Readiness for Enhanced

DEFINITION: A pattern of regulating and integrating into daily living a program for treatment of illness and its sequelae that is sufficient for meeting health-related goals and can be strengthened

SUGGESTED OUTCOMES:

Adherence Behavior
Compliance Behavior
Family Participation in Professional Care
Knowledge: Treatment Regimen

Participation in Health Care Decisions
Risk Control
Symptom Control
Treatment Behavior: Illness or Injury

ADDITIONAL ASSOCIATED OUTCOMES:

Adherence Behavior: Healthy Diet
Cardiac Disease Self-Management
Client Satisfaction
Client Satisfaction: Case Management
Client Satisfaction: Pain Management
Compliance Behavior: Prescribed Diet
Compliance Behavior: Prescribed Medication
Diabetes Self-Management
Energy Conservation
Health Beliefs: Perceived Ability to Perform
Health Promoting Behavior
Knowledge: Arthritis Management
Knowledge: Asthma Management
Knowledge: Cancer Management
Knowledge: Cancer Threat Reduction
Knowledge: Cardiac Disease Management
Knowledge: Congestive Heart Failure
    Management
Knowledge: Depression Management
Knowledge: Diabetes Management

Knowledge: Diet
Knowledge: Disease Process
Knowledge: Energy Conservation
Knowledge: Hypertension Management
Knowledge: Illness Care
Knowledge: Infection Management
Knowledge: Medication
Knowledge: Multiple Sclerosis
    Management
Knowledge: Pain Management
Knowledge: Pregnancy & Postpartum
    Sexual Functioning
Knowledge: Prescribed Activity
Knowledge: Treatment Procedure
Knowledge: Weight Management
Multiple Sclerosis Self-Management
Ostomy Self-Care
Risk Control: Infectious Process
Self-Care: Non-Parenteral Medication
Self-Care: Parenteral Medication

Thermoregulation, Ineffective

DEFINITION: Temperature fluctuation between hypothermia and hyperthermia

SUGGESTED OUTCOMES:

Risk Control: Hyperthermia
Risk Control: Hypothermia
Thermoregulation

Thermoregulation: Newborn
Vital Signs

ADDITIONAL ASSOCIATED OUTCOMES:

Burn Healing
Cardiopulmonary Status

Hydration
Neurological Status: Autonomic

ADDITIONAL ASSOCIATED OUTCOMES: CONT'D

Newborn Adaptation

Preterm Infant Organization

Respiratory Status

Symptom Severity: Perimenopause

Thought Processes, Disturbed

DEFINITION: Disruption in cognitive operations and activities

SUGGESTED OUTCOMES:

Cognition

Cognitive Orientation

Concentration

Decision-Making

Distorted Thought Self-Control

Identity

Information Processing

Memory

Neurological Status: Consciousness

ADDITIONAL ASSOCIATED OUTCOMES:

Acute Confusion Level

Agitation Level

Blood Glucose Level

Blood Loss Severity

Communication

Communication: Expressive

Communication: Receptive

Electrolyte & Acid/Base Balance

Fall Prevention Behavior

Fluid Balance

Hydration

Medication Response

Personal Safety Behavior

Respiratory Status: Gas Exchange

Risk Control: Alcohol Use

Risk Control: Drug Use

Safe Home Environment

Substance Withdrawal Severity

Tissue Integrity, Impaired

DEFINITION: Damage to mucous membrane, corneal, integumentary, or subcutaneous tissues

SUGGESTED OUTCOMES:

Allergic Response: Localized

Burn Healing

Tissue Integrity: Skin & Mucous Membranes

Wound Healing: Primary Intention

Wound Healing: Secondary Intention

ADDITIONAL ASSOCIATED OUTCOMES:

Burn Recovery

Fluid Overload Severity

Hydration

Immobility Consequences: Physiological

Infection Severity

Infection Severity: Newborn

Knowledge: Infection Management

Knowledge: Treatment Regimen

Nutritional Status

Ostomy Self-Care

Risk Control: Infectious Process

Self-Care: Hygiene

Sensory Function: Cutaneous

Thermoregulation

Thermoregulation: Newborn

Tissue Perfusion: Peripheral

Tissue Perfusion: Cardiopulmonary, Ineffective

DEFINITION: Decrease in oxygen resulting in the failure to nourish the tissues at the capillary level

SUGGESTED OUTCOMES:

Cardiac Pump Effectiveness
Circulation Status
Respiratory Status: Gas Exchange
Tissue Perfusion: Cardiac

Tissue Perfusion: Cellular
Tissue Perfusion: Pulmonary
Vital Signs

ADDITIONAL ASSOCIATED OUTCOMES:

Blood Coagulation
Blood Loss Severity
Burn Recovery
Cardiopulmonary Status
Electrolyte & Acid/Base Balance

Fluid Balance
Pain Level
Respiratory Status
Tissue Perfusion: Peripheral

Tissue Perfusion: Cerebral, Ineffective

DEFINITION: Decrease in oxygen resulting in the failure to nourish the tissues at the capillary level

SUGGESTED OUTCOMES:

Acute Confusion Level
Agitation Level
Cognition
Neurological Status
Neurological Status: Central Motor Control

Neurological Status: Consciousness
Seizure Control
Tissue Perfusion: Cellular
Tissue Perfusion: Cerebral

ADDITIONAL ASSOCIATED OUTCOMES:

Blood Coagulation
Circulation Status
Cognitive Orientation
Communication
Communication: Expressive
Communication: Receptive
Concentration

Coordinated Movement
Information Processing
Memory
Risk Control: Hyperthermia
Risk Control: Hypothermia
Swallowing Status
Tissue Perfusion: Peripheral

Tissue Perfusion: Gastrointestinal, Ineffective

DEFINITION: Decrease in oxygen resulting in the failure to nourish the tissues at the capillary level

SUGGESTED OUTCOMES:
Gastrointestinal Function
Tissue Perfusion: Abdominal Organs
Tissue Perfusion: Cellular

ADDITIONAL ASSOCIATED OUTCOMES:

Appetite	Hydration
Blood Coagulation	Nausea & Vomiting Severity
Blood Loss Severity	Nutritional Status
Bowel Elimination	Nutritional Status: Biochemical Measures
Cardiopulmonary Status	Nutritional Status: Energy
Circulation Status	Nutritional Status: Food & Fluid Intake
Electrolyte & Acid/Base Balance	Pain Level
Fluid Balance	Respiratory Status

Tissue Perfusion: Peripheral, Ineffective

DEFINITION: Decrease in oxygen resulting in the failure to nourish the tissues at the capillary level

SUGGESTED OUTCOMES:

Circulation Status	Tissue Perfusion: Cellular
Tissue Integrity: Skin & Mucous Membranes	Tissue Perfusion: Peripheral

ADDITIONAL ASSOCIATED OUTCOMES:

Blood Coagulation	Risk Control: Hypothermia
Cardiopulmonary Status	Sensory Function
Electrolyte & Acid/Base Balance	Vital Signs
Fluid Balance	Wound Healing: Primary Intention
Fluid Overload Severity	Wound Healing: Secondary Intention
Respiratory Status	

Tissue Perfusion: Renal, Ineffective

DEFINITION: Decrease in oxygen resulting in the failure to nourish the tissues at the capillary level

SUGGESTED OUTCOMES:

Circulation Status	Kidney Function
Electrolyte & Acid/Base Balance	Tissue Perfusion: Abdominal Organs
Fluid Balance	Tissue Perfusion: Cellular
Fluid Overload Severity	

ADDITIONAL ASSOCIATED OUTCOMES:

Blood Coagulation

Blood Transfusion Reaction

Cardiac Pump Effectiveness

Cardiopulmonary Status

Hydration

Respiratory Status

Urinary Elimination

Vital Signs

Transfer Ability, Impaired

DEFINITION: Limitation of independent movement between two nearby surfaces

SUGGESTED OUTCOMES:

Body Mechanics Performance

Body Positioning: Self-Initiated

Coordinated Movement

Mobility

Transfer Performance

ADDITIONAL ASSOCIATED OUTCOMES:

Ambulation

Ambulation: Wheelchair

Balance

Cognition

Discomfort Level

Endurance

Fatigue Level

Immobility Consequences: Physiological

Immobility Consequences: Psycho-Cognitive

Joint Movement: Hip

Joint Movement: Knee

Joint Movement: Shoulder

Joint Movement: Spine

Knowledge: Body Mechanics

Knowledge: Fall Prevention

Neurological Status

Pain Level

Self-Care: Bathing

Self-Care: Toileting

Skeletal Function

Vision Compensation Behavior

Trauma, Risk for

DEFINITION: Accentuated risk of accidental tissue injury (e.g., wound, burn, fracture)

SUGGESTED OUTCOMES:

Abuse Protection

Acute Confusion Level

Agitation Level

Balance

Community Risk Control: Violence

Community Violence Level

Coordinated Movement

Elopement Propensity Risk

Fall Prevention Behavior

Falls Occurrence

Knowledge: Child Physical Safety

Knowledge: Fall Prevention

Knowledge: Personal Safety

Parenting: Adolescent Physical Safety

Parenting: Early/Middle Childhood Physical
    Safety

Parenting: Infant/Toddler Physical Safety

Personal Safety Behavior

Physical Injury Severity

Risk Control

Risk Control: Alcohol Use

Risk Control: Drug Use

Risk Control: Sun Exposure

Risk Detection

Safe Home Environment

Safe Wandering

Substance Withdrawal Severity

Tissue Integrity: Skin & Mucous Membranes

Vision Compliance Behavior

Unilateral Neglect

DEFINITION: Impairment in sensory and motor response, mental representation, and spatial attention of the body and the corresponding environment characterized by inattention to one side and over attention to the opposite side. Left side neglect is more severe and persistent than right side neglect.

SUGGESTED OUTCOMES:

Adaptation to Physical Disability
Body Positioning: Self-Initiated

Coordinated Movement
Heedfulness of Affected Side

ADDITIONAL ASSOCIATED OUTCOMES:

Balance
Body Image
Body Mechanics Performance
Client Satisfaction: Functional Assistance
Client Satisfaction: Safety
Joint Movement: Passive
Knowledge: Fall Prevention
Neurological Status

Neurological Status: Peripheral
Personal Safety Behavior
Safe Home Environment
Self-Care: Activities of Daily Living (ADL)
Self-Care: Instrumental Activities of Daily
  Living (IADL)
Transfer Performance

Urinary Elimination, Impaired

DEFINITION: Dysfunction in urine elimination

SUGGESTED OUTCOMES:

Urinary Continence
Urinary Elimination

ADDITIONAL ASSOCIATED OUTCOMES:

Infection Severity
Kidney Function
Neurological Status: Spinal Sensory/Motor
  Function

Risk Control: Infectious Process
Self-Care: Toileting
Symptom Control
Symptom Severity

Urinary Elimination, Readiness for Enhanced

DEFINITION: A pattern of urinary functions that is sufficient for meeting eliminatory needs and can be strengthened

SUGGESTED OUTCOMES:

Motivation
Self-Care: Toileting

Urinary Continence
Urinary Elimination

ADDITIONAL ASSOCIATED OUTCOMES:

Compliance Behavior: Prescribed Medication
Health-Seeking Behavior
Hydration
Infection Severity
Kidney Function
Knowledge: Disease Process
Knowledge: Infection Management

Knowledge: Medication
Neurological Status
Nutritional Status: Food & Fluid Intake
Risk Control: Infectious Process
Symptom Control
Symptom Severity

Urinary Incontinence: Functional

DEFINITION: Inability of usually continent person to reach toilet in time to avoid unintentional loss of urine

SUGGESTED OUTCOMES:

Self-Care: Toileting
Symptom Severity

Urinary Continence
Urinary Elimination

ADDITIONAL ASSOCIATED OUTCOMES:

Acute Confusion Level
Agitation Level
Ambulation
Ambulation: Wheelchair
Cognition
Coordinated Movement
Medication Response

Mobility
Neurological Status: Spinal Sensory/Motor
 Function
Stress Level
Symptom Control
Transfer Performance
Vision Compensation Behavior

Urinary Incontinence: Overflow

DEFINITION: Involuntary loss of urine associated with overdistention of the bladder

SUGGESTED OUTCOMES:

Self-Care: Toileting
Symptom Severity

Urinary Continence
Urinary Elimination

ADDITIONAL ASSOCIATED OUTCOMES:

Knowledge: Disease Process
Knowledge: Medication

Medication Response
Tissue Integrity: Skin & Mucous Membranes

Urinary Incontinence: Reflex

DEFINITION: Involuntary loss of urine at somewhat predictable intervals when a specific bladder volume is reached

SUGGESTED OUTCOMES:

Neurological Status: Spinal Sensory/
   Motor Function
Symptom Severity

Urinary Continence
Urinary Elimination

ADDITIONAL ASSOCIATED OUTCOMES:

Caregiver Performance: Direct Care
Knowledge: Disease Process
Knowledge: Treatment Regimen
Neurological Status
Nutritional Status: Food & Fluid Intake

Self-Care: Hygiene
Self-Care: Toileting
Symptom Control
Tissue Integrity: Skin & Mucous Membranes
Treatment Behavior: Illness or Injury

Urinary Incontinence: Stress

DEFINITION: Sudden leakage of urine with activities that increase intra-abdominal pressure

SUGGESTED OUTCOMES:

Symptom Severity
Urinary Continence
Urinary Elimination

ADDITIONAL ASSOCIATED OUTCOMES:

Client Satisfaction: Symptom Control
Knowledge: Treatment Procedure
Knowledge: Treatment Regimen
Physical Aging
Self-Care: Hygiene

Self-Care: Toileting
Self-Esteem
Symptom Control
Tissue Integrity: Skin & Mucous Membranes

Urinary Incontinence: Total

DEFINITION: Continuous and unpredictable loss of urine

SUGGESTED OUTCOMES:

Symptom Severity
Tissue Integrity: Skin & Mucous Membranes

Urinary Continence
Urinary Elimination

ADDITIONAL ASSOCIATED OUTCOMES:

Acute Confusion Level
Adaptation to Physical Disability
Agitation Level

Client Satisfaction: Symptom Control
Cognition
Infection Severity

ADDITIONAL ASSOCIATED OUTCOMES: CONT'D

Knowledge: Treatment Procedure

Neurological Status: Spinal Sensory / Motor
   Function

Self-Care: Hygiene

Self-Care: Toileting

Self-Esteem

Symptom Control

Urinary Incontinence: Urge

DEFINITION: Involuntary passage of urine occurring soon after a strong sense of urgency to void

SUGGESTED OUTCOMES:

Self-Care: Toileting

Symptom Severity

Urinary Continence

Urinary Elimination

ADDITIONAL ASSOCIATED OUTCOMES:

Infection Severity

Knowledge: Disease Process

Knowledge: Treatment Regimen

Mobility

Nutritional Status: Food & Fluid Intake

Risk Control: Infectious Process

Self-Care: Hygiene

Self-Esteem

Symptom Control

Tissue Integrity: Skin & Mucous Membranes

Urinary Incontinence: Urge, Risk for

DEFINITION: At risk for involuntary loss of urine associated with a sudden, strong sensation or urinary urgency

SUGGESTED OUTCOMES:

Infection Severity

Knowledge: Medication

Knowledge: Treatment Regimen

Medication Response

Neurological Status: Spinal Sensory /
   Motor Function

Risk Control

Risk Control: Infectious Process

Risk Detection

Self-Care: Toileting

Stress Level

Urinary Continence

Urinary Elimination

Urinary Retention

DEFINITION: Incomplete emptying of the bladder

SUGGESTED OUTCOMES:

Symptom Severity

Urinary Elimination

ADDITIONAL ASSOCIATED OUTCOMES:

Knowledge: Disease Process
Knowledge: Medication
Knowledge: Treatment Regimen
Medication Response

Neurological Status: Spinal Sensory/
    Motor Function
Symptom Control

Ventilation, Impaired Spontaneous

DEFINITION: Decreased energy reserves result in an individual's inability to maintain breathing adequate to support life

SUGGESTED OUTCOMES:

Mechanical Ventilation Response: Adult
Respiratory Status: Gas Exchange

Respiratory Status: Ventilation
Vital Signs

ADDITIONAL ASSOCIATED OUTCOMES:

Allergic Response: Systemic
Anxiety Level
Anxiety Self-Control
Cardiopulmonary Status
Electrolyte & Acid/Base Balance
Endurance
Energy Conservation

Mechanical Ventilation Weaning Response:
    Adult
Neurological Status: Central Motor Control
Neurological Status: Consciousness
Post-Procedure Recovery
Respiratory Status

Ventilatory Weaning Response, Dysfunctional

DEFINITION: Inability to adjust to lowered levels of mechanical ventilator support that interrupts and prolongs the weaning process

SUGGESTED OUTCOMES:

Anxiety Self-Control
Mechanical Ventilation Weaning Response:
    Adult

Respiratory Status: Gas Exchange
Respiratory Status: Ventilation
Vital Signs

ADDITIONAL ASSOCIATED OUTCOMES:

Anxiety Level
Cardiopulmonary Status
Client Satisfaction: Technical
    Aspects of Care
Cognition
Electrolyte & Acid/Base Balance
Knowledge: Treatment Procedure

Mechanical Ventilation Response: Adult
Neurological Status: Consciousness
Pain Control
Post-Procedure Recovery Status
Respiratory Status
Sleep
Symptom Severity

Violence: Other-Directed, Risk for

DEFINITION: At risk for behaviors in which an individual demonstrates that he/she can be physically, emotionally, and/or sexually harmful to others

SUGGESTED OUTCOMES:

Abuse Cessation
Abuse Protection
Abusive Behavior Self-Restraint
Acute Confusion Level
Aggression Self-Control
Agitation Level
Cognition
Community Risk Control: Violence
Community Violence Level
Depression Self-Control

Distorted Thought Self-Control
Fear Level
Fear Level: Child
Hyperactivity Level
Impulse Self-Control
Risk Control
Risk Control: Alcohol Use
Risk Control: Drug Use
Risk Detection
Stress Level

Violence: Self-Directed, Risk for

DEFINITION: At risk for behaviors in which an individual demonstrates that he/she can be physically, emotionally, and/or sexually harmful to self

SUGGESTED OUTCOMES:

Acute Confusion Level
Adaptation to Physical Disability
Agitation Level
Cognition
Coping
Depression Level
Depression Self-Control
Distorted Thought Self-Control
Impulse Self-Control
Loneliness Severity

Mood Equilibrium
Quality of Life
Risk Control
Risk Control: Alcohol Use
Risk Control: Drug Use
Risk Detection
Self-Mutilation Restraint
Stress Level
Suicide Self-Restraint
Will to Live

Walking, Impaired

DEFINITION: Limitation of independent movement within the environment on foot

SUGGESTED OUTCOMES:

Ambulation
Balance
Coordinated Movement

Endurance
Mobility

ADDITIONAL ASSOCIATED OUTCOMES:

Body Mechanics Performance
Cardiopulmonary Status

Client Satisfaction: Functional Assistance
Client Satisfaction: Safety

ADDITIONAL ASSOCIATED OUTCOMES: CONT'D

Discomfort Level

Fall Prevention Behavior

Falls Occurrence

Hearing Compensation Behavior

Joint Movement

Joint Movement: Ankle

Joint Movement: Hip

Joint Movement: Knee

Joint Movement: Spine

Knowledge: Body Mechanics

Knowledge: Fall Prevention

Neurological Status: Central Motor Control

Pain Level

Physical Injury Severity

Respiratory Status

Safe Home Environment

Self-Care: Activities of Daily Living (ADL)

Skeletal Function

Vision Compliance Behavior

Wandering

DEFINITION: Meandering, aimless and/or repetitive locomotion that exposes the individual to harm; frequently incongruent with boundaries, limits, or obstacles

SUGGESTED OUTCOMES:

Elopement Propensity Risk

Safe Wandering

ADDITIONAL ASSOCIATED OUTCOMES:

Acute Confusion Level

Agitation Level

Anxiety Level

Cognition

Communication: Expressive

Depression Level

Elopement Occurrence

Fall Prevention Behavior

Hyperactivity Level

Memory

Rest

Safe Home Environment

Sleep

Linkages Between the Nursing Outcomes Classification and the International Classification of Functioning, Disability, and Health

The development of the standardized classification to measure consequences of care has gained more attention and parallels the emphasis on increasing the efficiency and effectiveness in health care. It has been suggested that the Nursing Outcomes Classification (NOC) and the International Classification of Functioning, Disability, and Health (ICF), as critical references for evaluating health care outcomes, be used to describe the results achieved within nursing care.[3] NOC is developed mainly to embrace the concepts and boundaries of nursing, while the ICF has been created for use in interdisciplinary care. Considering the growing demand for the development and refinement of classification systems that provide interdisciplinary as well as discipline-specific data, it is valuable to review both classifications. This section of the chapter presents results of the linkage between the ICF and NOC as a means to enable colleagues to become more knowledgeable of both classifications and to facilitate a distinctive view of nursing.

BACKGROUND

To assist nurses in describing nursing, standardized nursing languages such as NOC, the Nursing Interventions Classification (NIC), NANDA-International, and the International Classifications of Nursing Practice (ICNP), have been developed. These nursing languages have been recognized for their capacity to reflect nursing practice and are being used worldwide. However, the argument has been forwarded that nursing language initiatives contribute to the isolation of nurses from other health care professionals. Van Achterberg and colleagues[8] also contend that the nursing languages are not designed to facilitate the communication of patient data among disciplines, and this hinders the exchange of information in both patient care and knowledge development arenas. Therefore it has been suggested that exploring the use of an interdisciplinary classification, such as ICF, might facilitate the communication across all disciplines.

Rationales provided by other authors support exploring the use of ICF within nursing. Hassouneh-Phillips and Curry[2] suggest that when articulating the vision of nursing care for people with or without disabilities, it is necessary to reinforce an interdisciplinary practice to promote the health of people. Since ICF is in international use across disciplines, it can be expected that the use of ICF in nursing will strengthen this vision.[4]

Over the past number of years, papers have been written about the relevance of ICF to nursing. Authors note a variety of uses for ICF: as a predictor of the intensity of nursing care,[7] as a tool to classify nursing diagnoses,[9] as an assessment for nursing home resident-centered interventions,[1] as a tool for teaching undergraduate nursing students of patient assessments,[6] and as a means for nursing documentation systems (e.g., nursing assessment, diagnoses, nursing care plans, critical pathways, etc).[8] In an attempt to be responsive to the concern of standardized languages isolating nurses from other health professionals, but yet acknowledge the important contribution the ICF could make to nursing, this work evolved. It was suggested that linkage between the ICF and NOC may serve to facilitate use of both languages within an interdisciplinary system.

The linkage process may assist us to identify missing concepts in both classifications, to evaluate NOC from a different perspective, to view health care from the perspective of functioning and rehabilitation, and to detect core nursing concepts for measuring individual functions in daily life by identifying common terms across the two classifications. In addition, this exploration of the inner side of ICF will contribute to the identification of relevant concepts to promote language development in nursing.

The International Classification of Functioning, Disability, and Health (ICF)

Because our readers are very knowledgeable of NOC, the next section presents a brief overview of the ICF. ICF is "a multipurpose classification designed to provide a scientific basis for understanding and studying health and health-related states, outcomes, and determinants . . . and to establish a common language for describing health and health-related states in order to improve communication between different users (p. 5)."[10] The ICF is divided into two component parts: Part 1 covers Functioning and Disability with (a) Body Functions and Structures and (b) Activities and Participation; Part 2 deals with Contextual Factors with (a) Environmental Factors and (b) Personal Factors (currently not classified in the ICF). It is the contention of the developers that this structure allows practitioners to assess individuals comprehensively by addressing the interaction between the health condition and contextual factors.[10]

In addition to the component parts, ICF is organized into four levels with an alphanumeric coding system. First, the prefixes b, s, d, and e are used to denote each of the major components. For example, the b is for Body Functions, the s is for Body Structures, the d is for Activities and Participation, and the e is for Environmental Factors. These prefixes are followed by numeric codes that start with chapter number (one digit), followed by second level (two digits), and third and fourth levels (one digit each).[10] A specific example of this alphanumeric coding system would be "Chapter 1 Mental Functions" having a "b1" code at the first level of Body Functions; "b160 Thought Functions (b160)" represents a second-level item under "Mental Functions" while "b1603" represents a third-level item under Control of Thought. An example of the specific hierarchical structure of ICF is presented in Table 4-1.

In addition to this alphanumeric system, each coded item has a definition, inclusions, and exclusions to assist in the selection of the appropriate code. At the end of each embedded set of third- or fourth-level items, there are items coded as "other specified" and "unspecified" in order.

The Linkage Process and Operating Principles

The purpose of linking is to create relationships between terms, make suggestions for additional outcomes, and elucidate issues relevant to the process. In order to achieve this purpose, the authors reviewed the structures and definitions of the respective classifications. With careful attention to definitions across NOC and ICF, the consistency of terms between the outcome definitions at the third level of NOC and the ICF items at the third level was noted. In addition, the inclusion and exclusion statements of the ICF format were taken into account and attempts were made to include as many age groups and populations as possible. Other operating principles were as follows: (1) link the NOC

Table 4-1   COMPARISON OF CODING SYSTEM ACROSS CLASSIFICATIONS OF NOC AND ICF

NOC	Domains (I-VII)	Classes (A-Z) or (a-z)	Outcomes (4 digits)		Indicators (01-99)
Example	Psychosocial Health (III)	Self-Control (O) (IIIO)	Distorted Thought Self-Control (1403) (III 01403)		
ICF	Components (b, s, d, e)	Chapters (1 digit)	Items (2 digits)	Sub-items (1 digit)	
Example	Body Functions (b)	Chapter 1 Mental Functions (b1)	Thought Functions (b160)	Control of Thought (b1603)	

Table 4-2 EXAMPLE OF NOC LINKED TO THE ICF (IN BODY FUNCTIONS)

	ICF	NOC	
Level 1 Chapter	Chapter 1 Mental Functions	Physiological Health (II) Psychosocial Health (III) Energy Maintenance (A) Self Control (O)	**Level 1** Domain **Level 2** Class
Level 2 Item	b160 Thought Functions	Distorted Thought Self-Control (1403) Information Processing (0907)	**Level 3** Outcome
Level 3	b1600 Pace of Thought	Hyperactivity Level (0915) Psychomotor Energy (0006)	
	b1601 Form of Thought b1602 Content of Thought b1603 Control of thought	Abusive Behavior Self-Restraint (1400) Anxiety Self-Control (1402) Depression Self-Control (1409) Impulse Self-Control (1405) Suicide Self-Restraint (1408)	
	b1608 Thought functions, other specified b1609 Thought functions, unspecified		

outcome label to Level 2 of the ICF if the NOC label was repeated numerous times at the levels 3 and 4 of ICF; and (2) link the NOC outcome label if the NOC indicator(s) mirror(s) the word phases of the ICF item(s) at Level 3.[10]

Results

As illustrated in Table 4-2, the 7 domains and 31 classes of NOC were linked to Level 1 in the ICF, while the individual NOC outcomes were linked to Level 2 and 3 of the ICF. Generally, it appears that NOC outcomes linked mostly to ICF at Level 2 are more comprehensive than outcomes mapped to ICF at Level 3. For example, see the Distorted Thought Self-Control item in Table 4-2. The outcomes Distorted Thought Self-Control and Information Processing at Level 3 in NOC are linked not only to Thought Functions (b160) at Level 2 of ICF but also to all of specific functions items of Level 3 in the ICF (b1600-b1609). In the example of Pace of Thought (b1600), it was linked not only with NOC outcomes listed at the upper level but also with specific NOC outcomes: Hyperactivity Level (0915) and Psychomotor Energy (0006).

All classes of the NOC domains were linked to ICF. Of 330 NOC individual outcomes, 326 outcomes were linked to items of ICF (Table 4-3). All of the NOC outcomes were linked under Domain III (Psychosocial Health), Domain IV (Health Knowledge & Behavior), Domain V (Perceived Health), Domain VI (Family Health), and Domain VII (Community Health) (see Table 4-3).

An additional review noted that among all of the NOC outcomes linked to ICF, Child Development: 5 years, Neurological Status: Cranial Sensory/Motor Function, Self-Care: Instrumental Activities of Daily Living (IADL), and Social Involvement were most frequently linked, while four NOC outcomes were not linked at all. Domain I, Functional Health, had two outcomes of the class Growth & Development that could not be linked to any items of ICF: Fetal Status: Antepartum (0111) and Fetal Status: Intrapartum (0112). Under Domain II, Physiological Health, Bone Healing (1104) and Oral Hygiene (1100) could not be mapped to ICF.

While all but four outcome labels were able to be linked to ICF, some ICF items could not be linked to NOC. For example, the majority of items that could not be linked fell into the "Environmental Factors" section of the classification. One specific example is "Labor and Employment Services,

Table 4-3 NOC Outcomes Linked to ICF

Domains	Classes	Mapped/Total
Functional Health(I)	Energy Maintenance Growth & Development Mobility Self-Care	58/60
Physiologic Health(II)	Cardiopulmonary Elimination Fluid & Electrolyte Immune Response Metabolic Regulation Neurocognitive Nutrition Therapeutic Response Tissue Integrity Sensory Function	78/80
Psychosocial Health(III)	Psychological Well-Being Psychosocial Adaptation Self-Control Social Interaction	36/36
Health Knowledge & Behavior(IV)	Health Behavior Health Beliefs Health Knowledge Risk Control & Safety	76/76
Perceived Health(V)	Health & Life Quality Symptom Status Satisfaction with Care	31/31
Family Health(VI)	Family Caregiver Performance Family Member Health Status Family Well-Being Parenting	38/38
Community Health(VII)	Community Well-Being Community Health Protection	9/9
Total		326/330

Systems, and Policies (e590)," which is defined as services, systems, and policies related to finding suitable work for persons who are unemployed or looking for different work, or to support individuals already employed who are seeking promotion. In this particular instance, the reviewers believed these items were not within the realm of nursing.

Linking concepts is a valuable exercise to see the reflection of nursing practice in the ICF and vice versa. We were able to identify not only which areas were absent from both classifications, but also which concepts the classifications had in common. For classification in nursing to be complete, these types of comparisons are a critical step in the development of the language needed to capture the contributions of nursing.

References

1. Brush, J. A., Threats, T. T., & Calkins, M. P. (2003). Influences on perceived function of a nursing home resident. *Journal of Communication Disorders, 36*, 379-393.
2. Hassouneh-Phillips, D., & Curry, M. A. (2001). Re-thinking care for persons with disabilities: A vision for nursing. Paper presented at Global Conference on Rethinking Care. Retrieved from http://www.rethinkingcare.org
3. Heerkens, Y., van der Brug, Y., Napel, H. T., & van Ravensberg, D. (2003). Past and future use of the ICF (former ICIDH) by nursing and allied health professionals. *Disability and Rehabilitation, 25*(11-12), 620-627.
4. Kearney, P. M., & Pryor, J. (2004). The International Classification of Functioning, Disability and Health (ICF) and nursing. *Journal of Advanced Nursing, 46*(2), 162-170.
5. Moorhead, S., Johnson, M., & Maas, M. (Eds.). (2004). *Nursing Outcomes Classification (NOC)* (3rd ed.). St. Louis: Mosby.
6. Pryor, J., Forbes, R., & Hall-Pullin, L. (2004). Is there evidence of the International Classification of Functioning, Disability and Health in undergraduate nursing students' patient assessment? *Internal Journal of Nursing Practice, 10*, 134-141.
7. Tilquin, C., Michelon, P., D'hoore, W., Sicotte, C., Carillo, E., & Leonard, G. (1995). Using the handicap code of the ICIDH for classifying patients by intensity of nursing care requirements. *Disability and Rehabilitation, 17*, 176-183.
8. Van Achterberg, T., Holleman, G., Heijnen-Kaales, Y., van der Brug, Y., Roodbol, G., Stallinga, H. A., Hellema, F., & Frederiks, C. (2005). Using a multidisciplinary classification in nursing: the International Classification of Functioning, Disability and Health. *Journal of Advanced Nursing, 49*(4), 432-441.
9. Van Achterberg, T., Frederiks, C., Thien, N., Coenen, C., & Persoon, A. (2002). Using ICIDH-2 in the classification of nursing diagnoses: results from two pilot studies. *Journal of Advanced Nursing, 37*, 135-144.
10. World Health Organization. (2001). *International Classification of Functioning, Disability and Health.* (p. 5). Geneva: Author.

PART FIVE

Core Outcomes for Nursing Specialty Areas

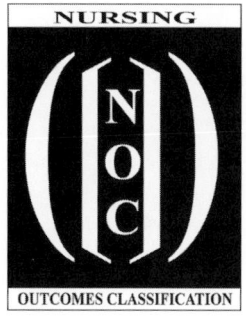

IDENTIFYING CORE OUTCOMES

Core outcomes were identified by 33 nursing organizations representing areas of nursing specialization and nurses representing eight areas of specialty practice in the third edition of NOC. Information to identify those core outcomes was collected from the organizations and specialty nurses through surveys sent in 1999 and 2000. Only 2nd edition NOC outcomes were used in the survey. Outcomes new to the third edition were not included in the survey since they were not part of the survey research. Since the surveys were sent, 76 new outcomes were added to the third edition and 58 new outcomes are added to this edition.

The survey methodology and results are discussed in the previous edition.[1] We have defined core outcomes as a concise set of outcomes that captures the essence of specialty practice by identifying the outcomes selected most frequently but is not comprehensive enough to include all outcomes used by nurses in that specialty. These outcomes provide a means to measure the effectiveness of practice and are one of the elements that direct the interventions nurses use in the specialty. The organizations and specialty nurses who responded to the survey included the following:

Specialty Organizations Responding to Survey

American Academy of Ambulatory Care Nursing
American Association of Nurse Anesthetists
National Consortium of Chemical Dependency Nurses
Association of Community Health Nursing Educators
American Association of Critical-Care Nurses
Dermatology Nurses Association
Emergency Nurses Association
Society of Gastroenterology Nurses and Associates, Inc.
International Society of Nurses in Genetics
Home Healthcare Nurses Association
Hospice and Palliative Nurses Association
Intravenous Nursing Society
National Association of Neonatal Nurses
American Nephrology Nurses Association
American Association of Neuroscience Nurses
Association of Operating Room Nurses, Inc.
American Society of Ophthalmic Registered Nurses, Inc.
National Association of Orthopaedic Nurses
Society of Otorhinolaryngology and Head-Neck Nurses, Inc.
American Society of Pain Management Nurses
Society of Pediatric Nurses
Association of Pediatric Oncology Nurses
American Society of PeriAnesthesia Nurses
Association of PeriOperative Registered Nurses
American College of Nurse Practitioners
Society for Education and Research in Psychiatric-Mental Health Nursing
American Radiological Nurses Association
Association of Rehabilitation Nurses
American Association of Spinal Cord Injury Nurses
Air and Surface Transport Nurses Association
Society of Urologic Nurses and Associates, Inc.
Society for Vascular Nursing
Association of Women's Health, Obstetric and Neonatal Nurses

Specialty Areas of Individual Nurses Responding to Survey
ANCC Cardiac Rehabilitation
ANCC Community Health
ANCC Gerontological
ANCC Home Health
ANCC Medical-Surgical
ANCC Pediatric
ANCC Psychiatric/Mental Health
ANCC School Nurse

The authors intend to interact with nursing organizations representing nurses in specialty practices to refine the core outcomes and include the 134 new outcomes since the survey was completed. More work is needed on outcome identification and development for specialty practice in the future to improve education and quality of patient care delivered by nurses. We need to debate and analyze the question: What is a reasonable number of core outcomes for each specialty to address? We need to identify methods to keep this work on core outcomes for specialty practice current and find ways to involve specialty organizations in the evolution and continued development of NOC outcomes. Efforts in this direction will allow for continued improvement in the nursing effectiveness efforts involving standardized languages and identify new outcomes for development.

In the meantime, we have revised the areas of core outcomes to represent major areas of nursing practice and have added the new outcomes to those areas of practice. Several new specialties were added, and content overlap between the two types of surveys are combined. The previously identified core outcomes were used as a basis for the identification of the core outcomes identified for each area of specialization. We elected to present the core outcomes in this way because we did not want to add outcomes to the ones previously identified by specialty organizations without their input. We appreciate any reaction, whether positive or negative, to the method we have chosen for this edition.

1. Moorhead, S., Johnson, M., & Maas, M. (Eds.). (2004). *Nursing Outcomes Classification (NOC)*. St. Louis: Mosby.

Air and Surface Transport

Acute Confusion Level
Agitation Level
Allergic Response: Systemic
Asthma Self-Management
Blood Coagulation
Blood Loss Severity
Blood Transfusion Reaction
Cardiopulmonary Status
Circulation Status
Client Satisfaction: Caring
Client Satisfaction: Pain Management
Client Satisfaction: Psychological Care
Client Satisfaction: Technical Aspects of Care
Cognition
Cognitive Orientation
Comfort Status
Communication
Concentration
Coping

Decision-Making
Electrolyte & Acid/Base Balance
Fluid Balance
Fluid Overload Severity
Hope
Hydration
Immune Hypersensitivity Response
Immune Status
Infection Severity: Newborn
Infection Severity
Information Processing
Kidney Function
Mechanical Ventilation Response: Adult
Medication Response
Memory
Nausea & Vomiting Severity
Neurological Status
Neurological Status: Autonomic
Neurological Status: Central Motor Control

Air and Surface Transport—cont'd

Neurological Status: Cranial Sensory/Motor Function
Neurological Status: Peripheral
Neurological Status: Spinal Sensory/Motor Function
Pain Level
Pain: Adverse Psychological Response
Physical Injury Severity
Respiratory Status
Respiratory Status: Airway Patency
Respiratory Status: Gas Exchange
Respiratory Status: Ventilation

Seizure Control
Symptom Severity
Thermoregulation
Thermoregulation: Newborn
Tissue Perfusion: Abdominal Organs
Tissue Perfusion: Cardiac
Tissue Perfusion: Cellular
Tissue Perfusion: Cerebral
Tissue Perfusion: Peripheral
Tissue Perfusion: Pulmonary
Vital Signs
Will to Live

Ambulatory Care

Acceptance: Health Status
Adherence Behavior
Adherence Behavior: Healthy Diet
Client Satisfaction: Case Management
Cognition
Compliance Behavior
Compliance Behavior: Prescribed Diet
Compliance Behavior: Prescribed Medication
Development: Late Adulthood
Development: Middle Adulthood
Development: Young Adulthood
Fatigue Level
Health Beliefs: Perceived Resources
Health Beliefs: Perceived Threat
Health Orientation
Health Promoting Behavior
Health Seeking Behavior
Knowledge: Health Behavior

Knowledge: Health Promotion
Knowledge: Health Resources
Knowledge: Treatment Procedure
Knowledge: Treatment Regimen
Medication Response
Motivation
Nutritional Status
Personal Health Status
Physical Aging
Post-Procedure Recovery
Pre-Procedure Readiness
Self-Care Status
Self-Care: Activities of Daily Living (ADL)
Self-Care: Instrumental Activities of Daily Living (IADL)
Vital Signs
Weight Maintenance Behavior
Weight: Body Mass

Anesthesia

Acute Confusion Level
Allergic Response: Systemic
Anxiety Level
Blood Coagulation
Blood Loss Severity
Blood Transfusion Reaction
Body Positioning: Self-Initiated
Cardiac Pump Effectiveness
Cardiopulmonary Status
Circulation Status
Client Satisfaction: Communication

Client Satisfaction: Protection of Rights
Client Satisfaction: Safety
Client Satisfaction: Technical Aspects of Care
Cognition
Cognitive Orientation
Comfort Status
Communication
Concentration
Decision-Making
Electrolyte & Acid/Base Balance
Fear Level

Continued

Anesthesia—cont'd

Fear Level: Child
Fetal Status: Antepartum
Fetal Status: Intrapartum
Fluid Balance
Fluid Overload Severity
Hydration
Immune Hypersensitivity Response
Information Processing
Knowledge: Treatment Procedure
Mechanical Ventilation Response: Adult
Medication Response
Memory
Nausea & Vomiting Severity
Neurological Status
Neurological Status: Autonomic
Neurological Status: Central Motor Control
Neurological Status: Consciousness
Neurological Status: Cranial Sensory/Motor
    Function
Neurological Status: Peripheral
Neurological Status: Spinal Sensory/Motor
    Function

Pain Level
Pain: Adverse Psychological Response
Participation in Health Care Decisions
Post-Procedure Recovery
Pre-Procedure Readiness
Respiratory Status
Respiratory Status: Airway Patency
Respiratory Status: Gas Exchange
Respiratory Status: Ventilation
Suffering Severity
Symptom Severity
Thermoregulation
Thermoregulation: Newborn
Tissue Integrity: Skin and Mucous
    Membranes
Tissue Perfusion: Abdominal Organs
Tissue Perfusion: Cardiac
Tissue Perfusion: Cellular
Tissue Perfusion: Cerebral
Tissue Perfusion: Peripheral
Tissue Perfusion: Pulmonary
Vital Signs

Cardiac Rehabilitation

Acceptance: Health Status
Adaptation to Physical Disability
Adherence Behavior
Ambulation
Balance
Cardiac Disease Self-Management
Cardiac Pump Effectiveness
Cardiopulmonary Status
Circulation Status
Client Satisfaction: Cultural Needs
    Fulfillment
Client Satisfaction: Pain Management
Client Satisfaction: Psychological Care
Client Satisfaction: Teaching
Compliance Behavior
Compliance Behavior: Prescribed Diet
Compliance Behavior: Prescribed Medication
Coping
Discomfort Level
Endurance
Energy Conservation

Family Support During Treatment
Fatigue Level
Fluid Overload Severity
Health Beliefs
Health Beliefs: Perceived Ability to Perform
Health Beliefs: Perceived Control
Health Beliefs: Perceived Resources
Health Orientation
Health Promoting Behavior
Health Seeking Behavior
Hope
Knowledge: Cardiac Disease Management
Knowledge: Congestive Heart Failure
    Management
Knowledge: Diet
Knowledge: Disease Process
Knowledge: Energy Conservation
Knowledge: Health Behavior
Knowledge: Health Resources
Knowledge: Hypertension Management
Knowledge: Medication

Cardiac Rehabilitation—cont'd

Knowledge: Prescribed Activity
Knowledge: Weight Management
Medication Response Mood Equilibrium
Participation in Health Care Decisions
Personal Health Status
Personal Resiliency
Personal Well-Being
Psychosocial Adjustment: Life Change
Quality of Life
Respiratory Status
Rest

Risk Control: Cardiovascular Health
Self-Care: Activities of Daily Living (ADL)
Self-Care: Instrumental Activities of Daily Living (IADL)
Self-Care: Non-Parenteral Medication
Sleep
Smoking Cessation Behavior
Stress Level
Tissue Perfusion: Cardiac
Vital Signs
Weight Maintenance Behavior

Chemical Dependency

Abuse Protection
Abuse Recovery
Abuse Recovery: Emotional
Abuse Recovery: Financial
Abuse Recovery: Physical
Abuse Recovery: Sexual
Agitation Level
Alcohol Abuse Cessation Behavior
Anxiety Level
Caregiver Emotional Health
Caregiver Lifestyle Disruption
Caregiver Performance: Direct Care
Caregiver Performance: Indirect Care
Caregiver Physical Health
Caregiver Role Endurance
Caregiver Stressors
Caregiver-Patient Relationship
Client Satisfaction: Communication
Client Satisfaction: Continuity of Care
Client Satisfaction: Protection of Rights
Client Satisfaction: Psychological Care
Client Satisfaction: Symptom Control
Comfort Status
Drug Abuse Cessation Behavior
Family Support During Treatment
Health Beliefs: Perceived Threat

Health Orientation
Knowledge: Depression Management
Knowledge: Health Resources
Knowledge: Medication
Knowledge: Personal Safety
Medication Response
Pain Level
Pain: Disruptive Effects
Personal Autonomy
Personal Health Status
Personal Resiliency
Quality of Life
Risk Control: Alcohol Use
Risk Control: Drug Use
Risk Control: Sexually Transmitted Diseases (STD)
Risk Control: Unintended Pregnancy
Seizure Control
Social Support
Spiritual Health
Stress Level
Substance Addiction Consequences
Substance Withdrawal Severity
Suffering Severity
Symptom Severity

Community Health

Alcohol Abuse Cessation Behavior
Ambulation
Comfort Status
Community Competence

Community Disaster Readiness
Community Disaster Response
Community Health Status
Community Health Status: Immunity

Continued

Community Health—cont'd

Community Risk Control: Chronic Disease
Community Risk Control: Communicable
    Disease
Community Risk Control: Lead Exposure
Community Risk Control: Violence
Community Violence Level
Compliance Behavior
Coping
Decision-Making
Drug Abuse Cessation Behavior
Family Coping
Family Functioning
Family Health Status
Family Integrity
Family Normalization
Family Participation in Professional Care
Family Resiliency
Family Social Climate
Family Support During Treatment

Health Beliefs
Health Beliefs: Perceived Ability to Perform
Health Beliefs: Perceived Control
Health Beliefs: Perceived Resources
Health Beliefs: Perceived Threat
Health Orientation
Health Promoting Behavior
Health Seeking Behavior
Immunization Behavior
Knowledge: Health Behavior
Knowledge: Health Promotion
Knowledge: Health Resources
Knowledge: Parenting
Personal Resiliency
Quality of Life
Smoking Cessation Behavior
Spiritual Health
Vital Signs

Critical Care

Acute Confusion Level
Allergic Response: Systemic
Anxiety Level
Blood Coagulation
Blood Loss Severity
Burn Healing
Burn Recovery
Cardiac Pump Effectiveness
Cardiopulmonary Status
Client Satisfaction: Pain Management
Client Satisfaction: Physical Care
Client Satisfaction: Technical Aspects of Care
Cognitive Orientation
Comfort Status
Comfortable Death
Dignified Life Closure
Discomfort Level
Electrolyte & Acid/Base Balance
Family Coping
Family Participation in Professional Care
Family Support During Treatment
Fear Level
Fear Level: Child
Fluid Overload Severity
Immobility Consequences: Physiological

Immobility Consequences: Psycho-Cognitive
Kidney Function
Mechanical Ventilation Response: Adult
Mechanical Ventilation Weaning Response:
    Adult
Medication Response
Nausea & Vomiting Control
Nausea & Vomiting: Disruptive Effects
Nausea & Vomiting Severity
Neurological Status: Autonomic
Neurological Status: Consciousness
Neurological Status: Cranial Sensory/Motor
    Function
Neurological Status: Peripheral
Neurological Status: Spinal Sensory/Motor
    Function
Nutritional Status
Nutritional Status: Biochemical Measures
Pain Control
Pain Level
Pain: Adverse Psychological Response
Pain: Disruptive Effects
Psychosocial Adjustment: Life Change
Respiratory Status
Respiratory Status: Airway Patency

Critical Care—cont'd

Risk Control: Cardiovascular Health
Stress Level
Swallowing Status
Symptom Severity
Tissue Perfusion: Cardiac
Tissue Perfusion: Cellular

Tissue Perfusion: Cerebral
Tissue Perfusion: Pulmonary
Urinary Elimination
Vital Signs
Wound Healing: Primary Intention
Wound Healing: Secondary Intention

Dermatology

Adherence Behavior
Allergic Response: Localized
Allergic Response: Systemic
Body Image
Burn Healing
Burn Recovery
Comfort Status
Communication
Compliance Behavior
Coping
Health Beliefs: Perceived Control
Health Promoting Behavior
Health Seeking Behavior
Information Processing
Knowledge: Cancer Management

Knowledge: Cancer Threat Reduction
Knowledge: Disease Process
Knowledge: Medication
Knowledge: Treatment Regimen
Medication Response
Personal Well-Being
Quality of Life
Risk Control: Sun Exposure
Self-Esteem
Social Involvement
Suffering Severity
Symptom Severity
Tissue Integrity: Skin & Mucous Membranes
Wound Healing: Primary Intention
Wound Healing: Secondary Intention

Emergency Care

Allergic Response: Systemic
Anxiety Level
Blood Loss Severity
Cardiopulmonary Status
Community Disaster Readiness
Community Disaster Response
Community Health Status
Community Risk Control: Communicable
    Disease
Compliance Behavior
Electrolyte & Acid-Base Balance
Fluid Overload Severity
Health Beliefs
Health Beliefs: Perceived Resources
Health Seeking Behavior
Knowledge: Health Behavior
Knowledge: Health Promotion

Knowledge: Health Resources
Knowledge: Illness Care
Knowledge: Medication
Knowledge: Personal Safety
Knowledge: Treatment Procedure
Knowledge: Treatment Regimen
Medication Response
Neurological Status
Pain Control
Participation in Health Care Decisions
Physical Injury Severity
Respiratory Status
Seizure Control
Skeletal Function
Treatment Behavior: Illness or Injury
Vital Signs

Gastroenterology

Acceptance: Health Status
Appetite
Blood Loss Severity
Comfort Status
Communication
Concentration
Decision-Making
Discomfort Level
Gastrointestinal Function
Health Promoting Behavior
Health Seeking Behavior
Infection Severity
Knowledge: Cancer Management
Knowledge: Disease Process
Knowledge: Health Promotion
Knowledge: Medication
Knowledge: Ostomy Care
Knowledge: Treatment Regimen
Knowledge: Weight Management
Medication Response
Nausea & Vomiting Control
Nausea & Vomiting Severity

Nausea & Vomiting: Disruptive Effects
Nutritional Status
Nutritional Status: Biochemical Measures
Nutritional Status: Food & Fluid Intake
Nutritional Status: Nutrient Intake
Ostomy Self-Care
Pain Level
Participation in Health Care Decisions
Post-Procedure Recovery
Pre-Procedure Readiness
Respiratory Status: Airway Patency
Sensory Function
Swallowing Status
Swallowing Status: Esophageal Phase
Swallowing Status: Oral Phase
Swallowing Status: Pharyngeal Phase
Symptom Control
Symptom Severity
Tissue Perfusion: Abdominal
Vital Signs
Weight Gain Behavior
Weight Maintenance Behavior

Genetics

Anxiety Control
Anxiety Level
Client Satisfaction
Client Satisfaction: Access to Care
Client Satisfaction: Case Management
Client Satisfaction: Psychological Care
Client Satisfaction: Teaching
Comfort Status
Communication
Compliance Behavior: Prescribed Diet
Coping
Decision Making
Family Coping
Family Functioning
Family Health Status
Family Integrity
Family Participation in Professional Care
Family Social Climate
Fear Control
Grief Resolution
Health Beliefs
Knowledge: Asthma Management

Knowledge: Cancer Management
Knowledge: Cancer Threat Reduction
Knowledge: Diet
Knowledge: Disease Process
Nutritional Status
Nutritional Status: Biochemical Measures
Participation in Health Care Decisions
Personal Autonomy
Personal Health Status
Personal Well-Being
Quality of Life
Risk Control: Cancer
Risk Control: Cardiovascular Health
Risk Control: Pre-Procedure Readiness
Risk Detection
Sensory Function: Hearing
Sensory Function: Vision
Social Support
Spiritual Health
Personal Well-Being
Will to Live

Gerontology

Acute Confusion Level
Adherence Behavior: Healthy Diet
Appetite
Body Mechanics Performance
Bowel Continence
Bowel Elimination
Cardiopulmonary Status
Cognition
Comfort Status
Comfortable Death
Communication
Compliance Behavior: Prescribed Diet
Compliance Behavior: Prescribed Medication
Coordinated Movement
Development: Late Adulthood
Dignified Life Closure
Discomfort Level
Elopement Occurrence
Elopement Propensity Risk
Endurance
Energy Conservation
Fall Prevention Behavior
Family Social Climate
Hydration
Joint Movement
Knowledge: Arthritis Management
Knowledge: Cardiac Disease Management
Knowledge: Congestive Heart Failure
    Management
Knowledge: Depression Management
Knowledge: Diabetes Management
Knowledge: Fall Prevention
Knowledge: Hypertension Management
Knowledge: Pain Management
Knowledge: Weight Management
Memory
Mobility
Neurological Status
Neurological Status: Autonomic
Neurological Status: Central Motor Control
Neurological Status: Consciousness
Neurological Status: Cranial Sensory/Motor
    Function
Neurological Status: Peripheral
Neurological Status: Spinal Sensory/Motor
    Function
Nutritional Status
Nutritional Status: Biochemical Measures
Nutritional Status: Energy
Nutritional Status: Food & Fluid Intake
Nutritional Status: Nutrient Intake
Oral Hygiene
Pain Control
Personal Health Status
Personal Resiliency
Personal Safety Behavior
Quality of Life
Respiratory Status
Rest
Safe Wandering
Self-Care Status
Self-Care: Activities of Daily Living (ADL)
Self-Care: Hygiene
Self-Care: Instrumental Activities of Daily
    Living (IADL)
Sensory Function
Sensory Function: Hearing
Sensory Function: Proprioception
Sensory Function: Taste & Smell
Sensory Function: Vision
Sleep
Social Involvement
Social Support
Swallowing Status
Tissue Integrity: Skin & Mucous Membranes
Tissue Perfusion: Cellular
Urinary Continence
Urinary Elimination
Vital Signs
Weight: Body Mass

Home Healthcare

Adherence Behavior: Healthy Diet
Ambulation
Body Mechanics Performance
Bowel Elimination
Burn Recovery
Caregiver Performance: Direct Care
Client Satisfaction
Client Satisfaction: Case Management

Continued

Home Healthcare—cont'd

Comfort Status
Comfort Status: Environment
Comfortable Death
Community Risk Control: Communicable
 Disease
Compliance Behavior: Prescribed Diet
Compliance Behavior: Prescribed Medication
Dignified Life Closure
Discomfort Level
Endurance
Fall Prevention Behavior
Family Resiliency
Family Support During Treatment
Fatigue Level
Health Beliefs
Health Beliefs: Perceived Ability to Perform
Health Beliefs: Perceived Control
Health Beliefs: Perceived Resources
Health Beliefs: Perceived Threat
Health Orientation
Joint Movement
Knowledge: Arthritis Management
Knowledge: Asthma Management
Knowledge: Cancer Management
Knowledge: Cancer Threat Reduction
Knowledge: Cardiac Disease Management
Knowledge: Congestive Heart Failure
 Management
Knowledge: Depression Management
Knowledge: Diabetes Management
Knowledge: Disease Process
Knowledge: Fall Prevention
Knowledge: Hypertension Management
Knowledge: Illness Care
Knowledge: Infection Management
Knowledge: Medication
Knowledge: Multiple Sclerosis Management
Knowledge: Ostomy Care

Knowledge: Pain Management
Knowledge: Personal Safety
Knowledge: Prescribed Activity
Knowledge: Treatment Procedure
Knowledge: Treatment Regimen
Knowledge: Weight Management
Medication Response
Mobility
Nutritional Status
Ostomy Self-Care
Personal Health Status
Personal Resiliency
Respiratory Status
Risk Control: Infectious Process
Safe Home Environment
Self-Care Status
Self-Care: Activities of Daily Living (ADL)
Self-Care: Bathing
Self-Care: Dressing
Self-Care: Eating
Self-Care: Hygiene
Self-Care: Instrumental Activities of Daily
 Living (IADL)
Self-Care: Toileting
Self-Care: Non-Parenteral Medication
Sensory Function
Smoking Cessation Behavior
Social Involvement
Social Support
Spiritual Health
Treatment Behavior: Illness or Injury
Urinary Continence
Urinary Elimination
Vital Signs
Weight Maintenance Behavior
Wound Healing: Primary Intention
Wound Healing: Secondary Intention

Hospice & Palliative Care

Acceptance: Health Status
Client Satisfaction: Pain
Client Satisfaction: Psychological Care
Client Satisfaction: Symptom Control
Comfort Status
Comfort Status: Psychospiritual

Comfortable Death
Communication
Community Competence
Community Health Status
Coping
Development: Late Adulthood

Hospice & Palliative Care—cont'd

Dignified Life Closure
Discomfort Level
Fall Prevention Behavior
Falls Occurrence
Family Coping
Family Health Status
Family Integrity
Family Normalization
Family Participation in Professional Care
Family Social Climate
Family Support During Treatment
Fatigue Level
Grief Resolution
Health Beliefs
Knowledge: Medication
Knowledge: Personal Safety
Medication Response
Oral Hygiene

Pain Level
Pain: Adverse Psychological Response
Pain: Disruptive Effects
Participation in Health Care Decisions
Personal Well-Being
Psychosocial Adjustment: Life Change
Quality of Life
Safe Home Environment
Safe Wandering
Self-Care Status
Self-Esteem
Social Support
Spiritual Health
Suffering Severity
Symptom Control
Symptom Severity
Tissue Integrity: Skin & Mucous Membranes

Intravenous Therapy

Blood Coagulation
Blood Transfusion Reaction
Caregiver Home Care Readiness
Circulation Status
Comfort Status
Electrolyte & Acid/Base Balance
Family Participation in Professional Care
Fluid Balance
Fluid Overload Severity
Hydration
Immobility Consequences: Physiological
Infection Severity
Knowledge: Infection Management
Knowledge: Medication
Knowledge: Prescribed Activity
Knowledge: Treatment Procedure

Medication Response
Nutritional Status: Biochemical Measures
Pain Level
Pain: Adverse Psychological Response
Pain: Disruptive Effects
Quality of Life
Risk Control: Infectious Process
Self-Care: Hygiene
Self-Care: Non-Parenteral Medication
Self-Care: Parenteral Medication
Symptom Severity
Tissue Integrity: Skin & Mucous Membranes
Tissue Perfusion: Cellular
Tissue Perfusion: Peripheral
Urinary Elimination
Vital Signs

Medical-Surgical

Acceptance: Health Status
Acute Confusion Level
Alcohol Abuse Cessation Behavior
Ambulation
Appetite
Balance
Blood Glucose Level

Blood Loss Severity
Blood Transfusion Reaction
Body Positioning: Self-Initiated
Bowel Elimination
Burn Healing
Burn Recovery
Cardiac Disease Self-Management

Continued

Medical-Surgical—cont'd

Cardiopulmonary Status
Client Satisfaction: Caring
Client Satisfaction: Communication
Client Satisfaction: Cultural Needs
    Fulfillment
Client Satisfaction: Functional Assistance
Client Satisfaction: Pain Management
Client Satisfaction: Physical Care
Client Satisfaction: Psychological Care
Client Satisfaction: Safety
Client Satisfaction: Symptom Control
Client Satisfaction: Teaching
Cognitive Orientation
Comfort Status
Communication
Compliance Behavior: Prescribed Diet
Compliance Behavior: Prescribed
    Medication
Development: Late Adulthood
Development: Middle Adulthood
Diabetes Self-Management
Discharge Readiness: Independent Living
Discharge Readiness: Supported Living
Discomfort Level
Drug Abuse Cessation Behavior
Elopement Occurrence
Elopement Propensity Risk
Endurance
Family Support During Treatment
Fatigue Level
Fluid Overload Severity
Gastrointestinal Function
Heedfulness of Affected Side
Hydration
Immune Hypersensitivity Response
Infection Severity
Joint Movement
Kidney Function
Knowledge: Arthritis Management
Knowledge: Cancer Management
Knowledge: Cancer Threat Reduction
Knowledge: Cardiac Disease Management

Knowledge: Congestive Heart Failure
    Management
Knowledge: Disease Process
Knowledge: Hypertension Management
Knowledge: Infection Management
Knowledge: Medication
Knowledge: Multiple Sclerosis Management
Knowledge: Ostomy Care
Knowledge: Weight Management
Mobility
Multiple Sclerosis Management
Neurological Status
Nutritional Status: Food & Fluid Intake
Ostomy Self-Care
Pain Level
Pain: Adverse Psychological Response
Participation in Health Care Decisions
Physical Aging
Post-Procedure Readiness
Pre-Procedure Readiness
Respiratory Status
Rest
Self-Care Status
Self-Care: Activities of Daily Living (ADL)
Self-Care: Bathing
Self-Care: Eating
Self-Care: Hygiene
Self-Care: Instrumental Activities of Daily
    Living (IADL)
Self-Care: Non-Parenteral Medication
Self-Care: Oral Hygiene
Self-Care: Toileting
Sleep
Smoking Cessation Behavior
Tissue Integrity: Skin & Mucous Membranes
Tissue Perfusion: Cellular
Tissue Perfusion: Peripheral
Transfer Performance
Urinary Elimination
Vital Signs
Wound Healing: Primary Intention
Wound Healing: Secondary Intention

Neonatology

Blood Coagulation
Blood Glucose Level

Bowel Elimination
Breastfeeding Establishment: Infant

Neonatology—cont'd

Cardiopulmonary Status
Child Development: 1 Month
Circulation Status
Comfort Status
Comfortable Death
Dignified Life Closure
Electrolyte & Acid/Base Balance
Family Participation In Professional Care
Family Support During Treatment
Fluid Balance
Gastrointestinal Function
Growth
Hydration
Immune Status
Infection Severity: Newborn
Knowledge: Parenting
Knowledge: Preterm Infant Care
Newborn Adaptation
Nutritional Status
Nutritional Status: Biochemical Measures
Nutritional Status: Energy

Nutritional Status: Food & Fluid Intake
Nutritional Status: Nutrient Intake
Pain Level
Parent-Infant Attachment
Parenting Performance
Preterm Infant Organization
Respiratory Status
Respiratory Status: Airway Patency
Respiratory Status: Gas Exchange
Respiratory Status: Ventilation
Thermoregulation: Newborn
Tissue Integrity: Skin & Mucous Membranes
Tissue Perfusion: Abdominal Organs
Tissue Perfusion: Cardiac
Tissue Perfusion: Cellular
Tissue Perfusion: Cerebral
Tissue Perfusion: Peripheral
Tissue Perfusion: Pulmonary
Urinary Elimination
Vital Signs
Weight Gain Behavior

Nephrology

Adherence Behavior
Body Image
Caregiver Home Care Readiness
Caregiver Lifestyle Disruption
Caregiver Performance: Direct Care
Caregiver Role Endurance
Caregiver Stressors
Caregiver-Patient Relationship
Cognition
Cognitive Orientation
Comfort Status
Compliance Behavior
Compliance Behavior: Prescribed Diet
Compliance Behavior: Prescribed Medication
Diabetes Self-Management
Discharge Readiness: Independent Living
Discharge Readiness: Supported Living
Family Coping
Fluid Balance
Fluid Overload Severity
Health Beliefs
Health Beliefs: Perceived Control

Health Beliefs: Perceived Threat
Health Promoting Behavior
Health Seeking Behavior
Hearing Compensation Behavior
Hemodialysis Access
Identity
Kidney Function
Knowledge: Diabetes Management
Knowledge: Diet
Knowledge: Disease Process
Knowledge: Energy Conservation
Knowledge: Health Resources
Knowledge: Hypertension Management
Knowledge: Personal Safety
Knowledge: Prescribed Activity
Knowledge: Treatment Procedure
Knowledge: Treatment Regimen
Leisure Participation
Loneliness Severity
Medication Response
Mood Equilibrium
Neurological Status

Continued

Nephrology—cont'd

Neurological Status: Autonomic
Neurological Status: Central Motor Control
Neurological Status: Consciousness
Neurological Status: Cranial Sensory / Motor Function
Neurological Status: Spinal Sensory / Motor Function
Nutritional Status
Nutritional Status: Biochemical Measures
Nutritional Status: Energy
Nutritional Status: Food & Fluid Intake
Nutritional Status: Nutrient Intake
Participation in Health Care Decisions
Personal Well-Being
Quality of Life
Risk Control: Cardiovascular Health
Self-Care: Activities of Daily Living (ADL)

Self-Care: Instrumental Activities of Daily Living (IADL)
Self-Care: Non-Parenteral Medication
Self-Esteem
Sensory Function: Cutaneous
Sexual Functioning
Social Interaction Skills
Social Involvement
Social Support
Spiritual Health
Suffering Severity
Symptom Control
Symptom Severity
Tissue Perfusion: Cellular
Treatment Behavior: Illness or Injury
Weight: Body Mass
Wound Healing: Primary Intention

Neuroscience

Activity Tolerance
Acute Confusion Level
Adaptation to Physical Disability
Agitation Level
Ambulation
Cognition
Comfort Status
Communication
Coordinated Movement
Coping
Discharge Readiness: Independent Living
Discharge Readiness: Supported Living
Elopement Occurrence
Elopement Propensity Risk
Endurance
Family Coping
Family Normalization
Family Participation in Professional Care
Family Resiliency
Family Support During Treatment
Heedfulness of Affected Side
Hope
Immobility Consequences: Psychological
Knowledge: Disease Process

Knowledge: Health Promotion
Knowledge: Illness Care
Knowledge: Multiple Sclerosis Management
Knowledge: Treatment Regimen
Medication Response
Mobility
Multiple Sclerosis Self-Management
Neurological Status
Neurological Status: Peripheral
Pain Level
Personal Resiliency
Psychomotor Energy
Respiratory Status
Quality of Life
Rest
Safe Wandering
Seizure Control
Sensory Function
Sleep
Social Support
Symptom Severity
Thermoregulation
Tissue Integrity: Skin & Mucous Membranes

Nurse Practitioner

Abuse Recovery
Adaptation to Physical Disability
Adherence Behavior
Adherence Behavior: Healthy Diet
Alcohol Abuse Cessation Behavior
Allergic Response: Localized
Anxiety Level
Appetite
Blood Glucose Level
Body Mechanics Performance
Bowel Elimination
Cardiac Disease Self-Management
Cardiac Pump Effectiveness
Cardiopulmonary Status
Circulation Status
Client Satisfaction: Case Management
Client Satisfaction: Communication
Client Satisfaction: Continuity of Care
Client Satisfaction: Cultural Needs
    Fulfillment
Client Satisfaction: Pain Management
Client Satisfaction: Protection of Rights
Client Satisfaction: Psychological Care
Client Satisfaction: Teaching
Cognition
Cognitive Orientation
Comfort Status
Comfortable Death
Communication: Expressive
Compliance Behavior
Compliance Behavior: Prescribed Diet
Compliance Behavior: Prescribed Medication
Coordinated Movement
Development: Late Adulthood
Development: Middle Adulthood
Development: Young Adulthood
Diabetes Self-Management
Drug Abuse Cessation Behavior
Family Coping
Family Functioning
Family Health Status
Family Integrity
Family Normalization
Family Participation in Professional Care
Family Resiliency
Family Support During Treatment
Fatigue Level
Fluid Balance

Gastrointestinal Function
Health Beliefs
Health Beliefs: Perceived Ability to
    Perform
Health Beliefs: Perceived Control
Health Beliefs: Perceived Resources
Health Promoting Behavior
Health Seeking Behavior
Hydration
Identity
Immune Hypersensitivity Response
Immunization Behavior
Infection Severity
Knowledge: Arthritis Management
Knowledge: Asthma Management
Knowledge: Cancer Threat Reduction
Knowledge: Cardiac Disease Management
Knowledge: Congestive Heart Failure
    Management
Knowledge: Diabetes Management
Knowledge: Diet
Knowledge: Energy Conservation
Knowledge: Health Behavior
Knowledge: Health Resources
Knowledge: Hypertension Management
Knowledge: Illness Care
Knowledge: Infection Management
Knowledge: Medication
Knowledge: Ostomy Care
Knowledge: Personal Safety
Knowledge: Pregnancy & Postpartum Sexual
    Functioning
Knowledge: Prescribed Activity
Knowledge: Treatment Procedure
Knowledge: Treatment Regimen
Knowledge: Weight Management
Medication Response
Mobility
Mood Equilibrium
Neurological Status
Neurological Status: Autonomic
Neurological Status: Central Motor Control
Neurological Status: Consciousness
Neurological Status: Cranial Sensory/Motor
    Function
Neurological Status: Spinal Sensory/Motor
    Function
Nutritional Status

Continued

Nurse Practitioner—cont'd

Nutritional Status: Energy
Nutritional Status: Nutrient Intake
Oral Hygiene
Ostomy Self-Care
Pain Level
Pain: Disruptive Effects
Personal Health Status
Personal Resiliency
Personal Safety Behavior
Personal Well-Being
Physical Fitness
Postpartum Maternal Health Behavior
Quality of Life
Respiratory Status
Risk Control
Risk Control: Cancer
Risk Control: Cardiovascular Health
Risk Control: Drug Use
Risk Control: Tobacco Use
Self-Care: Toileting
Self-Esteem

Sensory Function: Hearing
Sensory Function: Proprioception
Sensory Function: Vision
Skeletal Function
Smoking Cessation Behavior
Stress Level
Symptom Severity
Thermoregulation
Tissue Integrity: Skin & Mucous Membranes
Tissue Perfusion: Abdominal Organs
Tissue Perfusion: Cardiac
Tissue Perfusion: Cerebral
Tissue Perfusion: Peripheral
Tissue Perfusion: Pulmonary
Urinary Elimination
Vital Signs
Weight Gain Behavior
Weight Loss Behavior
Weight Maintenance Behavior
Weight: Body Mass

Oncology

Acceptance: Health Status
Activity Tolerance
Acute Confusion Level
Adaptation to Physical Disability
Adherence Behavior
Adherence Behavior: Healthy Diet
Anxiety Level
Anxiety Self-Control
Appetite
Body Image
Client Satisfaction
Client Satisfaction: Access to Care Resources
Client Satisfaction: Caring
Client Satisfaction: Case Management
Client Satisfaction: Communication
Client Satisfaction: Continuity of Care
Client Satisfaction: Pain Management
Client Satisfaction: Physical Care
Client Satisfaction: Protection of Rights
Client Satisfaction: Psychological Care
Client Satisfaction: Symptom Control
Client Satisfaction: Teaching
Client Satisfaction: Technical Aspects of Care

Comfort Status
Comfort Status: Environment
Comfort Status: Physical
Comfort Status: Psychospiritual
Comfort Status: Sociocultural
Comfortable Death
Communication
Compliance Behavior: Prescribed Diet
Compliance Behavior: Prescribed Medication
Coping
Decision-Making
Dignified Life Closure
Discharge Readiness: Independent Living
Discharge Readiness: Supported Living
Discomfort Level
Electrolyte & Acid/Base Balance
Endurance
Energy Conservation
Fall Prevention Behavior
Family Coping
Family Participation in Professional Care
Family Support During Treatment
Fatigue Level

Oncology—cont'd

Fear Level
Fear Level: Child
Fear Self-Control
Fluid Balance
Grief Resolution
Hope
Hydration
Immobility Consequences: Physiological
Immobility Consequences: Psycho-Cognitive
Infection Severity
Knowledge: Cancer Management
Knowledge: Cancer Threat Reduction
Knowledge: Diet
Knowledge: Disease Process
Knowledge: Energy Conservation
Knowledge: Health Behavior
Knowledge: Health Resources
Knowledge: Infection Management
Knowledge: Ostomy Care
Knowledge: Pain Management
Knowledge: Prescribed Activity
Knowledge: Treatment Procedure
Knowledge: Treatment Regimen
Medication Response
Memory
Nausea & Vomiting Control
Nausea & Vomiting Severity
Nausea & Vomiting: Disruptive Effects
Nutritional Status
Ostomy Self-Care
Pain Control

Pain Level
Pain: Adverse Psychological Response
Pain: Disruptive Effects
Participation in Health Care Decisions
Personal Autonomy
Personal Health Status
Personal Resiliency
Personal Well-Being
Psychosocial Adjustment: Life Change
Quality of Life
Respiratory Status
Risk Control: Cancer
Risk Control: Infectious Process
Risk Control: Sun Exposure
Self-Care Status
Self-Care: Activities of Daily Living (ADL)
Self-Care: Non-Parenteral Medication
Self-Care: Parenteral Medication
Sleep
Social Support
Spiritual Health
Stress Level
Suffering Severity
Symptom Control
Symptom Severity
Vital Signs
Weight Gain Behavior
Weight Loss Behavior
Weight Maintenance Behavior
Weight: Body Mass
Will to Live

Operating Room

Acute Confusion Level
Allergic Response: Systemic
Anxiety Level
Aspiration Prevention
Blood Coagulation
Blood Loss Severity
Cardiopulmonary Status
Circulation Status
Cognition
Cognitive Orientation
Comfort Status
Communication
Community Health Status: Immunity

Electrolyte & Acid/Base Balance
Family Coping
Family Participation in Professional Care
Fear Level
Fluid Balance
Fluid Overload Severity
Health Beliefs: Perceived Control
Health Beliefs: Perceived Resources
Hydration
Immobility Consequences: Physiological
Infection Severity
Joint Movement
Kidney Function

Continued

Operating Room—cont'd

Knowledge: Health Promotion
Knowledge: Treatment Regimen
Medication Response
Nausea & Vomiting Control
Nausea & Vomiting Severity
Pain Level
Participation in Health Care Decisions
Post-Procedure Recovery
Pre-Procedure Readiness
Psychomotor Energy
Respiratory Status
Respiratory Status: Airway Patency
Respiratory Status: Gas Exchange
Respiratory Status: Ventilation
Seizure Control
Sleep

Swallowing Status
Swallowing Status: Esophageal Phase
Swallowing Status: Oral Phase
Swallowing Status: Pharyngeal Phase
Symptom Severity
Thermoregulation
Tissue Integrity: Skin & Mucous Membranes
Tissue Perfusion: Abdominal Organs
Tissue Perfusion: Cardiac
Tissue Perfusion: Cellular
Tissue Perfusion: Cerebral
Tissue Perfusion: Peripheral
Tissue Perfusion: Pulmonary
Vital Signs
Wound Healing: Primary Intention

Ophthalmology

Decision-Making
Diabetes Self-Management
Health Beliefs
Knowledge: Disease Process
Knowledge: Health Behavior
Knowledge: Health Resources
Knowledge: Hypertension Management
Knowledge: Medication
Knowledge: Multiple Sclerosis Management
Knowledge: Personal Safety
Knowledge: Treatment Regimen
Neurological Status

Neurological Status: Cranial Sensory/Motor Function
Participation in Health Care Decisions
Physical Aging
Post-Procedure Recovery
Pre-Procedure Readiness
Risk Control
Risk Control: Sun Exposure
Risk Control: Visual Impairment
Sensory Function: Vision
Vision Compensation Behavior

Orthopaedics

Ambulation
Ambulation: Wheelchair
Adaptation to Physical Disabilty
Balance
Blood Coagulation
Body Mechanics Performance
Bone Healing
Caregiver Home Care Readiness
Caregiver Lifestyle Disruption
Cognition
Cognitive Orientation
Comfort Status

Communication
Coordinated Movement
Depression Level
Discharge Readiness: Independent Living
Discharge Readiness: Supported Living
Fall Prevention Behavior
Infection Severity
Joint Movement
Joint Movement: Ankle
Joint Movement: Elbow
Joint Movement: Fingers
Joint Movement: Hip

Orthopaedics—cont'd

Joint Movement: Knee
Joint Movement: Neck
Joint Movement: Passive
Joint Movement: Shoulder
Joint Movement: Spine
Joint Movement: Wrist
Knowledge: Body Mechanics
Knowledge: Fall Prevention
Knowledge: Infection Management
Mobility
Neurological Status: Consciousness
Neurological Status: Cranial Sensory/Motor
    Function
Neurological Status: Spinal Sensory/Motor
    Function
Nutritional Status: Biochemical Measures
Nutritional Status: Food & Fluid Intake
Pain Control
Pain Level

Pain: Adverse Psychological Response
Pain: Disruptive Effects
Participation in Health Care Decisions
Personal Well-Being
Physical Injury Severity
Respiratory Status
Safe Home Environment
Self-Care: Activities of Daily Living (ADL)
Self-Care: Instrumental Activities of Daily
    Living (IADL)
Self-Care: Toileting
Skeletal Function
Symptom Severity
Tissue Perfusion: Peripheral
Transfer Performance
Vital Signs
Wound Healing: Primary Intention
Wound Healing: Secondary Intention

Otorhinolaryngology and Head-Neck

Acceptance: Health Status
Activity Tolerance
Acute Confusion Level
Adaptation to Physical Disability
Ambulation
Appetite
Aspiration Prevention
Asthma Self-Management
Blood Loss Severity
Body Image
Comfort Status
Communication
Compliance Behavior
Coping
Electrolyte & Acid/Base Balance
Fluid Balance
Health Promoting Behavior
Health Seeking Behavior
Hearing Compensation Behavior
Hydration
Immobility Consequences: Physiological
Immobility Consequences: Psycho-Cognitive
Immune Status
Infection Severity
Knowledge: Health Promotion

Knowledge: Health Resources
Knowledge: Infection Management
Knowledge: Treatment Procedure
Knowledge: Treatment Regimen
Medication Response
Mobility
Neurological Status: Cranial Sensory/Motor
    Function
Nutritional Status
Nutritional Status: Biochemical Measures
Nutritional Status: Food & Fluid Intake
Nutritional Status: Nutrient Intake
Pain Control
Pain Level
Pain: Adverse Psychological Response
Participation in Health Care Decisions
Personal Resiliency
Personal Well-Being
Post-Procedure Recovery
Pre-Procedure Readiness
Quality of Life
Respiratory Status
Respiratory Status: Airway Patency
Respiratory Status: Gas Exchange
Respiratory Status: Ventilation

Continued

Otorhinolaryngology and Head-Neck—cont'd

Risk Control
Risk Control: Cancer
Risk Control: Hearing Impairment
Risk Control: Tobacco Use
Seizure Control
Self-Care Status
Self-Care: Activities of Daily Living (ADL)
Self-Care: Bathing
Sensory Function
Sensory Function: Hearing
Sensory Function: Taste & Smell
Smoking Cessation Behavior

Spiritual Health
Swallowing Status
Swallowing Status: Esophageal Phase
Swallowing Status: Oral Phase
Swallowing Status: Pharyngeal Phase
Symptom Control
Tissue Integrity: Skin & Mucous Membranes
Tissue Perfusion: Pulmonary
Vital Signs
Will to Live
Wound Healing: Primary Intention
Wound Healing: Secondary Intention

Pain Management

Burn Healing
Client Satisfaction: Pain Management
Cognitive Orientation
Comfort Status
Comfortable Death
Communication
Dignified Life Closure
Discomfort Level
Electrolyte & Acid/Base Balance
Family Support During Treatment
Fluid Balance
Information Processing
Knowledge: Pain Management
Nausea & Vomiting Control
Nausea & Vomiting Severity
Neurological Status: Consciousness
Pain: Adverse Psychological Response

Pain Control
Pain: Disruptive Effects
Pain Level
Personal Resiliency
Respiratory Status
Self-Care Status
Self-Care: Activities of Daily Living (ADL)
Self-Care: Bathing
Self-Care: Dressing
Self-Care: Instrumental Activities of Daily
    Living (IADL)
Skeletal Function
Thermoregulation
Tissue Perfusion: Cardiac
Vital Signs
Wound Healing: Primary Intention
Wound Healing: Secondary Intention

Parish Nursing

Abuse Recovery
Adaptation to Physical Disability
Adherence Behavior
Anxiety Level
Cardiac Disease Self-Management
Caregiver Adaptation to Patient
    Institutionalization
Caregiver Emotional Health
Caregiver Stressors
Caregiver Well-Being
Caregiver-Patient Relationship
Comfort Status: Psychospiritual

Compliance Behavior
Compliance Behavior: Prescribed Diet
Compliance Behavior: Prescribed Medication
Coping
Decision-Making
Dignified Life Closure
Discomfort Level
Family Coping
Family Functioning
Family Integrity
Family Normalization
Fear Level

Parish Nursing—cont'd

Grief Resolution
Health Beliefs
Health Orientation
Health Promoting Behavior
Health Seeking Behavior
Hope
Knowledge: Cancer Threat Reduction
Knowledge: Congestive Heart Failure
    Management
Knowledge: Diabetes Management
Knowledge: Diet
Knowledge: Health Behavior
Knowledge: Health Promotion
Knowledge: Health Resources
Knowledge: Hypertension Management
Knowledge: Medication
Knowledge: Weight Management
Leisure Participation
Loneliness Severity
Parenting: Adolescent Physical Safety
Parenting: Early/Middle Childhood Physical
    Safety
Parenting: Infant/Toddler Physical Safety
Participation in Health Care Decisions
Personal Health Status
Personal Well-Being
Quality of Life
Risk Control: Cancer
Risk Control: Cardiovascular Health
Risk Control: Tobacco Use
Risk Detection
Self-Care: Instrumental Activities of Daily
    Living (IADL)
Self-Care: Non-Parenteral Medication
Self-Esteem
Smoking Cessation Behavior
Social Involvement
Social Support
Spiritual Health
Stress Level
Suffering Severity
Symptom Severity
Weight Loss Behavior
Weight Maintenance Behavior

Pediatrics

Ambulation
Asthma Self-Management
Balance
Body Positioning: Self-Initiated
Breastfeeding Maintenance
Breastfeeding Weaning
Caregiver Adaptation to Patient
    Institutionalization
Caregiver Emotional Health
Caregiver Home Care Readiness
Caregiver Lifestyle Disruption
Caregiver Performance: Direct Care
Caregiver Performance: Indirect Care
Caregiver Personal Well-Being
Caregiver Physical Health
Caregiver Role Endurance
Caregiver Stressors
Caregiver-Patient Relationship
Child Adaptation to Hospitalization
Child Development: 1 Month
Child Development: 2 Months
Child Development: 4 Months
Child Development: 6 Months
Child Development: 12 Months
Child Development: 2 Years
Child Development: 3 Years
Child Development: 4 Years
Child Development: 5 Years
Child Development: Middle Childhood
Child Development: Adolescence
Comfort Status
Coping
Dignified Life Closure
Family Coping
Family Functioning
Family Health Status
Family Integrity
Family Normalization
Family Participation in Professional Care
Family Resiliency
Family Social Climate
Family Support During Treatment
Fear Level: Child
Grief Resolution

Continued

Pediatrics—cont'd

Growth
Health Promoting Behavior
Health Seeking Behavior
Immobility Consequences: Physiological
Immobility Consequences: Psycho-Cognitive
Immunization Behavior
Infection Severity: Newborn
Joint Movement
Knowledge: Asthma Management
Knowledge: Child Physical Safety
Knowledge: Disease Management
Knowledge: Health Behavior
Knowledge: Infant Care
Knowledge: Infection Management
Knowledge: Medication
Knowledge: Parenting
Knowledge: Personal Safety
Knowledge: Preterm Infant Care
Knowledge: Treatment Procedure
Knowledge: Treatment Regimen
Medication Response
Mobility
Newborn Adaptation
Nutritional Status
Oral Hygiene
Pain Level
Pain: Adverse Psychological Response
Pain: Disruptive Effects
Parent-Infant Attachment
Parenting Performance
Parenting: Adolescent Physical Safety
Parenting: Early/Middle Childhood Physical
   Safety
Parenting: Infant/Toddler Physical Safety
Parenting: Psychosocial Safety
Physical Fitness
Physical Injury Severity
Physical Maturation: Female
Physical Maturation: Male
Play Participation
Preterm Infant Organization
Psychosocial Adjustment: Life Change

Respiratory Status
Risk Control
Risk Control: Alcohol Use
Risk Control: Drug Use
Risk Control: Hyperthermia
Risk Control: Hypothermia
Risk Control: Sexually Transmitted
   Diseases (STD)
Risk Control: Sun Exposure
Risk Control: Tobacco Use
Risk Control: Unintended Pregnancy
Role Performance
Self-Care Status
Self-Care: Activities of Daily Living (ADL)
Self-Care: Bathing
Self-Care: Dressing
Self-Care: Eating
Self-Care: Hygiene
Self-Care: Non-Parenteral Medication
Self-Care: Oral Hygiene
Self-Care: Parenteral Medication
Self-Care: Toileting
Sexual Functioning
Skeletal Function
Smoking Cessation Behavior
Social Interaction Skills
Social Support
Spiritual Health
Student Health Status
Symptom Severity
Thermoregulation: Neonate
Tissue Integrity: Skin & Mucous Membranes
Tissue Perfusion: Pulmonary
Transfer Performance
Vital Signs
Weight: Body Mass
Weight Gain Behavior
Weight Loss Behavior
Weight Maintenance Behavior
Wound Healing: Primary Intention
Wound Healing: Secondary Intention

Pediatric Oncology

Activity Tolerance
Allergic Response: Systemic
Appetite

Blood Loss Severity
Body Image
Caregiver Performance: Direct Care

Pediatric Oncology—cont'd

Caregiver Performance: Indirect Care
Child Adaptation to Hospitalization
Comfort Status
Comfortable Death
Coping
Discomfort Level
Family Normalization
Family Participation in Professional Care
Family Resiliency
Family Support During Treatment
Fatigue Level
Fear Level: Child
Gastrointestinal Function
Hope
Immune Hypersensitivity Response
Kidney Function
Knowledge: Cancer Management
Knowledge: Disease Process
Knowledge: Health Promotion
Knowledge: Illness Care
Knowledge: Infection Management

Knowledge: Medication
Knowledge: Treatment Regimen
Nausea & Vomiting Control
Nausea & Vomiting Severity
Nutritional Status: Nutrient Intake
Pain: Adverse Psychological Response
Pain Level
Parenting Performance
Post-Procedure Recovery
Pre-Procedure Readiness
Respiratory Status
Skeletal Function
Social Support
Swallowing Status
Swallowing Status: Esophageal Phase
Swallowing Status: Oral Phase
Swallowing Status: Pharyngeal Phase
Symptom Severity
Will to Live
Weight Gain Behavior
Weight Maintenance Behavior

Perianesthesia

Acute Confusion Level
Allergic Response: Systemic
Anxiety Level
Aspiration Prevention
Blood Coagulation
Blood Glucose Level
Blood Loss Severity
Blood Transfusion Reaction
Bowel Elimination
Cardiac Pump Effectiveness
Cardiopulmonary Status
Child Adaptation to Hospitalization
Circulation Status
Client Satisfaction: Pain Management
Client Satisfaction: Symptom Control
Client Satisfaction: Technical Aspects of Care
Comfort Status
Discomfort Level
Fear Level
Fluid Balance
Fluid Overload Severity
Hydration
Immune Hypersensitivity Response

Immune Status
Infection Severity
Kidney Function
Knowledge: Disease Process
Knowledge: Energy Conservation
Knowledge: Infection Management
Knowledge: Medication
Knowledge: Personal Safety
Knowledge: Treatment Procedure
Knowledge: Treatment Regimen
Medication Response
Nausea & Vomiting Severity
Neurological Status: Peripheral
Pain Level
Pain: Adverse Psychological Response
Post-Procedure Recovery
Pre-Procedure Readiness
Respiratory Status
Respiratory Status: Airway Patency
Respiratory Status: Gas Exchange
Respiratory Status: Ventilation
Skeletal Function
Thermoregulation

Continued

Perianesthesia—cont'd

Thermoregulation: Newborn
Tissue Perfusion: Abdominal Organs
Tissue Perfusion: Cardiac
Tissue Perfusion: Cellular
Tissue Perfusion: Cerebral

Tissue Perfusion: Pulmonary
Vital Signs
Wound Healing: Primary Intention
Wound Healing: Secondary Intention

Perioperative Care

Acute Confusion Level
Allergic Response: Systemic
Anxiety Level
Aspiration Prevention
Blood Coagulation
Blood Glucose Level
Blood Loss Severity
Blood Transfusion Reaction
Cardiac Pump Effectiveness
Cardiopulmonary Status
Circulation Status
Client Satisfaction: Pain Management
Client Satisfaction: Protection of Rights
Communication
Coordinated Movement
Discomfort Level
Electrolyte & Acid/Base Balance
Family Coping
Family Participation in Professional Care
Fluid Balance
Fluid Overload Severity
Gastrointestinal Function
Hemodialysis Access
Hydration
Immune Hypersensitivity Response
Infection Severity
Joint Movement
Joint Movement: Passive
Kidney Function
Knowledge: Infection Management
Knowledge: Medication
Knowledge: Treatment Procedure
Knowledge: Treatment Regimen
Mechanical Ventilation Response: Adult
Medication Response
Nausea & Vomiting Severity

Neurological Status
Neurological Status: Autonomic
Neurological Status: Consciousness
Neurological Status: Cranial Sensory/Motor
    Function
Neurological Status: Peripheral
Neurological Status: Spinal Sensory/Motor
    Function
Nutritional Status: Food & Fluid Intake
Pain Control
Pain Level
Personal Resiliency
Physical Injury Severity
Post-Procedure Recovery
Pre-Procedure Readiness
Respiratory Status
Respiratory Status: Airway Patency
Respiratory Status: Gas Exchange
Respiratory Status: Ventilation
Seizure Control
Sensory Function: Cutaneous
Skeletal Function
Symptom Severity
Systemic Toxin Clearance: Dialysis
Thermoregulation
Thermoregulation: Newborn
Tissue Integrity: Skin & Mucous Membranes
Tissue Perfusion: Abdominal Organs
Tissue Perfusion: Cardiac
Tissue Perfusion: Cellular
Tissue Perfusion: Cerebral
Tissue Perfusion: Peripheral
Tissue Perfusion: Pulmonary
Urinary Elimination
Vital Signs
Weight: Body Mass

Psychiatric-Mental Health

Abuse Recovery
Acceptance: Health Status
Acute Confusion Level
Aggression Self-Control
Agitation Level
Alcohol Abuse Cessation Behavior
Anxiety Level
Client Satisfaction: Caring
Client Satisfaction: Communication
Client Satisfaction: Continuity of Care
Client Satisfaction: Protection of Rights
Client Satisfaction: Psychological Care
Client Satisfaction: Teaching
Cognition
Cognitive Orientation
Comfort Status: Psychospiritual
Communication
Communication: Expressive
Communication: Receptive
Concentration
Coping
Decision-Making
Depression Level
Depression Self-Control
Discharge Readiness: Independent Living
Distorted Thought Self-Control
Drug Abuse Cessation Behavior
Elopement Occurrence
Elopement Propensity Risk
Family Coping
Fatigue Level
Fear Level
Hope
Information Processing
Identity

Knowledge: Depression Management
Knowledge: Disease Process
Knowledge: Medication
Knowledge: Treatment Regimen
Loneliness Severity
Medication Response
Memory
Mood Equilibrium
Nutritional Status
Nutritional Status: Food & Fluid Intake
Oral Hygiene
Participation in Health Care Decisions
Personal Autonomy
Personal Resiliency
Personal Well-Being
Psychosocial Adjustment: Life Change
Rest
Safe Wandering
Self-Care: Activities of Daily Living (ADL)
Self-Care: Bathing
Self-Care: Dressing
Self-Care: Hygiene
Self-Care: Non-Parenteral Medication
Self-Esteem
Self-Mutilation Restraint
Sleep
Social Involvement
Social Support
Stress Level
Substance Withdrawal Severity
Suicide Self-Restraint
Symptom Control
Weight Gain Behavior
Weight Maintenance Behavior

Radiology

Acceptance: Health Status
Agitation Level
Anxiety Level
Balance
Blood Transfusion Reaction
Body Positioning: Self-Initiated
Cardiac Pump Effectiveness
Cardiopulmonary Status
Circulation Status

Client Satisfaction: Caring
Client Satisfaction: Communication
Client Satisfaction: Cultural Needs
    Fulfillment
Client Satisfaction: Pain Management
Client Satisfaction: Protection of Rights
Client Satisfaction: Psychological Care
Client Satisfaction: Teaching
Discomfort Level

Continued

Radiology—cont'd

Electrolyte & Acid/Base Balance
Family Support During Treatment
Fatigue Level
Fear Level
Fear Level: Child
Fluid Balance
Hope
Hydration
Immune Hypersensitivity Response
Immune Status
Infection Severity
Joint Movement
Knowledge: Cancer Management
Mobility
Nausea & Vomiting Severity
Neurological Status
Nutritional Status
Nutritional Status: Biochemical Measures
Nutritional Status: Nutrient Intake
Pain Control
Pain: Adverse Psychological Response

Post-Procedure Recovery
Pre-Procedure Readiness
Psychosocial Adjustment: Life Change
Respiratory Status
Rest
Sensory Function
Skeletal Function
Sleep
Social Support
Swallowing Status
Thermoregulation
Tissue Integrity: Skin & Mucous Membranes
Tissue Perfusion: Abdominal Organs
Tissue Perfusion: Cardiac
Tissue Perfusion: Cellular
Tissue Perfusion: Cerebral
Tissue Perfusion: Peripheral
Tissue Perfusion: Pulmonary
Transfer Performance
Vital Signs

Rehabilitation

Acute Confusion Level
Adaptation to Physical Disability
Ambulation
Ambulation: Wheelchair
Aspiration Prevention
Body Mechanics Performance
Bowel Continence
Bowel Elimination
Burn Recovery
Client Satisfaction: Access to Care Resources
Client Satisfaction: Case Management
Client Satisfaction: Continuity of Care
Client Satisfaction: Cultural Needs
    Fulfillment
Client Satisfaction: Functional Assistance
Client Satisfaction: Pain Management
Client Satisfaction: Protection of Rights
Client Satisfaction: Teaching
Cognition
Cognitive Orientation
Communication: Expressive
Communication: Receptive
Concentration

Coordinated Movement
Decision-Making
Discharge Readiness: Independent Living
Endurance
Fall Prevention Behavior
Fatigue Level
Family Participation in Professional Care
Heedfulness of Affected Side
Information Processing
Joint Movement
Joint Movement: Ankle
Joint Movement: Elbow
Joint Movement: Fingers
Joint Movement: Hip
Joint Movement: Knee
Joint Movement: Neck
Joint Movement: Passive
Joint Movement: Shoulder
Joint Movement: Spine
Joint Movement: Wrist
Knowledge: Arthritis Management
Knowledge: Body Mechanics
Knowledge: Energy Consulation

Rehabilitation—cont'd

Knowledge: Fall Prevention
Knowledge: Ostomy Care
Knowledge: Weight Management
Memory
Mobility
Neurological Status
Pain Level
Psychomotor Energy
Psychosocial Adjustment: Life Change
Self-Care Status
Self-Care: Activities of Daily Living (ADL)
Self-Care: Hygiene
Self-Care: Instrumental Activities of Daily
 Living (IADL)

Self-Care: Non-Parenteral Medication
Self-Care: Oral Hygiene
Self-Care: Toileting
Sleep
Swallowing Status
Swallowing Status: Esophageal Phase
Swallowing Status: Oral Phase
Swallowing Status: Pharyngeal Phase
Transfer Performance
Urinary Continence
Urinary Elimination

School Health

Activity Tolerance
Ambulation
Asthma Self-Management
Body Image
Cardiopulmonary Status
Child Development: Adolescence
Child Development: Middle Childhood
Client Satisfaction: Case Management
Cognitive Orientation
Communication
Compliance Behavior: Prescribed Diet
Compliance Behavior: Prescribed Medication
Concentration
Coordinated Movement
Diabetes Self-Management
Endurance
Fear Level: Child
Growth
Hope
Hyperactivity Level
Identity
Immunization Behavior
Information Processing
Knowledge: Asthma Management
Knowledge: Diabetes Management

Knowledge: Diet
Knowledge: Weight Management
Memory
Mood Equilibrium
Neurological Status
Nutritional Status
Oral Hygiene
Personal Autonomy
Physical Fitness
Play Participation
Respiratory Status
Risk Control: Alcohol Use
Risk Control: Drug Use
Risk Control: Sun Exposure
Risk Control: Tobacco Use
Self-Esteem
Sensory Function: Hearing
Sensory Function: Vision
Sleep
Smoking Cessation Behavior
Social Interaction Skills
Social Involvement
Student Health Status
Vital Signs

Spinal Cord Injury

Acceptance: Health Status
Activity Tolerance
Adaptation to Physical Disability
Adherence Behavior
Bowel Continence
Bowel Elimination
Cardiopulmonary Status
Client Satisfaction: Continuity of Care
Client Satisfaction: Functional Assistance
Client Satisfaction: Pain Management
Client Satisfaction: Physical Care
Client Satisfaction: Symptom Control
Comfort Status
Compliance Behavior
Depression Level
Discharge Readiness: Independent Living
Discharge Readiness: Supported Living
Discomfort Level
Endurance
Energy Conservation
Family Coping
Family Functioning
Family Health Status
Family Integrity
Family Normalization
Family Social Climate
Family Support During Treatment
Grief Resolution

Health Beliefs: Perceived Ability to Perform
Health Beliefs: Perceived Control
Kidney Function
Knowledge: Health Promotion
Knowledge: Health Resources
Knowledge: Illness Care
Knowledge: Medication
Knowledge: Personal Safety
Knowledge: Treatment Procedure
Knowledge: Treatment Regimen
Knowledge: Weight Management
Leisure Participation
Medication Response
Neurological Status: Autonomic
Neurological Status: Peripheral
Personal Resiliency
Physical Injury Severity
Psychomotor Energy
Psychosocial Adjustment: Life Change
Risk Control: Hyperthermia
Risk Control: Infectious Process
Self-Direction of Care
Skeletal Function
Social Support
Thermoregulation
Tissue Integrity: Skin & Mucous Membranes
Transfer Performance
Urinary Elimination

Urology

Acceptance: Health Status
Activity Tolerance
Acute Confusion Level
Bowel Continence
Bowel Elimination
Client Satisfaction: Access to Care Resources
Client Satisfaction: Continuity of Care
Client Satisfaction: Cultural Needs
  Fulfillment
Client Satisfaction: Pain Management
Client Satisfaction: Psychological Care
Client Satisfaction: Teaching
Cognition
Compliance Behavior: Prescribed Diet
Compliance Behavior: Prescribed Medication

Fatigue Level
Fluid Balance
Hydration
Kidney Function
Knowledge: Hypertension Management
Knowledge: Infection Management
Knowledge: Prescribed Activity
Knowledge: Sexual Functioning
Knowledge: Treatment Procedure
Knowledge: Treatment Regimen
Medication Response
Neurological Status: Central Motor Control
Psychosocial Adjustment: Life Change
Risk Control: Infectious Process
Self-Care: Toileting

Urology—cont'd

Sexual Identity
Sleep
Urinary Continence

Urinary Elimination
Vital Signs
Will to Live

Vascular

Activity Tolerance
Acute Confusion Level
Allergic Response: Systemic
Anxiety Level
Blood Glucose Level
Blood Transfusion Reaction
Cardiac Pump Effectiveness
Circulation Status
Client Satisfaction: Pain Management
Client Satisfaction: Physical Care
Client Satisfaction: Symptom Control
Client Satisfaction: Teaching
Cognition
Cognitive Orientation
Communication
Dignified Life Closure
Electrolyte & Acid/Base Balance
Fear Level
Fluid Balance
Grief Resolution
Hope
Hydration
Immune Hypersensitivity Response
Infection Severity
Kidney Function
Knowledge: Health Promotion
Knowledge: Illness Care
Knowledge: Treatment Procedure
Knowledge: Treatment Regimen
Neurological Status
Neurological Status: Autonomic
Neurological Status: Central Motor Control
Neurological Status: Consciousness
Neurological Status: Cranial Sensory/Motor
    Function
Neurological Status: Peripheral
Neurological Status: Spinal Sensory/Motor
    Function
Nutritional Status

Nutritional Status: Biochemical Measures
Nutritional Status: Energy
Nutritional Status: Food & Fluid Intake
Nutritional Status: Nutrient Intake
Pain Control
Pain Level
Pain: Adverse Psychological Response
Participation in Health Care Decisions
Psychomotor Energy
Psychosocial Adjustment: Life Change
Quality of Life
Respiratory Status
Rest
Risk Control: Sun Exposure
Self-Care: Eating
Sensory Function: Cutaneous
Sensory Function: Hearing
Sensory Function: Proprioception
Sensory Function: Taste & Smell
Sensory Function: Vision
Sleep
Spiritual Health
Suffering Severity
Symptom Severity
Thermoregulation
Tissue Integrity: Skin & Mucous Membranes
Tissue Perfusion: Abdominal Organs
Tissue Perfusion: Cardiac
Tissue Perfusion: Cellular
Tissue Perfusion: Cerebral
Tissue Perfusion: Peripheral
Tissue Perfusion: Pulmonary
Treatment Behavior: Illness or Injury
Urinary Elimination
Vital Signs
Weight: Body Mass
Wound Healing: Primary Intention
Wound Healing: Secondary Intention

Women's Health and Obstetrics

Activity Tolerance
Adherence Behavior: Healthy Diet
Blood Coagulation
Bowel Elimination
Breastfeeding Establishment: Maternal
Breastfeeding Maintenance
Breastfeeding Weaning
Circulation Status
Client Satisfaction: Communication
Client Satisfaction: Cultural Needs
    Fulfillment
Client Satisfaction: Pain Management
Client Satisfaction: Protection of Rights
Client Satisfaction: Teaching
Comfort Status
Community Health Status: Immunity
Community Risk Control: Communicable
    Disease
Community Risk Control: Lead Exposure
Development: Late Adulthood
Development: Middle Adulthood
Development: Young Adulthood
Discomfort Level
Family Coping
Family Functioning
Family Health Status
Family Integrity
Family Normalization
Family Participation in Professional Care
Family Social Climate
Fetal Status: Antepartum
Fetal Status: Intrapartum
Knowledge: Breastfeeding
Knowledge: Cancer Threat Reduction
Knowledge: Depression Management
Knowledge: Fertility Promotion
Knowledge: Health Promotion

Knowledge: Labor & Delivery
Knowledge: Postpartum Maternal Health
Knowledge: Preconception Maternal Health
Knowledge: Pregnancy
Knowledge: Pregnancy & Postpartum Sexual
    Function
Knowledge: Sexual Functioning
Knowledge: Weight Management
Medication Response
Nausea & Vomiting Control
Nausea & Vomiting Severity
Nutritional Status
Pain Level
Parent-Infant Attachment
Parenting: Infant/Toddler Physical Safety
Physical Fitness
Physical Maturation: Female
Postpartum Maternal Health Behavior
Prenatal Health Behavior
Respiratory Status
Rest
Risk Control: Sexually Transmitted Diseases
    (STDs)
Risk Control: Sun Exposure
Risk Control: Unexpected Pregnancy
Skeletal Function
Sleep
Smoking Cessation Behavior
Tissue Perfusion: Cardiac
Tissue Perfusion: Cerebral
Tissue Perfusion: Peripheral
Tissue Perfusion: Pulmonary
Urinary Continence
Weight: Body Mass
Weight Gain Behavior
Weight Loss Behavior
Weight Maintenance Behavior

PART SIX

Appendixes

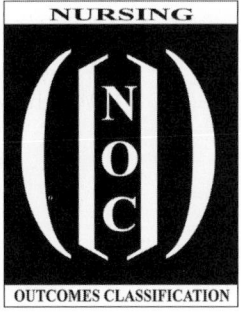

Outcomes: New, Revised, and Retired Since the Third Edition

Outcomes New to the Fourth Edition (**n** = 58)

0916	Acute Confusion Level	1834	Knowledge: Cancer Threat Reduction
1621	Adherence Behavior: Healthy Diet	1835	Knowledge: Congestive Heart Failure Management
1214	Agitation Level		
1629	Alcohol Abuse Cessation Behavior	1836	Knowledge: Depression Management
1106	Burn Healing	1837	Knowledge: Hypertension Management
1107	Burn Recovery		
0414	Cardiopulmonary Status	1842	Knowledge: Infection Management
3014	Client Satisfaction	1838	Knowledge: Multiple Sclerosis Management
3015	Client Satisfaction: Case Management		
3016	Client Satisfaction: Pain Management	1843	Knowledge: Pain Management
2008	Comfort Status	1839	Knowledge: Pregnancy & Postpartum Sexual Functioning
2009	Comfort Status: Environment		
2010	Comfort Status: Physical	1840	Knowledge: Preterm Infant Care
2011	Comfort Status: Psychospiritual	1841	Knowledge: Weight Management
2012	Comfort Status: Sociocultural	1631	Multiple Sclerosis Self-Management
2806	Community Disaster Response	0917	Neurological Status: Peripheral
1622	Compliance Behavior: Prescribed Diet	1309	Personal Resiliency
1623	Compliance Behavior: Prescribed Medication	1624	Postpartum Maternal Health Behavior
		1921	Pre-Procedure Readiness
0121	Development: Late Adulthood	0415	Respiratory Status
0122	Development: Middle Adulthood	1922	Risk Control: Hyperthermia
0123	Development: Young Adulthood	1923	Risk Control: Hypothermia
1630	Drug Abuse Cessation Behavior	1924	Risk Control: Infectious Process
2109	Discomfort Level	1925	Risk Control: Sun Exposure
1919	Elopement Occurrence	1926	Safe Wandering
1920	Elopement Propensity Risk	1625	Smoking Cessation Severity
0007	Fatigue Level	2108	Substance Withdrawal Status
1015	Gastrointestinal Function	0416	Tissue Perfusion: Cellular
0918	Heedfulness of Affected Side	1626	Weight Gain Behavior
1831	Knowledge: Arthritis Management	1627	Weight Loss Behavior
1832	Knowledge: Asthma Management	1628	Weight Maintenance Behavior
1833	Knowledge: Cancer Management		

Outcomes Revised for the Fourth Edition

LABEL NAME CHANGES (n=4)

Outcomes in this category have minor label name changes.

Third Edition Outcome	Change for Fourth Edition Outcome
2514 Abuse Recovery Status	2514 Abuse Recovery
2210 Caregiving Endurance Potential	2210 Caregiver Role Endurance
2303 Post-Procedure Recovery Status	2303 Post-Procedure Recovery
2405 Sensory Function Status	2405 Sensory Function

Definition Changes (n=30)

Outcomes in this category have minor changes in definition that clarify the concept and improve definition consistency within each scale.

1600 Adherence Behavior	1820 Knowledge: Diabetes Management
0704 Asthma Self-Management	1803 Knowledge: Disease Process
1002 Breastfeeding Maintenance	1818 Knowledge: Postpartum Maternal Health
1003 Breastfeeding Weaning	
1617 Cardiac Disease Self-Management	1812 Knowledge: Substance Use Control
2202 Caregiver Home Care Readiness	0411 Mechanical Ventilation Response: Adult
2210 Caregiver Role Endurance	2512 Neglect Recovery
2508 Caregiver Well-Being	1009 Nutritional Status: Nutrient Intake
3005 Client Satisfaction: Functional Assistance	1911 Personal Safety Behavior
3009 Client Satisfaction: Psychological Care	2002 Personal Well-Being
1601 Compliance Behavior	1906 Risk Control: Tobacco Use
1619 Diabetes Self-Management	0313 Self-Care Status
1912 Full Occurrence	2405 Sensory Function
2604 Family Normalization	1504 Social Support
2608 Family Resiliency	2005 Student Health Status
1830 Knowledge: Cardiac Disease Management	

Scale Changes (n=45)

0400 Cardiac Pump Effectiveness	1823 Knowledge: Health Promotion
2204 Caregiver-Patient Relationship	1806 Knowledge: Health Resources
0401 Circulation Status	1824 Knowledge: Illness Care
0600 Electrolyte & Acid/Base Balance	1819 Knowledge: Infant Care
1827 Knowledge: Body Mechanics	1817 Knowledge: Labor & Delivery
1800 Knowledge: Breastfeeding	1808 Knowledge: Medication
1830 Knowledge: Cardiac Disease Management	1829 Knowledge: Ostomy Care
	1826 Knowledge: Parenting
1801 Knowledge: Child Physical Safety	1809 Knowledge: Personal Safety
1821 Knowledge: Conception Prevention	1818 Knowledge: Postpartum Maternal Health
1820 Knowledge: Diabetes Management	
1802 Knowledge: Diet	1822 Knowledge: Preconception Maternal Health
1803 Knowledge: Disease Process	
1804 Knowledge: Energy Conservation	1810 Knowledge: Pregnancy
1828 Knowledge: Fall Prevention	1811 Knowledge: Prescribed Activity
1816 Knowledge: Fertility Promotion	1815 Knowledge: Sexual Functioning
1805 Knowledge: Health Behavior	1812 Knowledge: Substance Use Control

1814   Knowledge: Treatment Procedure
1813   Knowledge: Treatment Regimen
0411   Mechanical Ventilation Response: Adult
0412   Mechanical Ventilation Weaning
         Response: Adult
2102   Pain Level
0410   Respiratory Status: Airway Patency
0402   Respiratory Status: Gas Exchange

0403   Respiratory Status: Ventilation
2302   Systemic Toxin Clearance: Dialysis
0404   Tissue Perfusion: Abdominal Organs
0405   Tissue Perfusion: Cardiac
0406   Tissue Perfusion: Cerebral
0407   Tissue Perfusion: Peripheral
0408   Tissue Perfusion: Pulmonary

Outcomes in the Third Edition That Were Retired for the Fourth Edition (n = 4)

2100   Comfort Level
         Replaced with Discomfort Level
2607   Family Physical Environment
         Subsumed under Safe Home Environment
1807   Knowledge: Infection Control Replaced with Knowledge: Infection Management
1612   Weight Control
         Replaced with Weight Maintenance Behavior

Guidelines for Submission of a New or Revised Outcome
Nursing Outcomes Classification Review Form

The Nursing Outcomes Classification (NOC) research team is interested in feedback and submission of outcomes for review and potential addition to the NOC. Feedback may be organized in the following manner.

A. GENERAL COMMENTS ABOUT THE CLASSIFICATION

Comments about the classification in general are welcome, as are suggestions for outcomes that need to be developed. The outcome suggestions for development can be at the individual, family, or community level.

B. FEEDBACK ON AN OUTCOME

If the submission is a revision of an existing NOC outcome, provide a paragraph briefly describing the rationale for changes and note the changes on a copy of the existing outcome. Suggestions can include changes in the definition, indicators, or scale. Additional indicators and references can be suggested.

C. FEEDBACK ON A MEASUREMENT SCALE(S)

Comments on a particular scale are encouraged. Please briefly explain your suggestion and provide background on your experience in using the scale. Identify the outcome and provide a brief description of the patient populations(s) with which you are using the outcome.

D. GUIDELINES FOR OUTCOME SUBMISSION

Each submission of a proposed outcome must include a label, a definition, indicators, and a short list of references that support the outcome and document the indicators selected. You also may suggest a scale to use with the outcomes. A brief paragraph describing the rationale for adding the outcome to the NOC should be included. The rationale should note how the proposed outcome is different from outcomes already included in the NOC.

General Principles for Developing Outcomes

1. Define the outcome as a variable patient or client state, behavior, or perception that is responsive to nursing intervention(s).
2. Labels should be concise, stated in five or fewer words.
3. Colons can be used to make broader concepts more specific.
4. Labels should describe concepts that can be measured along a continuum.
5. Labels should be neutral and not stated as goals.
6. A set of indicators, more specific than the outcome, must be identified that can be used to determine the outcome status.
7. The definition should be a brief phrase that defines the concept and encompasses the indicators.

E. FEEDBACK ON LINKAGES TO NANDA INTERNATIONAL NURSING DIAGNOSES

Comments on linkages to nursing diagnoses are welcome. Please suggest additions or revisions with a brief rationale. For additions to the linkage list for a specific diagnosis, identify whether the NOC outcome should be listed as suggested or as an additional associated outcome.

F. FEEDBACK ON CORE OUTCOMES BY SPECIALTY

Comments on core specialty outcomes are welcome. Please send suggestions for additional outcomes, as well as any deletions you think are needed.

Comments and suggestions can be sent to:
Sue Moorhead
458 NB, College of Nursing
The University of Iowa
Iowa City, Iowa 52242
E-mail: sue-moorhead@uiowa.edu
Phone: (319) 335-7110
FAX: (319) 335-9990

Selected Publications

2006

Albers, C., Gloskey, D., Pahl, J., Kravutske, M. E., & Zuhcic, M. (2006). Methods of educating RNs to use the NOCs in their documentation. *International Journal of Nursing Terminologies & Classifications, 17*(1), 92-93.

Brier, J. (2006). NANDA, NIC, NOC care plans enhance communication among caregivers and improve measurable outcomes for patients and staff. *International Journal of Nursing Terminologies & Classifications, 17*(1), 61.

Brokel, J., & Nicholson, C. (2006). Care planning with electronic problem list and care set functions. *International Journal of Nursing Terminologies & Classifications, 17*(1), 21-22.

Burkhart, L. (2006). Integrating NNN into nursing education: A case study. *International Journal of Nursing Terminologies & Classifications, 17*(1), 22.

Burkhart, L. (2006). Measuring spiritual care in nursing practice. *International Journal of Nursing Terminologies & Classifications, 17*(1), 61.

Carlson, J. (2006). Consensus validation process: A standardized research method to identify and link the relevant NANDA, NIC, and NOC terms for local populations. *International Journal of Nursing Terminologies & Classifications, 17*(1), 23-24.

Carlson, J. (2006). Professional nursing latent tuberculosis infection standards of practice development using NANDA, NIC, and NOC. *International Journal of Nursing Terminologies & Classifications, 17*(1), 62.

Decker, S., & Roe, E. (2006). Using the nursing outcomes to define the role of the clinical nurse leader. *International Journal of Nursing Terminologies & Classifications, 17*(1), 30.

Franco de Carvalho, J. S., Fernandes Patelli, S. C., & Lima da Nobrega, M. M. (2006). Elaboration and validation of a systematic instrument for nursing care for the hypertensive client using NANDA, NOC, and NIC. *International Journal of Nursing Terminologies & Classifications, 17*(1), 50-51.

Garcia, T., Hansche, J., & Lobert, M. S. (2006). A user's guide to operationalizing NANDA, NIC, and NOC in a nursing curriculum. *International Journal of Nursing Terminologies & Classifications, 17*(1), 33-34.

Garutti Rodrigues, F. F., & Barros, A. (2006). NIC interventions and NOC outcomes in patients with activity intolerance. *International Journal of Nursing Terminologies & Classifications, 17*(1), 79.

Gloskey, D., Kravutske, M. E., & Zugcic, M. (2006). Do you need to educate RNs on how to document using the nursing outcome classification? *International Journal of Nursing Terminologies & Classifications, 17*(1), 34-35.

Johnson, M. (2006). Linking NANDA, NOC, and NIC. *International Journal of Nursing Terminologies & Classifications, 17*(1), 39-40.

Keenan, G. (2006). Revitalizing the care planning process with NANDA, NIC, and NOC using the HANDS method. *International Journal of Nursing Terminologies & Classifications, 17*(1), 87-88.

Lu, D-F., Park, H-T., Ucharattana, P., Konicek, D., & Delaney, C. (2006). Nursing outcomes classification (NOC) in SNOMED CT: A cross-mapping validation. *International Journal of Nursing Terminologies & Classifications, 17*(1), 43-44.

Kravutske, M. E., Zugcic, M., Gloskey, D., & Reed, D. (2006). Initial results from using NOCs in an acute care setting. *International Journal of Nursing Terminologies & Classifications, 17*(1), 93.

Lee, E. (2006). Analysis of nursing outcomes classification (NOC) used in neurosurgical units in Korea. *International Journal of Nursing Terminologies & Classifications, 17*(1), 73-74.

Lee, E. J. (2006). Analysis of nursing diagnoses and outcomes used in a respiratory unit in Korea. *International Journal of Nursing Terminologies & Classifications, 17*(1), 42.

Lunney, M. (2006). Helping nurses use NANDA, NOC, and NIC: Novice to expert. *Journal of Nursing Administration, 36*(3), 118-125.

Minthorn, C. (2006). Meeting Magnet research criteria with studies of NANDA, NIC, and NOC. *International Journal of Nursing Terminologies & Classifications, 17*(1), 46-47.

Moorhead, S. (2006). The importance of perspective and primary focus in choosing and measuring outcomes. *International Journal of Nursing Terminologies & Classifications, 17*(1), 91.

Pitcher, L., Strasser-Thomas, P., Hunt, P., Montgomery, M., & Daugherty, J. (2006). ECUIP your nurses—conducting NOC research in practice. *International Journal of Nursing Terminologies & Classifications, 17*(1), 88-89.

Reed, D. (2006). Characteristics of patients and settings related to the choice of indicators for Nursing Outcome Classification outcomes. *International Journal of Nursing Terminologies & Classifications, 17*(1), 90.

Sandholm, M. (2006). Teaching strategies for NANDA, NIC, and NOC from a BSN student's perspective. *International Journal of Nursing Terminologies & Classifications, 17*(1), 80.

Specht, J. P., Scherb, C. A., & Loes, J. (2006). Methodologic issues linking patient outcomes to individual nurse characteristics. *International Journal of Nursing Terminologies & Classifications, 17*(1), 54.

Swanson, E., Moorhead, S., Johnson, M., Maas, M., & Lee, M. Y. (2006). Using the model of mapping Nursing Outcomes Classification (NOC) to the International Classification of Functioning Disability and Health (ICF) to map NANDA, NIC and NOC. *International Journal of Nursing Terminologies & Classifications, 17*(1), 56-57.

Zugcic, M., Kravutske, M. E., & Gloskey, D. (2006). Relationship between utilization of selected NOCs and patient satisfaction. *International Journal of Nursing Terminologies & Classifications, 17*(1), 82.

2005

Behrenbeck, J. G., Timm, J. A., Griebenow, L. K., & Demmer, K. A. (2005). Nursing-sensitive outcome reliability testing in a tertiary care setting. *International Journal of Nursing Terminologies & Classifications, 16*(1), 14-20.

Caldwell, C. L., Wasson, D., Anderson, M. A., Brighton, V., & Dixon, L., 3rd. (2005). Development of the nursing outcome (NOC) label: Hyperactivity level. *Journal of Child and Adolescent Psychiatric Nursing, 18*(3), 95-102.

Romain, C. M. (2005). The nursing taxonomies, NANDA, NIC and NOC in hospital practice (Spanish). *Enfermeria Clinica, 15*(3), 163-166.

Von Krogh, G., Dale, C., & Naden, D. (2005). A framework for integrating NANDA, NIC, and NOC terminology in electronic patient records. *Journal of Nursing Scholarship, 37*(3), 275-281.

2004

Apalategui, M. U. (2004). Introduction to an operative structure that facilitates learning NNN. *NANDA, NIC, NOC 2004: Working together for quality nursing care: Striving toward harmonization.* Chicago, IL.

Arora, A., Pesco, J., & Krenz, M. (2004). Physical therapist modifications of the NOC to facilitate clinical accuracy in interdisciplinary computerized patient records. *NANDA, NIC, NOC 2004: Working together for quality nursing care: Striving toward harmonization.* Chicago, IL.

Baumberger, D., Sabbioni, S. B., Abderhalden, C., Staub, M. M., Schneider, C., Schweingruber, R., Vogel, D., & Widmer, R. (2004). NNN in the Bernese (Switzerland) clinical information system. *NANDA, NIC, NOC 2004: Working together for quality nursing care: Striving toward harmonization.* Chicago, IL.

Clarke, M. (2004). Diagnostic reasoning: How are our skills? *NANDA, NIC, NOC 2004: Working together for quality nursing care: Striving toward harmonization.* Chicago, IL.

Cox, T. (2004). Professional caregiver insurance risk and NNN: Risk theoretic models for predicting nursing services and costs. *NANDA, NIC, NOC 2004: Working together for quality nursing care: Striving toward harmonization.* Chicago, IL. Presented at *NANDA, NIC, NOC 2004: Working together for quality nursing care: Striving toward harmonization.*

da Silva Bastos, J., & de Almedia Lopes Monteiro da Cruz, D. (2004). Learning of scientific concepts and the development of higher mental functions according to Vygotsky. *NANDA, NIC, NOC 2004: Working together for quality nursing care: Striving toward harmonization.* Chicago, IL.

de Barros, A. L. B. L., de Lima Lopez, J., & Michel, J. L. M. (2004). NIC interventions and NOC outcomes in patients with the nursing diagnosis excess fluid volume. *NANDA, NIC, NOC 2004: Working together for quality nursing care: Striving toward harmonization.* Chicago, IL.

de Barros, A. L. B. L., Sabadini, A., & de Azevedo, S. R. (2004). Risk for infection: Nursing interventions and outcomes in hospitalized cardiac patients. *NANDA, NIC, NOC 2004: Working together for quality nursing care: Striving toward harmonization.* Chicago, IL.

Derks, A., Mooney, J., Fagerman, L., & Sterken, D. (2004). When NIC NOC does not mean child's play in a children's hospital. *NANDA, NIC, NOC 2004: Working together for quality nursing care: Striving toward harmonization.* Chicago, IL.

Espinosa, C., Mandico, R., Bros, M., & Serrano, P. (2004). NANDA-, NIC-, and NOC-based curriculum for basic nursing education. *NANDA, NIC, NOC 2004: Working together for quality nursing care: Striving toward harmonization.* Chicago, IL.

Falan, S., Keenan, G. M., & Yakel, E. (2004). Contrasting the results of two N3 language learning strategies with home care and school nurses. *NANDA, NIC, NOC 2004: Working together for quality nursing care: Striving toward harmonization.* Chicago, IL.

Ford, Y., & VanderKool, M. (2004). Implementing NANDA, NIC, and NOC in a multihospital system: Persuasion, planning, progress, and prognostication. *NANDA, NIC, NOC 2004: Working together for quality nursing care: Striving toward harmonization.* Chicago, IL.

Gabriel, R., & de Oliveira Campos, M. F. (2004). Outclinic nursing assistance for people living with HIV/AIDS. *NANDA, NIC, NOC 2004: Working together for quality nursing care: Striving toward harmonization.* Chicago, IL.

Gudmundsdottir, E., Delaney, C., Thoroddsen, A., & Karlsson, T.(2004). Translation and validation of the nursing outcomes classification labels and definitions for acute care nursing in Iceland. *Journal of Advanced Nursing, 46*(3), 292-302.

Head, B., & Androwich, I. (2004). NIC and NOC: Utility for community/public health nursing. *NANDA, NIC, NOC 2004: Working together for quality nursing care: Striving toward harmonization.* Chicago, IL.

Head, B. J., Aquilino, M., Johnson, M., Reed, D., Maas, M., & Moorhead, S. (2004). Content validity and nursing sensitivity of community-level outcomes from the nursing outcomes classification (NOC). *Journal of Nursing Scholarship, 36*(3), 251-259.

Heath, C. L., Keenan, G. M., & Yakel, E. (2004). Evaluating computer readiness of NOC indicators using the CPRI framework. *NANDA, NIC, NOC 2004: Working together for quality nursing care: Striving toward harmonization.* Chicago, IL.

Hernandez, A. M. G., & Curvo, S. D. (2004). Nursing training in NNN taxonomy. *NANDA, NIC, NOC 2004: Working together for quality nursing care: Striving toward harmonization.* Chicago, IL.

Hernandez, A. M. G., & Curvo, S. D. (2004). Results of a pilot experience with students in the first year of nursing studies using NNN taxonomy. *NANDA, NIC, NOC 2004: Working together for quality nursing care: Striving toward harmonization.* Chicago, IL.

Hoffman, L., & Blix, S. (2004). Strategies to implement NANDA, NIC, and NOC in Norwegian education. *NANDA, NIC, NOC 2004: Working together for quality nursing care: Striving toward harmonization*. Chicago, IL.

Jensen, G. A., Scherb, C., & Jones, L. (2004). NOC: Introducing a foreign language" to the clinic setting. *NANDA, NIC, NOC 2004: Working together for quality nursing care: Striving toward harmonization*. Chicago, IL.

Johnson, M., Lotegeluaki, J., & Schmidt, M. (2004). Utilizing the transtheoretical model of intentional behavior change: State-specific nursing diagnoses, interventions, and outcomes. *NANDA, NIC, NOC 2004: Working together for quality nursing care: Striving toward harmonization*. Chicago, IL.

Keenan, G. M., Yakel, E., Heath, C. L., Falan, S. L., & Stocker, J. (2004). The HANDS Project: Studying automated use of NANDA, NOC, and NIC under real-time clinical conditions. *NANDA, NIC, NOC 2004: Working together for quality nursing care: Striving toward harmonization*. Chicago, IL.

Kerr, P., Moorhead, S., Johnson, M., & Maas, M. (2004). Challenges of measuring construct validity of nursing outcomes. *NANDA, NIC, NOC 2004: Working together for quality nursing care: Striving toward harmonization*. Chicago, IL.

Killeen, M. B. (2004). Practical applications of NNN across the curriculum. *NANDA, NIC, NOC 2004: Working together for quality nursing care: Striving toward harmonization*. Chicago, IL.

Killeen, M. B., Keenan, G. M., Stocker, J., & Perry, A. (2004). Michigan Nurses Association awards for outstanding innovations in NNN use. *NANDA, NIC, NOC 2004: Working together for quality nursing care: Striving toward harmonization*. Chicago, IL.

Konrad, C., & Guebert, L. (2004). Nursing-sensitive outcomes in maternity nursing: A discussion of content validity. *NANDA, NIC, NOC 2004: Working together for quality nursing care: Striving toward harmonization*. Chicago, IL.

Kuiper, K. A., Kautz, D. D., & Pesut, D. J. (2004). Clinical reasoning, OPT, and NNN language: Evaluating structure, content, process and outcomes. *NANDA, NIC, NOC 2004: Working together for quality nursing care: Striving toward harmonization*. Chicago, IL.

Lee, B. (2004). Availability of NOC for the evaluation of quality of nursing care in Korea. *NANDA, NIC, NOC 2004: Working together for quality nursing care: Striving toward harmonization*. Chicago, IL.

Lobert, J. H., Kuzak, M., Garcia, T., & Schulte, K. E. (2004). The integration of NANDA, NIC, and NOC into an associate degree and practical nurse curriculum. *NANDA, NIC, NOC 2004: Working together for quality nursing care: Striving toward harmonization*. Chicago, IL.

Lunney, M., & Fiore, L. (2004). Nurses' use of standard terms in an electronic record with and without NNN. *NANDA, NIC, NOC 2004: Working together for quality nursing care: Striving toward harmonization*. Chicago, IL.

Lunney, M., Parker, L., Fiore, L., Cavendish, R., & Pulcini, J. (2004). Feasibility of studying the effects of using NANDA, NIC, and NOC on nurses' power and children's outcomes. *CIN: Computers, Informatics, Nursing, 22*(6), 316-325.

Matney, S., Androwich, I., Correia, C., Danko, A., Grobe, S., Harris, M., Haskell, R., Kennedy, R., & Russler, D. (2004). Developing methods to message domain knowledge using NANDA, NIC, and NOC coding systems. *NANDA, NIC, NOC 2004: Working together for quality nursing care: Striving toward harmonization*. Chicago, IL.

Moorhead, S., & Johnson, M. (2004). Diagnostic-specific outcomes and nursing effectiveness research. *International Journal of Nursing Terminologies & Classifications, 15*(2), 49-57.

Moorhead, S., Johnson, M., & Maas, M. (2004). *Iowa outcomes project: Nursing outcomes classification (NOC)*. St. Louis: Mosby.

Moorhead, S., Johnson, M., Maas, M., & Reed, D. (2004). Results of testing the nursing outcomes classification: Are the measurement scales reliable and do they capture change in patient status? *NANDA, NIC, NOC 2004: Working together for quality nursing care: Striving toward harmonization*. Chicago, IL.

Morgan, M. J. (2004). Integrating several standardized languages into advanced practice nursing education via a web-based clinical log. *NANDA, NIC, NOC 2004: Working together for quality nursing care: Striving toward harmonization*. Chicago, IL.

O'Connor, N., & Brenner, P. S. (2004). Exploring the inductive utility of NNN in a graduate health policy course. *NANDA, NIC, NOC 2004: Working together for quality nursing care: Striving toward harmonization*. Chicago, IL.

Ogasawara, C., Furuhashi, Y., Hasegawa, T., Kume, Y., Takahashi, I., Katayama, Y., Andou, M., Kuroda, M., Araki, Y., Yamamoto, Y., Okazaki, S., & Tanabe, M. (2004). Nursing diagnoses and nursing intervention in Japan for terminal stage breast cancer patients and admitted under differing care aims. *NANDA, NIC, NOC 2004: Working together for quality nursing care: Striving toward harmonization*. Chicago, IL.

Reed, D., Moorhead, S., Johnson, M., & Maas, M. (2004). Use of the indicators for selected core NOC outcomes: Similarities and differences across ten field settings. *NANDA, NIC, NOC 2004: Working together for quality nursing care: Striving toward harmonization*. Chicago, IL.

Ruiz, J. B., Krenz, M., Fallen, R., & Edson, D. (2004). Using NIC and NOC concepts and terminology to develop a computerized data collection. *NANDA, NIC, NOC 2004: Working together for quality nursing care: Striving toward harmonization*. Chicago, IL.

Smith, K. (2004). Interdisciplinary care planning and documentation using NIC and NOC. *NANDA, NIC, NOC 2004: Working together for quality nursing care: Striving toward harmonization*. Chicago, IL.

Stocker, J., Barkauskas, V., Keenan, G. M., & Hinshaw, A. S. (2004). Evaluating home care nursing outcomes with OASIS and NOC. *NANDA, NIC, NOC 2004: Working together for quality nursing care: Striving toward harmonization*. Chicago, IL.

Sweeney, S. (2004). Report of NNN conference March, 2004: Working together for quality nursing care: Striving toward harmonization. *ACENDIO Newsletter, 14*(11).

Thayer, A., & Coler, M. S. (2004). Implementing NNN in the documentation of a wellness center in a multicampus independent living facility for the elderly: Implications for intra/inter healthcare staff communication. *NANDA, NIC, NOC 2004: Working together for quality nursing care: Striving toward harmonization*. Chicago, IL.

Vieira, E. R., Michel, J. L. M., & Fonseca, S. M. (2004). Risk for bleeding and bleeding in hematological patients: Proposal of two nursing diagnoses. *NANDA, NIC, NOC 2004: Working together for quality nursing care: Striving toward harmonization*. Chicago, IL.

Von Krogh, G., & Dale, C. (2004). Developing a model for nursing documentation in the electronic patient record. *NANDA, NIC, NOC 2004: Working together for quality nursing care: Striving toward harmonization*. Chicago, IL.

2003

Ahern, C. (2003). Applying standardized nursing language to three cardiac and pulmonary rehabilitation programs in rural setting. *International Journal of Nursing Terminologies & Classifications, 14*(4), 32.

Cavendish, R. (2003). School nurses' use of NANDA, NIC, and NOC to describe children's abdominal pain. *International Journal of Nursing Terminologies & Classifications, 14*(4), 17-18.

Behrenbeck, J. G. (2003). Nursing-sensitive outcome implementation and reliability testing in a tertiary care setting. *International Journal of Nursing Terminologies & Classifications, 14*(4), 12.

Bjornsdottir, G., & Thorhallsdottir, I. (2003). An internet-based survey of Icelandic nurses on their use of and attitudes toward NANDA, NIC, and NOC. *International Journal of Nursing Terminologies & Classifications, 14*(4), 32-33.

Caldwell, C. L., Wasson, D., Brighton, V., Dixon, L., & Anderson, M. A. (2003). Personal autonomy: Development of a NOC label. *International Journal of Nursing Terminologies & Classifications, 14*(4), 12-13.

Calsinski de Assis, C., & Botura Leite de Barras, A. L. (2003). Evaluation of proposed interventions for fatigue in patients hospitalized with congestive heart failure. *International Journal of Nursing Terminologies & Classifications, 14*(4), 49.

Cox, R. (2003). Using NANDA, NIC, and NOC with Levine's conservation principles in a nursing home. *International Journal of Nursing Terminologies & Classifications, 14*(4), 41.

Demmer, K. (2003). NOC implementation and testing in a cardiac surgery ICU. *International Journal of Nursing Terminologies & Classifications, 14*(4), 13-14.

Finesilver, C. (2003). Use of standardized language in neuroscience nursing. *International Journal of Nursing Terminologies & Classifications, 14*(4), 52.

Finesilver, C., & Metzler, D. (2003). Use of NANDA, NIC, and NOC in a baccalaureate curriculum. *International Journal of Nursing Terminologies & Classifications, 14*(4), 34-35.

Flatt, M. (2003). Teaching systems transformation. *International Journal of Nursing Terminologies & Classifications, 14*(4), 35.

Frederick, J., & Watters, M. (2003). Integrating nursing acuity, NANDA, NIC, and NOC into an automated nursing documentation system. *International Journal of Nursing Terminologies & Classifications, 14*(4), 26.

Graiver, M., & Shannon, M., & Decker, S. (2003). Cognitive coherence: Use of nursing's standardized language. *International Journal of Nursing Terminologies & Classifications, 14*(4), 52.

Head, B. J., Maas, M., & Johnson, M. (2003). Validity and community-health-nursing sensitivity of six outcomes for community health nursing with older clients. *Public Health Nursing, 20*(5), 385-398.

Hughes, R. (2003). The use of NANDA, NIC, and NOC in the identification and measurement of problems, interventions, and outcomes in spinal cord injury. *International Journal of Nursing Terminologies & Classifications, 14*(4), 18-19.

Jenkins, P. (2003). Using Caretracker to validate NOC scores. *International Journal of Nursing Terminologies & Classifications, 14*(4), 53.

Johnson, M., Moorhead, S., Maas, M., & Reed, D. (2003). Evaluation of the sensitivity and use of the nursing outcomes classification. *Journal of Nursing Measurement, 11*(2), 119-134.

Johnson, M., Reed, D., Maas, M., & Moorhead, S. (2003). Clinical evaluation of NOC outcomes. *International Journal of Nursing Terminologies & Classifications, 14*(4), 14.

Keenan, G. (2003). Assessing the reliability, validity, and sensitivity of nursing outcomes classification in home care settings. *Journal of Nursing Measurement, 11*(2), 135-155.

Keenan, G., Barkauskas, V., Stocker, J., Johnson, M., Maas, M., Moorhead, S., & Reed, D. (2003). Establishing the validity, reliability, and sensitivity of NOC in an adult care nurse practitioner setting. *Outcomes Management, 7*(2), 74-83.

Keenan, G., Falan, S., Heath, C., & Treder, M. (2003). Establishing competency in the use of North American Nursing Diagnosis Association, nursing outcomes classification, and nursing interventions classification terminology. *Journal of Nursing Measurement, 11*(2), 183-198.

Keenan, G., Heath, C., Treder, M., Stocker, J., & Yakel, B. (2003). HANDS: Refining methods to generate comparable nursing data. *International Journal of Nursing Terminologies & Classifications, 14*(4), 28.

Keenan, G., Stocker, J., Barkauskas, V., Treder, M., & Heath, C. (2003). Toward collecting a standardized nursing data set across the continuum: Case of adult care nurse practitioner setting. *Outcomes Management, 7*(3), 113-120.

Keenan, G., Stocker, J., Barkauskas, V., Treder, M., & Heath, C. (2003). Toward integrating a common nursing data set in home care to facilitate monitoring outcomes across settings. *Journal of Nursing Measurement, 11*(2), 157-169.

Keenan, G. M., Barkauskas, V., Lee, J., Stocker, J., Treder, M., & Clingerman, E. (2003). Evaluation of NOC measures in home care nursing practice. *International Journal of Nursing Terminologies & Classifications, 14*(4), 50.

Killeen, M. (2003). Use of NANDA, NIC, and NOC as a framework for cyclic perimenstrual pain and discomfort. *International Journal of Nursing Terminologies & Classifications, 14*(4), 19-20.

Kol, Y., Jacobson, O., Wieler, S., Weiss, D., & Sadeh, Z. (2003). Evaluation of the nursing outcomes classification (NOC)—from theory to practice in Israel. *Outcomes Management, 7*(3), 121-128.

Krenz, M. (2003). The use of NOC to direct a competency-based curriculum. *International Journal of Nursing Terminologies & Classifications, 14*(4), 59.

Lippens, B. (2003). Use of NANDA, NIC, and NOC in infection control. *International Journal of Nursing Terminologies & Classifications, 14*(4), 20.

Lopes, J., & de Barros, A. L. B. L. (2003). Validation of priority NIC interventions and suggested NOC outcomes for fluid volume excess. *International Journal of Nursing Terminologies & Classifications, 14*(4), 50.

Lunney, M., & Parker, L. (2003). Effects of using NANDA, NIC, and NOC on health outcomes of schoolchildren: A pilot study. *International Journal of Nursing Terminologies & Classifications, 14*(4), 21.

Maas, M., Johnson, M., Moorhead, S., Reed, D., & Sweeney, S. (2003). Evaluation of the reliability and validity of nursing outcomes of classification patient outcomes and measures. *Journal of Nursing Measurement, 11*(2), 97-117.

McCloskey, J., & Johnson, M. (2003). Indicia. RE: Letter to editor in reference to review by Mary Ersek. *CIN: Computers, Informatics, Nursing, 21*(1), 10-11.

Moorhead, S., Johnson, M., Maas, M., & Reed, D. (2003). Testing the nursing outcomes classification in three clinical units in a community hospital. *Journal of Nursing Measurement, 11*(2), 171-181.

Morales, J., Azanon, R., Rodriguez, M., Palma, J., & Rodriguez, M. (2003). Implementing a standardized nursing language system in the prehospital emergency care setting. *International Journal of Nursing Terminologies & Classifications, 14*(4), 36-37.

Mrayyan, M. (2003). Nurse autonomy, nurse job satisfaction and client satisfaction with nursing care: Their place in nursing data sets. *Canadian Journal of Nursing Leadership, 16*(2), 74-82.

Nielsen, T., & Schutte, S. (2003). Linking nursing outcomes to long-term care quality indicators. *International Journal of Nursing Terminologies & Classifications, 14*(4), 55.

Pehler, S. R., & Bodenbender, K. (2003). Concept maps as a tool for learning standardized languages. *International Journal of Nursing Terminologies & Classifications, 14*(4), 39.

Porcella, A. (2003). Nursing outcomes across a surgical care episode. *International Journal of Nursing Terminologies & Classifications, 14*(4), 15.

Powelson, S., & Leiby, K. (2003). Implementation of standardized nursing language at a university. *International Journal of Nursing Terminologies & Classifications, 14*(4), 60.

Scherb, C. (2003). Describing nursing effectiveness through standardized nursing languages and computerized clinical data. *International Journal of Nursing Terminologies & Classifications, 14*(4), 29.

Scherb, C., & Cox-Kolek, M. (2003). Chemical dependency and standardized nursing language. *International Journal of Nursing Terminologies & Classifications, 14*(4), 56.

Scherb, C., Lehmkuhl, J., & Leasman, E. (2003). The use of standardized nursing language by physical therapy, occupational therapy, and speech pathology in acute care. *International Journal of Nursing Terminologies & Classifications, 14*(4), 44-45.

Scherb, C. A., & Bellinger, S. L. (2003). Validity surveys: Selected NOC physiologic outcomes. *International Journal of Nursing Terminologies & Classifications, 14*(4), 15-16.

Schifalacqua, M., Hook, M., & Lotegeluaki, J. (2003). Program, practice, and vision: Standardized nursing language and the computerized patient record. *International Journal of Nursing Terminologies & Classifications, 14*(4), 30.

Specht, J. P. (2003). Nursing outcomes for evaluations of caregiver outcomes in a rural Alzheimer demonstration project. *International Journal of Nursing Terminologies & Classifications, 14*(4), 51.

Torre, R., & Bertazzoni, G. (2003). Nursing Interventions Classification (NIC) and Nursing Outcome Classification (NOC) of Iowa University: A methods, tools, and contents description (Italian). *Professioni Infermieristiche, 56*(3), 143-158.

Van De Castle, B. (2003). Comparisons of NANDA/NIC/NOC linkages between nursing expert and nursing students. *International Journal of Nursing Terminologies & Classifications, 14*(4), 40.

Wasson, D., Dixon, L., Brighton, V., Caldwell, C., & Anderson, M. A. (2003). Hyperactivity level: Development of a nursing outcome label. *International Journal of Nursing Terminologies & Classifications, 14*(4), 16.

2002

Barros, A. L. B., Fakih, F. T., & Michel, J. L. M. (2002). The use of computers as a tool for nursing process implementation: The experience of Hospital Sao Paulo. *Revista Brasileira de Enfermagem, 55*(6), 714-719.

Keenan, G. M., Killeen, M. B., & Clingerman, E. (2002). NANDA, NOC, and NIC: Progress toward a nursing information infrastructure. *Nursing Education Perspectives, 23*(4), 162.

Johnson, M. R. (2002). Tools and systems for improved outcomes. Outcomes for an outcomes information system. *Outcomes Management, 6*(4), 143-145.

Johnson, M. R. (2002). Tools and systems for improved outcomes. Variables for outcome analysis. *Outcomes Management, 6*(3), 95-98.

Johnson, M. R. (2002). Tools and systems for improved outcomes. Institute of Medicine report on healthcare quality. *Outcomes Management, 6*(2), 45-48.

Johnson, M. R. (2002). Tools and systems for improved outcomes. Criteria for standardized languages. *Outcomes Management, 6*(1), 1-3.

Maas, M. L., Reed, D., Reeder, K. M., Kerr, P., Specht, J. P., Johnson, M., & Moorhead, S. (2002). Clinical adequacy of NOC outcomes: A report of field testing. In N. Oud (Ed.), Acendio 2002: *Proceedings of the special conference of the Association of Common European Nursing Diagnoses, Interventions, and Outcomes in Vienna* (pp. 45-64). Bern: Verlag Has Huber.

Maas, M. L., Reed, D., Reeder, K. M., Kerr, P., Specht, T., Johnson, M., & Moorhead, S. (2002). Nursing outcomes classification: A preliminary report of field testing. *Outcomes Management, 6*(3), 112-119.

Scherb, C. (2002). Outcomes research: Making a difference in practice. *Outcomes Management, 6*(1), 22-26.

Yom, Y.-H., Chi, S. A., & Yoo, H. S. (2002). Application of nursing diagnoses, interventions, and outcomes to patients undergoing abdominal surgery in Korea. *International Journal of Nursing Terminologies & Classifications, 13*(3), 77-87.

2001

Cavendish, R., Lunney, M., Kraynyak-Luise, B., & Richardson, K. (2001). The nursing outcomes classification: Its relevance to school nursing. *The Journal of School Nursing, 17*(4), 189-197.

Frederick, J., Scherb, C. A., Smith-Foreman, K., Witt, S., Quiram, J., Wagenaar, J., Slama, C., Bottema, K., Muilenburg, J., & Evans, K. (2001). Speaking a common language: Standardized nursing languages have increased the visibility of nursing practice at three facilities. *American Journal of Nursing, 101*(3), 2400-2403.

Head, B. (2001). Impaired home maintenance management. In M. Maas, K. Buckwalter, M. Hardy, T. Tripp-Reimer, M. Titler, & J. P. Specht (Eds.). *Nursing care of older adults: Diagnoses, outcomes and interventions* (pp. 64-74). St. Louis: Mosby.

Johnson, M., Bulechek, G., Dochterman-McCloskey, J. Maas, M., & Moorhead, S. (2001). *Nursing diagnoses, interventions, and outcomes: NANDA, NIC, and NOC linkages.* St. Louis: Mosby.

Legge, L. (2001). Measure of success: Southern Minnesota project documents nursing's effectiveness. *Nursing Minnesota, 6*(3), 8-13.

Maas, M. L., Buckwalter, K. C., Hardy, M D., Tripp-Reimer, T., Titler, M., & Specht, J. (Eds.). (2001). *Nursing care of older adults: Diagnoses, outcomes and interventions.* St. Louis: Mosby.

Maas, M., & Specht, J. (2001). Bowel incontinence. In M. Maas, K. Buckwalter, M. Hardy, T. Tripp-Reimer, M. Titler, & J. P. Specht (Eds.). *Nursing care of older adults: Diagnoses, outcomes and interventions* (pp. 238-251). St. Louis: Mosby.

Maas, M., & Specht, J. (2001). Impaired physical mobility. In M. Maas, K. Buckwalter, M. Hardy, T. Tripp-Reimer, M. Titler, & J. P. Specht (Eds.). *Nursing care of older adults: Diagnoses, outcomes and interventions* (pp. 337-365). St. Louis: Mosby.

Mastal, P. (2001). Ambulatory nursing outcomes. *AACN Viewpoint 23*(4), 6-7.

Moorhead, S., & V. Brighton. (2001). Anxiety and fear. In M. Maas, K. Buckwalter, M. Hardy, T. Tripp-Reimer, M. Titler, & J. P. Specht (Eds.). *Nursing care of older adults: Diagnoses, outcomes and interventions* (pp. 571-592). St. Louis: Mosby.

Schoenfelder, D. P., & Culp, K. (2001). Sleep pattern disturbance. In M. Maas, K. Buckwalter, M. Hardy, T. Tripp-Reimer, M. Titler, & J. P. Specht (Eds.). *Nursing care of older adults: Diagnoses, outcomes and interventions* (pp. 401-413). St. Louis: Mosby.

Specht, J., & Maas, M. (2001). Urinary incontinence: Functional, iatrogenic, overflow, reflex, stress, total and urge. In M. Maas, K. Buckwalter, M. Hardy, T. Tripp-Reimer, M. Titler, & J. P. Specht (Eds.). *Nursing care of older adults: Diagnoses, outcomes and interventions* (pp. 252-278). St. Louis: Mosby.

Swanson, E., & Drury, J. (2001). Sensory/Perceptual alteration. In M. Maas, K. Buckwalter, M. Hardy, T. Tripp-Reimer, M. Titler, & J. P. Specht (Eds.). *Nursing care of older adults: Diagnoses, outcomes and interventions* (pp. 476-491). St. Louis: Mosby.

Wakefield, B. (2001). Altered nutrition: less than body requirements. In M. Maas, K. Buckwalter, M. Hardy, T. Tripp-Reimer, M. Titler, & J. P. Specht (Eds.). *Nursing care of older adults: Diagnoses, outcomes and interventions* (pp. 145-157). St. Louis: Mosby.

Wakefield, B. (2001). Ineffective breathing pattern. In M. Maas, K. Buckwalter, M. Hardy, T. Tripp-Reimer, M. Titler, & J. P. Specht (Eds.). *Nursing care of older adults: Diagnoses, outcomes and interventions* (pp. 313-323). St. Louis: Mosby.

Wakefield, B., Mentes, J., et al. (2001). Acute confusion. In M. Maas, K. Buckwalter, M. Hardy, T. Tripp-Reimer, M. Titler, & J. P. Specht (Eds.). *Nursing care of older adults: Diagnoses, outcomes and interventions* (pp. 442-454). St. Louis: Mosby.

Weiler, K., & Moorhead, S. (2001). Self determination. In M. Maas, K. Buckwalter, M. Hardy, T. Tripp-Reimer, M. Titler, & J. P. Specht (Eds.). *Nursing care of older adults: Diagnoses, outcomes and interventions* (pp. 706-718). St. Louis: Mosby.

Williams, J., Skirton, H., Reed, D., Johnson, M., Mass, M., & Daack-Hirsch, S. (2001). Genetic counseling outcomes validation by genetics nurses in the UK and US. *Journal of Nursing Scholarship, 33*(4), 369-374.

2000

Aquilino, M., & Keenan, G. (2000). Having our say: Nursing's standardized nomenclatures. *American Journal of Nursing, 100*(7), 33-38.

Daly, J. (2000). Bowel elimination. In H. Harkreader (Ed.), *Fundamentals of nursing: Caring and clinical judgment* (pp. 846-883). Philadelphia: W.B. Saunders.

Daly, J. (2000). Planning for intervention. In H. Harkreader (Ed.), *Fundamentals of nursing: Caring and clinical judgment* (pp. 237-261). Philadelphia: W.B. Saunders.

Denehy, J. (2000). Measuring the outcomes of school nursing practice: Showing that school nurses do make a difference. *Journal of School Nursing, 16*(1), 2-4.

Dorr, G. G., Prophet, C. M., Gibbs, T. D., Porcella, A. A., & Clemons, D. K. (2000). *Implementation and evaluation of Standardized Nursing Languages (SNLs) in a Clinical Information System (CIS)* (183-189). Proceedings at the Nursing Informatics: One Step Beyond: The Evolution of Technology and Nursing. Auckland, New Zealand: Adis International.

Iowa Outcomes Project. M. Johnson, M. Maas & S. Moorhead (Eds.). (2000). *Nursing Outcomes Classification (NOC)* (2nd ed.). St. Louis: Mosby.

Kerr, P. (2000). Comparing two nursing outcomes reporting initiatives. *Outcomes Management for Nursing Practice, 4*(3), 144-149.

Maas, M., Moorhead, S., Specht, J., Schoenfelder, D., Swanson, E. A., Johnson, M., & Westra, B. L. (2000). Concept development of nursing-sensitive patient outcomes. In B. Rogers & K. Knafl (Eds.). *Concept analysis in nursing research* (pp. 387-400). New York: Springer Publishing.

McBeth, A. J., Weydt, A. P., Frederick, J. A., Scherb, C. A., & Foreman, K. M. (2000). Staffing challenges and opportunities in the rural setting. In M. F. Fralic (Ed.), *Staffing management and methods: Tools and techniques for nurse leaders* (AONE Management) San Francisco: Jossey-Bass.

Morrison, R. (2000). Evaluation of NOC instruments with chronically ill patients. *Southern Online Journal of Nursing Research 1*(1), 1-11.

Peters, R. M. (2000). Using NOC outcomes of risk control in prevention, early detection, and control of hypertension. *Outcomes Management for Nursing Practice, 4*(1), 39-45.

Prophet, C. M. (2000). The evolution of a clinical database: From local to standardized clinical languages. *Proceedings of the Annual Symposium of the American Medical Informatics Association (AMIA)* (pp. 660-664), Philadelphia: Hanley & Belfus.

Scherb, C. A. (2000). Measuring nursing effectiveness using standardized nursing languages. *Nursing Minnesota, 5*(9), 12.

Scherb, C. A., Frederick, J. (2000). Standardized nursing language: A necessity for computer information systems. *Clinical Data Management, 7*(1), 4-7, 12.

Scherb, C. A. (2000). Outcomes research: Making a difference in patient care. *Network News, 2*(5), 14.

Schoenfelder, D. P., Swanson, E. A., Specht, J. K. P., Johnson, M., & Maas, M. (2000). Outcome indicators for direct and indirect caregiving. *Clinical Nursing Research: An International Journal, 9*(1), 47-69.

Specht, J., Maas, M., Willit, S., & Meyers, N. (2000). Intermittent catheterization. In G. Bulechek & J. McCloskey (Eds.). *Nursing interventions: Treatments for nursing diagnoses* (3rd edition). Philadelphia: Saunders.

1999

Denehy, J., & Poulton, S. (1999). The use of standardized language in individualized healthcare plans. *The Journal of School Nursing, 15*(1), 38-45.

Heller, C., & Vlasses, F. (Eds.). (1999) Models of care for asthma. Chicago: Athena Healthcare Communications.

Johnson, M., & Maas, M. (1999). Nursing-sensitive patient outcomes: Development and importance for use in assessing health care effectiveness. In E. Cohen & V. DeBack (Eds.). *The outcomes mandate, case management in health care today* (pp. 37-48). St. Louis: Mosby.

Kinnaird, L. (1999). Patient education management: For nurse managers, education directors, case managers, discharge planners. *American Health Consultants, 6*(12), 133-135.

Maas, M., & Kerr, P. (1999). Risk adjustment in nursing effectiveness research. *Outcomes Management for Nursing Practice, 3*(2), 50-52.

Maas, M., & Specht, J. P. (1999). Context and patient outcomes in nursing homes. In A. S. Hinshaw & F. Feetham (Eds.), *State of the science in nursing research* (pp. 655-663). New York: Springer Publishing.

Poulton, S., & Denehy, J. (1999). Standardized languages in nursing: Integrating NANDA, NIC, and NOC into IHPs. In M. J. Arnold & C. K. Silkworth, *The school nurse's source book of individualized healthcare plans* (Vol. II, pp. 25-40). North Branch, MN: Sunrise River Press.

1998

Cox, R. (1998). Implementing nurse sensitive outcomes into care planning at a long-term care facility. *Journal of Nursing Care Quality, 12*(5), 41-51.

Denehy, J. (1998). Integrating Nursing Outcomes Classification in nursing education. *Journal of Nursing Care Quality, 12*(5), 73-84.

Donahue, M. P., & Brighton, V. (1998). Nursing Outcomes Classification: Development and implementation. *Journal of Nursing Care Quality, 12*(5), vii-viii.

Garand, L., Gerdner, L. A., Buckwalter, K. C., & Wakefield, B. (1998). Neuropsychiatric disorders. In M. A. Boyd & M. A. Nihart (Eds.). *Psychiatric mental health nursing* (pp. 612-666). Philadelphia: Lippincott.

Goode, C. (1998). About identifying nurse-specific cardiac outcomes. *Nursing Management, 29*(11), 72.

Hayewski, C., Maupin, J., Rapp, D., Sitterding, M., & Pappas, J. (1998). Implementation of Nursing Intervention Classification and Nursing Outcome Classification in a patient education plan. *Journal of Nursing Care Quality, 12*(5), 30-40.

Johnson, M., & Maas, M. (1998). The Nursing Outcomes Classification. *Journal of Nursing Care Quality, 12*(5), 9-20.

Johnson, M. (1998). Overview of the Nursing Outcomes Classification (NOC). *On-line Journal of Nursing Informatics, 2*(2). Retrieved from http://www.eaa-knowledge. Com/ojni/ni/dm/v2n2.html

Johnson, M., & Maas, M. (1998). Nursing Outcomes Classification. In J. J. Fitzpatrick (Ed.), *Encyclopedia of nursing research* (pp. 378-379). New York: Springer.

Johnson, M., & Maas, M. (1998). Implementing the Nursing Outcomes Classification in a practice setting. *Outcomes Management for Nursing Practice, 2*(3), 99-104.

Keenan, G. & Aquilino, M. (1998). Standardized nomenclatures: Keys to continuity of care, nursing accountability and nursing effectiveness. *Outcomes Management for Nursing Practice, 2*(2), 81-86.

Maas, M., Delaney, C., & Huber, D. (1998). Contextual variables and assessment of the outcome effects of nursing interventions. *Outcomes Management for Nursing Practice, 3*(1), 4-6.

Maas, M., & Head, B. (1998). Moving to measurement. *Outcomes Management for Nursing Practice, 2*(4), 139-142.

Maas, M. (1998). Structure and process constraints on nursing accountability. *Outcomes Management for Nursing Practice, 2*(2), 51-53.

Maas, M. (1998). Outcome data accountability. *Outcomes Management for Nursing Practice, 2*(1), 3-5.

Maas, M. (1998). Nursing's role in interdisciplinary accountability for patient outcomes. *Outcomes Management for Nursing Practice, 2*(3), 92-94.

McCloskey, J. C., & Maas, M. (1998). Interdisciplinary team: The nursing perspective is essential. *Nursing Outlook, 46*, 157-163.

Moorhead, S., Head, B., Johnson, M., & Maas, M. (1998). The nursing outcomes taxonomy: Development and coding. *Journal of Nursing Care Quality, 12*(6), 56-63.

Moorhead, S., Clarke, M., Willits, M., & Tomsha, K. (1998). Nursing Outcomes Classification implementation projects across the care continuum. *Journal of Nursing Care Quality, 12*(5), 52-63.

Prophet, C., & Delaney, C. (1998). Nursing Outcomes Classification: Implications for nursing information systems and the computer-based patient record. *Journal of Nursing Care Quality, 12*(5), 21-29.

Rankin, M., Donahue, P., Davis, K., Katseres, J., Wedig, J. A., Johnson, M., & Maas, M. (1998). Dignified dying as a nursing outcome. *Outcomes Management for Nursing Practice, 2*(3),105-110.

Scherb, C. A., Rapp, C. G., Johnson, M., & Maas, M. (1998). The Nursing Outcomes Classification (NOC): Validation by rehabilitation nurses. *Journal of Rehabilitation Nursing 23*(4), 174-191.

Timm, J., & Behrenbeck, J. (1998). Implementing the Nursing Outcomes Classification in a clinical information system in a tertiary care setting. *Journal of Nursing Care Quality, 12*(5), 64-72.

1997

Daly, J., Maas, M., & Johnson, M. (1997). Development of play and leisure nursing-sensitive patient outcomes. *Journal of Clinical Geropsychology, 3*(4), 267-273.

Daly, J., Maas, M., & Johnson, M. (1997). Nursing-sensitive Outcomes Classification (NOC): An essential element in data sets for nursing and health care effectiveness. *Computers in Nursing, 15*(2 Suppl.), S82-S86.

Head, B., Maas, M., & Johnson, M. (1997). Outcomes for home and community nursing in integrated delivery systems. *Caring Magazine, 16*(1), 50-56.

Iowa Outcomes Project. (1997). M. Johnson & M. Maas (Eds.). *Nursing Outcomes Classification (NOC).* St. Louis: Mosby.

Maas, M., & Johnson, M. (1997). Advancing nursing's accountability for outcomes. *Outcomes Management for Nursing Practice, 2*(1), 3-4.

Maas, M. (1997). Nursing-sensitive Outcomes Classification (NOC): Completing the essential comprehensive languages for nursing. Classification of Nursing Diagnosis: Proceedings of the 12th Conference North American Nursing Diagnosis Association (NANDA) (pp. 40-47) Pittsburgh, PA.

Prophet, C., Dorr, G. G., Gibbs, T. D., & Porcella, A. A. (1997). Implementation of standardized nursing languages (NIC, NOC) in on-line care planning and documentation (pp. 395-400). *Informatics: The Impact of Nursing Knowledge on Health Care Informatics.* Amsterdam: IOS Press.

Swanson, E., Jensen, D. P., Specht, J., Saylor, D., Johnson, M., & Maas, M. (1997). Caregiving: Concept analysis and outcomes. *Scholarly Inquiry for Nursing Practice: An International Journal, 11*(1), 65-76.

1996

Johnson, S. L., Brady-Schluttner, K., Ellenbecker, S., Johnson, M., Lassengard, E., Maas, M., Stone, J., & Westra, B. L. (1996). Evaluating physical functional outcomes: One category of the system. *MEDSURG Journal of Nursing, 5*, 157-162.

Maas, M., Johnson, M., & Kraus, V. (1996). Nursing-sensitive patient Outcomes Classification. In K. Kelly (Ed.), *Series on nursing administration: Outcomes of effective management practices* (Vol. 8, pp. 20-35). Thousand Oaks, CA: Sage Publications.

Maas, M., Johnson, M., & Moorhead, S. (1996). Classifying nursing-sensitive patient outcomes. *Image-Journal of Nursing Scholarship, 28*(4), 295-301.

1995-1992

Johnson, M., & Maas, M. (1995). Classification of nursing-sensitive patient outcomes. In N. M. Lang (Ed.). *Nursing Data Systems: The emerging framework* (pp. 177-183). Washington, DC: The American Nurses Association.

Delaney, C., Mehmert, M., Prophet, C., & Crossley, J. (1994). Establishment of the research value of nursing minimum data sets. *Nursing informatics: An international overview for nursing in a technological era* (pp. 169-173). Amsterdam: Elsevier.

Johnson, M., & Maas, M. (1994). Nursing-focused patient outcomes: Challenge for the nineties. In J. C. McCloskey & H. Grace (Eds.), *Current issues in nursing* (4th ed., pp. 136-142). St. Louis: Mosby.

Prophet, C. (1994). Nurses' orders in manual and computerized systems. In S. J. Grobe & E. S. P. Pluyter-Wenting (Eds.), *Nursing informatics: An international overview for nursing in a technological era* (pp. 286-289). Amsterdam: Elsevier.

Prophet, C. M., & Walker, K. P. (1993). Integration of systems applications: Computerized documentation of the patient discharge referral (pp. 185-196). Proceedings of the 1993 annual Healthcare Information and Management Systems Society (HIMSS) conference, San Diego, CA.

Prophet, C. (1993). Patient problem/nursing diagnosis form: A computer-generated chart document (pp. 326-330). Proceedings of the Seventeenth Annual Symposium on Computer Applications in Medical Care (SCAMC). Washington DC: McGraw-Hill.

Delaney, C., Mehmert, P., Prophet, C., Bellinger, S., Gardner-Huber, D., & Ellerbe, S. (1992). Standardized nursing language for healthcare information systems. *Journal of Medical Systems, 16*(4), 145-159.

APPENDIX D

Timeline and Highlights
of Nursing Outcomes Classification

1991

Nursing Outcomes research team is formed by Marion Johnson and Meridean Maas at the University of Iowa.

1992

Nursing Outcomes Classification (NOC) pilot work is funded by Sigma Theta Tau International with Marion Johnson and Meridean Maas as the principal investigators.

1993

The first *NIC Newsletter* is published at the University of Iowa (later changed to *The NIC Letter* and then to *The NIC/NOC Letter*).

NOC, with Marion Johnson and Meridean Maas as the principal investigators, is funded by NINR (Dec 1993-1997; extended to 1998).

1994

An institutional effectiveness grant for preparing pre- and postdoctoral students in effectiveness research, with Joanne McCloskey and Meridean Maas as directors, is funded at Iowa by NINR.

The Nursing Classifications Fund is established at the University of Iowa to provide ongoing financial support for the continued development and use of NIC and NOC.

The first publication about the *Nursing Outcomes Classification (NOC)* appears in print in *Current Issues in Nursing* (4th ed., pp. 136-142), published by Mosby.

1995

The Center for Nursing Classification at the University of Iowa is approved (December 13) by the Iowa Board of Regents (without funding) to facilitate the ongoing research and implementation of NIC and NOC. A fundraising advisory board for the Center is established and members appointed.

1996

The first journal article about the *Nursing Outcomes Classification (NOC)* appears in print in *Image—Journal of Nursing Scholarship.*

The first meeting of the Center's fundraising advisory board is held at the College of Nursing.

The first vendor (ERGO) signs licensing agreement for NIC and NOC.

1997

The first international NANDA, NIC, NOC Conference, focused on facilitating use of the languages, is held in St. Charles, Illinois, on November 1-9.

The first edition of *Nursing Outcomes Classification (NOC)* is published by Mosby.

The *NIC Letter* becomes *The NIC/NOC Letter.*

1998

The second outcomes research grant is funded by NINR (1998-2002) with three principal investigators: Marion Johnson, Meridean Maas, and Sue Moorhead.

NOC is recognized by the American Nurses Association.

NOC is added to the National Library of Medicine's Metathesaurus.

The Cumulative Index to Nursing and Health Care Literature (CINAHL) adds NOC to their index.

NIC and NOC submit information to American National Standards Institute Health Informatics Standards Board (ANSI HISB) for Inventory of Clinical Information Standards.

The NIC/NOC Letter is sponsored by Mosby-Year Book.

Multiple translations of NIC and NOC are processed/published (Dutch, Korean, Chinese, French, Japanese, and Spanish).

The Center for Nursing Classification receives 3 years of support from the College of Nursing (1998-2001) and is allocated space on the fourth floor of the College of Nursing. Joanne McCloskey is appointed director.

A monograph linking NIC interventions to NOC outcomes is published by the Center.

1999

The first Institute on Nursing Informatics and Classification is held at the University of Iowa, June 15-19.

NIC and NOC, along with other nursing language developers, give testimony about each language classification to a subcommittee of the National Committee on Vital and Health Statistics (NCHVS). The goal is to include nursing language into the standardized Patient Medical Record Information (PMRI).

NIC and NOC representatives participate in an invitational vocabulary conference at Vanderbilt University in Nashville, directed by Judy Osbolt with a goal of developing a reference terminology for nursing.

NIC and NOC representatives attend an invitational meeting of the SNOMED (Systematized Nomenclature of Medicine) Convergent Terminology group in Chicago, IL.

A second conference focused on NANDA, NIC, and NOC is held in New Orleans, Louisiana, April 14-17.

2000

The *Nursing Interventions Classification*, 3rd edition, and the *Nursing Outcomes Classification*, 2nd edition, are published by Mosby.

The NNN (3N) Alliance is created as a virtual organization to foster a working relationship between NANDA, NIC, and NOC, with Joanne McCloskey Dochterman and Dorothy Jones serving as co-chairs of the Alliance, along with a governing board including members of the NANDA Board and the Center for Classification Board at Iowa.

A monograph linking NIC and NOC with the Long Term Care Minimum Data Set Resident Assessment Instrument's (RAI) Resident Assessment Protocols (RAPs) is published by the Center.

A monograph linking NIC and NOC with OASIS (Outcome and Assessment Information Set) is published by the Center.

A monograph linking NOC with the Omaha classification is published by the Center.

The second Institute on Nursing Informatics and Classification is held at the College of Nursing on June 11-14.

2001

The first edition, authored by the NIC and NOC principal investigators, of *Nursing Diagnoses, Outcomes, Interventions: NANDA, NOC, and NIC Linkages* is published by Mosby.

A NNN Invitational Common Structure Conference is funded by the National Library of Medicine (Joanne McCloskey Dochterman and Dorothy Jones, principal investigators) and held in Utica, IL, in August.

An effectiveness grant is funded (by NINR and AHRQ) for large database research using NIC (Marita Titler and Joanne Dochterman, PIs). This is likely the first such grant to fund nursing effectiveness research using a clinical database with nursing standardized language.

NIC and NOC are registered in Health Level Seven (HL$_7$).

The Center for Nursing Classification receives 3 years of support from University of Iowa central administrative offices.

The third Institute on Nursing Informatics and Classification is held at the College of Nursing.

2002

The NNN Alliance holds an international conference on nursing language, classification, and informatics in Chicago, IL. NANDA's biennial conference becomes integrated into the 3N meeting. A White Paper on the Development of a Common Structure for NANDA, NIC, and NOC is presented to participants.

SNOMED (Systematized Nomenclature of Medicine) licenses NIC and NOC for inclusion in their database.

The Center for Nursing Classification expands its name to the Center for Nursing Classification and Clinical Effectiveness; its endowment reaches $600,000.

The fourth Institute on Nursing Informatics and Classification is held at the College of Nursing on June 23-26.

A 4-hour Web course, *NIC and NOC 101: The Basics,* is offered by the Center for Nursing Classification and Clinical Effectiveness at the University of Iowa.

A monograph, *Curriculum Guide for Implementation of NANDA, NIC, and NOC in an Undergraduate Nursing Curriculum,* authored by Cindy Finesilver and Debbie Metzler from Bellin College, is published by the Center.

A second institutional training grant for pre- and postdoctoral students in effectiveness research is funded at the University of Iowa by NINR, with Joanne McCloskey Dochterman and Martha Craft-Rosenberg as directors.

The position of Center Fellow is established (to assist in the ongoing development of NIC and NOC); approximately 30 people are appointed for 3-year terms.

2003

ANA publishes the Common Taxonomy of Nursing Practice in a monograph, *Unifying Nursing Languages: The Harmonization of NANDA, NIC and NOC* (edited by Joanne McCloskey Dochterman and Dorothy Jones).

The first meeting of the CNC Fellows is held on April 11 at the College of Nursing.

A NANDA, NIC, and NOC software program based on linkage book *Nursing Diagnoses, Outcomes, and Interventions: NANDA, NOC, and NIC Linkage—CD-ROM* is produced by Mosby.

The Center for Nursing Classification and Clinical Effectiveness receives the Sigma Theta Tau Board of Director's Award in recognition of established excellence in integrating knowledge and clinical experience to achieve exemplary practice.

The Fifth Institute on Nursing Informatics and Classification is held on June 9-12.

Elizabeth Swanson and Howard Butcher join the CNC Executive Board.

A Spanish version of the web course, *NIC and NOC 101: The Basics*, translated by Patricia Levi, is offered by the Center for Nursing Classification and Clinical Effectiveness at the University of Iowa.

2004

Nursing Interventions Classification (4th edition) and *Nursing Outcomes Classification* (3rd edition) are published by Mosby.

The second meeting of the CNC Fellows is held in April.

The NNN Alliance holds the second international conference on nursing language, classification, and informatics in Chicago, IL.

The first Annette Scheffel Fundraising event is held in the fall.

Joanne McCloskey Dochterman retires as director of the Center, and Sue Moorhead is appointed director effective July 1, 2004.

A monograph, *Guideline for Conducting Effectiveness Research in Nursing and Other Health Care Services*, authored by Marita Titler, Joanne McCloskey Dochterman, and David Reed, is published by the Center.

The Center for Nursing Classification and Clinical Effectiveness endowment reaches $700,000.

2005

NIC and NOC incorporated into GNIRC protocols.

The Sixth Institute on Nursing Informatics and Classification is held on June 13-15.

Center Fellows are reappointed for 3-year terms beginning July 1. Additional fellows are nominated and appointed.

The Center for Nursing Classification and Clinical Effectiveness celebrates its 10th anniversary in December.

The second Annette Scheffel Fundraising event is held December 2 with a reception and a silent auction.

2006

The second edition of *NANDA, NOC, and NIC Linkages: Nursing Diagnoses, Outcomes, Interventions* is published by Mosby.

The NNN Alliance holds the third international conference on nursing language, classification, and informatics in Philadelphia, PA.

Five new fellows are appointed at the annual meeting in April.

American Nurses Association (ANA) recognition of NIC and NOC is renewed.

In addition to the above events, NOC has been presented over the years at numerous national and international conferences. Presentations in other countries include those in Australia, Brazil, Canada, Denmark, England, France, Iceland, Ireland, Japan, Korea, Netherlands, Slovenia, Spain, Switzerland, Turkey, and Wales.

Index

The letter b indicates a box, t table, and f figure.